AN INTRODUCTION TO

GLOBAL
HEALTH

THIRD EDITION

AN INTRODUCTION TO

GLOBAL
HEALTH

THIRD EDITION

Michael Seear and Obidimma Ezezika

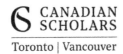

CANADIAN
SCHOLARS
Toronto | Vancouver

An Introduction to Global Health, Third Edition
by Michael Seear and Obidimma Ezezika

First published in 2017 by
Canadian Scholars
425 Adelaide Street West, Suite 200
Toronto, Ontario
M5V 3C1

www.canadianscholars.ca

Library and Archives Canada Cataloguing in Publication

Seear, Michael, 1950-
[Introduction to international health]
     An introduction to global health / Michael Seear and Obidimma Ezezika.
-- Third edition.

Previous editions published under title: An introduction to international
     health.
Includes bibliographical references and index.
Issued in print and electronic formats.
ISBN 978-1-77338-003-2 (softcover).--ISBN 978-1-77338-004-9 (PDF).--
ISBN 978-1-77338-005-6 (EPUB)

     1. World health--Textbooks. 2. Poverty--Developing countries--
Textbooks. 3. Public health--Developing countries--Textbooks. I. Ezezika,
Obidimma, author II. Title. III. Title: Introduction to international
health.

RA441.S43 2017   362.1   C2017-906629-3
                                                           C2017-906630-7

Cover and text design by Elisabeth Springate

17   18   19   20   21   5   4   3   2   1

Printed and bound in Canada by Webcom

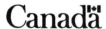

TABLE OF CONTENTS

ACKNOWLEDGEMENTS

I would like to thank the following people who have provided invaluable insights and comments on various chapters of the manuscript: Mark Brender, Trillium Chang, Jacqueline Ezezika, Jessica Oh, Vanessa Reddit, and Ken Simiyu.

—*Obidimma Ezezika*

PART I

WHAT IS GLOBAL HEALTH?

CHAPTER 1
An Overview of Global Health

There are two things which I am confident I can do very well: one is an introduction to any literary work, stating what it is to contain, and how it should be executed in the most perfect manner; the other is a conclusion showing from various causes why the execution has not been equal to what the author promised to himself and to the public.

—Samuel Johnson, 1775

OBJECTIVES

Global health is a rapidly evolving and exciting field with many huge opportunities to make a difference in the lives of millions. This chapter provides an overview of global health and how far the field has come in the last century.

- understand the scope of the subjects covered by the term "global health"
- understand how global health relates to the new Sustainable Development Goals (SDGs)
- understand the design and content of this book and how to get the most out of the material
- start to apply human faces and experiences to the broad concepts of poverty, malnutrition, and injustice

INTRODUCTION

> There is simply no good reason why in the 21st century, thousands of women and children in developing countries should be dying during childbirth and the early years of life.
>
> —*Hon. Aileen Carroll, Canadian Minister of International Cooperation, 2005*

Global health is, very broadly, the study of the health of populations in a global context. Although poor levels of health are common in many developing countries, it is important not to concentrate solely on diseases and to remember that they are just the most visible result of underlying social disruption. The need to study both the diseases and their causes means that global health covers a very wide range of subjects. These vary from tropical medicine and primary health care at one end of the spectrum to epidemiology and economics at the other end, with a great many stops in between. The solutions to these problems are, of course, no less complex than their underlying causes.

Despite widespread improvements in health and prosperity over the last few decades, malnutrition, poverty, and all the ills that stem from them are still very common around the world. In fact, to the newcomer, the statistics can be quite overwhelming. During a period when citizens of industrialized countries are healthier than at any time in history, hundreds of millions of people in the least developed countries still live lives of terrible deprivation. There is, of course, a natural human desire to assist people living under those conditions. Since the end of World War II, a complex mix of private, governmental, and international organizations has developed with the overall aim of improving the health of populations in developing countries. While the developing aid industry has had successes, it has also had its share of trials and considerable errors. Fortunately, the new millennium seems to have brought a renaissance in aid. Current developments—such as the Debt Relief Initiative, the Millennium Development Goals (MDGs, which have now been replaced with the SDGs), several successful disease eradication efforts, and serious attempts to improve the quantity and effectiveness of foreign aid—have all combined to bring a sense of great optimism to the field of aid.

Another development has been the growing popular interest in global health issues. When the world's seven richest countries first decided to hold annual meetings, about 30 years ago, it is unlikely that the average person paid much attention. This is in marked contrast to the period leading up to the 2005 Group of Eight (G8) Conference at Gleneagles, when it seemed as if the whole world was waiting for the latest word on debt relief. The health of developing populations (particularly the developing world debt) became a bandwagon that staggered under the weight of politicians, pop stars, and various other celebrities as they clambered aboard.

When Tony Blair announced general agreement on the Multilateral Debt Relief Initiative, there was a real sense of worldwide excitement. While the agreement may not quite have lived up to its billing, it cannot be denied that there is now widespread interest in the broad topic of global health.

This increased awareness of global health issues has probably been fashioned by events that were large enough to reach news reports. A lot has happened over the last 20 or 30 years—some of the international issues that caught public attention included a steady increase in political freedom (South Africa, eastern Europe), several widely reported famines (Ethiopia, Sudan), destructive civil wars (Rwanda, Bosnia), and natural disasters (Asian tsunami, Haitian earthquake). The current level of interest was exemplified by the spontaneous public response to the Asian tsunami. So much money was given by private citizens that the Red Cross actually asked people to stop sending any more, since it had enough!

Strangely enough, despite the increased demand for courses, books, and general information on the subject of global health, there is no clearly defined preparatory educational path for entry into the field. Degree and post-graduate courses in global health can be found in large centres, but there is still a surprisingly limited amount of educational material considering the level of interest. This book is designed to meet at least some of that demand by providing a broad overview of global health that nevertheless includes as much detail as possible on key topics, and by

Box 1.1 History Notes

Amartya Sen (1933–)

Amartya Sen is an Indian economist whose work has had a profound effect on the broad subject of global health. His early work on the origins of famine highlighted what everyone knew but few had articulated. Superficially "simple" population health problems such as famine are far more complex than they initially seem. He showed that starvation is not due just to lack of food any more than poverty is due only to lack of money. At the root of most complex problems lies inequity. His later work, *Development as Freedom*, is also widely quoted. Based on a wide range of his early research, he further develops his arguments in favour of political and economic freedom. He outlines five specific types of freedoms: political freedoms, economic facilities, social opportunities, transparency guarantees, and protective security, which are usually viewed as only the ends of development. However, he argues that such freedoms should be both the ends and the means of development.

Sen was born on a university campus established by the Indian philosopher and previous Nobel Prize winner, Rabindranath Tagore. He studied economics in India and England. After serving as master of Trinity College, Cambridge, he recently moved to Harvard University. He was awarded the Nobel Prize for Economics in 1998. Please follow the reference for more details: Nobelprize.org (2011).

considering other aspects of global health that are rarely given attention, such as poverty, wars, humanitarian disasters, and governance. Although the subject of global health is unavoidably medical in nature, this is not a medical textbook and is intended for readers with a wide range of interests. Whether you are a pure researcher tied to a laboratory bench, a nursing student planning a career in development work, or a fieldworker in a large aid agency, this book aims to provide a detailed introduction to global health and its inevitable companion, the modern aid industry. We would like to wish a warm welcome to anyone opening this book for the first time, and hope that it will help you find your way through the complex but fascinating subject of global health.

THE SCOPE AND DEFINITION OF GLOBAL HEALTH

> There can be no real growth without healthy populations. No sustainable development without tackling disease and malnutrition. No international security without assisting crisis-ridden countries. And no hope for the spread of freedom, democracy, and human dignity unless we treat health as a basic human right.
>
> —*Gro Brundtland, Director General of the World Health Organization, 2003*

Providing a concise, inclusive definition for a subject as varied as global health is a challenge. This is reflected in the common questions that newcomers ask: What is global health? How does it differ from international health? Where do tropical medicine, epidemiology, and public health fit in? An all-inclusive definition of global health would be similar to the description of an elephant by the blind philosophers—there are lots of parts, but no coherent whole. It is perhaps more useful to define the subject using its broad basic aims. Taking that approach, global health can be defined as a subject that tries to find practical answers to the following questions:

- Why is population health so poor in many developing countries?
- What is the extent of the problem?
- What can be done about it?

Those questions have dictated the general layout of this book and their answers will cover varied and interesting topics. Global health has been defined as "collaborative trans-national research and action for promoting health for all" (Beaglehole & Bonita, 2010). Global health has "health equity among nations and for all people" as its major objective (Koplan et al., 2009).

Before World War II, global health was largely the preserve of doctors and missionaries. As the industry has grown, ever-increasing numbers of new specialists have been added to the list. Investigating the causes and extent of ill health requires researchers, biostatisticians, and epidemiologists. Addressing the last question—What can be done about it?—requires a small army. Health initiatives may include economic interventions (economists, business specialists, agronomists, small-scale bankers, etc.), medical initiatives (doctors, nurses, pharmacists, nutritionists, etc.), and human rights initiatives (politicians, rights activists, and constitutional lawyers). Increasingly, standards of project management are improving, which requires accountants, project managers, and the full range of support staff associated with any large company. Finally, a large part of many aid projects consists of trying to get people to change their behaviour, so projects now also include psychologists, anthropologists, popular public figures, and even directors of soap operas. While a successful project certainly requires money and well-trained staff, it must always be remembered that the most important people in the whole process are the target population. No initiative stands a chance unless local people are included (and listened to) at every stage of planning and implementation.

FROM MILLENNIUM DEVELOPMENT GOALS TO SUSTAINABLE DEVELOPMENT GOALS

> Learn from the past, set vivid, detailed goals for the future, and live in the only moment of time over which you have any control: now.
>
> —*Denis Waitley*

Established following the Millennium Summit of the United Nations in 2000, the Millennium Development Goals (MDGs) helped guide the global health development community for 15 years. The eight MDGs were:

1. To eradicate extreme poverty and hunger
2. To achieve universal primary education
3. To promote gender equality
4. To reduce child mortality
5. To improve maternal health
6. To combat HIV/AIDS, malaria, and other diseases
7. To ensure environmental sustainability
8. To develop a global partnership for development

Important strides have been taken at the global level toward achieving many of the health-related MDGs. For example, the targets for both malaria and tuberculosis were met. In addition, substantial progress was made in reducing child under-nutrition, child mortality, and maternal mortality. There was also recorded progress in increasing access to improved sanitation (WHO, 2015).

While the MDGs have promoted increased health and well-being in many countries, progress toward reaching these goals has been uneven across countries. Studies have pointed out that the MDGs were prepared by only a few stakeholders without adequate involvement by developing countries and overlooked development objectives previously agreed upon and not appropriately adapted to national needs (Fehling et al., 2013).

Overall, the outcome of the MDGs has been incredible, particularly in the areas of poverty reduction, increased access to safe drinking water and education. For example, extreme poverty has declined significantly over the last two decades. In 1990, nearly half of the population in the developing world lived on less than US$1.25 a day; that proportion dropped to 14 percent in 2015. There has also been advancement on the three health goals and targets. For example, between 1990 and 2015, the global under-five mortality rate has declined by more than half, dropping from 90 to 43 deaths per 1,000 live births, and HIV, tuberculosis, and malaria epidemics were staved.

The transition from the MDGs to the Sustainable Development Goals (SDGs) is premised on building a sustainable world where environmental sustainability, social inclusion, and economic development are equally valued. There were a number of shortcomings or challenges in the MDGs that left out issues such as disasters, conflict situations, the epidemic of non-communicable diseases,

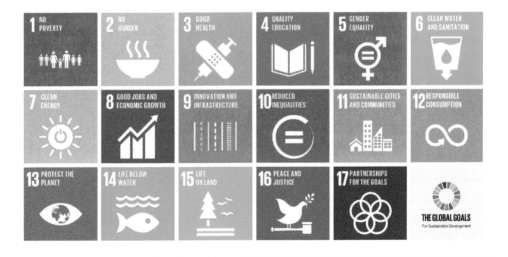

Photo 1.1: The Sustainable Development Goals

Source: Image courtesy of the Global Goals for Sustainable Development, www.globalgoals.org.

Table 1.1: Sustainable Development Goals

Goal 1	End poverty in all its forms everywhere
Goal 2	End hunger, achieve food security and improved nutrition and promote sustainable agriculture
Goal 3	Ensure healthy lives and promote well-being for all at all ages
Goal 4	Ensure inclusive and equitable quality education and promote lifelong learning opportunities for all
Goal 5	Achieve gender equality and empower all women and girls
Goal 6	Ensure availability and sustainable management of water and sanitation for all
Goal 7	Ensure access to affordable, reliable, sustainable, and modern energy for all
Goal 8	Promote sustained, inclusive and sustainable economic growth, full and productive employment and decent work for all
Goal 9	Build resilient infrastructure, promote inclusive and sustainable industrialization and foster innovation
Goal 10	Reduce inequality within and among countries
Goal 11	Make cities and human settlements inclusive, safe, resilient, and sustainable
Goal 12	Ensure sustainable consumption and production patterns
Goal 13	Take urgent action to combat climate change and its impacts
Goal 14	Conserve and sustainably use the oceans, seas and marine resources for sustainable development
Goal 15	Protect, restore and promote sustainable use of terrestrial ecosystems, sustainably manage forests, combat desertification, and halt and reverse land degradation and halt biodiversity loss
Goal 16	Promote peaceful and inclusive societies for sustainable development, provide access to justice for all and build effective, accountable and inclusive institutions at all levels
Goal 17	Strengthen the means of implementation and revitalize the Global Partnership for Sustainable Development

mental health disorders, and large inequalities in all parts of the world. The SDGs (Table 1.1) address many of these shortcomings and posit a new all-inclusive health goal ("Ensure healthy lives and promote well-being for all at all ages") with a broad set of targets (Table 1.2).

This book makes references to these SDGs (Photo 1.1), which are officially known as *Transforming Our World: The 2030 Agenda for Sustainable Development*. The SDGs are considered a successor to the MDGs. There are 17 SDGs and 169 core targets that relate to them. The goals are contained in *paragraph 55 United Nations Resolution A/RES/70/1 of 25 September 2015* (UN, 2015c).

The SDGs are far reaching and applicable to all countries. They also include a broad range of socio-economic environmental and equity objectives, and offer the prospect of more peaceful and inclusive societies. Issues like poverty eradication, health, education, and food security and nutrition remain priorities in the SDGs.

e 1.2: Targets for Goal 3: Ensure healthy lives and promote well-being for all at all ages

3.1	By 2030, reduce the global maternal mortality ratio to less than 70 per 100,000 live births
3.2	By 2030, end preventable deaths of newborns and children under 5 years of age, with all countries aiming to reduce neonatal mortality to at least as low as 12 per 1,000 live births and under-5 mortality to at least as low as 25 per 1,000 live births
3.3	By 2030, end the epidemics of AIDS, tuberculosis, malaria, and neglected tropical diseases and combat hepatitis, water-borne diseases and other communicable diseases
3.4	By 2030, reduce by one third premature mortality from noncommunicable diseases through prevention and treatment and promote mental health and well-being
3.5	Strengthen the prevention and treatment of substance abuse, including narcotic drug abuse and harmful use of alcohol
3.6	By 2020, halve the number of global deaths and injuries from road traffic accidents
3.7	By 2030, ensure universal access to sexual and reproductive health-care services, including for family planning, information and education, and the integration of reproductive health into national strategies and programmes
3.8	Achieve universal health coverage, including financial risk protection, access to quality essential health-care services and access to safe, effective, quality, and affordable essential medicines and vaccines for all
3.9	By 2030, substantially reduce the number of deaths and illnesses from hazardous chemicals and air, water and soil pollution and contamination
3.a	Strengthen the implementation of the World Health Organization Framework Convention on Tobacco Control in all countries, as appropriate
3.b	Support the research and development of vaccines and medicines for the communicable and noncommunicable diseases that primarily affect developing countries, provide access to affordable essential medicines and vaccines, in accordance with the Doha Declaration on the TRIPS Agreement and Public Health, which affirms the right of developing countries to use to the full the provisions in the Agreement on Trade-Related Aspects of Intellectual Property Rights regarding flexibilities to protect public health, and, in particular, provide access to medicines for all
3.c	Substantially increase health financing and the recruitment, development, training and retention of the health workforce in developing countries, especially in least developed countries and small island developing States
3.d	Strengthen the capacity of all countries, in particular developing countries, for early warning, risk reduction and management of national and global health risks

SDGS AND HEALTH

The 13 targets of the SDG goal on health are shown in Table 1.2. You will notice that some of the MDGs have been reflected in the SDG framework, such as maternal mortality (target 3.1), child mortality (target 3.2) and infectious diseases (target

Table 1.3: SDG targets related to health

1.3	Implement nationally appropriate social protection systems and measures for all, including floors, and by 2030 achieve substantial coverage of the poor and the vulnerable
2.2	By 2030, end all forms of malnutrition, including achieving, by 2025, the internationally agreed targets on stunting and wasting in children under five years of age, and address the nutritional needs of adolescent girls, pregnant and lactating women and older persons
4.2	By 2030, ensure that all girls and boys have access to quality early childhood development, care and pre-primary education so that they are ready for primary education
4.a	Build and upgrade education facilities that are child, disability and gender sensitive and provide safe, non-violent, inclusive, and effective learning environments for all
5.2	Eliminate all forms of violence against all women and girls in the public and private spheres, including trafficking and sexual and other types of exploitation
5.3	Eliminate all harmful practices, such as child, early and forced marriage and female genital mutilation
5.6	Ensure universal access to sexual and reproductive health and reproductive rights as agreed in accordance with the Programme of Action of the International Conference on Population and Development and the Beijing Platform for Action and the outcome documents of their review conferences
6.1	By 2030, achieve universal and equitable access to safe and affordable drinking-water for all
6.2	By 2030, achieve access to adequate and equitable sanitation and hygiene for all and end open defecation, paying special attention to the needs of women and girls and those in vulnerable situations
6.3	By 2030, improve water quality by reducing pollution, eliminating dumping and minimizing release of hazardous chemicals and materials, halving the proportion of untreated wastewater and substantially increasing recycling and safe reuse globally
10.4	Adopt policies, especially fiscal, wage and social protection policies, and progressively achieve greater equality
11.5	By 2030, significantly reduce the number of deaths and the number of people affected and substantially decrease the direct economic losses relative to global gross domestic product caused by disasters, including water-related disasters, with a focus on protecting the poor and people in vulnerable situations
16.1	Significantly reduce all forms of violence and related death rates everywhere
16.2	End abuse, exploitation, trafficking, and all forms of violence against and torture of children
16.6	Develop effective, accountable and transparent institutions at all levels
16.9	By 2030, provide legal identity for all, including birth registration
17.18	By 2020, enhance capacity-building support to developing countries, including for least-developed countries and small island developing States, to increase significantly the availability of high-quality, timely and reliable data disaggregated by income, gender, age, race, ethnicity, migratory status, disability, geographic location, and other characteristics relevant in national contexts

3.3). However, the SDG framework is expanded to include neonatal mortality and other infectious diseases beyond HIV/AIDS, such as hepatitis.

Due to increasing recognition of the burden of disease arising from non-communicable diseases, injuries, and other burdens beyond HIV/AIDS, malaria, and tuberculosis, the SDGs now include new targets on non-communicable diseases, mental health (target 3.4), substance abuse (target 3.5), injuries (target 3.6), and health impact from environmental pollution (target 3.9).

Although only Goal 3 directly concerns health, all other 16 SDGs are indirectly related to health. For instance, poverty and hunger as referred to in Goals 1 and 2, respectively, relate to health both as a cause of ill health and as a consequence of ill health. The goal of inclusive and equitable quality education and lifelong learning opportunities for all can only be possible if populations are well enough to enrol in classes, attend school, and have the capacity to learn. The aim of achieving gender equalities in Goal 5 is important to health issues that affect women globally and related to empowerment. Goal 6 on clean water and sanitation is an important element and cause of ill health and the spread of many infectious diseases. Employment, referred to in Goal 8, is an important social determinant of health

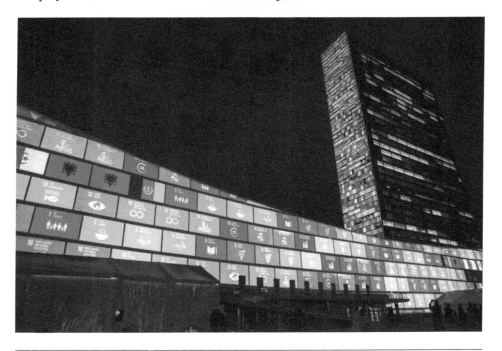

Photo 1.2: A 10-minute film introducing the Sustainable Development Goals is projected onto the UN Headquarters, 22 September 2015.

Source: UN Photo/Cia Pak, with kind permission of the UN Photo Library (www.unmultimedia. org/photo).

(i.e., a person's socio-economic status). The inequities referred to in Goal 10 are important in creating equitable health for all—and as you would see in the course of this book, health inequities are one of the major component challenges. Goals 11 and 12 deal with living conditions such as safety and health, while climate change impacts on health in Goal 13. Goals 14 and 15 refer to making ecosystems and environments more safe and preventing their distortion, which are important for population health. Goal 16 focuses on justice and peace, which in its absence leads to strife, civil wars, and wars. Finally, in order to "strengthen the means of implementation and revitalize the Global Partnership for Sustainable Development" as enunciated in Goal 17, different national and international partners must work collaboratively to help countries improve their health status.

Forming an idea of the standards of population health in developing countries, based purely on available statistics, is difficult; the numbers are simply too large to comprehend. However, no matter how bad health indicators might be today, they are all a great deal better than they used to be. In the six decades since the end of World War II, life expectancy in many countries has increased by over 25 years (Figure 1.1) and infant mortality rates have fallen steadily (Figure 1.2). The aid industry that grew during this same period can probably claim some credit for

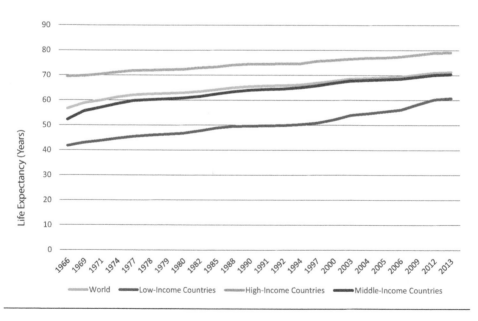

Figure 1.1: Global trends in life expectancy at birth with time

Source: World Bank. 2016a. Data from the World Bank. World Development Indicators: Life expectancy at birth, total (years). Retrieved from: http://data.worldbank.org/indicator/SP.DYN.LE00.IN/countries?display=graph (Accessed February 29, 2016).

these improvements (particularly due to immunizations and other public health interventions), but developed countries improved at much the same rate without receiving any aid, so some caution is required in drawing simple conclusions. The final report on the achievements of foreign aid is a mixed one (Easterly, 2006) and will be discussed in detail later in the book.

It must be remembered that global health statistics—typically Millennium Development Goals (MDGs)—are often expressed in reports as weighted average values based on results from studies in many different countries. Consequently, they are heavily influenced by public health improvements in the largest countries, particularly China and India. When poverty and health statistics are broken down by region, a more accurate view is obtained. For example, India and China have been able to elevate many of their people out of poverty. However, this obscures the point that other regions of the world, particularly sub-Saharan Africa, have seen little or no improvement over many years.

The term "developing world" covers a large range of countries in different regions of the world, with each country having its own complex mixture of social and economic challenges. Problems differ between countries and, as the HIV/AIDS epidemic has shown, new challenges also appear with time. While there is

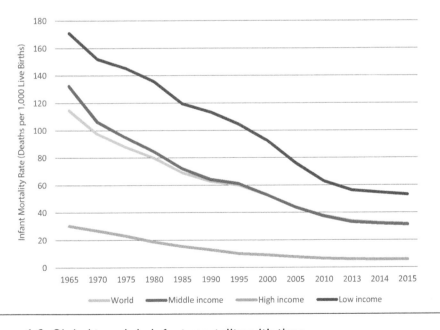

Figure 1.2: Global trends in infant mortality with time

Source: World Bank. 2016a. Data from the World Bank. World Development Indicators: Life expectancy at birth, total (years). Retrieved from: http://data.worldbank.org/indicator/SP.DYN.LE00.IN/countries?display=graph (Accessed February 29, 2016).

no simple cookie-cutter list of problems applicable to every one of these diverse areas, there are recurring themes. Of these, poverty and malnutrition stand out well above the crowd as both affect hundreds of millions of people around the world. It should always be remembered that wherever severe poverty and malnutrition are found, some form of serious injustice will always be close behind. When it comes to the spectrum of diseases affecting developing world populations, there have been profound changes over the last 20 years. The emergence of an increasingly prosperous global middle class has shifted the emphasis away from infectious diseases and more toward those associated with a "Western" lifestyle. Problems such as childhood obesity, motor vehicle accidents, smoking-related illnesses (particularly heart attacks and strokes), mental illness, and substance abuse are already at epidemic levels in some middle-income developing countries. Some of the major topics encountered within the subject of global health are listed below.

Poverty

Although global poverty has declined significantly over the past two decades and the MDG target for poverty was achieved ahead of the 2015 deadline, there are still about 836 million people who live in extreme poverty. The overwhelming majority of these people live in two regions—South Asia and sub-Saharan Africa—and they account for about 80 percent of the global total of extremely poor people (UN, 2015a). Poverty traps populations within a vicious cycle of poor education, limited job opportunities, and chronic ill health. Wherever there is widespread poverty, there will inevitably be inequity and injustice as two of the principal contributory causes.

Malnutrition

Although there have been slow improvements in global nutrition over time, the statistics concerning the extent of undernutrition are still startling. At a time of great prosperity for developed countries, there are currently 795 million people suffering from malnutrition, with the vast majority living in the developing regions (FAO, 2016). Increased food prices and global recession have combined to slow progress in reaching the MDGs for malnutrition. Again, global averages show a decline, but in Africa and parts of Asia, there has been little progress. Apart from areas of severe social chaos, large-scale famines are, fortunately, now much less common. Death from starvation has largely been replaced by the debilitating effects of chronic malnutrition, which sap the energy and the potential of huge numbers of the world's population. Through its effects on a child's immune response, malnutrition greatly increases mortality from diseases such as gastroenteritis and measles.

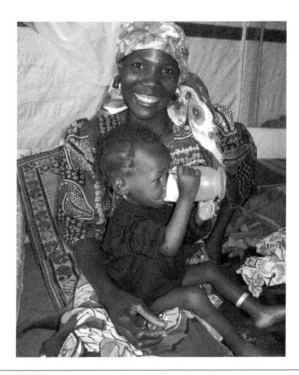

Photo 1.3: An undernourished child drinks a fortified milk formula at a feeding centre in Madaoua, Niger.

Source: Photo by Thorsten Muench, courtesy of the European Community Humanitarian Office (ECHO: http://ec.europa.eu/echo).

Childhood Illnesses

Child mortality from avoidable diseases is an area where there has been much progress (Figure 1.2), much of it attributable to aid. Since 1990, annual deaths of children under five have fallen from 12.4 million to 5.9 million. Many countries have seen mortality rates halved over that time. The leading causes of death include preterm birth complications (18 percent), pneumonia (15 percent), birth asphyxia and trauma (12 percent), and diarrhea (9 percent) (WHO, 2016). While this is great news, it is far too early for celebrations. Almost 6 million deaths still mean that 16,000 are occurring every single day, many of which strike babies that are not even a month old. These deaths leading to loss of human potential is made even worse by the fact that most of these children would have survived had they lived in a developed country. Not only are most of these cases treatable, but many are also completely avoidable with simple and affordable interventions. For example, roughly 100,000 children still die from measles every year, a disease for which there is a 99 percent effective vaccine costing roughly US$1 per child.

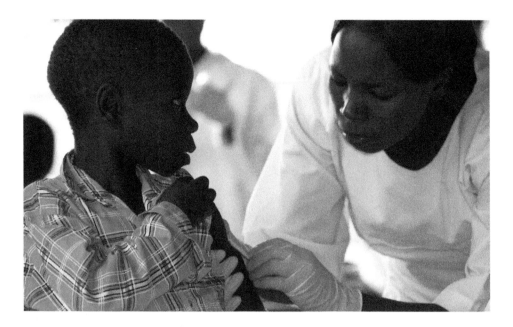

Photo 1.4: A young boy receives a meningitis vaccine in Nigeria.

Source: Photo by Claire Barrault, courtesy of the European Community Humanitarian Office (ECHO: http://ec.europa.eu/echo).

Pregnancy-Related Deaths

It is only within the last decade that serious attention has been paid to the health of women around the world. Prior to this time, the best available estimates suggest that well over 500,000 women died each year from pregnancy-related causes (WHO, 2010); 99 percent of these occurred in developing countries.

In 2015, developing regions still accounted for approximately 99 percent (302,000) of the global maternal deaths, with sub-Saharan Africa alone accounting for roughly 66 percent (201,000), followed by South Asia (66,000) (WHO, 2016). Almost all of these deaths are completely avoidable with improved standards of care. For example, a quarter of the total simply bled to death (Say et al., 2014). Until the impetus of the MDGs in 2000, there was a great deal more talk than action, but latest figures suggest that deaths are finally falling. However, in some areas of the world, women still face a 1–2 percent chance of dying with every delivery and a nearly 10 percent lifetime risk of dying from a pregnancy-related cause. Although statistics are not accurately collected, it is widely believed that for every woman who dies, 10 times that number are left with disabling injuries such as bowel or bladder fistulas, chronic infection, or permanent pain. This statistic can only be improved by provision of better maternal health care.

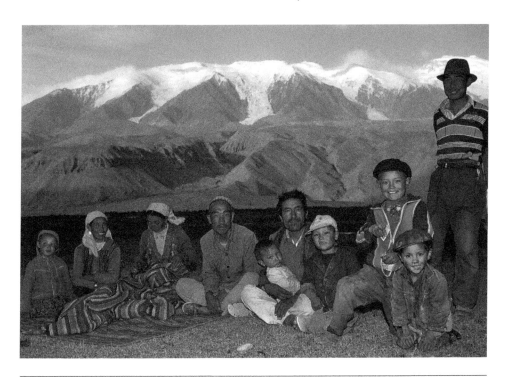

Photo 1.5: Members of a Kirghiz family living at the foot of the Kongur Mountains in Xinjiang, China. They are 1 of nearly 50 Indigenous minority groups living in China.

Source: Photo/F. Charton, with kind permission of the UN Photo Library (www.unmultimedia.org/photo).

Indigenous Health

From Canadian Inuit in the North to Australian Aboriginals in the South, there are roughly 370 million Indigenous peoples around the world that form at least 5,000 separate groups in over 90 countries (Photo 1.5). Although their backgrounds are widely diverse, they frequently share a history of conquest and varying degrees of subsequent discrimination (UNPFII, 2010). As a result of this poor treatment, Indigenous peoples also share surprisingly common health problems that often include high rates of substance abuse, diabetes, family violence, and suicide. Wherever records are available, Indigenous health lags far behind the average levels of the dominant population. For example, life expectancy is usually at least 5 to 10 years shorter than national averages. The non-binding UN Declaration on the Rights of Indigenous Peoples, signed in 2007, has improved the visibility of such minority groups. After a very long time, Indigenous peoples are finally gaining an international voice, particularly in the area of self-determination.

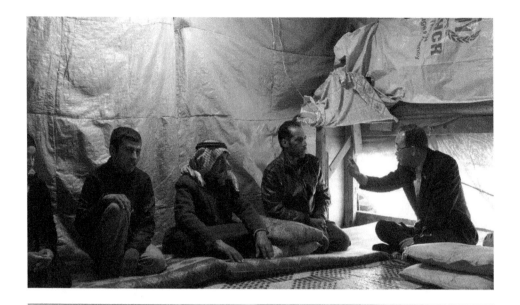

Photo 1.6: Former Secretary-General Ban Ki-moon (on the right) visits a Syrian family that has been living in a refugee camp in the Beqaa Valley of eastern Lebanon for five years, 25 March 2016.

Source: UN Photo/Mark Garten, with kind permission of the UN Photo Library (www.unmultimedia.org/photo).

War

From Bosnia to Guatemala and from Somalia to Sudan, modern war has changed. Fighting between countries has largely been replaced by internal wars marked by high levels of violence against civilian populations, usually further complicated by progressive economic and social collapse. This situation has given rise to the term "humanitarian disaster." Apart from the millions of people who have been killed over decades of war, there is also an incalculable cost for the survivors in terms of land mine injuries, the terrible legacy of child soldiers, confinement to a refugee camp, and the destruction of a country's entire socio-economic structure (Chen et al., 2007). For example, the current civil war in Syria has led to at least 300,000 deaths as of September 2016 and has displaced millions of people, with civilians bearing the brunt of the on-going violence and with rising numbers of people killed or injured (SOHR, 2016).

Natural Disasters

Natural catastrophes, such as earthquakes, hurricanes, and volcanoes, are not rare. During the last decade, the world has witnessed two of the most lethal disasters in

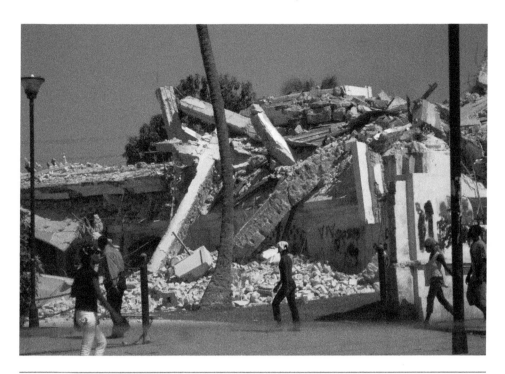

Photo 1.7: Devastated area of Port au Prince after Haiti's 2010 earthquake.

Source: Phuong Tran/Integrated Regional Information Network photo library (www.irinnews. org/photo).

history (the Asian tsunami and the Haitian earthquake) and also the most costly disasters in history (Hurricane Katrina and the Kobe earthquake). As the world population grows, more and more people live in vulnerable areas of the world, so death rates from disasters climb steadily each decade (Guha-Sapir et al., 2010). Apart from the immediate loss of life, the cost for survivors is enormous in terms of property destruction and loss of livelihood (Photo 1.7). Although disasters cannot be prevented, their effects can be mitigated by planning and preparation. The United Nations' recent International Strategy for Disaster Reduction is an attempt to improve the preparedness of developing world communities to face unexpected disasters.

Human Rights Abuses

Abuses of basic human rights are not confined to the developing world; they can be found, to some degree, in almost every country. However, the worst examples of abuse are found in developing countries, particular those in the very poorest areas of the world. Examples include discrimination and oppression based on gender (e.g., female genital mutilation, exclusion of girls from school) or violence against

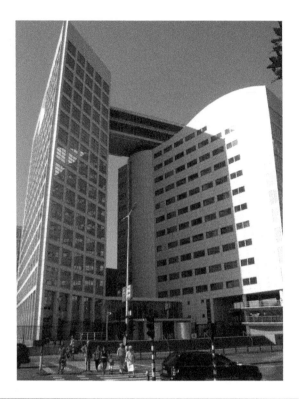

Photo 1.8: The International Criminal Court in the Hague

Source: Photo by Hanhil, courtesy of Wikimedia Commons.

---

particular ethnic and religious groups (some examples include the Rwandan geno-cide, the humanitarian crisis in Darfur, and the collapse of the former Yugoslavia). The full list is, unfortunately, a very long one. In the past, human rights have been looked on as a separate issue that stands on its own, but with the establishment of the International Criminal Court in 2002 (Photo 1.8), this attitude has changed. It is now realized that peace and prosperity (and also successful aid projects) depend on a fundamental foundation of benign governance that respects the rights of individuals (Annan, 2005). Beneficial changes in human rights are increasingly being included as a central feature of large-scale aid projects.

NOTES ABOUT THE THIRD EDITION

There must be an ideal world, a sort of mathematician's paradise where everything happens as it does in textbooks.

—*Bertrand Russell, 1914*

Using This Book

Global health is a rapidly changing subject even at the best of times. Yet, over the last decade that pace of change has accelerated. This third edition has been rewritten in light of the emerging health trends and ongoing discussions on the attainment of the new SDGs. New graphs have been added throughout the textbook, and new pedagogical tools such as discussion questions and chapter summaries have been included at the end of each chapter that further provide readers with feedback and discussion points.

As we have already seen, global health covers a wide range of subjects; it does not lend itself to a neat, linear narrative. That has not changed in the last few years, so while the book has been well updated, the basic form of the first edition has been maintained. Chapters are still grouped into sections based on their relevance to the three main questions set at the beginning of this introduction: Why is population health so poor in developing countries? What is the extent of the problem? What can be done about it? The final section of the book is devoted to other aspects of global health such as refugees, disasters, and Indigenous health. Finally, advice is given on the planning requirements needed for a successful project and also on working effectively in overseas partnerships. Although the subject matter is often medical in nature, it should be stressed that this is not a medical text and is written for a mixed audience (no previous medical training is necessary).

Enough information has been included within the text to allow readers to gain a good grasp of the subject without the need for extra research. However, for those who are interested in further information on particular subjects, there are over 1,000 references and recommended books spread throughout the chapters. Tables and graphs are often used to illustrate points, and references are added for the original data sources. Conventional notation is used for books (author, date, title, publisher) and scientific journals (authors, date, title, volume, pages):

CDC. 2005. *Health information for international travel, 2005–2006.* Pub: Elsevier Press.

Jha, P., et al. 2006. Low male-to-female sex ratio of children born in India: National survey of 1.1 million households. *The Lancet,* 367: 211–218.

Other references will include websites for large organizations that are likely to remain unchanged:

National Aboriginal Health Organization (NAHO) website. Retrieved from: www.naho.ca/english/.

Some reports, manuals, and booklets can be obtained by downloading them from the relevant websites:

Lavizzari, L. 2001. *A guide for project management and evaluation: Managing for impact in rural development.* May be downloaded from International Fund for Agricultural Development website at: www.ifad.org/evaluation/guide/.

The modern aid industry has a reasonably long history and has, as a result, accumulated its own share of interesting characters. Under the heading "History Notes," each chapter includes a brief mention of someone who has made a major contribution to the field of global health. Finally, in the modern world, the rich are so rich and the poor are so poor that it is fairly simple to find incongruous examples of the differences in the lives lived by these two groups. In order to give some insight into the harsh reality of life in a developing country, most chapters include an example under the heading "Moment of Insight." Although some of the comparisons may seem surprising, they are all true (original information sources are provided).

Check Your Sources

> For my part, I consider that it will be found much better by all parties to leave the past to history, especially as I propose to write that history myself.
>
> —*Winston Churchill, speech to the House of Commons, 1948*

Whether you prefer Churchill or the blunter style of Henry Ford ("History is more or less bunk"), the message is the same: do not believe everything you read, particularly when it comes to complex social problems. Modern communications

---

Box 1.2 Moment of Insight

Amount of revenue generated at the domestic box office within five days for the movie *Star Wars Ep. VII: The Force Awakens*:	Cost of smallpox eradication program, 1967–1979 (total, not annual):
US $300 million	**US $300 million**
(The movie set the record for fastest to reach this milestone.)	
Source: www.the-numbers.com/movie/records/Fastest-to-300-million-at-the-Box-Office	*Source:* Glynn, I., & Glynn, J. 2004. *The life and death of smallpox.* Pub: Cambridge University Press.

provide us with unprecedented access to endless sources of unedited information that must be used carefully. Unfortunately, when you ask the question, "Why are these people sick?" the answer is frequently some form of injustice. Trying to understand the roots of that injustice and simply getting to the truth of the story will present difficulties, particularly for those with a trusting nature. There is no substitute for detailed research followed by careful and thoughtful analysis. The point of this section is not to push a particular political agenda, but simply to stress that easy access to unedited information carries with it the obligation to check those sources carefully.

The history of any conflict is usually written by the victors. It would be interesting to compare schoolbooks written during the apartheid regime in South Africa to those currently available. To an outsider it might even be difficult to imagine that they are describing the same events. A less extreme example might be found in the portrayal of Native peoples in the school texts of North American history. Contemporary events are no different. Research into the events following the disintegration of Yugoslavia would also be strongly dependent on the source. Without getting involved in the issues, it is fair to say that Croatian Muslims, Albanian Macedonians, or Serbs from Kosovo would all have widely different interpretations of recent history. Equally, the prospect of writing a summary of recent events in the Middle East that was acceptable to all involved parties is difficult to imagine.

Examples of inequity and injustice are not difficult to find; any student of global health will constantly meet controversial topics. For example, anyone studying the health of poor labouring classes in India will soon discover the economic and social results of an ancient caste system that relegates Dalits, or "untouchables," to a life of drudgery and abuse. This is a complex and inflammatory subject. The Indian government will point out that Dalits have a vote and their position in society is slowly improving. The Dalit class is less impressed by this opinion. Initiatives based on superficial research (particularly when combined with political or religious biases) are quite likely to make matters worse. Whether you are studying the suicide rate among Inuit teens or worsening health indicators of infants in Iraq, Sudan, North Korea, or southern Lebanon, the causes are complex (as are the solutions) and require serious study before leaping to conclusions.

SUMMARY

Global health is essentially the blending together of various disciplines and professions along the journey toward health equity. These disciplines include medicine, primary health care, public health epidemiology, economics, sociology, development studies, anthropology, cultural studies, law, and others. Global health is premised on the fact that the economic and social conditions in which people live have an important impact on their health. Global health as a subject seeks to understand why population health is so poor in many developing countries and what can be done about it. There is no doubt that a great deal of progress has been made in improving health status in the last 50 years in many countries as indicated by a number of health indicators, such as life expectancy. However, hundreds of millions of people in the least developed countries still live lives of terrible deprivation. Since the end of World War II, a complex mix of private, governmental, and international organizations has developed with the overall aim of improving the health of populations in developing countries. While the developing aid industry has had successes, it has also had its share of trials and considerable errors. The current SDGs, several successful disease eradication efforts, and serious attempts to improve the scale and effectiveness of foreign aid have all combined to bring a sense of great optimism to the field of global health.

DISCUSSION QUESTIONS

1. How might one define global health? Why study global health?
2. What are some examples of global health issues? Which ones do you think are the most critical?
3. What are the SDGs and how do they relate to health? How would you improve on the SDGs?
4. How do the SDGs differ from the MDGs?
5. What is health equity? How does accomplishing the SDGs help to achieve health equity?
6. What is the relationship between poverty and health?
7. What key factors determine your personal health?
8. How do human rights abuses relate to global health?
9. Why is malnutrition considered an element of global health?
10. Why is population health so poor in many developing countries?

RECOMMENDED READING

Collier, P. 2007. *The bottom billion: Why the poorest countries are failing and what can be done about it*. Pub: Oxford University Press.
Katz, J. M. 2014. *The big truck that went by: How the world came to save Haiti and left behind a disaster*. Pub: St. Martin's Griffin.
Riddell, R. 2008. *Does foreign aid really work?* Pub: Oxford University Press.

REFERENCES

Annan, K. 2005. In larger freedom: Towards security, development, and human rights for all. Retrieved from: www.un.org/largerfreedom/.

Beaglehole, R., & Bonita, R. 2010. What is global health? *Global Health Action*, 3: 5142.

Chen, S., et al. 2007. The aftermath of civil war. *The World Bank Economic Review*, 22(1): 63–85.

Chen, S., et al. 2008. The developing world is poorer than we thought, but no less successful in the fight against poverty. World Bank Policy Research Working Paper no. 4703. Retrieved from: https://openknowledge.worldbank.org/bitstream/handle/10986/6322/WPS4703.pdf?sequence=1.

De Onis, M., et al. 2004. Methodology for estimating regional and global trends of child nutrition. *International Journal of Epidemiology*, 33: 1260–1270.

Easterly, W. 2006. *The white man's burden.* Pub: Penguin Press.

FAO (Food and Agriculture Organization). 2010. The state of food insecurity in the world. Retrieved from: www.fao.org/docrep/013/i1683e/i1683e.pdf.

FAO. 2016. The state of food insecurity in the world. Meeting the 2015 international hunger targets: Taking stock of uneven progress. Retrieved from: www.fao.org/3/a-i4646e.pdf.

Fehling, M., et al. 2013. Limitations of the Millennium Development Goals: A literature review. *Global Public Health*, 8(10): 1109–1122.

Glynn, I., & Glynn, J. 2004. *The life and death of smallpox.* Pub: Cambridge University Press.

Guha-Sapir, D., et al. 2010. Annual disaster statistical review. Retrieved from: www.cred.be/sites/default/files/ADSR_2010.pdf.

Koplan, J. P., et al. 2009. Towards a common definition of global health. *The Lancet*, 373: 1993–1995.

Merson, M. H., et al. 2006. International public health: Diseases, programs, systems, and policies (2nd ed.). Pub: Jones and Bartlett Publishers.

Millennium Development Goals. Retrieved from: www.un.org/millenniumgoals/.

Nobelprize.org. Amartya Sen autobiography. Retrieved from: nobelprize.org/nobel_prizes/economics/laureates/1998/sen-autobio.html.

Say, L., et al. 2014. Global causes of maternal death: A WHO systematic analysis. *Lancet Global Health 2014*, 2: e323–333.

SOHR. 2016. Syrian Observatory for Human Rights. Retrieved from: http://www.syriahr.com/en/?p=50612. UN. 2015a. The Millennium Development Goals report 2015. Retrieved from: www.un.org/millenniumgoals/reports.shtml.

UN. 2015b. Transforming our world: The 2030 Agenda for Sustainable Development. Retrieved from: https://sustainabledevelopment.un.org/post2015/transformingourworld/publication.

UN. 2015c. United Nations Resolution 70/1, Transforming our world: The 2030 Agenda for Sustainable Development, A/RES/70/1 (25 September 2015). Available from: undocs. org/A/RES/70/1.

UNdata (United Nations Data Retrieval System). Retrieved from: http://data.un.org.

UNPFII. 2010. UN Permanent Forum on Indigenous Peoples report. Retrieved from: www. un.org/esa/socdev/unpfii/en/sowip.html.

WHO (World Health Organization). 2010. Trends in maternal mortality: 1990 to 2008. Retrieved from: http://whqlibdoc.who.int/publications/2010/9789241500265_eng.pdf.

WHO. 2015. Trends in maternal mortality: 1990 to 2015. Estimates by WHO, UNICEF, UNFPA, World Bank Group and the United Nations Population Division. Retrieved from: www. who.int/reproductivehealth/publications/monitoring/maternal-mortality-2015/en/.

WHO. 2016. Global Health Observatory Data Repository: Mortality and global health estimates. Retrieved from: http://apps.who.int/gho/data/node.main. CM3002015REGWORLD?lang=en (Accessed July 6, 2016).

World Bank. 2016a. Data from the World Bank. World Development Indicators: Life expectancy at birth, total (years). Retrieved from: http://data.worldbank.org/indicator/SP.DYN.LE00.IN/ countries?display=graph (Accessed February 29, 2016).

World Bank. 2016b. Data from the World Bank. World Development Indicators: Mortality rate, infant (per 1,000 live births). Retrieved from: http://data.worldbank.org/indicator/SP.DYN. IMRT.IN (Accessed February 20, 2016).

CHAPTER 2

A History of International Aid

... and not flatter me at all; but remark all these roughness, pimples, warts, and everything as you see me.

—Oliver Cromwell, 1658

OBJECTIVES

Starting from small beginnings after World War II, foreign aid has grown into a multi-billion-dollar industry. In the absence of any guiding authority, each donor country's aid policy developed in response to its own set of external influences. The final result has been a complicated framework of differing agencies and policies that, not surprisingly, has had its ups and downs over the years. Much good has been achieved but, equally, many mistakes have been made. It is important to understand the long history of experimentation, success, and failure that has led to the currently revitalized aid industry with its exciting plans for the future. After completing this chapter, you should be able to:

- understand the broad trends that have shaped the modern aid industry since its start after World War II
- understand the origins of the principal foreign aid institutions and organizations
- gain insight into the long history of trial and error that lies behind the current large-scale foreign aid initiatives
- appreciate the rapidly changing world of aid in the new millennium

INTRODUCTION

Those who cannot remember the past are condemned to repeat it.

—*George Santayana, The Life of Reason, 1906*

It should be stressed that this chapter is not a polemic against aid. There is a long history of such criticism, from Hancock's well-known book, *Lords of Poverty* (1989), to Moyo's *Dead Aid* (2009). These two books (and many others during the intervening two decades) have emphasized major problems with the past and present results of foreign aid. It's not a difficult task—there is no shortage of suitable targets to choose from the last five or six decades of foreign aid. However, dwelling on past problems without considering the very real (one could almost say, revolutionary) changes that are currently taking place risks giving a rather limited view of a very complex undertaking. It is important to understand the past; after all, it was a knowledge of past failures that stimulated current initiatives in aid effectiveness and improved funding. However, it is also important not to remain stuck in the past, fighting old battles that have largely been won. Foreign aid isn't a waste of time, but neither is it the saviour of the poor. It is a complex and difficult undertaking, planned and managed by humans. It certainly could have been done a lot better in the past, but judged by current developments, it will certainly be done a lot better in the future.

Box 2.1 Moment of Insight

Net worth of the world's three richest people in 2015:	Annual GDP of the world's low-income countries in 2015:
Bill Gates: US$79.2 billion Carlos Slim: US$77.1 billion Warren Buffett: US$72.7 billion	from no. 194 Tuvalu: US$0.038 billion to no. 135 Armenia: US$11.64 billion
Total assets held by the three richest people in 2015:	Total annual GDP of the world's 60 poorest countries in 2015:
US$229 billion	**US$229 billion**

Source: Forbes. 2015. The world's billionaires. Retrieved from: www.forbes.com/sites/chasewithorn/2015/03/02/forbes-billionaires-full-list-of-the-500-richest-people-in-the-world-2015/#467eaf8716e3.

Source: World Bank. 2016. World development indicators database. Retrieved from: http://data.worldbank.org/indicator/NY.GDP.MKTP.CD.

At first glance, a history of the aid industry might seem to be a fairly dry subject. The newcomer could be forgiven for thinking that it has just been a long story of well-meaning governments giving money for worthwhile causes. Sadly, that is not even close to reality. If you want to understand the aid industry, you need to study it "warts and all." This expression certainly applies to the developing stages of the aid industry. From its start in the early postwar years, it rolled along, slowly gathering layer upon layer of government and private agencies. Uncoordinated, unanswerable to its constituents, and governed only by passing political and economic fads, it took a long time before the industry started to learn from its mistakes.

There has never been a central planning authority to guide the development of foreign aid. The current multi-billion-dollar industry grew in response to numerous external factors that might have suited the donors, but often had little to do with the best interests of the poor. Its management framework and the philosophical and theoretical reasons behind current development initiatives have all changed significantly with time. The final structure has been fashioned by experiences gained from many years of trial and error and painfully learned lessons (mainly painful to the recipients). The contemporary major debate over aid effectiveness is a broad response to that accumulated experience. In order to understand the modern aid industry and its ambitious plans for the next few decades, it is important to understand the details of the industry's history.

The modern global development industry is still relatively young; it traces its roots mostly to the reconstruction efforts in Europe following World War II. The framework of the industry, and its broad ideas about the best ways to improve population health, have all changed considerably since then. During the subsequent five or six decades, it has been fashioned by unavoidable external forces, such as the Cold War, the end of colonialism, the 1980s economic crisis, the HIV epidemic, and, most recently, by the Millennium Development Goals, plus the moves toward improved funding and aid effectiveness stimulated by that international agreement. Internally, the industry has been influenced by widely varying philosophies ranging from the Washington economic consensus on the right to primary health care enthusiasts on the left. The aid industry might now be approaching calmer maturity, but it certainly had a very difficult childhood!

Before embracing the orthodoxies of the day, it should be remembered that the aid industry has a long history of transient enthusiasms for new initiatives. Few people now remember the Global Initiative for Health for All by 2000, and fewer still can recall the announcement of the New International Economic Order. More importantly, who remembers past failures such as early disease eradication efforts, the structural adjustment era, or the use of aid for geopolitical advantage or economic gain? If these are just swept under the carpet or called unavoidable growing pains, future planners will not learn the available lessons.

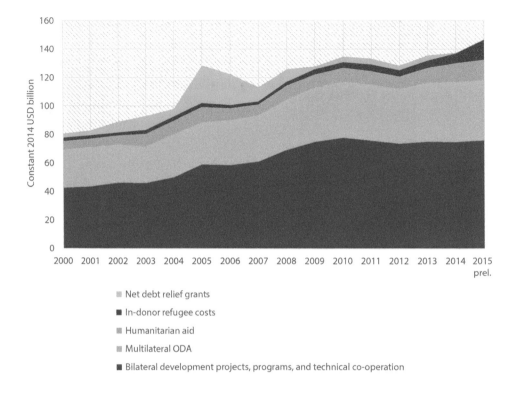

Figure 2.1: Components of DAC donors' net official development assistance

Source: OECD. 2016a. Retrieved from: www.oecd.org/dac/financing-sustainable-development/development-finance-data/.

The widespread adoption and subsequent support of the SDGs is a very promising sign that the aid industry has learned some important lessons about the best way to do business. After passing through a period in the 1990s when the relevance of aid was seriously questioned, the industry's future is looking much brighter. Increasing volumes of foreign aid, combined with a fundamental focus on the needs of the poor and the use of published outcome measurements, all give very real hope that the wealth and influence of the richest countries can make a substantial contribution toward that most optimistic goal set almost 40 years ago at Alma Ata—health for everyone, not just rich people, but everyone.

THE DEVELOPMENTAL STAGES OF FOREIGN AID

Foreign Aid before World War II

> I regard many of our Colonies as being in the condition of undeveloped estates and estates which can never be developed without Imperial assistance.
>
> —*Joseph Chamberlain, secretary of state for the colonies, 1895*

If poverty could be cured by words, it would have been solved long ago. Since writing began, numerous pious platitudes have been written about charity and the poor. There are plenty of examples from secular and religious literature. Ancient laws protecting the poor were carved on a stone stele under Hammurabi (Goldman Law Library, 2008) and scratched on parchment with quill pen 30 centuries later under the first Queen Elizabeth (Bloy, 2002). Despite this, a great deal of history passed before humans reached the point where a group of prosperous countries could consider giving aid to less fortunate ones. Some of the laws and practices introduced during the more benign periods of the Roman Empire could be considered as the earliest attempts at public health initiatives. The introduction of clean water (Rome's Trevi fountain is still fed by one of those early aqueducts), public baths, and toilets meant that the largest cities in the Roman Empire had standards of health that were little worse than those in London during the early days of Queen Victoria's rule.

Although foreign aid was very slow to develop, the elements of the modern system, including the rudiments of military intervention, humanitarian assistance, and, of course, the first aid agencies, can all be dated to the 19th century. The first recognizable aid project was conducted by the Spanish roughly 200 years ago. In response to the devastation caused by smallpox in the Spanish colonies, Charles IV sent Xavier de Balmis to spread the newly discovered vaccination process throughout Spanish holdings. In the absence of refrigeration, the vaccine was kept alive by sequential vaccination among a group of "volunteers" taken from La Coruna Orphans Home. The expedition, which left in 1803, vaccinated an estimated 100,000 people in areas ranging from the Caribbean, South and Central America to as far north as Texas, and subsequently in the Philippines, Macao, and Canton. They arrived back in Spain three years later (Aldrete, 2004). Whether this work was motivated by general altruism or just a pragmatic desire for healthier slaves is not recorded.

Direct financial assistance for poor areas of the world was a particularly late development. The main colonial countries, such as Britain and France, tended to view their colonies as sources of money during the 19th century. Roads, railways, and ports were built, but the benefits were intended for the colonial masters, not the local poor. Local schooling and health care was usually provided either by missionaries or large landowners, but certainly not in any organized fashion by the imperial authorities. Chamberlain's quote above shows that they made some attempt at developing the colonies, but it was all rather late in the day. Britain's first efforts at planned development started with the British Colonial Development Act in 1929. Not only did this leave little time before the moves toward independence, but the departing colonial countries also gave the newly independent governments a bill for the work done! More on this when we come to study the origins of the developing world debt.

The development of large health agencies was stimulated by the spread of steam-powered rail and sea transport during the 19th century. Then, as now, rapid transportation had the effect of increasing the spread of epidemics. Waves of infectious diseases spread through all the large cities, particularly the major ports. Smallpox, bubonic plague, yellow fever, and cholera were all common illnesses in North American port cities—no different from the spread of SARS or avian influenza today (Tatem et al., 2006). Responses to this new challenge were slow. After intermittent meetings in the late 19th century, the first international Sanitary Bureau was established in 1902 and included the United States and others from South America. This later grew into the Pan American Health Organization (PAHO). The notion of a truly international health agency followed much the same course as the development of PAHO. The concept was first discussed at various international sanitary conferences from 1851 onward, but

Box 2.2 History Notes

Francisco Xavier de Balmis (1753–1819)

Born into a medical family, he first worked as a military surgeon in Spain's North African colonies. He later worked in Mexico as head of the Amor de Dios Hospital. He gained a reputation through his writing, particularly his translation of a French book on vaccination. When it was decided to spread the benefits of smallpox vaccination throughout the Spanish Empire, he was chosen as head of the project. In the absence of refrigeration, the vaccine was kept alive by sequential inoculation of 20 orphans taken along for the trip. The expedition left Spain in 1803, sailing for Venezuela, Mexico, and Cuba. He then sailed on to China, the Philippines, and finally home after over three years of travelling. Follow the reference for more information: Aldrete (2004).

it was not until 1907 that the Office International d'Hygiène Publique (OIHP) was first formed. Those early roots can be traced through the subsequent health section of the League of Nations and finally to the formation of the World Health Organization (WHO) in 1948.

The roots of humanitarian aid principally lie in the early responses to famines. The best known, but by no means the largest, was the Irish famine in the years around 1850. The response was slow, but the famine went on for so long that eventually money and food were donated on an international scale—even from as far away as the Ottoman Empire. There were, of course, a great many others during this period that received little attention, particularly recurrent famines in India and largely unrecorded but enormous loss of life in China. An early success story was the British response to famine in Bihar in 1873. Importation and distribution of rice from Burma greatly minimized mortality. The organizer, Sir Richard Temple, was heavily criticized for wasting money. The United States has a long history of donating agricultural surpluses as food aid (Hanrahan, 2006). The first congressional grant for food aid was directed to Venezuela as early as 1812. Other large programs included food aid to Europe in 1919 and Russia in 1920. The program was formalized by Public Law 480 in 1954 and still continues to provide large volumes of food aid despite considerable controversy about the potential harm of donated food (US Government Accountability Office, 2011).

Given 19th-century attitudes toward colonization (at least, those of the colonizers), it is not surprising that a serious emphasis on human rights did not appear until the middle of the following century with the formation of the United Nations. However, some advances were made—the most obvious success was the abolition of slavery—but progress was glacial. Britain banned slave trading in 1807, but did not stop slave ownership until 1833. In the US, it took a civil war before slavery was finally banned by the 13th Constitutional Amendment in 1865. The related topic of military intervention to remove tyrannical rulers also has a long history. The recent NATO-led military support of the civilian uprising in Libya can be traced back to the combined military support by France, Britain, and Russia, which helped end Turkish control of Greece around 1830.

The battle of Solferino between Austria and a joint French and Italian army in 1859 was the unlikely starting point for the first international aid agency, the International Committee of the Red Cross (ICRC). A travelling Swiss businessman, Henri Dunant, arrived in Solferino on the evening after the battle. He was horrified by the sight of wounded men who were simply left to die. He organized local women to nurse the wounded, paid for tents to be set up, and negotiated the release of Austrian doctors held by the French. The book he wrote describing the chaos was well received and helped him spread his ideas for improving the care of wounded soldiers. In 1863, the International Committee of the Red Cross was formed. The following year, the first Geneva convention was signed by 12 states. War was also the stimulus for one of the earliest NGOs, Save the Children. It was formed in 1919 in response to the starvation induced by World War I (Save the Children, 2017).

These slow steps toward today's international organizations needed to be supported by advances in the young sciences of epidemiology and tropical medicine. The need for well-trained doctors for the British colonial service prompted the establishment of the first schools of tropical medicine in Liverpool in 1898 and in London the following year. Both have aged well and they remain acknowledged leaders in their field.

Table 2.1: Major events in the history of health aid

Year	Event	Year	Event
1803	De Balmis's international smallpox vaccination expedition	1978	Alma Ata meeting (start of PHC era)
		1979	Smallpox eradicated
1844	Engels's *Condition of the Working Class in England*	1980s	First case reports of HIV/AIDS; steady spread of HIV south through Africa; child survival revolution
1848	Chadwick's report of the labouring classes of Britain		
		1987	Movement toward "Adjustment with a human face"
1851	First International Sanitary Conference		
		1992	WHO/UNICEF introduce IMCI initiative
1854	John Snow removes pump handle during cholera outbreak	1993	WDR report (*Investing in Health*) starts strong move toward health sector reform
1863	International Committee of Red Cross forms		
		1999	Roll Back Malaria Program
1898	First tropical medicine research centres in Liverpool and London	2000	Global Alliance for Vaccines and Immunizations
1902	Pan American Sanitary Bureau (becomes PAHO in 1949)	2002	GFATM (new approaches to health funding)
1919	League of Nations, International Health Section	2003	SARS epidemic; President's emergency fund for HIV/AIDS
1942	UN Relief and Rehabilitation Administration	2008	First longitudinal reports confirming falling malaria and maternal mortality rates
1946	UNICEF formed		
1948	UNRRA merges with WHO	2011	Steady progress against neglected diseases such as filariasis, leishmaniasis, and schistosomiasis
1950s	Export of Western-style health care; first eradication campaigns (yaws, leprosy, TB, malaria)		
		2013	West African Ebola virus epidemic (the most widespread epidemic of Ebola in recorded history)
1961	UNICEF report (Children of the Developing Countries)		
1965	UNICEF awarded Nobel Peace Prize	2015	17 Sustainable Development Goals (SDGs) is established (2016–2030) and adopted by the 193 countries of the UN General Assembly.
1967	Smallpox eradication program starts		

1940s and 1950s

> Fourth, we must embark on a bold new program for making the benefits of our scientific advances and industrial progress available for the improvement and growth of under-developed areas.
>
> *—President Harry S. Truman, inaugural speech, 1949*

To understand the development of the aid industry, it is important to appreciate the major events of this period. The war had brought devastation to many countries, but it had also catalyzed unstoppable social movements. For example: India became independent in 1947, Israel was created in 1948, and Mao came to power in China in 1949; the times were certainly changing. Between about 1945 and 1990, the countries of the Eastern and Western blocs increasingly split apart, separated by an ideological and, in some places, physical barrier. In fact, it was the Soviet blockade of West Berlin that prompted one of the earliest large-scale aid initiatives. During 1948 and 1949, the United States, Britain, and France supplied the population of West Berlin entirely by air, shifting 2.3 million tons of food, coal, and other supplies (Cold War Museum, n.d.). This was also an early example of foreign aid and foreign policy becoming entangled (Photo 2.1).

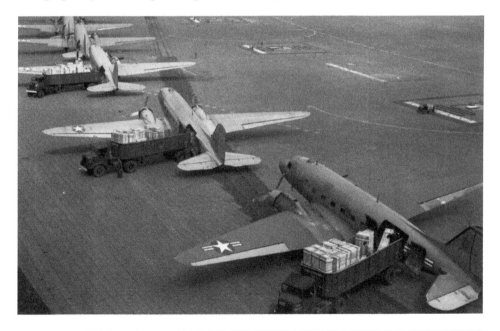

Photo 2.1: A 1948 photograph of transport aircraft being unloaded at Berlin's Tempelhof airport. At the height of the airlift, a plane landed at West Berlin's main airport every 90 seconds.

Source: National Museum of the US Air Force, courtesy of Wikimedia Commons.

Around the same time, a wave of nationalism swept the world from Africa to Asia. As the colonial masters shuffled out the back door, the two ideological blocs would spend the next few decades squabbling for influence over these newly independent states. Financial aid and military assistance were the tools used by both sides to gain political influence. In the process, foreign aid money was wasted shamelessly on a succession of tyrants from Marcos to Sesi Seko, while the poor of those countries were viewed as little more than pawns in the great game.

A quote from President Truman's much-quoted "four-point" inaugural speech in 1949 is given at the beginning of this section. Many date the start of modern aid from this speech—subsequent initiatives based on this promise were often included within what was called the "Point Four Program." While it was an important milestone, it was, in fact, preceded by a large aid project run during the war years called the Lend Lease Program, which began in 1941. Under that agreement, the United States provided food and military hardware to war allies, principally Great Britain, Russia, and China. By the end of the war, the United States had lent over US$45 billion worth of supplies. In a forgotten lesson for the future, the allied countries were also allowed to repay the loans at below market interest rates.

Poor agricultural and industrial recovery following the war produced starvation and malnutrition in several European countries. The United States proposed a scheme for European reconstruction named after President Truman's then secretary of state, George Marshall (USAID, 2002). The administration of the plan is worth noting because it has many lessons for the future of aid. Most importantly, it was a true joint venture, with complete planning and administration of the money left in the hands of the European countries. America's role was largely to provide the cash. European countries formed the Organisation for European Economic Co-operation (OEEC) to run the project. This later grew to become the OECD and also formed the seeds of the future European common market.

Over a four-year period beginning in 1947, over US$13 billion worth of aid was distributed. The result was a rapid rebuilding of Europe and two decades of unbroken economic growth. Apart from being allowed to administer the projects themselves, it is also important to note that many European countries were given low-interest loans (without conditionality clauses) and were allowed to maintain their own protective trade barriers. Several were later granted outright debt forgiveness. Many of those countries are now major creditors and seem to have forgotten those early lessons! Much of the money was spent on American goods and contributed to the US economic recovery. A strong Europe also helped limit the westward expansion of the new Soviet bloc.

This early successful program greatly influenced the development planners of the time. Broadly speaking, aid was already separating into two camps (Tarp, 2000):

- *Aid directed toward economic growth:* Examples include balance of payments assistance, agriculture and industrial investment, investment in infrastructure (ports, railways, power stations, roads, etc.), and, much later, poverty alleviation and debt relief.
- *Aid directed toward improved population health:* Examples include projects within the broad topic of health (from clean water and food to immunization and hospitals), but also education and, later, gender equity, human rights, democracy support, ecology, etc.

Around this time, the major international agencies that supported those development aims were also established—the start of an ever-enlarging list of large agencies. Following a meeting at Bretton Woods in 1944, the International Monetary Fund and World Bank were both established. They were initially intended to help rebuild larger Western countries and also stabilize international exchange rates. Both later concentrated more on economic development for poor countries. The General Agreement on Tariffs and Trade was started at the same time and later changed to the World Trade Organization in 1994 (Bretton Woods Committee, 2011).

The United Nations was established in 1945 after an initial proposal by Roosevelt in 1942. It replaced the earlier, short-lived League of Nations, but inherited some of its institutions, such as the International Labour Organization. Numerous health-related UN bodies have subsequently been formed, including: the Food and Agriculture Organization in 1945, the UN International Children's Emergency Fund in 1946 (which since 1953 has been the UN Children's Fund, but it retains its original acronym), the World Health Organization in 1948, and the UN High Commissioner for Refugees in 1950 (originally the UN Relief and Rehabilitation Administration).

Economic and health-related projects of the 1940s and 1950s were based on the optimistic feeling that technology and money could be used to eradicate poverty and ill health as they had in Europe. The "big push" was the order of the day. Economic programs were based on the theories attributed to Harrod and Domar. Growth was dependent on money—all you had to do was supply investment and infrastructure, and then growth would naturally follow. Unfortunately, neither theory nor practice resulted in economic growth (Easterly, 1997). This was in the early days of aid, so implementation was influenced by old colonial attitudes. In particular, the practical lessons from the Marshall Plan were not heeded. Recipient countries were not included in the planning and implementation process, so aid money disappeared like water poured on sand—with about the same results. No matter how well intentioned those projects might have been, it took many more

Table 2.2: Major Events in the History of Economic Aid

1800s	Widely varying investments in colonized countries	1975	Lome Convention (EU aid framework)
1929	British Colonial Development Act	1980s	First structural adjustment loans; collapse of numerous developing economies
1941	Lend Lease Program		
1947	Marshall Plan, OEEC forms	1990s	Increasing criticism of IMF/WB economic policies; end of Cold War
1948	Berlin airlift		
1950s	Big projects (dams, roads, railways)	1994	World Trade Organization forms
1950	Colombo Plan (British Commonwealth aid framework)	1996	HIPC initiative
		1999	EHIPC initiative
1954	US Public Law 480 (Food for Peace)	2000	Millennium Development Goals
1955	Bandung meeting (start of non-aligned movement)	2001	Doha round of international trade talks
1960s	Start of NGO expansion; Green Revolution	2002	Monterrey consensus on increased aid funding
1960	OPEC forms	2003	Paris consensus on aid effectiveness; failed Cancun talks, G20 formed
1961	OECD forms and its development arm, DAC; US Foreign Assistance Act (separates military and non-military aid)	2005	Hong Kong trade talks, tentative agreements; Gleneagles G8; Multilateral Debt Relief Initiative
1964	First UNCTAD meeting		
1969	Pearson Commission (0.7 percent of GDP goal)	2008	Geneva, collapse of Doha talks
1972	McNamara reorganizes the World Bank and emphasizes focus on the poor	2011	Annual financial aid climbs over US$120 billion, double the 1995 total
1974	Declaration of New International Economic Order	2013	Spending on development assistance for health (DAH) peaks at $38 billion

years of trial and error before the benefits of true aid partnerships were realized. However, for those who wanted to look, the lessons were there—imposed programs, even ones that look great on paper, will produce no benefit without active involvement of the target population.

In the field of health, optimism seemed to be justified based on the discoveries of effective drugs and insecticides stimulated by the demands of war. Examples included penicillin, chloroquine, and DDT. During the 1950s, top-down eradication programs were announced against a range of diseases (UNICEF, 1996a). Newly discovered penicillin worked well against yaws, a disfiguring chronic infection of skin and bones common in Africa and Asia. Over a million people were treated in Thailand alone. Other programs were started against malaria (based on chloroquine, proguanil, and DDT), tuberculosis (based on streptomycin, PAS, and isoniazid), leprosy (based on promin and dapsone), and trachoma (a chronic eye infection treated with newly developed antibiotic ointments). Despite some successes, all those early eradication efforts ultimately foundered on the same shoals—the solid and immovable rocks of human nature and limited resources. Treating yaws is not too difficult. The response to treatment is quick and obvious, so people are prepared to co-operate. Unfortunately, most diseases are not so easily interrupted (certainly not tuberculosis, malaria, or HIV). Modern drugs are only one part of the eradication of most diseases. The full program must include education, changes in personal behaviour, and better living conditions. There are no quick fixes for the complexities of infectious diseases.

Modern HIV/AIDS researchers have had to relearn epidemiological lessons established decades ago (Henderson, 1999). Effective disease control requires co-ordinated programs aimed at multiple levels of intervention. The disease reservoir must be identified and treated, transmission must be interrupted (often at more than one level), and infectious contacts must be traced and treated. This all takes money, organization, and long-term changes in human behaviour. Of all these obstacles, the need to change human behaviour is probably the biggest.

So, the stage is set for the next phase of the industry's development. The early years following World War II saw the aid industry grow up from a tangled set of roots that included lessons derived from the reconstruction of postwar Europe, a desire for Cold War political advantage, a need for an economic return for all that money, and lastly, some measure of altruism (Hjertholm et al., 2000).

1960s and 1970s

To those peoples in the huts and villages of half the globe struggling to break the bonds of mass misery, we pledge our best efforts to help them help themselves.

—*President John F. Kennedy, inaugural speech, 1961*

The start of the 1960s was declared the "first decade of development" by the United Nations and was ushered in by another much-quoted speech by an American president on the future of development aid. The period began with growing enthusiasm for the "big plan" approach to development and also witnessed the continuing process of decolonization—17 newly independent African states were formed in 1960 alone. These young countries needed help with their early economic and social development, so aid was naturally directed toward them. More money available for more new countries could lead only to one thing—more bureaucrats. An endless succession of agencies was needed to feed this growing industry.

In 1960, the International Development Association was established within the World Bank to coordinate interest-free loans to poor countries. The European agency set up to administer the Marshall Plan aid was expanded in 1961 to become an international organization (Organisation of Economic Co-operation and

Development). The following year, its Development Assistance Committee was established. In 1965, the UN Development Program was formed from two earlier bodies in order to help developing countries use aid more effectively. The following year the UN Industrial Development Organization was formed specifically to help developing world industries. To add to the abbreviations, individual countries started their own bilateral aid agencies around this time (USAID, Britain's DFID, Europe's ECHO, etc.). Finally, non-governmental organizations were formed in the thousands, from Oxfam (1942) to the Jubilee 2000 Coalition (1996).

Newly independent countries were not prepared to continue their colonial attitudes. Their collective voice slowly started to affect the aid debate, but their limited economic muscle made this a slow process. The non-aligned movement grew out of a conference at Bandung in 1955. It ultimately represented over 100 countries that wanted to enter the development debate, but were not prepared to align themselves with either of the great powers. Its main architects were Jawaharlal Nehru (India's first prime minister), Sukarno (Indonesia's first president), Gamal Abdel Nasser (Egypt's second president), Kwame Nkrumah (Ghana's first president) and Josip Broz Tito (president of the former Yugoslavia). By the early 1960s, their combined voice persuaded the UN to call its first UN Conference on Trade and Development (UNCTAD) in 1964.

Despite regular four-year meetings, UNCTAD had little or no influence on international trade. The sense of frustration of non-aligned countries grew to such a level that in 1973, the UN called a meeting of the General Assembly to discuss development and international trade. The result was the declaration of a New International Economic Order, which was accepted by the UN in 1974 (Johnson, 1978). It contained 18 clauses covering a range of issues from increased aid to trade liberalization that looks very similar to contemporary aid thinking currently celebrated as being brand new.

Forty years later, it is hard to understand the high expectations surrounding the New Order—who remembers it now? Hopefully, the same fate does not lie in store for the Doha Development Round. The declaration was not legally binding and the developing bloc lacked significant influence to impose a serious development debate. Inevitably, the process generated much debate (labelled "the North-South debate" at the time), but little action. The oil-rich elites of the developing world had formed the Organization of the Petroleum Exporting Countries (OPEC), their own pressure group, in 1960, but this influence was used sparingly. However, not everything was wasted; the ghosts of UNCTAD and the New Order live on. They are easily seen today, drifting through the failure of the Doha round of trade talks and the collapse of the World Trade Organization (WTO) into various developing world pressure groups. The arguments are exactly the same, but the countries making them now have enough economic influence to get themselves heard.

Apart from early aid-funded benefits of agricultural advances (subsequently known as the Green Revolution), the 1960s brought little help to the absolute poor—you have to own some land before you can benefit from improved crops. The initial postwar enthusiasm for aid was also declining. In 1962, developed countries gave roughly 0.5 percent of their GDP in aid. The 1969 Pearson Commission on Aid used available mathematical models (plus a bit of guesswork) to arrive at the widely quoted recommendation that countries should give 0.7 percent of GDP as aid. By 1972, the Development Assistance Committee (DAC) average was about 0.3 percent. It later fell to a low of 0.22 percent in the 1990s, but has now risen back above 0.3 percent in response to the demands of the MDGs.

Health aid had few major successes in the 1960s. The push to import Western-style medical services was not successful, but no clear alternative was yet available. An influential multi-agency report on the health of children in 1961 (*Children of the Developing Countries*) helped raise the profile of children's health needs and also of UNICEF. This ultimately led to UNICEF being awarded the Nobel Peace Prize

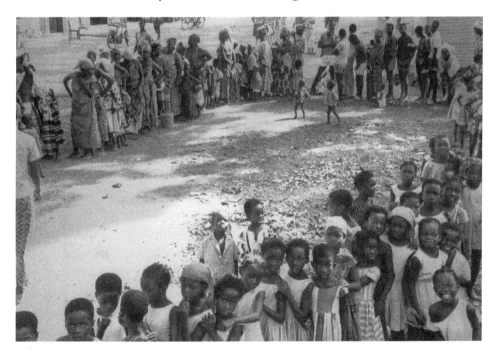

Photo 2.2: A 1969 image from the early days of the smallpox eradication program showing adults and children in Niger, West Africa, queueing for their vaccination. Only 10 years after this picture was taken, smallpox was declared completely eradicated from the world.

Source: Photo courtesy of the CDC's Public Health Image Library (PHIL: http://phil.cdc.gov/phil/home.asp).

in 1965 (UNICEF, 1996b). Just as early eradication efforts from the 1950s were being cancelled, the WHO decided to have one more try. The smallpox eradication program was announced in 1967 under the direction of Donald Henderson (Fenner et al., 1989). This remains one of the most striking examples of the successful use of foreign aid. Smallpox was declared eradicated from the world in 1978 (Photo 2.2).

In a triumph of hope over experience, the United Nations introduced the second development decade with even more ambitious goals than they had declared for the first. These did, at least, produce some significant changes in guiding principles behind foreign aid. The 1970s started with some signs that the poor would be included in the debate—the decade also included the famous Alma Ata meeting on primary health care. Ultimately, these hopeful advances were overwhelmed by the steady economic decline induced by falling commodity markets and rising oil prices. Unfortunately, a specific emphasis on the needs of the poor was lost in this period of worsening economic news. In 1973, Robert McNamara, then president of the World Bank, made an influential speech encouraging aid donors and developing world governments to redesign their policies to meet the needs of the poorest 40 percent of the population and relieve their poverty directly (Milobsky et al., 1995). But it would take another 20 years before this approach was adopted by World Bank economists.

The need for a new approach was also becoming obvious in the field of health aid. It was becoming clear that Western-style medical care, typified by a modern urban hospital, packed with high-technology equipment, was not as useful as it might have first appeared. Apart from being out of reach of the rural poor, the cost of running such an institution could consume a significant portion of a small country's health budget (Morley et al., 1983). Growing dissatisfaction with the poor results of health development made it obvious that change was necessary; the experience gained by a few developing countries (particularly China's approach) attracted a great deal of attention. The "great leap forward" in 1958 had responded to rural health needs by developing local clinics staffed by medical orderlies, subsequently known as barefoot doctors. The reality was not as perfect as the political propaganda would suggest, but this basic needs approach did seem to offer an alternative model for development. The culmination was the Alma Ata Summit in 1978 and the subsequent Health for All Strategy that emerged from it (Perin et al., 2003). Primary health care and services at the village level now supplanted the previous emphasis on shiny new hospitals.

The end of these two decades of development saw health aid and economic aid moving in two very different directions. The health debate, with all its imperfections, did at least base its programs on what was best for the poor. Unfortunately, the organizers of economic aid responded to the debt crisis of the time by imposing conditional aid, the main aim of which was to make countries more prosperous so they could keep up with their debt obligations. It was expected that some of that prosperity would subsequently trickle down, but the poor were very much a secondary issue behind economic growth. It would be some time before common ground could be found between these two approaches.

1980s and 1990s

Rather than requiring several generations of effort and astronomical economic resources, it is now actually possible to provide virtually every man, woman, and child on earth with adequate food, clean water, safe sanitation, primary health care, family planning, and basic education—by the end of the century and at an affordable price.

—*James Grant, director, UNICEF, 1993*

The United Nations' optimistic call for a third development decade in 1980 was out of touch with reality. By the end of the 1980s, fieldworkers who had battled the effects of developing world debt, structural adjustment policies (SAPs), deepening crisis in sub-Saharan Africa, and the onset of HIV/AIDS epidemic referred to this period as the lost decade. The failure of Mexico to meet its debt repayments in 1982 heralded the start of the developing world debt crisis. The solution of the day was ideologically based economic therapies (often called the Washington Consensus), which included privatization of state industries, trade liberalization, and reduction in social spending on health, education, and food subsidies for the poor (Williamson, 2000). These economic interventions were collectively known as structural adjustment policies. In the late 1980s, it was already becoming clear that their effects were disastrous for the health of the poor. UNICEF published a report demanding action to protect children from the worst effects of the economic crisis (Cornia et al., 1987). Its influence slowly took effect through the 1990s.

At the start of the second United Nations decade in 1972, the General Assembly had defined 24 countries as "least developed"; by 1991, this number had almost doubled to 47 countries. Despite 20 years of economic interventions, agreements, and binding resolutions, more countries than ever before were overwhelmed by debt. It was not until the 1990s that the World Bank and the International Monetary Fund (IMF) responded to criticism of their policies by taking a new approach to poverty alleviation and debt relief. The Highly Indebted Poor Countries (HIPC) Initiative in 1996, their second try in 1999 (enhanced HIPC), and recent initiatives aimed at absolute debt relief are the current results of that debate (Oxfam, 2005).

The primary health care (PHC) era, which started at Alma Ata, and the subsequent Health for All Declaration meant that health aid began the decade with great optimism. Under the leadership of James Grant, UNICEF introduced targeted care for poor children in a program known as the "child survival revolution" (UNICEF, 1996c). This involved a package of cost-effective therapies known by the acronym GOBI (growth monitoring, oral rehydration, breastfeeding, and immunization). Women's health later received more emphasis when family spacing, female education, and food supplements during pregnancy were added (GOBI-FFF). In 1992, the program was expanded in a joint WHO/UNICEF initiative called the Integrated Management of Childhood Illnesses (IMCI). This treatment approach has been widely adopted in developing countries, but has encountered criticism concerning its effectiveness (IMCI, 2010). Two related events at the end of the decade included the Convention on the Rights of the Child in 1989, and the World Summit for Children held the following year. The goal-oriented methods proposed at this meeting were the foundations for the Millennium Development Goals.

Although real advances were made, particularly the expanded vaccine initiative, PHC did face significant problems. Financial considerations and a great deal of in-fighting limited its implementation to a narrower focus than its initial originators intended. After all the squabbling was over, the watered-down version remaining was called "selective PHC" (Hall, 2003). We'll never know what might have happened if the initial plans had been carried out. But even selective PHC had its successes. The GOBI-FFI program was of value to women and children, but it was limited in its scope. What a rural subsistence farmer might want (care for his aching back)

Table 2.3: Major events in human rights and humanitarian aid

Year	Event	Year	Event
1698	English Bill of Rights	1978	Helsinki Watch founded, later Human Rights Watch
1789	French Declaration of the Rights of Citizens	1979	UN Convention eliminating gender discrimination
1791	US Bill of Rights	1987	UN Convention banning torture
1812	Food aid to Venezuela	1982	Carter Centre founded
1850s	Slow response to Irish potato famine	1989	UN Convention on the Rights of the Child
1863	13th Amendment to US Constitution banning slavery	2002	International Criminal Court established
1873	Successful Bihar famine relief	2004	Asian tsunami
1919	Fight the Famine Council, the precursor of Save the Children	2005	UN Human Rights Council formed to replace dysfunctional predecessor
1919	League of Nations founded	2007	UN Declaration on the Rights of Indigenous Peoples
1920	Food aid to Russia		
1925	League of Nations' Declaration on children's rights	2010	Haitian earthquake response
1945	United Nations established	2011	Pakistan earthquake
1948	UN Universal Declaration of Human Rights	2011	Japanese earthquake/tsunami
1961	Amnesty International founded	2014	West Africa Ebola outbreak

and what he gets with selective PHC (breastfeeding advice, immunization for his children, and a lecture on safe sex) are not at all the same thing. Basically, people everywhere want the same thing—a well-equipped clinic run by well-trained staff who will meet their broad health needs. Immunizations and breastfeeding are measurably beneficial, but they do not match up to expectations in isolation.

The delivery of health services has, of course, continued to change since the PHC era, but it has not been replaced by a single philosophy. Current moves toward health sector reform usually date back to an influential 1993 World Development Report and a subsequent World Health Report in 2000 (World Bank, 1993; WHO, 2000). Changes obviously vary with region, but they include decentralization of health services, various forms of community financing, provision of a cost-effective package of services, and varying degrees of privatization. Primary health care slowly disappeared from view and is hardly mentioned in the current debate. The 1993 report also marked a reunification of the two arms of development assistance since it emphasized the absolute need for economic growth combined with improved health; both are fundamental human needs. If they head in opposite directions, the only losers are the poor; it is now generally accepted that you cannot have one without the other.

The classification of development initiatives into health aid and economic aid is obviously an oversimplification, but it is of some value when giving a broad overview of the period. During the 1980s and 1990s, health aid did fairly well. The implementation of the Alma Ata Accord was patchy and slow, but even immunization and oral rehydration on their own saved millions of lives. Economic aid responded to the challenge of world recession by concentrating on economic growth incentives, even when some of those initiatives were demonstrably harmful to the poor. By the end of the 1990s, many hard lessons had been learned, and economic planners had learned to include the poor in the solutions to their own problems. Aid had passed through a period when many thought it was no longer relevant. The approaching new millennium brought a sense of optimism that the time was right for real change.

The New Millennium

> Reflecting on the MDGs and looking ahead to the next 15 years, there is no question that we can deliver on our shared responsibility to end poverty, leave no one behind and create a world of dignity for all.
>
> —*Ban Ki-moon, 8th Secretary-General of the United Nations*

At the beginning of each decade, the UN announced optimistic hopes for the first, second, third, and fourth development decades. Unfortunately, reality always lagged far behind those optimistic projections. However, the start of the new millennium coincided with very real hopes that the future of the aid industry would be increasingly bright. There have been several promising developments, particularly an increasing emphasis on the poor. It is also encouraging to see the two separate arms of the industry (economic aid and health projects) being merged into common projects with shared aims.

To some extent, the aid industry is just about back where it started in the 1940s and 1950s. The end of World War II has been replaced by the end of the Cold War. The "big plan" approach to infrastructure projects of 40 or 50 years ago has now been replaced by or is mirrored in some aspects of the MDGs and can certainly be seen in Sachs's approach to development (Sachs, 2005). Early vertical eradication programs, once heavily criticized as remnants of colonialism, have been replaced by large initiatives targeted at specific diseases such as Roll Back Malaria (RBM). The term "vertical eradication program" is no longer used in polite circles, but current projects against HIV/AIDS, tuberculosis, and malaria show their roots in those early eradication efforts of the 1950s and 1960s.

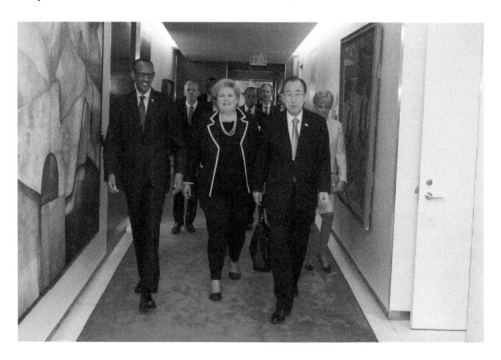

Photo 2.3: Former Secretary-General Ban Ki-moon (right) with the co-chairs of his Millennium Development Goals (MDG) Advocacy Group, Erna Solberg (centre), prime minister of Norway, and Paul Kagame, president of Rwanda, 29 September 2015.

Source: UN Photo/Eskinde Debebe, with kind permission of the UN Photo Library (www. unmultimedia.org/photo).

The aid industry is currently going through a period of revival, largely triggered by the financial and administrative demands of the MDGs and the new SDGs, plus a broad consensus that the old ways of doing business need to change. Foreign aid donations have almost doubled compared to the mid-1990s, and major attempts are being made to harmonize the efforts of multiple agencies and improve the effectiveness of aid. The involvement of highly successful business leaders has brought new ideas for organization and fundraising from within the aid industry, while the growth of large non-DAC donors such as China, India, and Brazil now provides competition from without. Foreign aid has travelled a bumpy road during the last 60 years. There is now a sense that the industry has matured and learned some lessons, which can only be a good thing for the future of aid and, obviously, for the people it is intended to benefit.

MDGs and Foreign Aid

The launch of the MDGs catalyzed major increases in development assistance as evidenced by the 66 percent jump in official development assistance (ODA) between 2000 and 2014, when it reached an unprecedented US$135 billion (Figure 2.2).

More aid has flowed into education and public health while also being directed toward poorer countries to supplement the increases in domestically sourced development finance (OECD, 2010). The influence on donor policies and practices and—more variably—on governments in the developing world has been considerable. For instance, the MDGs (specifically, MDG 6) were integral considerations in the policy formation of the Global Fund to Fight AIDS, Tuberculosis, and Malaria (Global Fund), which was created in 2002. The MDGs have gone a long way toward changing the way we think and talk about the world, shaping the international discourse and debate on development, and stimulating popular awareness of moral imperatives such as achieving gender equality and ending poverty and starvation. The new SDGs are bound to continually shape the foreign aid industry with more focus on metrics, impact, and equity.

Emerging Donors

DAC has been a part of the OECD since 1961 and provides a forum for (bilateral and multilateral) donors to come together for harmonizing their aid activities in order to decrease poverty and realize the Millennium Development Goals. The DAC works on issues like aid effectiveness, collecting aid statistics, and the evaluation of the development process (OECD, 2010). Countries like the United States, Australia, the UK, Japan, and the EU have been the

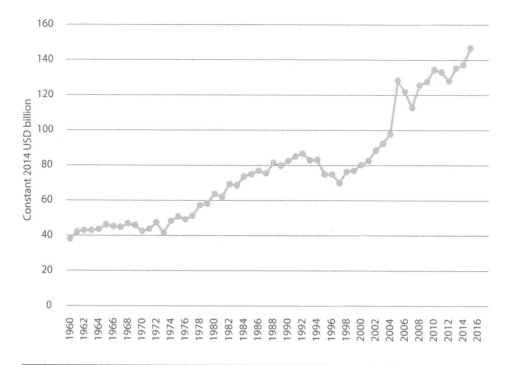

Figure 2.2: Share of total ODA going to least developed countries

Source: OECD. 2016b. Development Co-operation Report 2016: The Sustainable Development Goals as business opportunities. Retrieved from: www.oecd-ilibrary.org/development/development-co-operation-report-2016_dcr-2016-en.

long-standing donors and part of the DAC, but that is changing with the increasing value of international aid from emerging donors such as China, India, Brazil, Turkey, and South Africa. By scaling up their aid budgets these nations are growing their international influence. For example, in 2006, about 7–10 percent of total aid flows was provided by emerging donors, and in 2012 this had risen to 25 percent of the total official development assistance (OECD CRS, 2014). In the 1990s, over 90 percent of development assistance came from the DAC countries (Manning, 2010), and developed countries dominated international development co-operation. However, since 2000 the number of non-DAC donors has risen significantly, reaching 30 in number (Smith et al., 2010).

We also have non-state actors, such as the Bill and Melinda Gates Foundation, a development NGO, which are filling the gap in areas like vaccination, agriculture, and pursuing innovative projects that government donors find hard to do.

SUMMARY

Foreign aid is a multi-billion-dollar industry which has grown in response to numerous external factors that might have suited donor countries, but often had little to do with the best interests of the poor. Its management framework and the philosophical and theoretical reasons behind current development initiatives have all transformed significantly with time. The final structure has been fashioned by experiences gained from the industry's history, which has resulted in a complicated framework of differing agencies and policies that have vacillated over the years. The aid industry is currently going through a period of revival, largely triggered by the financial and administrative demands of the MDGs and the new SDGs, plus a broad consensus that the old ways of doing business need to change. There has also been a focus on metrics to improve the efficiency of the impact of foreign aid and to harmonize the efforts of multiple agencies in improving the effectiveness of aid.

DISCUSSION QUESTIONS

1. What are the key events that have shaped the modern aid industry? How has aid changed between World War II and now?
2. What would you consider the major successes in the history of foreign aid? What are some of the key factors that led to those successes?
3. Why was the start of the 1960s declared the first decade of "development" by the United Nations?
4. How have the MDGs and new SDGs shaped foreign aid?
5. What were some of the key factors that led to the eradication of smallpox? How would you apply some of these factors in global health?
6. If you were in charge of a major multilateral agency such as the World Bank, how would you make foreign aid more effective?
7. If you were in charge of a major bilateral agency such as Global Affairs Canada or the Department for International Development, what structures would you put in place to ensure that international aid is not wasted by corrupt governments?
8. Do you believe the views that official aid might be harming countries, creating dependency, and fostering corruption? Why or why not?
9. How important is the aid industry in global health? Should international aid end? Why or why not?
10. What can donors (including bilateral and multilateral agencies) do to improve foreign aid to better alleviate poverty and improve health outcomes?

RECOMMENDED READING

Acemoglu, D., & Robinson, J. 2013. *Why nations fail: The origins of power, prosperity, and poverty*. Pub: Crown Business.

Annan, K. 2013. *Interventions: A life in war and peace*. Pub: Penguin Books.

Banerjee, A., & Duflo, E. 2011. *Poor economics: A radical rethinking of the way to fight global poverty*. Pub: Public Affairs.

Chan, S. 2013. *The morality of China in Africa: The Middle Kingdom and the Dark Continent*. Pub: Zed Books.

Collier, P. 2007. *The bottom billion: Why the poorest countries are failing and what can be done about it*. Pub: Oxford University Press.

Foreman, J. 2013. *Aiding and abetting: Foreign aid failures and the 0.7% deception*. Pub: Civitas.

Munk, N. 2013. *The idealist: Jeffrey Sachs and the quest to end poverty*. Pub: Anchor.

Rist, G. 2008. *The history of development: From Western origins to global faith*. Pub: Zed Books.

Studwell, J. 2014. *How Asia works: Success and failure in the world's most dynamic region*. Pub: Grove Press.

Watson, L. 2014. *Foreign aid and emerging powers: Asian perspectives on official development assistance*. Pub: Routledge.

REFERENCES

Aldrete, J. 2004. The travels of Francisco Xavier de Balmis. *Southern Medical Journal*, 97: 375–378.

Bloy, M. 2002. The 1601 Elizabethan Poor Law. Retrieved from: www.victorianweb.org/history/poorlaw/elizpl.html.

Bretton Woods Committee. 2011. Retrieved from: www.brettonwoods.org/.

Cold War Museum. n.d. The Berlin Blockade. Retrieved from: www.coldwar.org/articles/40s/berlin_blockade.asp.

Cornia, G., et al. 1987. *Adjustment with a human face*. Pub: Oxford University Press.

Easterly, W. 1997. The ghost of the financing gap: How the Harrod-Domar growth model still haunts development economics. World Bank Development Research Group, paper 1807. Retrieved from: http://ideas.repec.org/p/wbk/wbrwps/1807.html.

Fenner, F., et al. 1989. *Smallpox and its eradication. History of Public Health* (Vol. 6). Pub: World Health Organization. Retrieved from: whqlibdoc.who.int/smallpox/9241561106.pdf.

Forbes. 2015. The world's billionaires. Retrieved from: www.forbes.com/sites/chasewithorn/2015/03/02/forbes-billionaires-full-list-of-the-500-richest-people-in-the-world-2015/#467eaf8716e3.

Goldman Law Library. 2008. The code of Hammurabi. Retrieved from: avalon.law.yale.edu/subject_menus/hammenu.asp.

Hall, J., et al. 2003. Health for all beyond 2000: The demise of the Alma Ata Declaration and primary health care in developing countries. *Medical Journal of Australia*, 178: 17–20.

Hancock, G. 1989. *Lords of poverty: The power, prestige, and corruption of the international aid business*. Pub: Atlantic Monthly Press.

Hanrahan, C. 2006. Agricultural export and food aid programs. Retrieved from: www.usembassy.it/pdf/other/IB98006.pdf.

Henderson, D. 1999. Eradication: Lessons from the past. *Morbidity and Mortality Weekly Review*, 48: 16–22. Retrieved from: www.cdc.gov/mmwr/preview/mmwrhtml/su48a6.htm.

Higgins, K. Reflecting on the MDGs and making sense of the Post-2015 Development Agenda. Ottawa: North-South Institute; 2013. Retrieved from: www.nsi-ins.ca/wp-content/uploads/2013/05/2013-Post-2015.pdf (Accessed September 16, 2015).

Hjertholm, P., et al. 2000. Survey of foreign aid: History trends and allocation. Institute of Economics, University of Copenhagen. Retrieved from: www.econ.ku.dk/wpa/pink/2000/0004.pdf.

ICRC. International Committee of the Red Cross. Retrieved from: www.icrc.org/eng/.

IMCI. 2010. Integrated management of childhood illnesses. Retrieved from: www.who.int/child_adolescent_health/topics/prevention_care/child/imci/en.

Johnson, H. 1978. The new international economic order. University of Chicago selected paper no. 49. Retrieved from: www.chicagogsb.edu/research/selectedpapers/sp49.pdf.

Kenny, C., & Sumner, A. 2011. More money or more development: What have the MDGs achieved? Working paper no. 278. Centre for Global Development. Retrieved from: www.cgdev.org/sites/ efault/files/1425806_file_Kenny_Sumner_MDGs_FINAL.pdf (Accessed September 16, 2015).

Manning, R. 2010. The impact and design of the MDGs: Some reflections. In A. Sumner and C. Melamed (Eds.), The MDGs and beyond. *International Development Studies (IDS) Bulletin*, 41(1): 7–14.

MDGs. UN Millennium Development Goals. Retrieved from: www.un.org/millenniumgoals.

Milobsky, D., et al. 1995. The McNamara bank and its legacy 1968–1987. *Business and Economic History*, 24(2): 167–195. Retrieved from: www.h-net.org/~business/bhcweb/publications/BEHprint/v024n2/p0167-p0196.pdf.

Morley, D., et al. 1983. *Practicing health for all*. Oxford: Oxford University Press.

Moyo, D. 2009. *Dead aid: Why aid is not working and how there is a better way for Africa.* Pub: Farrar, Strauss, and Giroux.

OECD. 2010. Inside the DAC. A Guide to the OECD Development Assistance Committee 2009–2010. Retrieved from: www.oecd.org/dac/40986871.pdf (Accessed May 28, 2016).

OECD. 2014. Query Wizard for International Development Statistics. Retrieved from: www.oecd.org/dac/stats/crsguide.htm (Accessed May 28, 2016).

OECD. 2016a. Retrieved from: www.oecd.org/dac/financing-sustainable-development/development-finance-data/.

OECD. 2016b. Development Co-operation Report 2016: The Sustainable Development Goals as business opportunities. Retrieved from: www.oecd-ilibrary.org/development/development-co-operation-report-2016_dcr-2016-en.

Oxfam. 2005. Beyond HIPC: Debt cancellation and the Millennium Development Goals. Oxfam briefing paper no. 78. Retrieved from: www.oxfam.org.uk/what_we_do/issues/debt_aid/downloads/bp78_hipc.pdf.

Perin, I., et al. 2003. Trading ideology for dialogue: An opportunity to fix international aid for health? *The Lancet*, 361: 1216–1219.

RBM. Roll back malaria. Retrieved from: www.rollbackmalaria.org.

Sachs, J. 2005. *The end of poverty: Economic possibilities for our time.* Pub: Penguin Press.

Save the Children. 2017. Our Story. Retrieved from: www.savethechildren.net/about-us/our-story.

Smith, K., Fordelone, T. Y., & Zimmermann, F. 2010. Beyond the DAC. The welcome role of other providers of development co-operation. DCD Issues Brief, OECD Development Cooperation Directorate.

Tarp, F. 2000. *Foreign aid and development: Lessons learned and directions for the future.* London: Routledge.

Tatem, A., et al. 2006. Global transport networks and infectious disease spread. *Advances in Parasitology*, 62: 293–343.

UNICEF. 1996a. The 1950s: Era of the mass disease campaign. Retrieved from: www.unicef.org/sowc96/1950s.htm.

UNICEF. 1996b. The 1960s: Decade of development. Retrieved from: www.unicef.org/sowc96/1960s.htm.

UNICEF. 1996c. The 1980s: Campaign for child survival. Retrieved from: www.unicef.org/sowc96/1980s.htm.

US Government Accountability Office. 2011. International food assistance: Report to Congress. Retrieved from: www.gao.gov/new.items/d11636.pdf.

USAID. 2002. Marshall Plan home page. Retrieved from: www.usaid.gov/multimedia/video/marshall/.

Williamson, J. 2000. What should the World Bank think about the Washington consensus? *World Bank Research Observer*, 15(2): 251–264. Retrieved from: www.iie.com/publications/papers/paper.cfm?researchid=351.

World Bank. 1993. World development report 1993: Investing in health. Retrieved from: http://econ.worldbank.org/external/default/main?pagePK=64165259&theSitePK=469382&piPK=64165421&menuPK=64166093&entityID=000009265_3970716142319.

World Bank. 2016. World Development Indicators database. Retrieved from: http://data.worldbank.org/indicator/NY.GDP.MKTP.CD.

WHO (World Health Organization). 2000. World health report 2000. Health systems: Improving performance. Retrieved from: www.who.int/whr/2000/en/whr00_en.pdf.

PART II

WHY ARE POOR POPULATIONS LESS
HEALTHY THAN RICH ONES?

CHAPTER 3

The Basic Requirements for a Healthy Life

We might free ourselves from innumerable diseases, both of the body and of the mind, and perhaps even from the infirmity of old age, if we had sufficient knowledge of their causes and of all the remedies that nature has provided.

—René Descartes, 1637

OBJECTIVES

In this second section of the book, we will look at the significant challenges faced by many of the people living in developing countries. The basic aim of the section can be summed up by the seemingly simple question, "Why are poor people less healthy than rich people?" Before examining the answers to that question, it is a good idea to begin by studying the basic requirements that people need in order to lead a long, healthy life. The answers are not as obvious as many would assume. The full story behind the steady improvement in population health over the last century is complex. Although prosperity and health care are important factors, several less tangible variables must be included. If your aim is to help improve the health of poor people, it is important to understand why they got sick in the first place—the answers will guide subsequent initiatives. After completing this chapter, you should be able to:

- understand the principal requirements for a healthy life, particularly the contributions of income, medical care, and social equity
- appreciate some of the complex determinants of health that appear once the basic needs have been met
- understand that a knowledge of the major determinants of health is an essential foundation for anyone interested in designing effective development strategies

INTRODUCTION

Of course, everyone wants to be healthy. The amusing thing is no one's really sure how to do it.

—*Jerry Seinfeld, 1995*

No matter what methods are used, the basic aim of any aid project is to improve the health of people living in poor regions. Clearly, before trying to improve population health, it is important to know why the people got so sick in the first place; it is better to define a diagnosis before rushing in with a cure. This is not as obvious as it sounds—the aid industry has a history of following treatment trends that subsequently proved to have had little benefit, particularly for the rural poor. A clear understanding of health determinants prevents money from being wasted on initiatives that are unlikely to have widespread advantages. For example, in the early years of the aid industry, too much emphasis was placed on curative medical treatment as the first response to widespread ill health. It took over 20 years before it was finally realized that Western medical care had little ability to control epidemic diseases caused by poverty and social chaos. It was finally agreed at the 1978 Alma Ata meeting that far greater benefits could be gained for a given aid budget if the basic determinants of health were attended to first. These include clean water, sanitation, housing, nutrition, and peace. Health care is surprisingly far down the list of cost-effective strategies. Think of the money that was wasted in the 20 years it took to learn that simple lesson.

Once the basic needs for existence are met, a wide range of less tangible factors appear. Humans are complex creatures; once their social conditions have improved beyond the level of bare survival, it is unlikely that the determinants of their health will be simple. Humans need to love and be loved. They need stable, peaceful societies and close social ties with family and friends. They need to feel they have control over their professional lives and, above all, that there is a sense of equity and fairness within their society. When these features are in place, a society can reach the final goal of population health, which is when mortality gradients no longer exist between social classes and the poorest in a country have the same mortality as the rich. When this happens, life expectancy for that country is probably as high as it will get. Some countries, such as Sweden, are close to this point, but it will be a long time before most of the world is anywhere near such a goal.

When Chadwick first studied the effects of social class on mortality in Victorian England (Figure 3.1), he found that life expectancy at birth for the most privileged classes was 44 years and the infant mortality rate was above 100 per 1,000 live births. The poor of Dickensian London or Victor Hugo's Paris lived lives that were

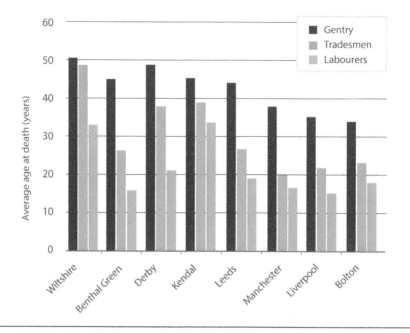

Figure 3.1: Average age at death calculated by Chadwick for three social classes in mid-19th-century England

Source: Chadwick, E. 1842. Spartacus Schoolnet. Retrieved from: www.spartacus.schoolnet.co.uk/PHchadwick.htm.

not essentially different from those who live in the shantytowns of today. Whatever it was that improved their health in the past probably has relevant application today. The health of the world's population has greatly improved since Chadwick's time, even among the poorest nations. During the 20th century, this trend accelerated. In the last 100 years, human life expectancy at birth has nearly doubled in some countries. The average American newborn in 1900 could expect to live 49 years. By 2000, that average baby could expect to live for 77 years (Figure 3.2). This is the greatest improvement in human health in history, but it is neither widely appreciated nor fully understood. The newcomer might assume that these improvements were most likely due to advances in medical care, but even a cursory examination shows this is not the explanation. Mortality rates from major killers such as tuberculosis in adults (Figure 3.3) and measles in children fell steadily decades before specific therapies were discovered. Clearly, other mechanisms were involved.

There is vast literature on the subject of health determinants. Although there is inevitable controversy, the major variables have been identified and health care is less prioritized. Below a certain level of per capita income, health is governed by money and access to basic human needs. However, after a country's GDP per

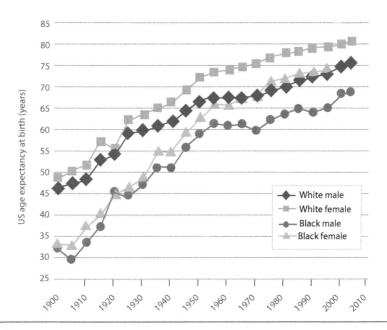

Figure 3.2: Historical trends in life expectancy at birth for the United States

Source: Shrestha, L. 2006. Life expectancy in the United States. Retrieved from: http://aging.senate.gov/crs/aging1.pdf.

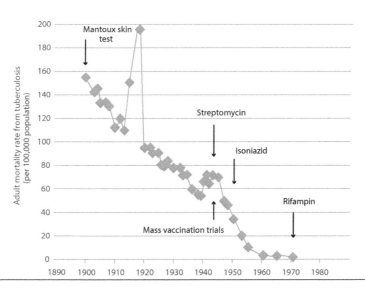

Figure 3.3: Age-standardized adult death rate from tuberculosis for England and Wales; the timing of advances in diagnosis and treatment are indicated with arrows

Source: Vynnycky, E., et al. 1999. Interpreting the decline in tuberculosis. *International Journal of Epidemiology*, 28: 327–334.

capita rises above approximately US$4,000, the relationship is completely lost and other variables gain in importance, such as social cohesion, income distribution, education, and social class. This is a fascinating subject that has great relevance for the design of modern aid projects.

HISTORY OF BASIC NEEDS STUDIES

> Battles are only the terminal operations engaged in by those remnants of the armies which survived the camp epidemics.
>
> —*Hans Zinsser, Rats, Lice, and History, 1934*

The Egyptian civilization lasted roughly 3,000 years before it finally gave way to British rule—not bad when you consider that the Canadian federation is barely 150 years old. During all that time, the population survived without the benefits of anaesthesia, antibiotics, or any knowledge of microbiology. Other early civilizations in Central America, the Indus and Yangtze River valleys, Rome, and Greece thrived for centuries even though their physicians had little more than primitive surgery and a handful of effective drugs (Nutton, 2004). It is likely that these early civilizations based their knowledge of population health on the experience gained from military campaigns. Once a large group of humans is

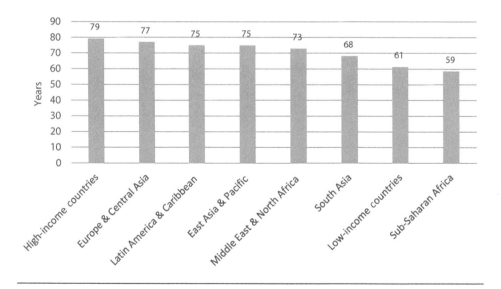

Figure 3.4: Life expectancy at birth, by World Bank region and for high- and low-income countries, 2014

Source: World Bank. 2016a. Data from the World Bank. Life expectancy, total (years). Retrieved from: http://data.worldbank.org/indicator/SP.DYN.LE00.IN.

crammed together with minimum attention to clean water and waste disposal, it soon becomes very obvious to an intelligent observer that some basic rules of hygiene are necessary. It is probable that more armies have been stopped by infection than by combat (Peterson, 1995).

Some armies took longer than others to learn these lessons on hygiene. As recently as the American Civil War, deaths among soldiers from infections such as typhoid, cholera, smallpox, and malaria (roughly 250,000) were nearly as high as those due to combat (roughly 350,000) (American Civil War Story, 2016). Help arrived in the unlikely form of a society gardener called Frederick Law Olmsted. He had gained such a reputation for organization while landscaping Central Park in New York that he was placed in charge of the US Sanitary Commission during the Civil War. In this position, Olmsted's Committee of Enquiry into military health slowly forced the US Army to improve living conditions and medical care for its soldiers (Frederick Law Olmsted, 2011). The standards of hygiene in the British Army (and the subsequent mortality) would have horrified any of the campaigning generals from ancient times. Long after Pacini's discovery of the bacterial cause of cholera (in fact, after his death from old age), the British Army still persisted in the belief that a flannel body wrap was the best way to prevent cholera. The "cholera belt" was a standard part of army issue in the tropics until 1920 (Renbourn, 1957)!

Archaeological evidence of existing Roman military camps shows clear evidence of their knowledge of the essentials of public health. Tents and cooking areas were placed well away from latrines and waste disposal. These ideas probably influenced early city design. Excavations at the middle-class holiday resort of Pompeii showed that all but the poorest houses had running water and central sewage disposal (Pompei, 2011). Today, any visitor to the slums of Dhaka in Bangladesh or Accra in Ghana would not take long to sort out why the inhabitants are unhealthy—probably less healthy than an average Roman citizen 2,000 years ago. There is clearly a minimum set of standards (e.g., clean water, shelter, food) that must be in place before any sort of restful, healthy life is possible.

As an exercise, it is well worth debating what basic features are required for a healthy society and then setting them in some sort of order. Ideas will vary, but the lists given in the first column of Table 3.1 combine published opinions with the result of a debate among medical and resident students in Vancouver, Canada. Whatever results your own debate produces, one point will be common to all: medical treatments do not appear until well down the list. It is important to remember that we are discussing population health rather than individual health. Anyone with a treatable emergency such as appendicitis or pneumonia will be very happy to have access to good-quality medical care. However, on a population level, as we will discuss later in this chapter, medical care does not have a big impact on population mortality rates,

Table 3.1: Basic requirements for a healthy life, listed in order of importance, from four sources

VANCOUVER MEDICAL STUDENTS (2010)	CLARK ET AL. (2005)	DOYAL ET AL. (1991)	MASLOW (1943)
• Peace	• Housing or shelter	• Nutritious food and clean water	• Basic physiological needs
• Easy access to clean water	• Food	• Protective housing	• Safety
• Comfortable shelter	• Water	• Safe work environment	• Belonging and love
• Adequate food supply	• Work/jobs	• Safe physical environment	• Esteem
• Employment with fair pay	• Money/income	• Safe birth control and child-bearing	• Need to know and understand
• Education for all	• Clothes	• Appropriate health care	• Aesthetic needs
• Stable judiciary/police force	• Education and schools	• A secure childhood	• Self-actualization
• Immunization	• Health/health care	• Significant primary relationship	• Transcendence
• Good-quality obstetric care	• Electricity/energy	• Physical security	
• Democratic government structure	• Safety/security	• Economic security	
• Free press and freedom of speech	• Transport/car	• Appropriate education	
	• Family and friends		
	• Sanitation		
	• Infrastructure		
	• Leisure/leisure facilities		

particularly when it is compared to the provision of the basic needs of food, shelter, water, and absence of war. In fact, in a large review of what happens when doctors go on strike, it was clearly shown that death rates usually decrease (Cunningham et al., 2008), mainly because of decreased surgery being done on older patients.

Over the last three to four decades, there has been growing literature on the subject of population health (See "Recommended Reading"). It has become increasingly apparent that this is a very complicated topic. Some of the major determinants, such as clean water, shelter, and food, as mentioned earlier, are quite apparent, but others are far less intuitive. For example, the health benefits of a free press or democracy are not immediately clear, but, as the economist Amartya Sen pointed out in his famous study on the origins of famine (Sen, 1983), their benefits are measurable. His research prompted the famous statement that there has never been a famine in a functioning democracy or in a country with a free press. The health effects of these and other, even more intangible determinants—such as social cohesion—are difficult to analyze, but their effects are very real (Lynch et al., 2001).

At first glance, the basic needs for health are much the same as your grandmother's advice: eat your greens, take some exercise, go to bed early, and do not

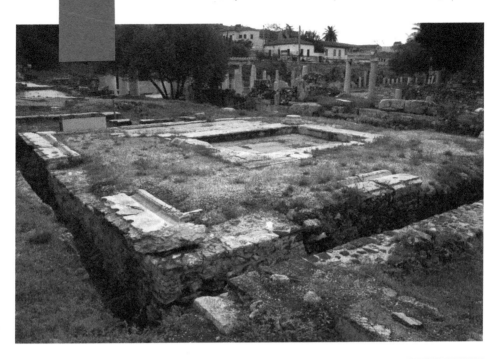

Photo 3.1: Ruins of the first-century public toilet built by the Romans in the main Athens marketplace. It is served by running water and drained by a sewer system. Roman standards of public hygiene were not reached again until the late stages of Queen Victoria's reign, nearly 2,000 years later.

Source: Photo by G. Dall'Orto, courtesy of Wikimedia Commons.

misbehave. On a population basis, your grandmother's advice scales up to clean water, good nutrition, shelter, peace, and acceptable behaviour. An American psychologist, Abraham Maslow, proposed a rather more complex list, ranging from absolutely basic needs up to less definable requirements such as self-actualization and transcendence (Maslow, 1943). Despite this, the base of his pyramid (commonly known as "Maslow's hierarchy of needs") contains much the same essentials as those compiled by the Vancouver students (Table 3.1). Similarly, the 11 basic needs summarized by Doyal et al. (1991) and the essentials of life defined by poor communities in South Africa (Clark et al., 2005) all come to the same general conclusions: human societies have much the same basic hopes and dreams no matter where they live.

So far, we have defined the first few rungs of the ladder that populations must climb to reach a safe, happy life; those steps include clean water, peace, food, shelter, fair employment, education, and a safe and stable community (Table 3.1). This is, of course, much neater and simpler in theory than in practice. In later chapters we will examine the practical problems of implementation (not least of which is the

money needed to pay for the initiatives). However, despite these practical difficulties, the widespread introduction of basic human needs is the most cost-effective
way to spend aid money. Not surprisingly, many of the United Nations SDGs are
based on such initiatives (UN, 2016).

Interestingly, the first of the SDGs addresses poverty: "End poverty in all its
forms everywhere." Eradicating poverty in all its forms remains one of the greatest
challenges of our times. One in five people in developing regions still live on less
than US$1.25 a day. Malnutrition, discrimination, lack of clean drinking water
and basic sanitation, limited access to education, and social discrimination are a
few of the many manifestations of poverty. While the number of people living in
extreme poverty (currently measured as people living on less than US$1.25 a day as
set by the World Bank) has dropped in the last 30 years, the drop has been limited
to South Asia and sub-Saharan Africa, which account for 80 percent of the global
total of those living in extreme poverty.

The first core goal of ending poverty in all its forms everywhere includes five
associated objectives:

1. By 2030, eradicate extreme poverty for all people everywhere, currently mea-
    sured as people living on less than US$1.25 a day.
2. By 2030, reduce at least by half the proportion of men, women and chil-
    dren of all ages living in poverty in all its dimensions according to national
    definitions.
3. Implement nationally appropriate social protection systems and measures for
    all, including floors, and by 2030 achieve substantial coverage of the poor and
    the vulnerable.
4. By 2030, ensure that all men and women, in particular the poor and the vul-
    nerable, have equal rights to economic resources, as well as access to basic
    services, ownership and control over land and other forms of property, inher-
    itance, natural resources, appropriate new technology and financial services,
    including microfinance.
5. By 2030, build the resilience of the poor and those in vulnerable situations
    and reduce their exposure and vulnerability to climate-related extreme
    events and other economic, social and environmental shocks and disasters.
    (UN, 2015)

Although the specific targets related to ending poverty might seem too ambitious, they are feasible (Sachs, 2015).

THE EFFECTS OF MONEY ON POPULATION HEALTH

I've been rich and I've been poor. Rich is better.

—Sophie Tucker, 1955

It would seem to be a logical assumption that the health of a population is reasonably correlated with its average income. This holds true for low- and middle-income countries whose per capita GDPs fall below about US$4,000 (Wilkinson, 1996). The average life expectancy for high-income countries is almost 20 years higher than the life expectancy for low-income countries (Figure 3.4). These lower-income countries and their populations are the ones where well-planned health initiatives are likely to produce the greatest cost-effective benefits. The introduction of clean water, sanitation, or improved housing can all help to move people as quickly as possible up the steep part of the health-wealth curve. Life expectancy is an imprecise marker of population health, but, whether the indicator is maternal mortality or under-five mortality, the relationship is identical: mortality rates improve rapidly as income increases, but then flatten off at the same level of GDP per capita (Figure 3.5). After that point, variables other than income dominate the picture.

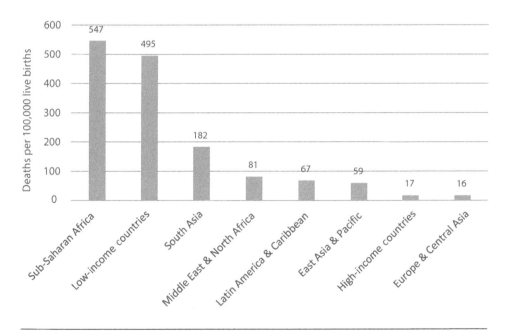

Figure 3.5: Maternal mortality ratio, by World Bank region and for high- and low-income countries, 2015

Source: World Bank. 2016b. Data from World Bank. Data: Maternal mortality ratio. Retrieved from: http://databank.worldbank.org/data/reports.aspx?source=2&country=&series=SH.STA.MMRT&period=.

Oddly enough, above the annual GDP per capita level of US$4,000, the clear beneficial relationship between health and wealth breaks down. Some relatively poor areas of the world manage to maintain healthy populations despite low incomes. For example, although Georgia and Swaziland have similar GDPs per capita (roughly US$3,500), the average person in Georgia lives 26 years longer! The difference is partially due to the effects of HIV/AIDS, but the full explanation is far more complex. These mortality differences also exist within countries. Some rich countries, such as the United States, have disadvantaged populations whose life expectancy can only be considered that of a developing country. There is a 20-year gap in life expectancy between Whites in the healthiest areas of the US and Blacks in the least-healthy areas (Kaplan et al., 1996). This is equivalent to the difference in life expectancy between Japan and the worst parts of Bangladesh, so there is clearly a great deal more to health than simply money (Diez Roux, 2001). This disparity between the poorest and the richest is particularly marked in rapidly growing economies like Brazil, China, and India.

The relationship between health and wealth is fairly obvious and has been known about for a long time. Edwin Chadwick published his careful study of disease and mortality in Victorian London. When it was published in 1842, it shocked the Victorian middle classes. He showed clear health and mortality gradients between the five defined social classes, ranging from level one (the gentry) to level five (unskilled labourers) (Figure 3.1). A typical quote from the report describes the poverty, overcrowding, filth, and disease common in London at that time:

> Shepherd's Buildings consist of two rows of houses with a street seven yards wide between them; each row consists of what are styled back and front houses—that is two houses placed back to back. There are no yards or out-conveniences; the privies are in the centre of each row, about a yard wide; over them there is part of a sleeping-room; there is no ventilation in the bedrooms; each house contains two rooms, viz., a house place and sleeping room above; each room is about three yards wide and four long. In one of these houses there are nine persons belonging to one family, and the mother on the eve of her confinement. (Chadwick, 1842)

The relationship between life expectancy and income noted by Chadwick 170 years ago is applicable to any developing country today. At one time in their history, all countries have witnessed increasing life expectancy in relation to increasing wealth. However, as countries grew richer, it became clear that there was a limit to this relationship—increasing wealth does not produce ever-increasing life expectancy. At some point there is an upper limit. The health-wealth transition point has likely always existed, although the inflection point obviously moves up and to the right with increasing global health and prosperity. It is important to remember that this is an average for many countries. As we shall see later, social gradients still exist within every society no matter how high its average income. The richest and most influential always seem to be healthier than those who have less than they do—even in countries where "less" still represents great wealth.

Once basic needs have been met and a country has turned the corner on the graph, the relationship between health and income becomes more complex and generates plenty of controversy. Slowly rising prosperity increasingly allows people to buy the basic necessities to live a healthy life, but each of those factors comes with a price. When this progress is combined with enlightened government health policies, the proportion of deaths due to infectious diseases falls and the number of children reaching their fifth birthday starts to rise.

The health transitions noted in more developed countries have attracted considerable research. The analysis of methods used by successful countries has relevance for the planning of health interventions in high-mortality areas. For example, over the last 50 years, Tunisia has managed to reduce its infant mortality from 150 per 1,000 down to 26.2 per 1,000, while life expectancy has increased by nearly 50 percent (50 years to 72 years) (Ben Hamida et al., 2005). How did they manage to do that? Can those lessons be applied in other countries? So far, a combination of money and basic needs implementation has helped our population move about halfway up the health-wealth curve. From here on, the story gets a lot more complicated.

Box 3.1 Moment of Insight

Chance of an Afghan baby dying before its fifth birthday: 250 per 1,000	Chance of getting tails twice in a row when tossing a coin:
1 in 4	1 in 4

Source: UNICEF. 2009. Childinfo. Retrieved from: www.childinfo.org.

THE EFFECTS OF MEDICAL CARE ON POPULATION HEALTH

> Medicine is a collection of uncertain prescriptions, the results of which, taken collectively, are more fatal than useful to mankind. Water, air, and cleanliness are the chief articles in my pharmacopeia.
>
> *—Napoleon Bonaparte*

No one who has received high-quality treatment in a modern hospital would argue that medical care is of no value. Although it may be a comforting service at a personal level, does the enormous expense and complexity of modern medicine make any measurable difference at a population level? We know that money and basic needs move a population up the health-wealth curve, but does the addition of medical care add any further significant benefits?

Modern medicine is a huge and ever-growing beast. Over the last two decades, every developed country has had to deal with the problem of trying to control it, but until quite recently, research into outcomes and efficiency was mainly aimed at the financial costs of treatment. Illich's critical review of health care in 1976 helped to trigger a more useful debate about whether medical treatments actually achieve anything useful (Relman, 1988). Topics such as waiting lists, wide variations in use of procedures, and medical errors now attract serious attention, but it is still surprisingly difficult to tell how much value the industry actually produces for all that money.

In historical terms, medical advances did little to improve health during the first half of the 20th century; tuberculosis is a good example. As McKeown (1979) pointed out, the death rate from tuberculosis in all developed countries fell steadily decades before the discovery of effective drugs in the late 1940s and the use of surveillance programs and BCG (*Bacillus Calmette-Guérin*) vaccination in the 1950s (Figure 3.3). These programs were vital and helped remove TB as a public health problem, but much of the disease had already disappeared by the time they started. Population surveys using tuberculosis skin tests in Britain during the 1940s and 1950s showed that most adults had still been exposed to the bacillus, but far fewer of them were contracting the disease. An increasingly healthy and prosperous population appeared to be able to resist TB, but what was the mechanism? As mentioned above, early diagnosis and treatment were not the explanation—clearly other factors were involved. Medical care is certainly a major part of modern tuberculosis control programs, but the eradication of this infection from a community requires social as well as medical interventions.

Similar patterns are found with other major infectious diseases. For example, acute rheumatic fever and rheumatic heart disease were the most common causes of death for Canadian children in 1900 (English, 1999). One hundred years later, the disease has almost disappeared even though the causative agent, group A Streptococcus (GAS), can still be found in the throats of 5 to 10 percent of children after a 10-day course of antibiotics (Pichichero, 1999). Antibiotics did not cause the decline in rheumatic fever because the bacterial cause still exists. Decreasing bacterial virulence is also not an explanation because GAS remains a common cause of invasive bacterial disease at all ages (Davies et al., 1996). Similarly, the death rate from whooping cough (pertussis) had already fallen from 1,400 per million in 1860 to 100 per million in 1950, when effective vaccination was introduced. Over the same period, the death rate from measles fell from 1,200 per million down to 10 per million—again in the absence of any specific medical treatment.

People just seemed to get steadily stronger over the last century. There has to be a rational explanation, but just what was going on? As infectious diseases became less important causes of mortality (even with the advent of the HIV epidemic),

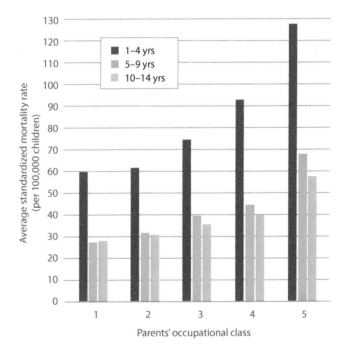

Figure 3.6: Three age-standardized childhood mortality rates plotted by social class: occupational class 1 (professional) to occupational class 5 (labourer)

Source: Black Report: Inequalities in Health, 1982.

it was argued that medical treatment would play an increasingly important part in the health of modern societies. Deaths from cancer, atherosclerosis, and other diseases of an aging population might not be governed by the same variables as infectious diseases, so all that money might finally be making a measurable change in modern life expectancy. However, subsequent studies showed this to be incorrect. It turns out that it does not matter what is wrong with you, whether you have cancer or measles; case fatality remains strongly affected by social class. The first large-scale report to study the question of medical care and population health was commissioned by the British government in 1980. It was led by Sir Douglas Black and is commonly called the Black Report. It represented a revolution in thought concerning the place of health care, but was very unpopular with the prevailing government attitudes of the day. Despite limited publicity, its conclusions were very influential. Its findings were repeatedly confirmed by subsequent government reports on the same subject—the Whitehead Report in 1987, the Acheson Report in 1998, and the most recent in 2010, led by Sir Michael Marmot (Marmot, 2010).

Black's committee studied mortality rates in five defined socio-economic classes among the British population; complete data stretched back to 1911. Predictably, the data showed clear mortality differences between the social classes. His data on child mortality (Figure 3.6) was essentially no different than Chadwick's findings from over a century earlier (Figure 3.1): mortality rates were roughly twice as high in social class 5 compared to social class 1. The most shocking result was that this relationship had not changed over time. In particular, Black showed that there had been no narrowing of the class mortality gap following the introduction of free health care for all classes with the introduction of the National Health Service (NHS). In fact, gradients had worsened slightly (Figure 3.7). The report concluded that class-related differences in mortality had little to do with failings of the NHS but were likely the result of social inequities in education, housing, diet, work conditions, and income. The need for social programs to combat these problems, rather than simply giving more money to the NHS, is a valuable lesson for those planning population health initiatives. It also failed to make the report popular with the Thatcher government of the day.

Mackenbach et al. (1990) looked at studies of disease outcome in medical conditions that should have been completely treatable with modern health care (such as acute appendicitis). Even when medical care ought to have had the dominant effect, these studies showed that outcomes were still more heavily influenced by socio-economic factors than by medical treatment. A review article that depended on well-informed estimates rather than measurements (Bunker et al., 1994) concluded that modern medicine (including screening tests, medical treatment, and immunization) explained only about 20 percent of the observed improvement in American

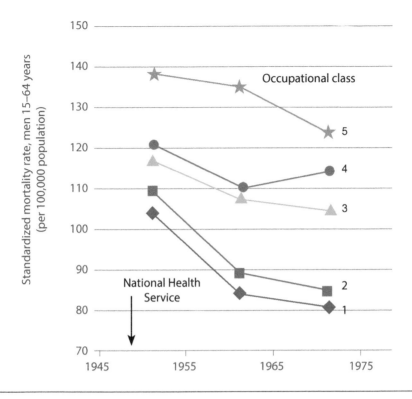

Figure 3.7: Changes in the adult mortality rate, classified by occupational class, for the 20 years following the establishment of the National Health Service in Britain: occupational class 1 (professional) to occupational class 5 (labourer)

Source: Black Report: Inequalities in Health, 1982.

life expectancy. Finally, there have been several doctors' strikes in various countries. Studies of mortality rates during these strikes are available, particularly for two strikes in Israel (Siegel-Itzkovitch, 2000). On both occasions, observed mortality rates fell during the strike, then worsened again when the doctors resumed work.

The average person living in a modern Canadian city probably does not think much about why he or she did not catch tuberculosis, typhoid, or smallpox during a working day even though all those diseases were common in Canada in the early 20th century. The health of a population is largely determined by economic and social variables; medical care is in the difficult position of simply trying to tidy up the mess when something goes wrong. It cannot do much to improve population health, but it is certainly a valuable asset at a individual level. A perfect example is given by the effect of contaminated water on population health in the prosperous town of Walkerton, Ontario, Canada. Widespread fecal contamination of the town's water supply caused seven deaths and hundreds to get sick (Ali, 2004). Medical care, with the amazing advances in dialysis and intensive care, certainly saved the lives of many infected individuals. However, the simple and cost-effective public health provision of clean water would have prevented the problem altogether.

THE EFFECTS OF SOCIAL INEQUALITY ON HEALTH

> Class differences in health represent a double injustice: life is short where its quality is poor.
>
> —*Richard Wilkinson, Class and Health, 1986*

So far, the combination of money and basic needs (plus a little help from medical care) has dragged our hypothetical population out of the Middle Ages. It is now well into the 21st century, with life expectancy around 60–70 years and per capita income of US$5,000–$10,000. What are the variables that now determine whether a population can slowly reach the life expectancies in Japan, Sweden, and Australia—which are near the top of the list with life expectancies over 80 years? One thing is certain: the variables we have examined so far are not the full story. For example, Americans (78.1 years) and Portuguese (78.2 years) have almost exactly the same life expectancy at birth, yet America's GDP per capita is over twice that of Portugal (US$45,989 versus $21,903). Clearly, above a certain level, more money does not necessarily buy more health. Similarly, most of the points

Box 3.2 History Notes

Sir Edwin Chadwick (1800–1890)

Chadwick was born in Manchester in 1800. While studying law, he earned extra money as a journalist writing review articles for London newspapers. His early work on poverty, sanitation, and the poor was widely read, and this set the course for the rest of his long life. Although he never believed in the existence of bacteria, his work and studies led to major advances in the eradication of infectious diseases in urban areas. To his dying day, he (and his friend Florence Nightingale) believed that infections arose spontaneously among dirt. He made significant contributions to public health and Poor Law reform, particularly with the establishment of official public health inspectors. His *Report on the Sanitary Condition of the Labouring Population* is widely considered to be the start of modern epidemiology and public health. Along with Engels in his report on the health of English labourers and Virchow in his report on the health of the poor in Silesia, Chadwick was one of the first people to link poverty to ill health. He was a famously difficult man to deal with and was described as a bore, a prig, and a fanatic. Despite this, he made major contributions to the health of England's population (Porter, 1990).

on the flat part of the health-wealth curve represent wealthy OECD countries. They have all provided basic health care for their populations for decades and, with the exception of the US, all have some form of national insurance to ensure easy access to health care for every level of society. Despite this, life expectancy still varies greatly both within and among these countries. It is time to search for other variables influencing the health of wealthy populations.

The Black Report, discussed above, gave some early insights into this problem. The findings confirmed what Chadwick had found in Victorian England—that there are health gradients in every society that run from rich to poor. In some strange and complex manner, social class is strongly related to health outcomes. A significant socio-economic mortality gradient is a universal finding. It affects all age groups and is present in every country studied (Leon et al., 1992; Wilkins et al., 1990). One of the extraordinary findings is that this mortality difference persisted from the first data measurements in 1921 (Wilkinson, 1989). Even though the basic causes of mortality changed greatly over this time period (from tuberculosis to atherosclerosis), social class mortality gradients persisted. As mentioned earlier, there was also no change in the mortality gradient even after the introduction of free health care for all.

These points need emphasizing. When tuberculosis was common, it killed the poor more than the rich even though all levels of society were exposed to the bacillus. Later in the century, when cancer and atherosclerosis displaced infectious diseases, the rich still did far better than the poor. The only plausible explana- tion is that some factor associated closely with social hierarchies is bad for health. Even though this factor is expressed in terms of disease mortality, it seems to be independent of the type of disease, and it also appears to be unaffected by medical care. No matter what type of disease is prevalent, its burden will always fall more heavily upon the poor.

It is not difficult to imagine that there is a mortality difference between the richest and the very poorest people in a given country. However, many subsequent studies have shown that mortality gradients also exist within each of the broadly defined social classes. In fact, it looks as if human societies can be broken down into smaller and smaller levels, each with its own mortality gradient. Sergeants, on average, are not as healthy as majors, who, in turn, are not as healthy as generals. Poverty is not sufficient to explain these differences. In two famous long-term studies named Whitehall 1 (Marmot et al., 1978) and Whitehall 2 (Marmot et al., 1991), Marmot et al. limited the number of variables by studying mortali- ty gradients within a single industry. They chose the British civil service, where clearly defined occupational grades were used as an approximation of social class. They found that coronary heart disease mortality varied greatly between these civil service grades. Men in the lowest category had a three times higher mortality rate when compared to administrators in the highest grade. Differences in blood pressure, smoking rates, and cholesterol levels also differed significantly between the grades, but these explained only a small proportion of the observed difference in mortality rates. Clearly, other causes were operating.

Members of all these grades had sufficient money to meet basic needs, so poverty was not an issue. Attention turned to the stress and lack of control associated with lower social positions. Another well-known study in Alameda County, California, offered some clues (Berkman et al., 1979). The study showed that complex social interactions can have a significant effect on health. People without social ties had significantly higher mortality rates compared to those who had broad social interactions. There was also a significant gender difference. Marriage was more beneficial for men, while contacts with friends, relatives, and membership in community groups was more important for women.

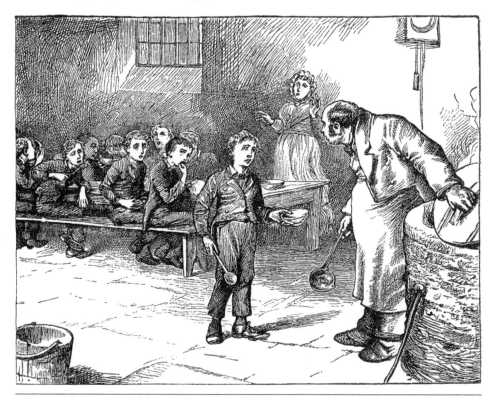

Photo 3.2: There is nothing new about the concept of basic needs and the connection between social conditions and health. Any child currently living in poverty would have no trouble recognizing the characters described by Dickens.

Source: Photo courtesy of Wikimedia Commons.

A joint study of Japanese men living in Japan, Hawaii, and California (Marmot et al., 1975) showed that as Japanese men lost their traditional contact with Japanese society, there was an increasing mortality from coronary heart disease as they moved from Japan to Hawaii and then to California. This mortality gradient existed even after controlling for risk factors such as cholesterol, blood pressure, and smoking. In fact, although men in Japan smoked heavily, their rate of smoking-related diseases was relatively low. Something about traditional ties offers a health protection. British civil servants are not the only mammals with strict rules governing social behaviour. Studies of baboons, both in the wild and in captivity, show that low-status animals suffer the greatest stress and mortality (Sapolsky, 1993). Captive vervet monkeys examined after death have been shown to have multiple gastric ulcers, bite marks, and other injuries that probably all reflected their lower position in the local social hierarchy of the troop.

While it is clear that social and cultural environments have an impact upon health, human societies are so complex that it is difficult to identify the principal variables affecting population health. Concepts such as "social cohesion" or "social capital" are useful descriptive terms for the strength of cultural interactions, but they are difficult things to measure. More importantly, although they can be understood as determinants of health, they cannot be easily applied to a given society. Aid projects can provide clean water or immunizations, but how do you go about improving health variables such as social cohesion in any country, let alone in grindingly poor developing world populations (Government of Canada, 2006)?

It is becoming increasingly apparent that the physiological effects of chronic social stress are major determinants of health in humans. The stress induced by the chronic deprivation of poverty is easy to understand, but it seems that even when someone has enough money, being at the bottom of the local pecking order is still enough to induce harmful physiological results. Adverse effects on the immune system and the endocrine system have received particular attention as possible final common pathways linking stress to increased mortality, in both animals and humans (Cohen et al., 1996). But it is, perhaps, the common feeling of lacking control over one's own destiny that starts the harmful stress response rolling. The final result is a mortality gradient that exists for almost every disease in every social category regardless of other personal risk behaviours.

Another source of stress that has attracted considerable research interest is the degree of income distribution within a country (Wilkinson, 1996). This is a topical issue, since one of the commonly quoted explanations for the recent riots in Britain has been the steady worsening of income distribution in that country. Being poor is bad enough, but being poor in a country where others are very rich appears to be a factor that exacerbates the effects of poverty on health. Rodgers

(1979) was the first to show a relationship between life expectancy and income distribution. Numerous other studies have supported this original work both between countries and within countries. In a large US study (Kaplan et al., 1996) it was also shown that a clear relationship exists between income distribution and mortality within the 50 states.

As discussed earlier in this chapter, the major determinants of population health are clearly defined. Communities lacking access to water, peace, shelter, and food will indeed suffer from poor health. However, once these basic needs are met, there are still clear and measurable health differences among outwardly similar populations. Thus, there are other, less obvious factors determining health in more prosperous communities. Although the story is complex, a picture is slowly emerging. Inequalities in social position, lack of cultural and social cohesion, plus the added strain of unequal income distribution, have all been shown to be correlated with life expectancy. It is at least a plausible explanation that the final common pathways linking these variables to health are the adverse physiological effects of stress.

SUMMARY

There is no doubt that there has been progress in increasing life expectancy in all regions of the world over the last seven decades. However, it is also clear that basic health indicators such as maternal and child mortality are much worse in sub-Saharan Africa and Asia. There are basic requirements that people need in order to lead long, healthy lives. An understanding of these basic requirements helps prioritize resources that can advance the health of populations. This was the basis of the 1978 Alma Ata meeting, where it was agreed that far greater benefits could be realized for a given aid budget if the basic determinants of health were attended to first. These basic requirements include clean water, sanitation, housing, nutrition, and peace. Health care is surprisingly far down on the list of cost-effective strategies. In the early years of the aid industry, too much emphasis was placed on curative medical treatment as the first response to widespread ill health. It took over 20 years before it was finally realized that Western medical care had little ability to control epidemic diseases caused by poverty and social chaos. Since meeting basic human needs is the most cost-effective way to spend aid money, it is not surprising that many of the United Nations SDGs aim to do just that. Income, a key determinant of health, is included in the first SDG to "End poverty in all its forms everywhere." Reaching this goal in eradicating poverty by 2030 and other goals related to the social determinants of health would not be easy, but is critical for the overall health of populations.

DISCUSSION QUESTIONS

1. How is income related to the health of populations?
2. How do the SDGs relate to the social determinants of health? Which of the SDGs has the strongest relationship to the social determinants of health? Why?
3. Why is knowledge of the major determinants of health important when designing effective development strategies?
4. What are the complex determinants of health that appear once the basic needs have been met?
5. Why is health care not a significant or major determinant of health?
6. Recall in the chapter a reference to a report that concluded that class-related differences in mortality had little to do with failings of the NHS but were likely the result of social inequities in education, housing, diet, work conditions, and income. Do you consider these results to be valid? Why or why not?
7. What are the factors that would determine the health of poor populations?
8. Are there any other factors you would add to Table 3.1 on the basic requirements for a healthy life?
9. What are the most common measures of social differences?
10. Give some examples of the link between economic factors and health. Is there evidence for the relationship between life expectancy and income distribution?

RECOMMENDED READING

Davidson, A. 2014. *Social determinants of health: A comparative approach*. Pub: Oxford University Press.

Evans, R., Barer, N., & Marmor, T. 1994. *Why are some people healthy and others not?* Pub: Aldine De Gruyter.

Farmer, P. 2001. *Infection and inequalities: The modern plagues*. Pub: University of California Press.

Keating, D., & Hertzman, C. (Eds.). 1999. *Developmental health and the wealth of nations: Social, biological, and educational dynamics*. Pub: The Guildford Press.

Marmot, M., & Wilkinson, R. 2005. *Social determinants of health* (2nd ed.). Pub: Oxford University Press.

McKeown, T. 1979. *The role of medicine: Dream, mirage, or nemesis?* Pub: Basil Blackwell.

Raphael, D. 2015. *Social determinants of health: Canadian perspectives* (3rd ed.). Pub: Canadian Scholars Press Inc.

Sen, A. 1983. *Poverty and famines: An essay on entitlement and deprivation*. Pub: Oxford University Press.

Wilkinson, R. 1996. *Unhealthy societies: The affliction of inequality*. Pub: Routledge.

REFERENCES

Ali, S. 2004. A socio-ecological autopsy of the E. coli 0157:H7 outbreak in Walkerton, Ontario, Canada. *Social Science and Medicine*, 58: 2601–2612.

American Civil War home page. Retrieved from: sunsite.utk.edu/civil-war.

Ben Hamida, A., et al. 2005. Health transition in Tunisia over the past 50 years. *East Mediterranean Health Journal*, 11: 181–189.

Berkman, L., et al. 1979. Social networks, host resistance, and mortality: A nine-year follow-up study of Alameda County residents. *American Journal of Epidemiology*, 109: 186–204.

Black report: Inequalities in health. 1982. Pub: Penguin Books.

Bunker, J., et al. 1994. Improving health: Measuring effects of medical care. *Millbank Quarterly*, 72: 225–258.

Central Intelligence Agency. 2011. The world factbook. Retrieved from: www.cia.gov/cia/publications/factbook/index.html.

Chadwick, E. 1842. *Report on the Sanitary Condition of the Labouring Population of Great Britain*. Retrieved from: www.deltaomega.org/documents/ChadwickClassic.pdf.

Clark, D., et al. 2005. Core poverty, basic capabilities, and vagueness. Global Poverty Research Group working paper no. 26. Retrieved from: www.gprg.org/pubs/workingpapers/pdfs/gprg-wps-026.pdf.

Cohen, S., et al. 1996. Health psychology: Psychological factors and physical disease from the perspective of human psycho-neuro-immunology. *Annual Review of Psychology*, 47: 113–142.

Cunningham, S., et al. 2008. Doctors' strikes and mortality: A review. *Social Science and Medicine*, 67: 1784–1788.

Davies, H., et al. 1996. Invasive group A streptococcal infections in Ontario, Canada. *New England Journal of Medicine*, 335: 547–554.

Diez Roux, A. 2001. Neighborhood of residence and incidence of coronary heart disease. *New England Journal of Medicine*, 345: 99–106.

Doyal, L., et al. 1991. *A theory of human need*. Pub: MacMillan Press.

English, P. 1999. *Rheumatic fever in America and Britain: A biological, epidemiological, and medical history*. Pub: Rutgers University Press.

Frederick Law Olmsted. 2011. Retrieved from: www.fredericklawolmsted.com.

Government of Canada. 2006. Social capital as a public policy tool. Retrieved from: policyresearch.gc.ca/page.asp?pagenm=rp_sc_index.

Kaplan, G., et al. 1996. Income inequality and mortality in the United States. *British Medical Journal*, 312: 999–1003.

Leon, D., et al. 1992. Social class differences in infant mortality in Sweden: A comparison with England and Wales. *British Medical Journal*, 305: 687–691.

Liu, Q., et al. 2015. Poverty reduction within the framework of SDGs and Post-2015 Development Agenda. *Advances in Climate Change Research*, 6(1): 67–73.

Lynch, J., et al. 2001. Income inequality, the psychosocial environment, and health: Comparisons of wealthy nations. *The Lancet*, 358: 194–200.

Mackenbach, J., et al. 1990. Avoidable mortality and health services: A review of aggregate data studies. *Journal of Epidemiology and Community Health*, 44: 106–111.

Marmot, M. 2010. The Marmot report: Fair society, healthy lives. Retrieved from: www.marmotreview.org/.

Marmot, M., et al. 1975. Epidemiological studies of coronary heart disease and stroke in Japanese men living in Japan, Hawaii, and California. *American Journal of Epidemiology*, 102: 514–525.

Marmot, M., et al. 1978. Employment grade and coronary heart disease in British civil servants: Whitehall I study. *Journal of Epidemiology and Community Health*, 32: 244–249.

Marmot, M., et al. 1991. Health inequalities among British civil servants: Whitehall II study. *The Lancet*, 337: 1387–1393.

Maslow, A. 1943. A theory of human motivation. *Psychological Review*, 50: 370–396.

McKeown, T. 1979. *The role of medicine: Dream, mirage, or nemesis?* Pub: Basil Blackwell.

Nutton, V. 2004. *Ancient medicine*. Pub: Routledge.

Peterson, R. 1995. Insects, disease, and military history: The Napoleonic campaigns and historical perception. *American Entomologist*, 41: 147–160.

Pichichero, M., et al. 1999. Variables influencing penicillin treatment outcome in streptococcal tonsillpharyngitis. *Arch Dis Adolesc Med*, 153: 565–570.

Pompei. 2011. World Heritage Convention. Retrieved from: http://whc.unesco.org/en/list/829/gallery/.

Porter, D. 1990. The ghost of Edwin Chadwick. *British Medical Journal*, 301: 252–255.

Raphael, D., et al. 2004. Researching income and income distribution in Canada. Retrieved from: www.gpiatlantic.org/clippings/mc_incomehealth.pdf.

Relman, A. 1988. Assessment and accountability: The third revolution in medical care. *New England Journal of Medicine*, 319: 1220–1222.

Renbourn, E. 1957. The history of the flannel binder and cholera belt. *Medical History*, 1: 211–225.

Rodgers, G. 1979. Income and inequality as determinants of mortality: An international cross-section analysis. *Population Studies*, 33: 343–351.

Sachs, J. D. 2015. Achieving the Sustainable Development Goals. *Journal of International Business Ethics*, 8(2): 53–62, 66.

Sapolsky, R. 1993. Endocrinology alfresco: Psycho-endocrine studies of wild baboons. *Recent Progress in Hormone Research*, 48: 437–468.

Sen, A. 1983. *Poverty and famines: An essay on entitlement and deprivation*. Pub: Oxford University Press.

Shrestha, L. 2006. Life expectancy in the United States. Retrieved from: http://aging.senate.gov/crs/aging1.pdf.

Siegel-Itzkovitch, J. 2000. Doctors' strike in Israel may be good for health. *British Medical Journal*, 320: 1561.

UN. 2010. United Nations. Global strategy for women's and children's health. Retrieved from: www.who.int/pmnch/activities/advocacy/fulldocument_globalstrategy/en.

UN. 2015. United Nations Resolution 70/1, Transforming our world: The 2030 Agenda for Sustainable Development, A/RES/70/1 (25 September 2015). Available from: undocs.org/A/RES/67/97.

UN. 2016. United Nations Sustainable Development Goals. Retrieved from: https://sustainabledevelopment.un.org/sdgs.

UNICEF. 2009. Childinfo. Retrieved from: www.childinfo.org.

Vynnycky, E., et al. 1999. Interpreting the decline in tuberculosis. *International Journal of Epidemiology*, 28: 327–334.

Wilkins, R., et al. 1990. Changes in mortality by income in urban Canada from 1971 to 1986. *Statistics Canada Health Reports*, 1: 137–174.

Wilkinson, R. 1989. Class mortality differentials, income distribution, and trends in poverty 1921–1981. *Journal of Social Policy*, 18: 307–335.

Wilkinson, R. 1996. *Unhealthy societies: The affliction of inequality*. Pub: Routledge.

World Bank. 2016a. Data from the World Bank. Life expectancy, total (years). Retrieved from: http://data.worldbank.org/indicator/SP.DYN.LE00.IN (Accessed May 2, 2016).

World Bank. 2016b. Data from the World Bank. Maternal mortality ratio. Retrieved from: http://databank.worldbank.org/data/reports.aspx?source=2&country=&series=SH.STA.MMRT&period= (Accessed May 2, 2016).

CHAPTER 4
War and Civil Unrest

Every gun that is made, every warship launched, every rocket fired, signifies in the final sense a theft from those who hunger and are not fed, those who are cold and are not clothed.

—Dwight D. Eisenhower, "A Chance for Peace," 1953

OBJECTIVES

When it comes to analysis, war can be viewed exactly as it is—an endemic human disease that has likely affected humans as long as they have existed. It has an epidemiology, a financial cost, and, of course, a considerable mortality. To a limited extent, some clear causes can be defined and effective preventive therapies have been developed. It is the perfect example of a condition where an ounce of prevention is worth a ton of cure. The inclusion among the SDGs of a goal to "promote just, peaceful and inclusive societies" highlights the significance of peace in the context of the global development agenda over the next decade and a half. After completing this chapter, you should be able to:

- understand how wars have changed in type and number since the end of World War II
- understand conflicting theories about the causes of civil war
- understand the mechanisms available to prevent wars
- understand the growing place of military intervention in unstable developing countries

INTRODUCTION

The most persistent sound which reverberates through men's history is the beating of war drums.

—*Arthur Koestler*

Throughout the changes of history, war has remained a dependable constant. It seems fair to assume that humans have been fighting each other for as long as there have been humans. For example, when the "Ice man" was discovered in a glacier on the border of northern Italy in 1991, his body was dated to 5,300 years ago. After extensive examination, it was discovered that he had been beaten up and shot in the shoulder with an arrow, possibly as a member of an early unsuccessful raiding party. He wasn't the first victim of war and, by uncountable numbers, he certainly wasn't the last. Like malnutrition and poverty, war is a social ill that developed countries went through surprisingly recently. Rich countries should help poor ones get through this predictable stage in development, not out of a sense of superiority but out of a sense of shared past history.

Modern communications allow pictures of war to be shown in our homes every night. Given all these images of terror and violence, the average person may well form the idea that war is now more common than it has ever been. The good news is that this impression is wrong. The next section on the epidemiology of war will show that there has been a steady decrease in the number of wars, and also a decrease in the number of people killed in wars since the mid-1990s. If war is defined as an armed conflict that causes 1,000 or more battle deaths each year, the number of wars has declined sharply since the end of the Cold War. The bad news is that there is still plenty of fighting going on, including signs of a recent upturn in conflicts during the last few years (Figure 4.1). There were 40 armed conflicts recorded for 2014, out of which 11 were defined as wars, that is, conflicts generating 1,000 or more battle-related deaths in one calendar year (UCDP, 2016).

Direct wars within and between developed countries have become increasingly rare since the end of World War II, although proxy wars exist. Several of these wealthy countries are now involved as combatants in countries such as Afghanistan, Iraq, and Syria, but the burden of violence now falls disproportionately upon poor countries. Since they are the countries least able to sustain the associated social and economic costs, it remains a mystery why so many poor countries spend so much money on their military rather than pursuing other means of resolving conflicts. Eight of the 10 countries at the bottom of the list of GDP per capita have active or recent violent conflicts. Of the two peaceful countries (Malawi and Niger), Niger had a recent military coup in 2010. War and conflict are clearly an important part of any study of global health.

It is necessary to interpret the literature on war with some caution. In that respect it is quite similar to the research literature concerning poverty and economic growth. The technical jargon is confusing, contradictory points of view are common, and much of the work on the causes of war is based on cross-country regression analysis, which, as discussed in the chapter on poverty, is open to considerable potential error. It should be remembered that war is the final result of complex social and economic problems, all further complicated by the unpredictability of human nature. Understanding the causes of unrest and predicting those high-risk situations that will suddenly go from argument to violence are difficult tasks. After nearly 100 years, the origins of World War I are still not settled, so simple answers and quick fixes for modern wars should be examined carefully.

There are, of course, broad patterns in the development of wars since the end of World War II, but these should not be overinterpreted. Post–World War II fighting began with colonial wars of independence that finally ended in the 1970s. These were followed by post-independence power struggles and internal conflicts between right and left, supported by the opposing sides of the Cold War. Violence declined steadily from the mid-1990s after the stimulus of the Cold War was removed. This also coincided with a period of greatly increased external peacekeeping and mediation. That decline shows recent signs of reversal with the upsurge of unrest in Islamic countries and the fighting stimulated by the so-called "war on terror." The measurable reduction in wars secondary to mediation and the removal of financial

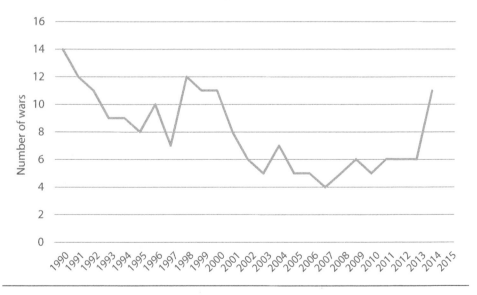

Figure 4.1: Number of wars between 1990 and 2014

Source: Pettersson, T., & Wallensteenet, P. 2015. Armed conflicts, 1946–2014. *Journal of Peace Research,* 52(4): 536–550.

and military support from opposing factions give some hope for the future. War should not be viewed as an inevitable and uncontrollable part of human behaviour. With early recognition, mediation, targeted interventions, and even, in some circumstances, military intervention, active fighting can be stopped. If caught early enough, it can be avoided altogether. The returns from effective peacekeeping, in terms of improved prosperity and health, are substantial and well worth pursuing.

THE EPIDEMIOLOGY OF WAR

> War, to be abolished, must be understood. To be understood, it must be studied.
> —Quincy Wright, *A Study of War*, 1942

Everyone knows that the first victim of war is truth, so when it comes to statistical data concerning wars, it is important to define the sources carefully. The data in this section are obtained principally from the most recent Human Security Report (2013). This is a regular publication of the Human Security Report Project, which is an independent research centre affiliated with Simon Fraser University, Vancouver, Canada (Human Security Report, 2013). Their research and analysis is based mainly on data from the Uppsala Conflict Data Program (UCDP, 2016). This is a widely used source of statistical information on all aspects of conflict; it is generated by researchers within the Department of Peace and Conflict Research, University of Uppsala, Sweden (DPCR, 2011).

The Pattern of Wars

Since the end World War II, there have been identifiable patterns in war that are, to some extent, guided and driven by external forces such as the end of colonialism and the start of the Cold War. Sixty years ago, the most common forms of war were colonial struggles for independence and wars between countries—civil wars were relatively uncommon. With time, colonial wars have disappeared and interstate wars have become increasingly rare (Figure 4.2). For example, since 2000, there have been fewer than one interstate conflict per year on average, compared to three during the 1980s. At present, the only form of conflict is civil war within a state—either with the government as one combatant or between two other groups within the country (non-state conflicts). The murder of civilians by armed groups (one-sided violence) is not strictly a war, but these terrible events kill a lot of people, so they are included in this section. The newest development has been the increasing use of external military force to intervene in a civil war. These five types of conflict are discussed in more detail below.

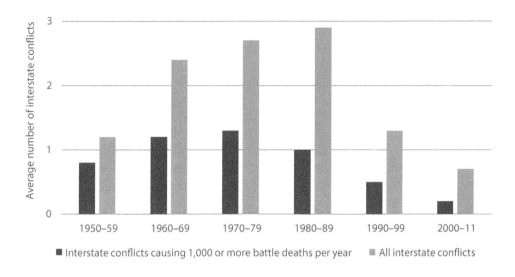

Figure 4.2: Average number of interstate conflicts per year per decade

Source: Human Security Report. 2013. Retrieved from: www.hsrgroup.org/human-security-reports/2013/overview.aspx.

Colonial Wars of Independence

> The wind of change is blowing through this [African] continent and, whether we like it or not, this growth of national consciousness is a political fact. We must all accept it as a fact, and our national policies must take account of it.
>
> *—Harold MacMillan, British prime minister, 1960*

The period in history when it was accepted that a rich, powerful country could colonize a weaker one finally ended in 1999, when Portugal handed over control of Macau to China. This was an appropriate way to end because Macau had been one of the first European colonies and spanned the whole period of colonialism. Moves toward self-rule came from the original inhabitants (Vietnam, South Africa), from settlers of the colonial country (America), or from slaves or indentured workers used by the colonists (Haiti). The first large-scale fight for independence was mounted by the young American state against Britain. It was successful in 1783. Haiti was another country granted early independence—by France following a successful slave revolt in 1804. For the majority of colonies, it took a long time before they had accumulated the necessary leadership, financial support, and weapons to support a successful fight for self-rule. Despite the obvious differences between the colonial powers and various independence groups, most wars were ultimately won by the local independence movements.

Box 4.1 History Notes

United Nations' Peacekeeping Force

One of the fundamental reasons behind the foundation of the United Nations in 1945 was the prevention of future wars between nations. The founding charter allows UN-sanctioned forces to intervene as peacekeepers and also allows the use of military force under some circumstances. This is just as well because both would be tested within the first five years of the UN's existence. Unarmed observers were first posted in 1947 (Indo-Pakistan war and Yugoslavia) and then 1948 (Arab-Israeli war). The first large-scale test was in support of South Korea after the invasion by North Korea in 1950. At the height of the war, the multinational UN army consisted of over a million men.

Following the Suez crisis in 1956, the Canadian prime minister, Lester Pearson, suggested the establishment of an armed UN emergency force that would principally be for peacekeeping, but would be able to defend itself if necessary. He was awarded a Nobel Prize for this and other humanitarian work. The UN peacekeeping force was awarded the Nobel Peace Prize in 1988. There has been no shortage of work in the intervening years, particularly after the internal antagonism within the UN was reduced at the end of the Cold War. Since then, UN Emergency Force detachments have acted as peacekeepers around the world, including another military action to remove Iraqi forces from Kuwait. Given the volatile circumstances within which the peacekeepers work, there have inevitably been criticisms and perceived failures to do enough to prevent deaths, particularly concerning missions in Darfur, Rwanda, and Bosnia. At time of writing, UN peacekeepers continue to contribute to the maintenance of peace, with 16 missions around the world, including multinational air support for the civilian uprising against the Gaddafi regime in Libya. For further information, follow the reference: UN (2011).

World War II acted as a major catalyst for self-rule. Many colonies had contributed considerable resources toward the war and felt they had now earned their independence—certainly this was the case with Australia, Canada, and India. Probably more importantly, times and attitudes had simply changed to the point that colonialism was not simply viewed as an anachronism, but was actually illegal under international law. The establishment of the United Nations and widespread ratification of the Declaration of Human Rights meant that the writing was on the wall. Unfortunately, many colonial powers didn't go without a fight. The result was a constant series of struggles that were harmful to both sides. Some, such as Portugal's wars against Mozambique and Angola or France's wars against Vietnam and Algeria, were so expensive and damaging that they caused political unrest and revolution in their own countries. This late and unlamented period of war ended in the 1970s.

Wars between Countries

The League is very well when sparrows shout, but no good at all when eagles fall out.

—Mussolini, 1938

Peace agreements between previously warring states are recorded in hieroglyphics of Egypt and cuneiform of Assyria and are essentially no different from the complex treaties and agreements formed in response to later threats from the forces of Napoleon, Bismarck, or Hitler. They all had roughly the same success rates. World War I was supposed to be the war to end all wars, but it took another catastrophic global conflict before it became clear that it was time to try other ways of resolving disagreements. The League of Nations was started after World War I in order to maintain world peace, but it was ahead of its time and collapsed because of its failure to alter the onset of World War II. It was not until the establishment of the United Nations that serious international efforts were made to prevent fighting and also to mediate an end to established wars.

While interstate conflicts are unusual, they have been by far the worst in terms of civilian and military deaths. The wars between Iran and Iraq, the two Vietnams, and the two Koreas all produced more than a million deaths. Endless social theories have been devised to explain the decline in conflicts between countries, but none is fully accepted. The simple fact is that societal attitudes change with time. War has become increasingly unfashionable for the same reasons that slavery was abolished and heretics are no longer burned in public—society slowly, at a glacial pace, does actually improve with time. It is hoped that this trend will catch on. However, in recent years, there have been upsurges in both the number and severity of conflicts (Figure 4.1). Syria and Ukraine accounted for most of the worsening trend in armed conflict in 2014. For example, the four new armed conflicts which erupted in 2014 were all in Ukraine, where one was fought over the control of government and the others related to the status of territories in eastern Ukraine, which included Donetsk, Lugansk, and Novorossiya (Pettersson and Wallensteenet, 2015).

Civil War

For many countries liberated from colonial rule, it was a case of "jumping out of the frying pan and into the fire." Some countries, like Uganda, Zimbabwe, Cambodia, and Burma, simply swapped one set of dictators for others that were often even worse. In other countries, such as Nicaragua, Guatemala, and Honduras, loose alliances that were formed during the independence struggle soon collapsed into increasingly complicated factional fighting that dragged on for decades. The main protagonists of the Cold War greatly exacerbated these conflicts by arming and financing whichever faction best served the political aims of the day. In this way, some truly terrible tyrants were supported by aid money. Such was the complexity of these arrangements that the heroes of one decade (Saddam Hussein's war against Iran) could become the villains of the next (Saddam Hussein's invasion of Kuwait).

The opposing ideologies behind the Cold War not only perpetuated struggles by supporting the opposing sides, they also paralyzed any serious attempts within the United Nations to interfere. This incredibly wasteful and unproductive period ended with the formal dissolution of the Soviet state on Christmas Day in 1991. The effects of removing financial and military supports are easily seen in the subsequent steady decline in civil wars. That trend has recently been reversed, at least in part, by unrest within Islamic countries and the results of the "war on terror," but levels still remain well below the peak reached at the end of the 1980s. The reduction in tensions between the Cold War adversaries also allowed the United Nations to work more efficiently. With arguments and vetoes removed, the international community began trying to control conflicts surprisingly quickly after 1991. This is reflected in the rapid increase in peacekeeping operations and also in the rapidly growing number of imposed sanctions throughout the 1990s.

Non-state Civil War

The term "non-state civil war" refers to civil war between rebel groups within a country, neither of which is the government, that results in at least 25 deaths

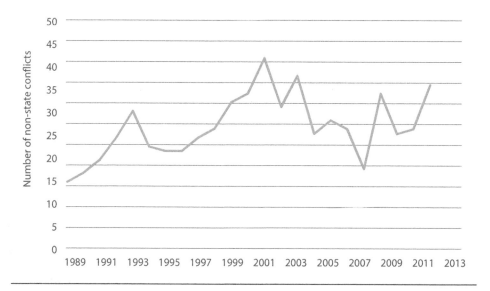

Figure 4.3: Global trends in non-state conflicts, 1989–2011

Source: Human Security Report. 2013. Retrieved from: www.hsrgroup.org/human-security-reports/2013/overview.aspx.

in a year. These may be between tribal groups, as in Kenya in 2008, or between powerful drug cartels, as in Colombia and Mexico. Statistics are usually gathered on state-based violence. Only within the last few years has the Human Security Report Project/Uppsala Conflict Data Program been publishing data (Figure 4.3) on this subject (Human Security Report, 2013). Compared to civil wars where the government is a combatant, non-state conflicts are usually of shorter duration (less than one year) and less lethal. Such conflicts are largely, but not entirely, confined to countries in sub-Saharan Africa and reflect the effects of poor central authority. The number of non-state armed conflict has been increasing since 2010, with 38 conflicts in 2011 (Figure 4.3).

From 1991 to 2009, battle deaths from non-state armed conflict were concentrated in sub-Saharan Africa, mostly in Somalia, Ethiopia, Sudan, Nigeria, the Democratic Republic of Congo, and Kenya. However, in 2010, conflicts between drug cartels led to an increase in the death toll in the Americas. Nearly 60 percent of the global battle-death total in 2010 was recorded in the Americas. On the other hand, sub-Saharan Africa had the lowest recorded battle deaths compared to past years (Human Security Report, 2013). Unfortunately, Saharan Africa is witnessing a rise in battle deaths due to the resumption of two non-state conflicts, one between ethnic groups in Sudan and the other between Christians and Muslims in Nigeria.

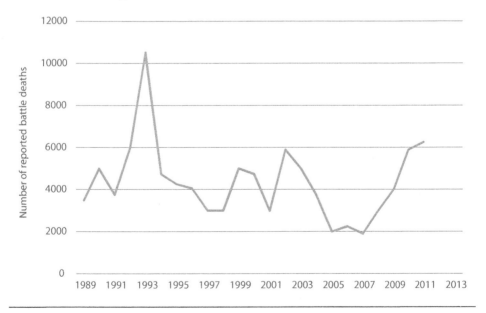

Figure 4.4: Trends in battle deaths from non-state conflicts, 1989–2011

Source: Human Security Report. 2013. Retrieved from: www.hsrgroup.org/human-security-reports/2013/overview.aspx.

One-Sided Violence

One-sided violence refers to massacres of unarmed civilians by armed groups. The term is used to avoid more contentious names such as genocide or ethnic cleansing, although why we must worry about upsetting people capable of such horrors is a mystery. This is another area where organized data collection has been a recent development. The details of many atrocities against civilians are covered up, only to have them come to light years later through the work of forensic pathologists, so accurate data is impossible to collect. The difficulties in determining the death toll in Tiananmen Square is a good example. The largest example of postwar, one-sided violence was the slaughter of civilians in Rwanda (Figure 4.5). If that terrible death toll is removed from the analysis, there are signs of reducing mortality in recent years (Figure 4.6). While one-sided violence is most common in sub-Saharan Africa, it occurs in every region of the world. Although the death toll seems to be falling, there is no clear reduction in the numbers of these events.

THE EFFECTS OF WAR

> A great war leaves the country with three armies—an army of cripples, an army of mourners, and an army of thieves.
>
> —*German proverb*

Mortality

The most obvious effect of war is casualties. In keeping with the drop in numbers of wars and also their shorter duration, reported battlefield deaths have fallen to a fraction of their levels in the 1980s. Modern civil wars are often confined to a relatively small part of the country, so the main business of the country can continue. For those within the affected areas, life is brutal, but for those in the rest of the country, there may be few signs that a war is in progress. This was the case during fairly recent wars in Sri Lanka and Uganda. In some countries, the fighting becomes so widespread that the business of the country almost ceases—civil wars in Liberia and Sierra Leone are good examples.

Figures for civilian casualties are not accurate due to limited reporting and highly contentious arguments about the "true" numbers generated by each side of any conflict. The first survey sample of deaths in Iraq illustrates these points (Roberts et al., 2004). Their estimate of excess deaths due to the war was 98,000, but their confidence limits for this value varied between 8,000 and 194,000. They were heavily criticized by both poles of opinion—far too low by one and far too high by the other. The available figures can never be considered as anything more than rough estimates

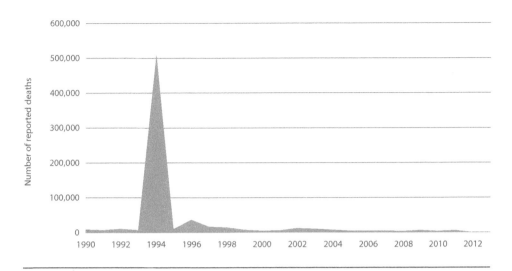

Figure 4.5: Global deaths from one-sided violence

Source: Human Security Report. 2013. Retrieved from: www.hsrgroup.org/human-security-reports/2013/overview.aspx.

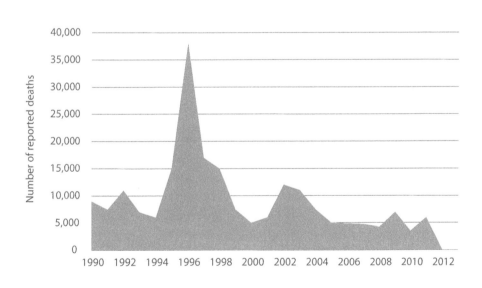

Figure 4.6: Global deaths from one-sided violence, excluding the Rwandan genocide

Source: Human Security Report. 2013. Retrieved from: www.hsrgroup.org/human-security-reports/2013/overview.aspx.

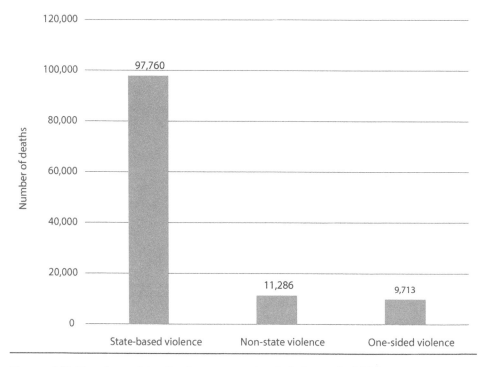

Figure 4.7: Number of deaths from organized violence in 2015

Source: UCDP. 2016. Uppsala Conflict Data Program. Retrieved from: www.pcr.uu.se/research/UCDP/.

(Human Security Report, 2013), but they do at least show a steady decrease with time. Given the greatly improved standards of care for those affected by violent conflict, the decreasing number of wars, and also the increasing proportion of foreign aid directed toward humanitarian crises, this seems a reasonable conclusion. Any claims about the ratio of civilian to military deaths suffer from the same unreliability (Roberts, 2010), but it is probably still safe to say that civilians bear an unfair proportion of the economic and military burdens of modern wars.

In addition, there are fatalities due to organized violence. In 2014, more than 130,000 people were killed in organized violence, and in 2015 this figure had decreased to close to 118,000 (Figure 4.7). The year 2014 was the second-worst year in the post–Cold War period in terms of fatalities, and 2015 was the third (UCDP, 2016).

Population Health

During periods of war, population health statistics will likely be gathered from safer parts of the country. Determining the health effects of civil war on a population will be underestimated if too much reliance is placed on average or selective figures (Agadjanian et al., 2003). While it is true that child health statistics often continue

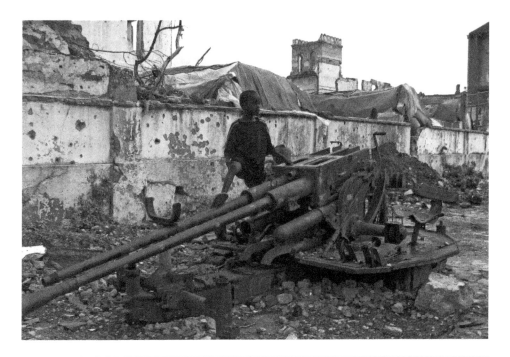

Photo 4.1: A child plays with a rusting anti-aircraft gun in the Shangani district of Mogadishu. Decades of recurrent violence have destroyed the social and economic structures of the region.

Source: Mohamed Amin/Integrated Regional Information Network photo library (www.irinnews.org/photo).

to improve even during prolonged conflicts (Human Security Report, 2011), these figures do not apply to the whole country. For example, during the civil war in Sri Lanka, child survival rates in Colombo were probably not indicative of health standards among children living in the war zone. For those directly affected, the adverse health effects of war are considerable. A recent empirical study highlighted the association between peace and life expectancy at birth as an outcome measure of the population health (Yazdi et al., 2015). Some of the health aspects that are often not considered include:

- disabling mental illness among survivors, particularly in women, children, and the elderly (Murthy et al., 2006)
- a terrible legacy of continuing injuries from land mines and other unexploded munitions (Mines Action Canada, 2006)
- the long-term results of gender-specific atrocities such as rape as a means of war, forced prostitution, sexual slavery, and other forms of violence against women (Ward et al., 2006)

- the long-term physical and mental effects among children forced to fight as soldiers (Child Soldiers, 2008)

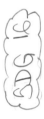

Developing countries are increasingly separating into two camps. Those with the benefits of peace and steadily growing economies are forming a global middle class. The second group consists of fragile states that are increasingly falling behind the rest of the world, largely because of the destructive effects of chronic violence. At least 20 percent of the world's population live under such conditions (Photo 4.1). In recognition of the impact of violence and insecurity on health and development, the 2030 Agenda includes SDG 16, to "promote just, peaceful and inclusive societies." The goal includes 12 associated objectives: (1) Significantly reduce all forms of violence and related death rates everywhere. (2) End abuse, exploitation, trafficking and all forms of violence against and torture of children. (3) Promote the rule of law at the national and international levels and ensure equal access to justice for all. (4) By 2030, significantly reduce illicit financial and arms flows, strengthen the recovery and return of stolen assets and combat all forms of organized crime. (5) Substantially reduce corruption and bribery in all their forms. (6). Develop effective, accountable and transparent institutions at all levels. (7) Ensure responsive, inclusive, participatory and representative decision-making at all levels. (8) Broaden and strengthen the participation of developing countries in the institutions of global governance. (9) By 2030, provide legal identity for all, including birth registration. (10) Ensure public access to information and protect fundamental freedoms, in accordance with national legislation and international agreements. (11) Strengthen relevant national institutions, including through international cooperation, for building capacity at all levels, in particular in developing countries, to prevent violence and combat terrorism and crime. (12) Promote and enforce non-discriminatory laws and policies for sustainable development (UN 2016).

The Trap of Perpetual Violence and Poverty

You can build a throne with bayonets, but you can't sit on it for long.

—Boris Yeltsin, 1993

Once the conflict is over, those armed young men who were once so important in the war now have nothing to do, and they also have an automatic rifle in the closet. Not surprisingly, one of the legacies of war is high levels of post-conflict violence. This becomes so widespread that some countries live in a limbo that is not quite war, but certainly isn't peace. The situation is recent enough and sufficiently widespread that older data and predictions may hav▮▮▮▮▮evance in the modern world of fragile states. The forms that this pot▮▮▮▮▮violence ultimately take will vary from place to place. Post-conflict st▮▮▮▮as South Africa, El Salvador, Guatemala, and the Democratic Republic of Congo have very high levels of violence with homicide rates far above 10 per 100,000 population per year. In other areas, such as Western Balkans, Northern Ireland, and Afghanistan, gangs of ex-combatants have moved into a postwar life of crime (Newman et al., 2007). As recent political violence in Kenya has shown, gangs may also hire themselves out to political groups to help the electorate make up their minds at election time.

The adverse economic results of violence are substantial both within and outside affected countries. Within countries, Collier's research suggests that civil war reduces economic growth by 2.3 percent per year of war (Collier, 2006). This effect does not end just because a ceasefire is signed. If the war did not result in more benign governance (which is, unfortunately, the most likely result), that economic drag on the economy may last for years. It has been estimated that if the violence in Jamaica and Haiti could be reduced to the levels found in Costa Rica, each country would increase its growth rate by over 5 percent (UNODC, 2007). As an example of the indirect costs of instability to the external community, the bill for policing ex-combatants who now operate as pirates in the Gulf of Aden is measured in billions of dollars. The combination of high levels of violence and slow economic recovery, often in a setting of poor governance, is an obvious recipe for trouble. As we'll see in the next section, the cumulative risk of a post-conflict country slipping back into further violence is considerable.

THE CAUSES OF WAR

To estimate the probability of war at any time involves, therefore, an appraisal of the effect of current changes upon the complex of intergroup relationships throughout the world.

—*Quincy Wright, 1965*

Check the Data

If you torture the data long enough, it will eventually confess.

—*Ronald Coase, Nobel Prize for Economics, 1991*

Quincy Wright was a prolific researcher and writer on the subject of war. His two-volume book, *A Study of War*, is considered a classic on the subject. Throughout his work he emphasized that opinions about war should be based on careful study. Unfortunately, subsequent researchers in this field have not always followed that advice. One source of conflict data is based on qualitative studies. Unfortunately, wars are terrible events that generate strong emotions among observers and commentators, which is a poor basis for objective interpretation. It is easy to find descriptions of the same group of fighters that vary from heroes to villains, motivated by everything from self-sacrifice to sadism. Don't forget that we are talking about the same group of fighters—it's just the opinions about their complex motivations that change. Some might conclude that a particular war was caused by a selfless desire to help the oppressed, while others may feel this was just a pretence to allow the rebel group to gain control of the country's mineral resources. The lengthy debate about whether fighting is triggered by "greed or grievance" is one example out of dozens of such debates (Collier et al., 2004). Similar arguments are held about the influence of ethnic diversity, oppression of a minority, form of governance, and even the significance of mountainous terrain (Human Security Report, 2011).

While there is a long history of quantitative studies of war, research into developing world civil conflicts is quite a recent development. War is bad for business, whether national or international, so it is not surprising that the first large-scale studies of civil war were started by the World Bank's Economics of Civil War, Crime, and Violence project in 2000, under the leadership of Paul Collier, and its importance is also reflected in the World Development Report's focus on security and development (World Development Report, 2011). As mentioned earlier, conflict research is similar to economic research—it is primarily based on large cross-country studies. Unfortunately, neither economics nor war is a simple subject—there are always many ways to explain why a given country is poor or why another is at war. As a rough rule of thumb in statistics, there should be 5 to 10 measured points for each variable that is being studied. If the true number of variables were known, then most country analyses likely have more variables than measurements. Under these circumstances, erroneous associations and unreliable conclusions are a real possibility. In statistical terms, the results are not robust. For example, in a recent review of 46 different studies of the causes of civil war (Dixon, 2009), the authors found more than 200 explanatory variables used. There was some agreement on 30 of them, but good consensus was found in only 7.

It is important not to push the research results further than they are willing to go. In particular, they cannot be viewed as accurate predictive indicators. Attempts have been made to predict wars using the combination of a few variables (Goldstone et al., 2010), but theory lags much too far behind fact to allow such equations to have any practical value (Ward et al., 2010). Apart from any other inaccuracies, the vagaries of human nature, such as hatred, jealousy, and revenge, are hard to understand and even harder to measure. The results of conflict research should be viewed as preliminary guides for long-term policy-making.

The Principal Predisposing Factors behind Civil Wars

The field of civil war research is only a decade old, so it is a bit early to expect widespread agreement. Competing theories abound, which makes the available literature both extensive and contradictory. For those willing to take on the challenge, the following detailed studies and reviews are worthwhile: Blattman et al. (2010), Collier et al. (2004), Dixon (2009), Fearon et al. (2003), and Hegre et al. (2006). Most readers will probably find the titles in the "Recommended Reading" list an easier place to start, particularly Paul Collier's popular book, *The Bottom Billion*. Despite all the disagreement, the following factors are widely accepted as major contributors to the development of civil wars.

Chronic Poverty and Disgruntled Young Men

Poverty is at least one area of agreement. Rich democracies gave up fighting 60 years ago; current conflicts are confined to grindingly poor countries. However, this is simply an observation, and many questions about the mechanism remain. There are plenty of poor countries, but they don't all go to war. Figure 4.8 plots a measure of instability against per capita income. Levels of governance and endemic violence are often terrible in poor countries, but the data are widely spread—some equally poor countries have quite high scores, so poverty on its own is only a part of the explanation. Another problem is determining cause or effect. The complex results of poverty predispose a country to war, but chronic war can also ruin an economy so that it also produces poverty. The two are certainly connected, but what is the main mechanism?

This is a good time to move away from arguments over rough terrain, density of roads, and degrees of democracy, and rely more on qualitative data, perhaps even using common sense as a guide. At the core of any war is young men. They are the essential fuel that keeps any conflict burning. Any theory of war must include their motivations as a central issue. Poverty reduces access to education and usually worsens the distribution of income within a country. There is a strong association between conflict and poor access to education, particularly for males (Dixon, 2009). There are weaker associations between violence and unequal distribution of money (vertical inequality), and also much debated and weaker links between violence and group inequalities (horizontal inequality) (Stewart, 2002). Taking this as a starting point, it is not difficult to construct some likely scenarios that centre on poverty.

Uneducated, unemployed men, dissatisfied with a life of poverty and frustrated by the obvious inequalities within their country, are an easy target for leaders able to manipulate and exaggerate ethnic or religious differences to the point that people will actually fight. Perhaps some of the rank-and-file actually believe these stories

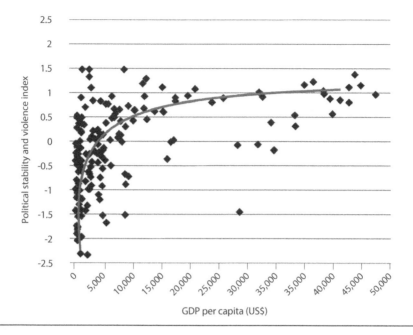

Figure 4.8: The World Bank's index of political stability and absence of violence plotted against GDP per capita for all countries below US$50,000 per head. The index varies from −2.5 (unstable and violent) to +2.5 (stable and peaceful).

Source: WGI. 2010. World Bank's world governance indicators. Retrieved from: http://info.worldbank.org/governance/wgi/sc_country.asp.

as they go off to war, but the evidence would suggest that their leaders are more often motivated by power or the possibility of loot such as blood diamonds in Sierra Leone or minerals in the Democratic Republic of Congo (Collier et al., 2004).

Endemic Violence

The effects of war are bad enough when they happen only once. In many developing countries, the end of one war is unfortunately soon followed by the start of another. Collier et al.'s (2007) concept of countries trapped in an endless cycle of violence and poverty is a powerful image. Despite all the efforts at preventing conflict since the end of the Cold War, the evidence suggests that the five-year relapse rate is increasing with time. As some countries manage to climb out of this destructive cycle, it leaves behind a smaller hard core of fragile states that increasingly diverge from the rest of the world's slowly growing prosperity. In a country of poor governance and weak policing, it takes only a relatively small number of armed young men to perpetuate a state of violence. Unfortunately, in such countries, it doesn't cost much to arm and feed a thousand men, particularly if oil or diamonds are the source of funding.

The evidence would suggest that it isn't difficult to find suitable volunteers. Unless such fragile, war-torn states are given substantial economic and social assistance, they are unlikely to emerge from this chaos using their own resources.

Bad Governance

The effects of bad governance are like those of poverty—they are frequently associated with conflict, but not in an easily predictable manner. Many countries have bad governments without civil war. The governments of countries like Haiti, Sudan, Zimbabwe, and Burma are so bad that if they simply did nothing, it would be an improvement. Citizens expect their governments to organize the country in a safe, prosperous manner. If this unwritten contract is broken, then authority is lost and a degree of anarchy results, a situation that isn't helped by the usual associated weakness of policing and peacekeeping abilities of the state. One particular element of government authority that is a source of trouble is the management of valuable resources. In a typical fragile state, the population hasn't a clue where the money from minerals or oil resources finally goes—they only know that it doesn't seem to go to them.

Lootable Resources

Valuable resources are associated with so many potential problems that they are often referred to as a "resource curse" (Pegg, 2005). The curse refers to the observation that resource-rich countries frequently perform far below their expected economic level. The presence of valuable reserves is also associated with an increased risk of internal conflict. Diamonds and oil are particularly closely related with violence. As usual, several mechanisms are proposed, including weakening of the economy through artificial strengthening of the currency so that exports fall (Dutch disease), a source of easily convertible loot for rebel groups, and a trigger for violence following boom and bust shocks to the local economy, which are common in single-resource–based economies. There have been recent moves to improve the levels of management of mineral resources (Oxfam, 2009).

Neighbourhood

In 1776, Adam Smith pointed out that the landlocked areas of Central Asia and Africa were the poorest parts of the world. This situation hasn't changed and is still one that affects all parts of the globe. Examples include Bhutan, Laos, Bolivia, and Zambia.

Once again, the relationship isn't straightforward since there are countries like Botswana and Switzerland that manage to be prosperous and peaceful despite being far from international ports. The difference is due to the type of neighbourhood. If surrounding countries are peaceful, they are customers for products, not simply a road to the outside world. Whether the roads and railways are repaired, whether trucks can pass without being looted, and whether exports can be sold locally all depend on the peace and stability of the surrounding states. Unless the whole region can be helped, there is little chance for one small country in the middle.

PREVENTING WAR

> Peace is an equilibrium among many forces. It is unlikely to come about by itself. It must be organized in order to bring it about, to maintain it thereafter, and to restore it after it has broken down.
>
> *—Quincy Wright, 1942*

War should not be viewed as an intractable problem without any solution. Asia serves as a good example of a region that, in only 20 years, has gone from experiencing the horrors of multiple major and minor wars to becoming one of the most peaceful regions in the world. Peacemaking is possible. Results don't happen overnight, but solutions do exist. Although there is considerable debate concerning the causes of conflict, there is enough agreement to guide major policies. Some of the areas open to intervention raised in the section on the causes of war include economic growth, peacekeeping, education, open management of resources, and assistance with exports.

Economic Growth

The risk of conflict increases as poverty worsens. This risk is slowly reversed by rising incomes (Figure 4.9). Aid clearly has a part to play, but the quantity, timing, and type of aid are all important. Paul Collier's work in this area has had a significant effect on policy. His team has shown that prior to conflict, aid appears to have little effect on the risk of civil war, but, for unexplained reasons, it seems to increase the chance of a coup. In the post-conflict period, the picture is very different. Under those circumstances, aid can have significant benefits for economic growth, but it must be phased in slowly as local capacity to absorb aid improves (Collier et al., 2002). Clearly, technical assistance for institutional capacity building is also essential during this early period. The peak effect of aid appears to be roughly five years after the ceasefire, so external agencies should accept that investment in post-conflict countries requires a graded input, a long investment period (at least seven years), and a large cumulative total of cash. Compared to the total costs of collapse back into civil war, the investment is highly cost-effective.

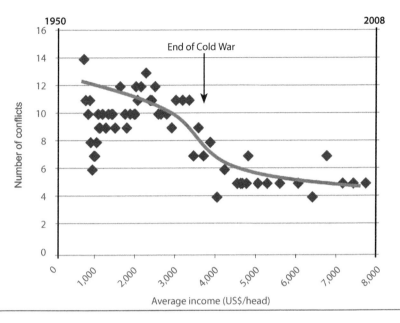

Figure 4.9: Trend in numbers of state-based armed conflicts in East Asia, plotted against rising personal income, between 1950 and 2008

Source: Human Security Report. 2011. Retrieved from: www.hsrgroup.org/human-security-reports/20092010/overview.aspx.

Reducing the Resource Curse

Income from resources is far bigger than aid for the poorest countries. The problem is that governments never say what happened to the cash, so much ends up diverted to personal gain, bribes, and commissions. If governments and the resource companies could be persuaded to open their accounting practices, the results would only be good for the poorest. The first initiative toward openness in resource profits was taken by Tony Blair in 2002, when he suggested the establishment of the Extractive Industries Transparency Initiative (EITI, 2011). This obliges countries and companies to publish regular audited accounts of their income and payments. Despite initial cynicism, the initiative has prospered and now includes 35 mineral- and oil-rich countries. A similar response was started by the United Nations in 2003 to prevent rebels from using profits from private sales of diamonds. The initiative is called the Kimberley Process. Member states must ensure that no diamonds from their countries end up financing wars (Kimberley Process, 2011).

Peacekeeping

Despite its internal problems, the United Nations remains the natural body to take on the role of international peacekeeping because of its broad representation of world states (Photo 4.2). When operations began in the 1940s, the world was a very different place. Initially unarmed and later lightly armed, UN detachments worked around the world as non-aggressive observers. With the end of the Cold War, the number of peacekeeping missions increased rapidly. During the early 1990s, the UN authorized 20 new missions, and the number of peacekeepers rose from 11,000 to 75,000 troops. As at April 2016, the total Uniformed personnel contributed by UN operations was approximately 106,000, with the majority coming from Africa and Asia (Figure 4.10). Unfortunately, these forces had not

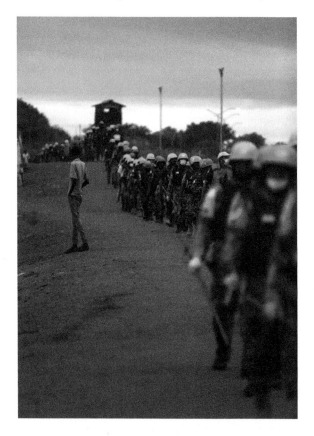

Photo 4.2: Peacekeepers and UN police officers with the UN Mission in South Sudan conduct a search for weapons and contraband in Protection of Civilians (POC) Site III, near the Jebel area of Juba, 19 July 2016.

Source: UN Photo/Eric Kanalstein, with kind permission of the UN Photo Library (www. unmultimedia.org/photo).

adapted to the new reality of brutal civil wars fought by people with absolutely no respect for any authority other than force. While there has been an increase in the number of ceasefires and peace agreements, there have also been some spectacular disasters, including the failure to prevent the massacres in Rwanda, the slaughter of civilians in the UN safe haven of Srebrenica, and the failed intervention and withdrawal from Somalia. The subsequent enquiries revealed that the causes were quite obvious—the peacekeepers were poorly trained, poorly equipped, and inadequately supported.

The UN has responded to these crises and is currently in the middle of greatly reformed and renewed peacekeeping efforts. Following the Brahimi report in 2000 (UN Reform, 2010), the peacekeeping process has been overhauled, first with the establishment of the UN Peacebuilding Commission in 2006 (UNPC, 2011) and now with the New Partnership Agenda plotting a clear policy course for the future (UN, 2010). Although protracted conflicts in Iraq and Afghanistan have made countries reluctant to use military force without clear end points, the overwhelming success of the British intervention in Sierra Leone has acted as a counterpoint. The NATO bombing campaign against the former Yugoslavia and the more recent air support of the Libyan uprising show that military force is an option under clearly defined circumstances.

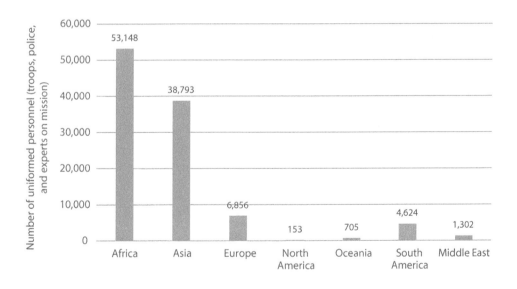

Figure 4.10: Total Uniformed personnel contributed by UN operations by UN region, 2016

Source: GPOR. 2016. Global Peace Operations Review. Retrieved from: http://peaceoperationsreview.org/featured-data/#Uniform.

Reducing Military Spending

The world spends startling amounts of money on the military. From a post–Cold War low of about US$800 billion in 1998, that total had more than doubled by 2011. Why foreign aid is still given to some of the biggest spenders, such as China, India, Brazil, and Indonesia, remains a mystery. The poorest fragile states make up only a tiny fraction of this total, but this money represents around 3 percent (often much more) of their GDPs. Not only would this money be far better spent on health, Collier's research suggests that military spending doesn't even achieve its main aim—increasing military spending does not act as a deterrent to the development of civil war (Collier, 2006). The challenge, of course, is reducing military spending in a coordinated fashion across a region so that no single country emerges as a local power. The allocation of foreign aid and peacekeeping forces will have a part to play. Harsh experience has shown that aid conditionality often does not work. Unexpectedly, this may not be the case with military spending. It has been shown that aid is not significantly lost by diversion to the military (Collier, 2007), so conditions might be working in this area. The combination of regional aid conditionality concerning military spending, backed up by properly trained observers and the necessary investment in demobilization and disarmament costs, will hopefully be a model for the future. The UK government-funded Global Facilitation Network for Security Sector Reform is an example of moves toward a coordinated approach to improvements in regional security (GFN-SSR, 2007). The OECD's section on Security Sector Reform produces a similar handbook (OECD, 2007).

Box 4.2 Moment of Insight

2009 military spending by African countries:	2009 total aid for Africa: US$47.6 billion
North Africa: US$17.3 billion sub-Saharan Africa: US$10.1 billion	Fraction used for social and economic programs: 57 percent
Total military spending in Africa in 2009:	Total economic and social aid for Africa in 2009:
US$27.4 billion	**US$27.4 billion**

Source: SIPRI. 2010. Stockholm International Peace Research Institute. Yearbook 2010. Retrieved from: www.sipri.org/.

Source: OECD-DAC. 2010. OECD development database on aid. Retrieved from: www.oecd.org/document/33/0,2340,en_2649_34447_36661793_1_1_1_1,00.html.

SUMMARY

Throughout human history, war has remained a constant; however, since the end of the Cold War, the number of conflicts has declined sharply and the nature of conflicts has changed. Seventy years ago, the most common conflicts were colonial struggles for independence and wars between countries—civil wars were relatively uncommon. At present, the only form of conflict is civil war within a state—either with the government as one combatant or between two other groups within the country (non-state conflicts). Factors influencing civil wars include chronic poverty and disgruntled young men, endemic violence, bad governance, and presence of lootable resources. Wars within and between developed countries have been increasingly rare since the end of World War II. While several of these wealthy countries are now involved as combatants in countries such as Afghanistan and Iraq, the burden of violence now falls disproportionately upon poor countries. War and conflict are clearly an important part of any study of global health.

War should not be viewed as an intractable problem without a solution. Peacemaking is possible. Some interventions include economic growth, peacekeeping, education, open management of resources, and assistance with exports. With early recognition, mediation, targeted interventions, and even, in some circumstances, military intervention, active fighting can be stopped. If caught early enough, it can be avoided altogether. The returns from effective peacekeeping, in terms of improved prosperity and health, are substantial and well worth pursuing. It is for this reason that promoting peace and justice is one of 17 global Goals that make up the 2030 Agenda for Sustainable Development—specifically, to "promote just, peaceful and inclusive societies." A specific target of the goal is to "reduce all forms of violence and related death rates everywhere by 2030."

DISCUSSION QUESTIONS

1. What are the most significant causes of wars?
2. Can you foresee a time when wars would no longer exist? Why or why not?
3. What does civil unrest mean to you? What is an interstate conflict?
4. What is the SDG related to war and civil unrest? What you think about its associated SDG targets and how would you change, modify, or add to the current targets to foster peace?
5. Why does the risk of conflict increase as poverty worsens?
6. What are the mechanisms available to prevent wars? Which do you think has the most impact?
7. What is the relationship between peace and health?

8.   Do you think a reduction in military spending can prevent war? Why or why not?
9.   What is one-sided violence? Why do you think wars and conflicts have increased in developing countries?
10.   What is the "resource curse" and how does it generate internal conflict?

RECOMMENDED READING

Collier, P. 2007. *The bottom billion*. Pub: Oxford University Press.

Human Security Report Project. 2013. *Human security report 2013: The decline in global violence: Evidence, explanation, and contestation*. Pub: Human Security Press. Retrieved from: www.hsrgroup.org/human-security-reports/2013/overview.aspx.

OECD. 2015. *States of fragility 2015: Meeting post-2015 ambitions*. Pub: OECD Publishing, Paris. DOI: http://dx.doi.org/10.1787/9789264227699-en.

Pegg, S. 2005. Can policy intervention beat the resource curse? Evidence from the Chad-Cameroon pipeline project. *African Affairs*, 105: 1–25.

Pinker, S. 2011. *The better angels of our nature: Why violence has declined*. Pub: Viking Books.

World Development Report. 2011. Conflict, security, and development. Retrieved from: http://wdronline.worldbank.org/includes/imp_images/book_pdf/WDR_2011.pdf.

REFERENCES

Agadjanian, V., et al. 2003. Civil war and child health: Regional and ethnic dimensions of child immunization and malnutrition in Angola. *Social Science and Medicine*, 56: 2515–2527.

Blattman, C., et al. 2010. Civil war. *Journal of Economic Literature*, 48: 3–57.

Child Soldiers. 2008. Global Report. Retrieved from: www.childsoldiersglobalreport.org/.

Collier, P. 2006. War and military expenditure in developing countries and their consequences for development. *The Economics of Peace and Security Journal*, 1: 10–13.

Collier, P. 2007. *The bottom billion*. Pub: Oxford University Press.

Collier, P., et al. 2002. Aid, policy, and growth in post-conflict societies. World Bank Policy Research working paper no. 2902. Retrieved from: www.csae.ox.ac.uk/conferences/2002-UPaGiSSA/papers/Hoeffler-csae2002.pdf.

Collier, P., et al. 2004. Greed and grievance in civil war. *Oxford Economic Papers*, 56: 563–595.

Collier, P., et al. 2007. Unintended consequences: Does aid promote arms races? *Oxford Bulletin of Economics and Statistics*, 67: 1–26.

Dixon, J. 2009. What causes civil wars? Integrating quantitative research findings. *International Studies Review*, 11: 707–735.

DPCR. 2011. Department of Peace and Conflict Research, University of Uppsala, Sweden. Retrieved from: www.pcr.uu.se/research/ucdp/program_overview/about_ucdp/.

EITI. 2011. Extractive Industries Transparency Initiative. Retrieved from: http://eiti.org.

Faye, M., et al. 2004. The challenges facing landlocked countries. *Journal of Human Development*, 5: 31–68.

Fearon, J., et al. 2003. Ethnicity, insurgency, and civil war. *American Political Science Review*, 97: 75–90.

GFN-SSR. 2007. A beginner's guide to security sector reform. Retrieved from: www.ssrnetwork.net/documents/GFN-SR_A_Beginners_Guide_to_SSR_v2.pdf.

Goldstone, J., et al. 2010. A global model for forecasting political instability. *American Journal of Political Science*, 54: 190–208.

GPOR. 2016. Global peace operations review. Retrieved from: http://peaceoperationsreview.org/featured-data/#Uniform.

Harbom, L., et al. 2010. Armed conflicts, 1946–2009. *Journal of Peace Research*, 47: 501–509.

Hegre, H., et al. 2006. Sensitivity analysis of empirical results on civil war onset. *Journal of Conflict Resolution*, 50: 508–535.

Human Security Report Project. 2011. *Human security report 2009/2010: The causes of peace and the shrinking costs of war.* Pub: Oxford University Press. Retrieved from: www.hsrgroup.org/human-security-reports/20092010/overview.aspx.

Human Security Report Project. 2013. *Human security report 2013: the decline in global violence: Evidence, explanation, and contestation.* Pub: Human Security Press. Retrieved from: www.hsrgroup.org/human-security-reports/2013/overview.aspx.

Kimberley Process. 2011. Retrieved from: www.kimberleyprocess.com/home/index_en.html.

Mines Action Canada. 2006. Landmine monitor report. Retrieved from: www.the-monitor.org/index.php/publications/display?url=lm/2006.

Murthy, R., et al. 2006. Mental health consequences of war: A brief review of research findings. *World Psychiatry*, 5: 25–30.

Newman, E., et al. 2007. Criminal legacies of war economies. *Journal of Peacebuilding and Development*, 3: 49–62.

OECD. 2007. The OECD-DAC handbook on security system reform (SSR). Retrieved from: www.oecd.org/dataoecd/43/25/38406485.pdf.

OECD. 2015. *States of fragility 2015: Meeting post-2015 ambitions.* Pub: OECD Publishing, Paris. DOI: http://dx.doi.org/10.1787/9789264227699-en.

OECD-DAC. 2010. OECD development database on aid. Retrieved from: www.oecd.org/document/33/0,2340,en_2649_34447_36661793_1_1_1_1,00.html.

Oxfam. 2009. Lifting the resource curse: How poor people can and should benefit from the revenues of extractable industries. Oxfam briefing paper no. 134. Retrieved from: www.oxfam.org/sites/www.oxfam.org/files/bp134-lifting-the-resource-curse-011209.pdf.

Pegg, S. 2005. Can policy intervention beat the resource curse? Evidence from the Chad-Cameroon pipeline project. *African Affairs*, 105: 1–25.

Pettersson, T., & Wallensteenet P. 2015. Armed conflicts, 1946–2014. *Journal of Peace Research*. 2015, 52(4): 536–550.

Roberts, A. 2010. Lives and statistics: Are 90% of war victims civilians? *Survival: Global Politics and Strategy*, 52: 115–136.

Roberts, L., et al. 2004. Mortality before and after the 2003 invasion of Iraq: Cluster sample survey. *The Lancet*, 364: 1857–1864.

SIPRI. 2010. Stockholm International Peace Research Institute. Yearbook 2010. Retrieved from: www.sipri.org/.

Stewart, F. 2002. Root causes of violent conflict in developing countries. *British Medical Journal*, 324: 342–345.

UCDP. 2016. Uppsala Conflict Data Program. Retrieved from: www.pcr.uu.se/research/UCDP/.

UN. 2010. The New Horizon initiative. Progress report no. 1. Retrieved from: www.un.org/en/peacekeeping/documents/newhorizon_update01.pdf.

UN. 2011. United Nations peacekeeping. Retrieved from: www.un.org/en/peacekeeping/.

UN. 2016. United Nations Sustainable Development Goals. Retrieved from: https://sustainabledevelopment.un.org/sdgs.

UN Reform. 2010. Peacekeeping reform: The Brahimi report. Retrieved from: www.un.org/en/peacekeeping/operations/reform.shtml.

UNODC. 2007. Crime, violence, and development: Trends, costs, and policy options. UN Office on Drugs and Crime. Report no. 37820. Retrieved from: www.unodc.org/pdf/research/Cr_and_Vio_Car_E.pdf.

UNPC. 2011. United Nations Peacebuilding Commission. Retrieved from: www.un.org/peace/peacebuilding/.

Ward, J., et al. 2006. Sexual violence against women and girls in war and its aftermath. UNFPA briefing paper. Retrieved from: www.unfpa.org/emergencies/symposium06/docs/finalbrusselsbriefingpaper.pdf.

Ward, M., et al. 2010. The perils of policy by p-value: Predicting civil conflicts. *Journal of Peace Research*, 47: 363–375.

WGI. 2010. World Bank's world governance indicators. Retrieved from: http://info.worldbank.org/governance/wgi/sc_country.asp.

World Development Report. 2011. Conflict, security, and development. Retrieved from: http://wdronline.worldbank.org/includes/imp_images/book_pdf/WDR_2011.pdf.Yazdi, F. V., et al. 2015. The association between peace and life expectancy: An empirical study of the world countries. *Iranian Journal of Public Health*, 44(3): 341–351.

CHAPTER 5
Poverty and Developing World Debt

Living poor is like being sentenced to exist in a stormy sea in a battered canoe, requiring all your strength simply to keep afloat; there is never any question of reaching a destination. True poverty is a state of perpetual crisis, and one wave just a little bigger or coming from an unexpected direction can and usually does wreck things.

—Moritz Thomsen

OBJECTIVES

Poverty and its inevitable companions, injustice and malnutrition, form a brutal trio that terrorize the developing world. You will never find one of them without the other two. A good understanding of each of these three issues is an essential foundation for anyone interested in global health. This chapter will examine poverty (and its big brother, developing world debt). Although debt and poverty can be analyzed separately, in practice they are so closely interrelated that it is better to deal with them together. After completing this chapter, you should be able to:

- appreciate the full range of adverse effects that poverty imposes on a population
- understand the controversies surrounding the definition and measurement of poverty
- understand the unfair historical origins of the current developing world debt
- understand the magnitude of the debt and the adverse health effects that result from excessive debt repayments

INTRODUCTION

Poverty is the worst form of violence.

—Mahatma Gandhi

Along with malnutrition and social injustice, poverty is one of the major contributing factors to the widespread ill health found in developing countries. A detailed knowledge of all three is essential for any serious study of global health. No matter what measuring system is used, at a personal level, enormous numbers of people around the world live lives of absolute discomfort, eking out a precarious and uncomfortable existence. Depending on the measurement methodology, 15–20 percent of the world's population live without access to even the most basic essentials of a dignified and decent life.

Like malnutrition, poverty is a subject that is commonly oversimplified. In practice, poverty is a complex issue with different presentations, different measurement techniques, and, of course, different solutions according to the underlying contributory causes. Even the seemingly simple task of comparing degrees of poverty is a challenge. What research method can adequately compare a family of pavement dwellers in Calcutta with a nomadic tribe in northeastern Iran? Apart from having little or no money, their lives are otherwise very different. Various measures of well-being have been devised that allow such comparisons to be made. These range from the World Bank's original US$1 per day calculation (Ravallion et al., 1991) to complex composite measures of living standards that combine scores for income, health, and education, such as the Human Development Index (HDI, 2016). Although it is essential to have a unified measure of world poverty for monitoring and planning purposes, it is important to remember that different definitions produce different estimates of numbers of poor, and also that all are open to significant measurement error.

The use of combined scoring systems reflects the fact that poverty is a vast and complex subject. It is not, of course, simply a lack of money. If that were the case, all you would have to do is hand out cash and shut down the aid agencies, which has been tried, as we shall see later. Low wages and lack of adequate land resources are usually associated with many other problems, such as insecurity of employment, illiteracy, bad housing, large families, and exploitation (Sen, 1981). Poverty is not an ennobling experience. Its effects on morale and expectations, combined with exhaustion from overwork and poor nutrition, imprison people within an endless cycle of hopelessness. The health effects of poverty begin to operate from the moment of conception and continue throughout the child's life (Feuerstein, 1997). The intrauterine environment of an undernourished mother who may have conceived too young or too

Box 5.1 Moment of Insight

Amount of money spent on clothes by the average American family in 2015:	Average income of all people living in Zimbabwe in 2015:
US$1,700	**US$1,700**
Source: Johnson, E. 2015. The real cost of your shopping habits. *Forbes*. Retrieved from: www. forbes.com/sites/emmajohnson/2015/01/15/the-real-cost-of-your-shopping-habits/#7070b1d921ae.	*Source:* Gross national income per capita 2015, Atlas method and PPP. Retrieved from: http://databank.worldbank.org/data/download/GNIPC.pdf.

often—combined with a crowded home environment without clean water, a family broken up by migrant labour or social stress, a school without desks or qualified teachers, a neighbourhood ruled by gangs of violent youths, and an economy offering few, poorly paid jobs—all limit children's health and standard of living.

No matter which measurement method is used, the statistics regarding the extent and magnitude of poverty are staggering. At a time when people in developed countries live lives of great prosperity, more than a billion people in developing regions live lives of absolute poverty, existing on less than US$1 each day. The enormous debt burden carried by many developing countries is not the only cause of this poverty, but it is a significant contributory factor. The need for regular debt repayments means that a great number of developing countries must divert limited resources away from essential services such as health and education, ultimately worsening life for the poorest in that country. Some countries are so heavily indebted that they have no possibility of ever paying off their debt. Recent moves toward debt cancellation for the most heavily indebted countries are long overdue, particularly when it is considered that much of that debt was imposed under very unfair conditions.

It should be emphasized that unfairness is not just a feature of developing world debt. It is a constant factor that is found wherever there is poverty and it greatly complicates the task facing those who wish to alleviate poverty. Until the inevitable underlying injustice is addressed, the chance of finding a long-term solution to the associated poverty is small. For example, attributing the health problems of Aboriginal Canadians living on the Labrador coast simply to lack of money, without considering the complex underlying social problems, would not be a firm foundation for a long-term solution. Whether you are a humanitarian who wants universal health and prosperity or a manufacturer who wants a bigger market for gadgets, it does not matter. Poverty eradication and all the benefits that stem from it must form the basis of your plan (Sachs, 2005).

Box 5.2 History Notes

J. M. Keynes (1883–1946)

Whether you are studying national debt, poverty, unemployment, or the Bretton-Woods Institutions, you will soon hear about J. M. Keynes. After studying economics and politics at Cambridge, he became one of the most famous economists of his day. Apart from his influential books and teaching, his talents were in demand in several other areas. He was the Treasury representative to the Versailles peace treaty in 1919, and accurately predicted that harsh reparations would cause social chaos in Germany. He was later the chairman of the World Bank Commission and played an important part in the establishment of the Bretton-Woods Institutions. He also found time to be an active member of the Bloomsbury group of artists and intellectuals. His theories affected international economic policies well after his death. He was openly gay during his youth at a time when such a lifestyle risked severe penalties, but in later life, he married a Russian ballerina. If you hear people talking of "Keynesian money theory" and you suspect they don't have a clue what they are talking about, you may be right. Follow the reference to learn more: Friedman (1997).

Over the last 10 or 15 years, there has been an increasing emphasis upon the needs of the poor. True substantive improvements have been made in the culture and organization of foreign aid that have now made those needs a central focus of the aid industry. Despite methodological measurement problems, progress has been made—not as fast as earlier optimistic claims, but progress nonetheless (Chen et al., 2008). There is now a sense of optimism that something can finally be done about the scandal of poverty in a time of prosperity. However, it is always important to be aware that poverty assessments are open to considerable potential errors. Final results can be changed simply by altering the basic definitions. For example, the target of reducing extreme poverty rates by half was met five years ahead of the 2015 deadline.

More than 1 billion people have been lifted out of extreme poverty since 1990. However, it should be noted that average measures of global poverty are heavily influenced by rapid improvements in China and India. There are still areas of the world where only very slow progress has been made against poverty. The problem is far from over.

POVERTY IN DEVELOPED COUNTRIES

No arts; no letters; no society; and which is worst of all, continual fear and danger of violent death; and the life of man, solitary, poor, nasty, brutish, and short.

—*Thomas Hobbes, Leviathan, 1651*

The concept of providing universal prosperity for everyone (or at least the provision of some basic minimal standards) is a surprisingly recent one. Scientific and agricultural advances in the decades following World War II have led to unprecedented prosperity for a growing number of people. It is easy to forget that life for generations as recent as our grandparents was, in many cases, a great deal harder than standards we have today (Geremek, 1997). Poverty is not something that happens only in tropical countries. All the current developed countries have been through times when conditions for the poor were every bit as bad as any that can be found in today's developing world.

When Queen Victoria took the throne in mid-19th-century England, the Industrial Revolution was a century old, but the social benefits of steam power and agricultural innovation were very slow to come. Standards of waste disposal and clean water supply in Victorian London were little better than those that had existed in Rome 2,000 years previously. The richest maintained a health advantage secondary to improved nutrition and housing, but everyone was exposed to

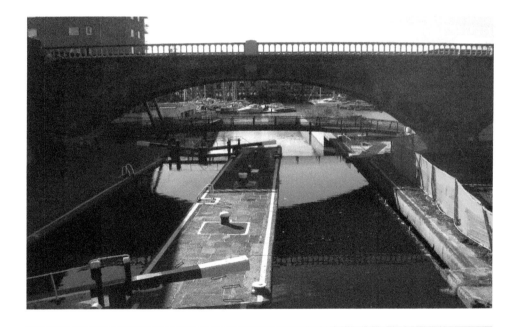

Photo 5.1: The final lock gate on the Regent's Canal before it enters Limehouse Basin in London. When the railways took cargo traffic away from London's port in the 19th century, Limehouse was described by Dickens as a black hole of poverty. It is now a marina filled with expensive boats surrounded by equally expensive apartment blocks. Every currently developed country has passed through a period where poverty was common.

Source: Photo by Edward Betts.

infectious diseases that are nowadays associated with only the poorest of developing countries. Tuberculosis remained the most common single cause of death until well into the 20th century. Water-borne diseases of poverty, such as cholera and typhoid, were a constant threat—in fact, Queen Victoria's husband died of typhoid he contracted while living in a palace!

The dreadful working conditions associated with the early factories (Blake's "dark satanic mills") produced an extensive underclass of working poor. Their lives are well documented in the works of Dickens, particularly *Oliver Twist*. These conditions were not confined to England but were widespread throughout the slowly developing countries of Europe and the squalid ghettos of America, such as the Bowery and Hell's Kitchen in 19th-century New York. Clearly, there is nothing new about poverty. Ever since humans started to gather in cities, life for those at the fringes of society has been harsh. Though they may choose to forget history, all the currently prosperous developed countries passed through a period when poverty was as severe as any that can be found today in developing countries (Photo 5.1).

As societies grew larger and more sophisticated, it became clear that some support for the poor was necessary. These supports included workhouses, almshouses, and care for abandoned children and the destitute (Geremek, 1997). Distinction was made between the worthy poor, who were prepared to work for charity, and the unworthy poor, who were not (and who also faced severe penalties). The first British Poor Laws date back to Elizabeth I's reign in the 16th century. They were prompted by the results of a severe economic decline. Those laws were slowly improved and updated with time until they were finally replaced by the new laws of the welfare state after World War II (EH Net, 2010). Britain's attitude to caring for the poor was far ahead of other European countries' and serves as an example of the beneficial impact of social legislation on population health.

The social implications of widespread poverty were taken more seriously from the end of the 19th century onward. This had been known about for a long time, but, apart from England's Poor Laws, not much had been done about it at a government level. With the steady growth of the population in Europe, care of the poor could no longer be left to charity. Poverty was bad for the business of a country, so its alleviation slowly became a government responsibility. For example, during World War I, the British government was shocked to discover that significant numbers of the country's young men were so unhealthy from tuberculosis, chronic malnutrition, and rheumatic fever that they were not even fit enough to serve as cannon fodder. Moves toward financial support for poor families and some form of national health care date back to the first part of the 20th century in most large European countries. However, despite the social advances in Europe since that time, there is still to this day a marked difference in mortality rates between the poorest areas of Europe and the richest (Elo, 2009). In the poorer European countries, mortality rates among the poor are still twice those of the rich.

When the foreign aid industry started after World War II, poverty was not a distant collective memory in developed countries as it is now. Apart from a few history lessons, today's Canadian schoolchildren have little idea of the reality of life faced by average people only three generations ago. Even in our grandparents' early lives there were no antibiotics, no immunizations, little anaesthesia, no social supports, and primitive standards of dentistry and obstetric care. Epidemics of polio happened well within the memory of people alive today. All the major European donor countries have been through a period of poverty and national debt equivalent to that of current developing countries. They were provided with low-interest grants from America after World War II and were later granted debt cancellation. It is hoped that policy-makers in developed countries have longer memories than their children, and that their foreign aid plans reflect that past shared experience. Aid should not be given as cold charity from the rich to the poor, but rather as a helping hand through a predictable stage in a country's development.

THE EFFECTS OF POVERTY

Poverty is a weapon of mass destruction.

—Dennis Kucinich, 2003

The adverse effects of poverty are so pervasive that there will likely be a graphical relationship between poverty and any chosen measure of well-being. For example, children in poverty are unhealthy, but which came first? Lack of education reduces employment opportunities, which contributes to poverty, but poverty also reduces access to education, and so it goes round. This circular argument can be applied to a host of other social variables and is the reason that studies talk of populations being trapped within a perpetual cycle of social ills that cause poverty, but are themselves also exacerbated by poverty. In reality, this isn't an either/or argument. The variables are so mixed together that they cannot be analyzed separately and are better viewed as associations rather than cause and effect. Bearing in mind that poverty is endlessly complex, the following associations are worth examining.

Poverty and Inequity

No matter what statistical games can be played with the data, poverty is not the fault of the poor. Leaving aside the effects of acute disasters, most poverty cycles continue

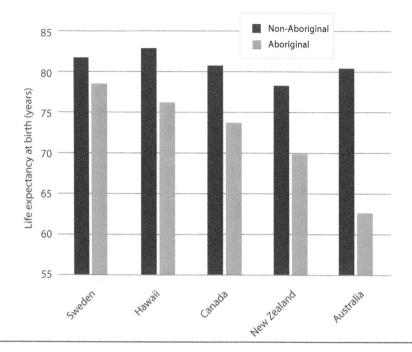

Figure 5.1: Life expectancies for Indigenous peoples compared to those of the dominant national group in various countries around the world

Sources: ABS, 2011; Braun et al., 1996; Hausler et al., 2005; StatsCan, 2011; Bramley et al., 2004.

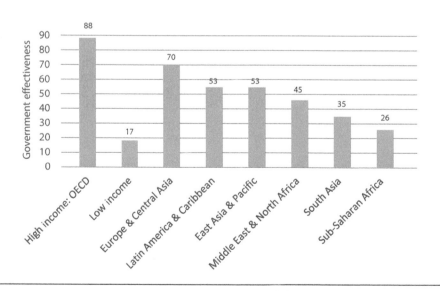

Figure 5.2: Measure of government effectiveness by region

Source: WGI. 2016. Worldwide governance indicators (government effectiveness). Retrieved from: http://info.worldbank.org/governance/wgi/index.aspx#reports.

because of the effects of unfairness on a large scale perpetuated by poor governance. Wherever there is endemic poverty, there will always be endemic injustice very close by. If there is a single cause-and-effect argument applicable to poverty, it is that of injustice and poverty. Poor people may well be unable to prevent injustice, but they certainly don't cause it. A perfect example of the adverse effects of inequity is the widespread poverty of Indigenous peoples. As we shall see later in the book (Chapter 17), Indigenous groups have a depressingly common history of relative poverty based on discrimination and often far worse. As a result, their health outcomes are invariably worse than those of the dominant group (Figure 5.1).

The widespread belief that aid works best in a supportive environment has stimulated the development of several scoring systems used to measure the degree of government corruption (CPI, 2015) and government effectiveness (WGI, 2015). While these are not direct measures of injustice, it is likely that widespread injustice will be more possible and more likely in countries with weak and corrupt governments. As seen in Figure 5.2, regions with the lowest per capita income are also

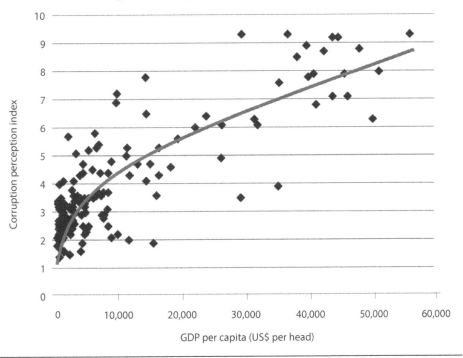

Figure 5.3: Plot of Corruption Perception Index against GDP per capita for countries below US$60,000 per head. Corruption Index runs from 0 (bad corruption) to 10 (honest government).

Sources: CPI. 2010. Transparency International's Corruption Perception Index. Retrieved from: www.transparency.org/policy_research/surveys_indices/cpi/2010; World Bank. 2011. Global economic prospects: Maintaining progress amid turmoil. Retrieved from: http://go.worldbank.org/PF6VWYXS10.

the places with the worst measures of governance. Interestingly, the income point associated with improved governance and falling corruption is around US$4,000 per capita. As discussed in Chapter 3, this is also the income level where measures of maternal and child health start to improve and the health-wealth curve flattens off.

Poverty and Nutrition

The relationship between poverty and nutrition is a close one. As we'll discuss in the chapter on nutrition, there are many causes of malnutrition (lack of food, lack of education, poor living standards, etc.). Each of these variables is closely interrelated with poverty. For example, early severe malnutrition often causes permanent limitations in a child's physical and neurological development that ultimately limit that child's employment opportunities as an adult. When this is scaled up to a population level, early malnutrition has a measurable effect on a country's economic output, which, in turn, worsens poverty, and so the cycle

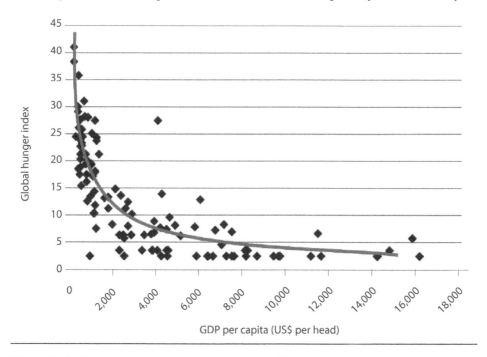

Figure 5.4: Compound measure of nutrition (Global Hunger Index) plotted against GDP per capita. The index is an open-ended scale where 0 represents no significant malnutrition.

Sources: IFPRI. 2010. International Food Policy Research Institute: Global Hunger Index report. Retrieved from: www.ifpri.org/sites/default/files/publications/ghi10.pdf; World Bank. 2011. Global economic prospects: Maintaining progress amid turmoil. Retrieved from: http://go.worldbank.org/PF6VWYXS10.

continues (World Bank, 2006). Not surprisingly, there is a close cross-country relationship between measures of poverty and the extent of childhood malnutrition (Figure 5.4). In fact, the relationship is close enough that some studies use malnutrition rates as a proxy measure for poverty in an attempt to rule out the effects of inflation over time. There are several measures of malnutrition—the one chosen for Figure 5.4 was a compound measure of child nutrition called the Global Hunger Index (IFPRI, 2010).

Poverty and Education

Once again, there is a tight and complex relationship between poverty and education, much of it probably mediated by poverty's effects on nutrition. Poorly nourished children miss far more school time due to illness. Even when they attend school, their ability to concentrate and learn is compromised. Lack of parental education (itself a result of poverty) reduces the emphasis on the need for education,

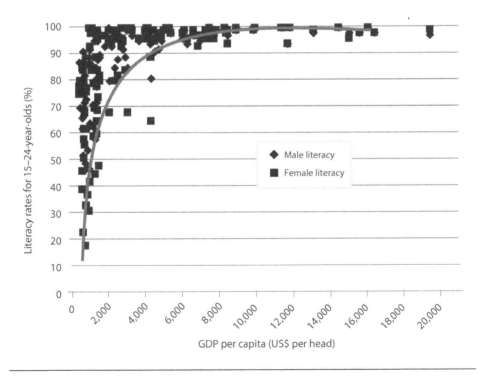

Figure 5.5: Literacy rates for 15–24-year-olds plotted against GDP per capita for all countries less than US$20,000 per head

Sources: UNICEF. 2010. Childinfo. Retrieved from: www.childinfo.org/index.html; World Bank. 2011. Global economic prospects: Maintaining progress amid turmoil. Retrieved from: http://go.worldbank.org/PF6VWYXS10.

and all these variables are further complicated by lack of schools and gender disparities that are frequently found in the poorest countries. The plot of GDP per capita against literacy again shows a distinct improvement around US$3,000 to $4,000 per head (Figure 5.5).

Poverty and Health

Everyone understands that health and money are connected, but of all the relationships, this is the most complex. The health differences between rich and poor countries are a global scandal. In Afghanistan, out of every 1,000 children born alive, over 200 of them will be dead before their fifth birthday. In Canada, fewer than 5 per 1,000 will die before their fifth birthday. Libraries could be filled with books explaining the causes of ill health, and many of those variables will, in some way, be the result of poverty. Clearly, there will be a correlation between the two, but it's not going to be a straight line. There are some exceptions. For example, the health system in Cuba not only outperforms other low- and medium-income countries, but in some cases also outperforms high-income countries; surprisingly, although Cuba spends US$817 per head per year compared with the United States' $9,403, Cuba still has the lower infant mortality rate of the two, and life expectancy in both countries is comparable (World Bank, 2016).

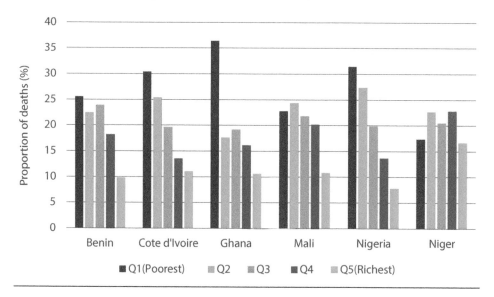

Figure 5.6: Relationship between income quintile and under-five mortality within six developing countries

Source: Bado, A. R., & Appunni, S. S. 2015. Decomposing wealth-based inequalities in under-five mortality in West Africa. *Iranian Journal of Public Health*, 44(7): 920–930.

While there are obvious health differences between rich and poor countries, there are also demonstrable health gradients between different social groups within each country. This is demonstrated in Figure 5.6, in which under-five mortality is plotted by income quintile for five developing countries. In all but one, there is a clear reduction in mortality as income rises. There is also a marked difference between the average national values for each of these countries.

DEFINING AND MEASURING POVERTY

We are not concerned with the very poor. They are unthinkable, and only to be approached by the statistician or the poet.

—*E. M. Forster, Howard's End, 1910*

The Western concept of poverty (having little or no money) is not sufficient to deal with the broader reality of poverty in developing countries. Lack of money is a part of the picture, but as the World Bank's revolutionary study titled "Conversations with the Poor" revealed, poverty is also closely tied to social and cultural isolation, lack of education, marginalization, and absence of power (Narayan et al., 1999). This does not mean that all poor people are vulnerable to ill health (any more than all vulnerable people are poor). If economically poor agricultural communities are given access to the basics of good health—such as schooling, immunization, clean water, and sanitation—then it is possible for them to lead generally healthy lives without access to high incomes (Sen, 1999). This has clearly been demonstrated in many parts of the world, such as the Indian province of Kerala, where population health measures are far better than per capita income figures would suggest (Michael et al., 2003).

The issue of poverty is too complex to resolve itself into a single descriptive phrase. The common definition, "Poverty is the state in which an individual or family has to spend more than 80 percent of their income on food," does not apply in many situations. How can the health and income of a hunter-gatherer Amerindian family from Venezuela be compared with those of an unemployed Inuit family living in the North of Canada? Clearly, before tackling the problem, it is necessary to understand there are different types of poverty that may require different solutions. In her 1997 book, *Poverty and Health*, Dr. Feuerstein outlines several forms of poverty:

Economic poverty: This is caused by low productivity and a poor resource base. It is reflected in low income, poor nutrition, and, inevitably, poor health. Typical examples include rural smallholders dependent on adequate rainfall. The children have nothing to inherit and few opportunities, so they are caught in an unending cycle of poverty.

Instant and temporary poverty: Sudden hazards such as earthquakes, drought, and war can cause instant poverty in an area. Some of these may be relatively short-lived. Conditions may improve following a permanent ceasefire or improved rains. In the same way, migration and population pressures may overwhelm an area that was previously reasonably prosperous, forming an overcrowding poverty.

New poor: Imposed national austerity measures or high inflation may precipitate poverty in a significant percentage of a country by eroding income and savings.

Hidden poverty: Examples include retirees living on small pensions who might have adequate shelter and food, but who lack sufficient extra income to heat their houses or seek health care.

Absolute poverty: Such people are deprived of all the elements necessary to make an adequately healthy life. They lack access to safe water, shelter, or security and are more likely to remain in that condition despite improvements in society brought on by better market conditions.

The debate surrounding the definition and measurement of poverty is not simply a sterile academic argument, since the approach used to reduce poverty depends greatly on the definitions and explanations used to define that poverty. The World Bank, not surprisingly, has concentrated on a financial definition of poverty. It first defined the US$1 per day measurement in its 1990 World Development Report (Ravallion et al., 1991). In an updated form, this measurement has also been adopted as the scoring system for the Millennium Development Organization's goal of poverty alleviation. Enthusiasts of "a dollar a day" analysis took the approach that emphasizing economic growth was the quickest way to reduce poverty. They implemented various economic recovery programs and structural adjustment policies that tended to concentrate on economic growth at the expense of the poor. The widely acknowledged failure of these structural adjustment programs was, in fact, one of the principal catalysts for debate in this area.

The United Nations Development Programme (UNDP) took a very different attitude toward poverty assessment and alleviation. It adopted a much broader approach to poverty measurement based on the Nobel Prize–winning work of the

Indian economist Amartya Sen, and the leadership of the late Pakistani economist Mahbub Ul-Haq. They developed a more comprehensive composite scoring system for classifying and measuring poverty based on variables such as health, education, gender equality, and political freedom. The best-known examples are the Human Development Index and the Multidimensional Poverty Index (Alkire et al., 2010), which has replaced the older Human Poverty Index. Results are published in the UNDP's annual Human Development Report (UNDP, 2015). Global poverty estimates have been updated to reflect a re-estimated international poverty line of US$1.90 a day, based on 2011 purchasing power parity (PPP) (World Bank & IMF, 2016).

Following the failure of the structural adjustment policies of the 1980s and early 1990s, even the World Bank and International Monetary Fund (IMF) realized that there was more to poverty alleviation than imposed economic restructuring plans that had often actually made life worse for the poor. With the introduction of the Enhanced Heavily Indebted Poor Countries (EHIPC) Initiative in 1999, the World Bank and IMF shifted to a rather gentler set of economic interventions that no longer required the abolition of price supports on essential foods or steep reductions in spending on health and education. The process is guided by national poverty plans called Poverty Reduction Strategy Papers (PRSPs) that are developed by the target country. The development of a national PRSP has to include that country's poor at every level of planning. It takes time for a country to pass through the debt relief process, but early experience has been cautiously optimistic (IMF, 2008).

Benjamin Seebohm Rowntree (1910) was the first person to establish a baseline poverty level (called a "poverty line") by studying the cost of a minimum diet for a family of six for one week in the city of York. After adding a factor for shelter, clothing, fuel, and others, he arrived at a poverty line of 26 shillings per week for a family of six. At that time, 10 percent of the population fell below this line. His final conclusion was that poverty was due to poor wages. This went against the opinion of the day, which generally blamed the poor for their own misfortunes. There are, of course, many other ways to measure poverty. Each has its own methodological problems and errors. Simply put, there is no single measure or definition of poverty that reliably tracks the magnitude and extent of poverty under all circumstances around the world. The best approach is obviously to use different scores and measures in order to get a general idea of the progress of poverty reduction.

The commonly used measures of poverty are either based on a family's income or on an assessment of some of the services that money can buy (summarized in Table 5.1). Income is used for purchases such as food, education, and health care. Those purchases have results in terms of health, nutrition, education, and employment.

The final outcome is, hopefully, healthy, educated children who become productive, happy adults. There are reasonable correlations between these variables, but they are far from perfect. For example, it is possible to have money and yet still be poor in some other aspect of your life, such as nutrition, health, or happiness (Sen, 1999).

It is important to have an understanding of some of the common poverty indices because there are wide differences and considerable arguments between proponents of the various methods. Each of the measures has methodological problems, potential errors, and plenty of critics (Reddy et al., 2005). Sometimes, the criticism of various poverty measures can almost become an end in itself (Saith, 2005). There is a danger of forgetting that no matter what technique is used, vast numbers of people live lives of wretchedness on a daily basis (Photo 5.2). The main measurement methods come under the following headings.

Income analysis (Sillers, 2002): The US$1 per day measure, popularized by the World Bank, seems superficially simple but is based on a complex chain of calculations that is open to considerable error. The basic income data depend on household surveys from a wide range of developed countries. Even this first step alone is open to criticism since trying to compare different surveys done at different times in different countries has obvious difficulties. The second step involves deriving a

Table 5.1: Different aspects of poverty, from income to income inequality, and their associated poverty indicators

	INCOME	PURCHASES	RESULTS OF PURCHASES	FINAL SENSE OF WELL-BEING	INCOME INEQUALITY
Examples	• Wages • Crops • Welfare	• Food • Education • Fuel • Transport • Shelter • Clothes • Health care	• Nutrition levels • Health • Safe childbirth • Diplomas, degrees • Employment • Safety	Degree of: • Safety • Vulnerability • Powerlessness • Happiness • Optimism or hope	• Range from richest to poorest • Distribution of wealth
Poverty Indicators	• US$1/day • US$2/day • GDP/capita • Percentage of standard-ized national income	• Cost of basic needs analysis • Standard bag of groceries, plus non-food essentials	• Composite scores of health, nutrition, etc.—Human Development Index (HDI) and Human Poverty Index (HPI)	• Open-ended discussions and subjective reports— Voices of the Poor • Gender Empowerment Measure (GEM)	• Lorenz Curve • Gini Index • Poverty Gap Index

standard currency so that the different incomes can be universally compared. This process is based on regular five-year estimates of Purchasing Power Parity (PPP) from the World Bank's International Comparison Program (ICP, 2011).

This international dollar is intended to compare economic performances between different countries. It differs greatly from the official quoted exchange rate. Average per capita income in 2000 for India was US$450. When placed in international PPP dollars, the average income rises to US$2,340. To complicate matters further, the initial US$1 cut-off point was based on 1985 prices. It was updated to US$1.08 in 1993 and, more recently, to US$1.25 in 2005. Each change generates new estimates of the number of people below that line (Chen et al., 2008) and opens the technique to significant criticism from either side. Some argue the method greatly underestimates the number of poor in the world (Reddy et al., 2005). Others claim it greatly overestimates the number of poor and that the MDGs have already been met (Pinkovskiy et al., 2009). Although this second group uses

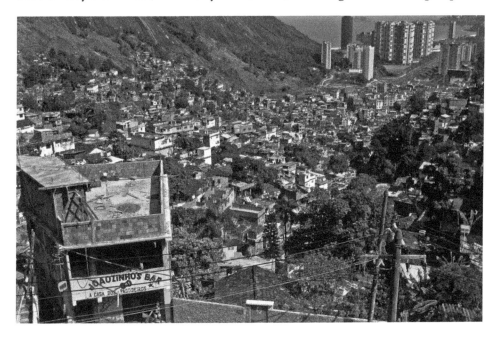

Photo 5.2: Technical arguments about poverty measures should not obscure the fact that hundreds of millions of people around the world live under terrible conditions. The picture shows the Favelha Rocinha, an overcrowded slum that exists right next to the modern high-rises of Brazil's Rio de Janeiro. Residents live in shacks with limited access to electricity, clean water, or sewage disposal.

Source: UN Photo/McGlynn, with kind permission of the UN Photo Library (www.unmultimedia.org/photo).

the US$1 per day terminology, they arrive at the calculation using different techniques—grounds for yet another disagreement! The US$1 per day measure is the most widely used poverty line despite its potential errors.

Consumption analysis (Deaton, 2003): Household surveys of income have been shown to be less reliable than questions based on family consumption. The numbers appear to be more representative of a family's economic position over time. Inevitably, different countries have very different views on what constitutes a bare minimum when it comes to food and non-food essentials. Poverty lines based on these calculations are higher in richer countries because of greater expectations. Comparison between countries consequently can become difficult. The non-food component of the budget also varies between countries. Indonesia sets its poverty line assuming that families spend 80 percent of their income on food, while the United States assumes that food represents only one-third of a poor household's expenditure. Significant variations also exist within a country. Bare minimum requirements vary significantly between rural and urban settings such that different rural and urban poverty lines may be set for a single country.

Multidimensional analysis (OPHI, 2010): The UNDP in particular has concentrated on measuring compound indicators of poverty. The Human Development Index (HDI) consists of three components (education, average income, and life expectancy at birth). The more recently introduced Multidimensional Poverty Index is based on scores of longevity, educational achievement, and various measures of a decent standard of living, such as access to clean water. Both indices are published in the UNDP's annual Human Development Report (UNDP, 2011).

Sense of well-being (Narayan et al., 1999): Conventional measures of poverty are commonly based on the information obtained in household surveys. This more or less quantifiable information is used to provide various indices of poverty. Some researchers have taken this process further to include more detailed questions about the daily reality of the lives of the poor. The results have given greater insight into the adverse effects of poverty. In particular, there is now a better understanding of the sense of vulnerability, fear, and powerlessness that are constant companions of poor people.

Relative poverty indicators (World Bank, 2010): Absolute poverty measures, such as US$1 per day, can be used to calculate the population fraction or absolute numbers of people living below a minimum poverty line (Ravallion, 2003). More recently, there has been increased interest in measures of relative poverty that assess the extent of maldistribution of income between the richest and the poorest in a country. The methods used are technical—distribution is often plotted using Lorenz lines and the degree of dispersion is summarized in a single number called the Gini coefficient. The higher the Gini coefficient, the worse the distribution.

MAGNITUDE AND TRENDS OF POVERTY

As discussed in Chapter 3, poverty in all its forms remains one of the key social determinants of health. While the number of people living in extreme poverty has dropped by more than half, there are too many that are still struggling for the most basic human needs. One of the targets of the SDG goal on poverty is "By 2030, eradicate extreme poverty for all people everywhere." The SDG 1 targets highlight that there are different ways to measure poverty. The World Bank has updated international poverty lines (based on 2011 PPP), which incorporate new information on differences in the cost of living between countries. Extreme poverty is defined as living on a household per capita income of less than US$1.90 PPP per day. Moderate poverty is defined as living on between $1.90 PPP and $3.10 PPP per capita per day. ILO estimates suggest that nearly US$10 trillion is needed to eradicate extreme and moderate poverty by 2030 (ILO, 2016).

Judging whether that goal will be reached is a challenge. As we have just seen, all poverty measures have errors and the US$1 per day measure is no different—this should always be remembered when interpreting poverty statistics. Quite apart

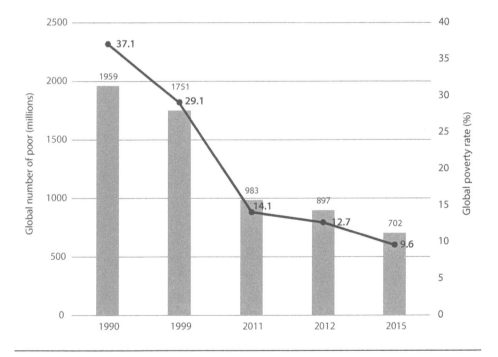

Figure 5.7: Global number of poor and poverty rate since 1990

Source: WorldBank & IMF. 2016. Development goals in an era of demographic change. Global Monitoring report, 2015/2016. Retrieved from: http://pubdocs.worldbank.org/en/503001444058224597/Global-Monitoring-Report-2015.pdf.

from the problem of research methods, the arguments around poverty trends can also become heated because the results are used by both sides of the globalization debate to support differing views about the effects of economic growth on the poor (Ravallion, 2003).

While global average values for poverty do seem to be decreasing, that progress is not evenly spread across different regions. Expressed as an average for the whole world, poverty levels have reduced, but on closer analysis, most of that progress has occurred in China and India. In sub-Saharan Africa and Latin America, progress has been much slower.

DEVELOPING WORLD DEBT

> The history of Third World debt is the history of a massive siphoning off by international finance of resources of the most deprived people. This process is designed to perpetuate itself, thanks to a diabolic mechanism whereby debt replicates itself on an ever greater scale, a cycle that can be broken only by canceling the debt.
>
> —*E. H. Guissé, UN Subcommittee on Human Rights, 2004*

For almost 50 years, the poorest countries of the world have been consistently held back by the need to service an ever-increasing financial debt owned by the richest countries in the world. At a time in world history of unprecedented prosperity, the foot-dragging and failure of these wealthy countries to forgive the debt of the poorest nations is difficult to explain (Millet et al., 2005). At the G8 summit meeting in 2005, a well-publicized effort was made to take debt relief seriously. The decision to forgive US$40 billion of debt for the world's 18 poorest countries, and the Multilateral Debt Reduction Initiative that stemmed from the meeting, was a good start, and substantive progress has subsequently been made, but there is still a long way to go.

Tony Blair and George Bush might be claiming credit for the developed world's change of heart toward debt, but it is quite likely that growing popular pressure from events such as the Live 8 Concert let them know that their voters were expecting changes (Live 8, 2006). Inevitably, popular stars such as Bono and Bob Geldof have been criticized for using this event for personal gain. Whatever their motivations might be, most would agree that the enthusiastic support of millions of potential voters in the world's richest countries probably had a major influence on the G8 leaders. One thing is certain—popular stars understand popular culture. They have an enormous fan base and ready access to news media. The subsequent debate can become heated, with hurriedly prepared facts recycled through newspapers, television, and radio. In the middle of all this, the details about debt relief can be elusive.

The Third World debt developed in three distinct stages. The first was the arbitrary imposition of debt onto newly independent countries by their previous colonial masters. The second was a decade of indiscriminate lending of vast amounts of money to poorly prepared dictatorships, money that was subsequently wasted and pillaged by corrupt governments, with little or no benefits for their people. The third was a period of financial collapse secondary to rising interest rates and falling commodity prices. If recent developments become sustainable, then we are now hopefully entering a fourth stage: debt forgiveness.

Phase One: Colonial Legacy

> Colonies do not cease to be colonies because they are independent.
>
> *—Benjamin Disraeli*

African countries did not ask to be colonized. The benefits of colonization were, at best, questionable, so the ultimate imposition of debt by the departing colonizers should not automatically be accepted as legal (*South Bulletin*, 2004). A good example was Indonesia. After accumulating a debt caused by fighting Indonesian rebels for four years, the Dutch government left and then imposed that debt upon the very people they had been fighting. In a similar way, the enforcement of apartheid in South Africa cost a great deal of money. The government of the day had to raise money to pay for a large military machine. Its purpose was simply to enforce an evil system onto most of the country's population. It is difficult to see why the new South African government should pay the debts accumulated in their subjugation. It is rather like asking President Mandela to pay rent for his 25 years in jail!

There is plenty of historical precedent to justify refusal of unfair colonial loans. Ironically, the earliest example involved Britain and the United States. Following its war with Britain, the newly independent United States flatly refused to accept any imposed debt from its recent colonial master. Many other examples exist:

- 1867: Mexico, under President Juarez, repudiated debts imposed by the departing Hapsburg Empire.
- 1898: The US supported Cuba in its fight against Spain's imposition of debts. This was the first application of the principal of "odious debt," since it was claimed that the debts were enforced by arms without consent of the people of Cuba.
- 1923: Loans by the Royal Bank of Canada to President Tinoco of Costa Rica were deemed illegal since they were used to oppress the independence movement.

- 1925: After much debate, newly independent Syria, Lebanon, and Iraq were deemed completely new countries and were not automatically responsible for any of the debt incurred by the Ottoman Empire.
- 1983: The Vienna Convention on Succession of State Property agreed that "debt of the predecessor state does not automatically pass to the newly independent state." Unfortunately, this convention has not been ratified by enough countries to carry sufficient legal weight.
- Present day: Division of Yugoslavia's debts among the new post-conflict republics is a topic of considerable current debate.

Succession of the liabilities of the colonial masters should be approached legally rather than financially, since many feel that those original debts were illegal. By 1960, arbitrary impositions of colonial debt had already risen to US$59 billion. The situation was worsened by the exorbitant 14 percent interest rate. Before these new countries had time to organize themselves, the debt burden rapidly grew out of control.

Phase Two: Indiscriminate Lending

> If a despotic power incurs a debt not for the needs or in the interest of the State but to strengthen its despotic regime ... this debt is odious for the populations of all the State.
>
> —*Alexander Sack, 1927*

The second cause of the debt mainly occurred during the decade of the 1970s. In this period, a rapid increase in oil prices produced huge profits for countries in the Middle East. This money was deposited with Northern banks for investment. At that time, Europe was in a recession because of the effects of high energy costs, so banks looked to the developing world for their customers. It is just possible that some of the banks and consultants from the World Bank actually persuaded themselves they were doing a useful service. Borrowing cheap money seemed, at least on the surface, to be a good way of generating much-needed development. Unfortunately, it was an absolute disaster.

It is easy to blame tyrants and corrupt officials, but it would be more sensible to blame the people who made the loans. Why was money given to people like Mobutu or Marcos? Even without the benefit of hindsight, it is obvious that money given to such people would be ultimately wasted and probably never repaid. Sometimes money was lent simply out of greed. The 2004 book *Confessions of an Economic Hit Man*, by John Perkins, gives some insight into this area. Loan salesmen competed with each other to see who could give the largest loans to the biggest tyrants. Their approach was utterly callous; they were indifferent to the purposes for which these loans were used. At other times, aid was used as a tool of foreign policy. The competition between East and West to extend their influence in the developing world meant that tyrannical regimes were supported with aid by the West simply because they were seen as the only feasible option to Soviet, Chinese, or Cuban communist alternatives.

With this background, it is hardly surprising that much of the money was stolen for personal use or wasted on the military or grandiose projects where failure was inevitable; there is no shortage of examples. A significant proportion of the borrowed money—as high as 20 percent, according to the International Peace Research Institute in Stockholm (Hess, 1989)—was spent on arms. These arms allowed dictators to terrorize and murder their own people. Increased weapons sales boosted profits for the major players in the arms industry (the US, Britain, the USSR, France, Germany), who were also the major aid donors.

The list of four-lane highways to nowhere or of steel-and-glass presidential palaces is endless, but perhaps the greatest of all these fiascos is the Bataan nuclear power station. President Marcos of the Philippines was allowed to build a nuclear power station with international loans. Westinghouse (of Three Mile Island fame) was the chosen contractor. What could possibly go wrong? Charges of corruption are the least of the project's problems. Westinghouse admitted paying a friend of President Marcos a 5 percent commission in order to confirm selection. Westinghouse admits paying this US$17.3 million simply as a "commission." No one knows how many millions more were looted by Marcos. Unfortunately, it gets worse. The project was eventually completed at a total of US$2.2 million. It was built near Mount Pinatubo in a volcanic region. It was so close to a major geological fault line that it was considered unsafe to operate. The plant has never been used and it sits, shiny and useless, as a wonderful monument to the endless corruption of that decade of loans. The latest plan is to turn it into a tourist attraction (CNN, 2011).

Money wasted on useless projects is one problem; outright corruption and theft is another. Again, evidence is easy to find since the largest examples were so flagrant that they prompted major enquiries. Of the US$64 billion raised by Iraqi oil sales, an estimated US$10 billion was skimmed off by Saddam Hussein (UN Resolution 1538, 2004). Of the US and IMF loans given to bail out Russia's economy in the 1990s, US$10 billion found its way to various people, including Boris Yeltsin's daughter and the Russian Mafia! How much more sits in bank accounts of ex-dictators such as Baby Doc Duvalier? The prevailing morality of the Cold War allowed normal ethical considerations to be ignored. Loans were made for political and strategic reasons to a range of dictators and thugs, many of whom would have been jailed under the laws of the lending country; the final list is a long one.

Loans were made to support Brazil's military dictatorship, Mobutu's tyranny over the Congo, and Marcos's corruption in the Philippines. Private banks even lent money to apartheid South Africa in the face of global opposition to that regime.

The term "odious debt" can be applied to much of the money that was loaned to developing countries during the 1970s. This is a legal concept developed by Alexander Sack, who was a professor of international law (Adams, 1991). The concept is summarized by the quotation at the beginning of this section. Since the loan was of benefit only to the dictatorial regime, there is no reason that it should be paid off by subsequent governments: "This debt is not an obligation for the nation; it is a regime's debt, a personal debt of the power that has incurred it, consequently it falls with the fall of this power."

In cases where the borrowed money was used against the people's interest, with the knowledge of creditors, the creditors can be said to have colluded in a hostile act against the people, so the creditors should not legitimately expect to get their money back.

Phase Three: Financial Collapse

> Today we spend more on debt interest than we currently do on running schools in England plus climate change plus transport.
>
> —*David Cameron, UK prime minister, 2010*

Unfortunately, around 1980, a number of events conspired to make a bad situation much worse. The era of Thatcher and Reagan coincided with rising interest rates and consequent increases in the size of debt repayments. In May 1981, the US prime rate peaked at 21.5 percent (Figure 5.8). Most of the loans were borrowed at variable rates, given at 1 percent above the US prime; such interest rates could be considered usurious. In addition, the rising oil price (Figure 5.9), which had originally caused the decade of easy loans, now triggered a global recession with a sharp drop in the commodity prices that supported much of the exports of developing countries. The combination of falling commodity prices and rising interest rates meant that developing countries found themselves having to pay more with diminishing revenues. At time of writing, the rich developed nations are going through a similar debt crisis and are getting a crash course on the realities of uncontrolled debt.

Private banks in the north refused grants for new loans until previous ones had been repaid. The end of the Cold War and collapse of the Soviet state also had adverse effects. Financial support was reduced for many developing countries in the Soviet sphere. It was no longer felt necessary to support unjust tyrants against the threat of a communist "menace." Consequently, supplies of easy loans to a range of

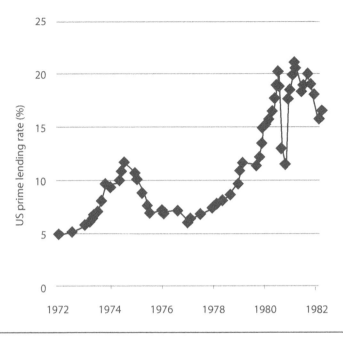

Figure 5.8: Prime US lending rate in the years leading up to the developing world financial crisis of the 1980s

Source: Wall Street Journal. 2011. US prime rate history. Retrieved from: www.wsjprimerate.us/wall_street_journal_prime_rate_history.htm.

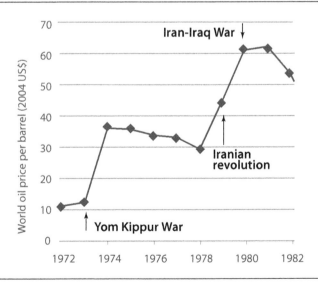

Figure 5.9: World oil price in 2004 US$ in the years leading up to the developing world financial crisis of the 1980s

Source: WTRG Economics. 2009. Oil price history and analysis. Retrieved from: www.wtrg.com/prices.htm.

countries dried up (Patterson, 1997). The economies of developing countries were often shaped largely by one or two commodities, either mineral or agricultural. They did not have the flexibility to respond to the new economic demands, so failure of debt repayment became inevitable.

In August 1982, Mexico became the first country to threaten default on its debt repayments. Obviously, other countries were not far behind. Financial crises followed in Thailand, Russia, Brazil, Turkey, and Argentina, to mention some of the major ones. For insight into this chaotic period, two books are essential reading: *Globalization and Its Discontents* (Stiglitz, 2002) and *The Chastening* (Blustein, 2003). The IMF and leading industrialized capitalist countries put up new loans and enabled the private banks to recover their initial outlay and avoid a series of international bank failures. Donor and multilateral institutions (particularly the IMF and World Bank) used their financial leverage to impose financial adjustment policies upon the debtors. Those refusing to implement adjustments ran the risk of being cut off from any further credit. The subject of Structural Adjustment Policies (SAPs) and subsequent developments will be discussed in detail later.

Magnitude of Developing World Debt

> When a government is dependent upon bankers for money, they and not the leaders of the government control the situation, since the hand that gives is above the hand that takes.
>
> —*Napoleon Bonaparte, 1815*

Under the influence of the factors noted above, the debt of the developing world rose steadily from US$59 billion in 1960 to numbers that are now too big to conceive. The total passed through US$2.5 trillion in 2004 and is now well over US$3.5 trillion! About a quarter is owed by low-income countries, while the remainder is owed by heavily indebted middle-income countries such as Mexico, Venezuela, Argentina, and Brazil. The original loans have all been paid off, but, thanks to the wonders of compound interest, the total keeps on rising. Until about 1990, the bulk of the debt was in the form of either official government loans (bilateral debt), loans from international financial institutions such as the IMF and the World Bank (multilateral debt), or long-term loans from large private banks (private debt). The debt relief mechanisms that have received so much recent publicity apply to multilateral debt held by the IMF, the World Bank, and the African Development Bank. While debt forgiveness in billions is important for those heavily indebted countries, it is still only a small part of the total developing world debt measured in trillions.

After the financial crisis of the late 1980s and early 1990s, the types of loan changed. Many developing countries could no longer get access to long-term bank loans, so they substituted bond financing in place of bank credit. In order to finance trade, some are also able to obtain higher-interest short-term loans. Some countries are also now retiring external debt by raising internal bonds. This total receives little attention, but it is substantial (Panizza, 2008). The mix of credit varies widely depending on the country. Private banks will extend credit to countries holding strategic assets such as gold or oil. Consequently, the debts of Venezuela and South Africa are weighted toward private lenders. However, many poor countries can obtain loans only from the IMF and the World Bank, so these institutions hold the bulk of loans from the poorest countries.

As the debt grew, the debt repayments also rose. Over the last 20 years, debt service payments from developing countries have steadily increased in relation to the foreign aid given back to these countries (Figure 5.10). For example, in 2008, developing countries transferred over US$510 billion to banking institutions in the richest countries. It is worth remembering that in that same year, those rich countries very generously gave US$118 billion back in overseas aid. Despite all the generosity of rich countries, we should note that the developing world gives five times more money to us than we give to them! It should be stressed that this is an average value for all developing countries—the picture is not so bad for the very

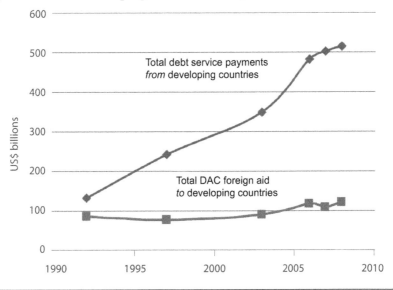

Figure 5.10: Total debt service payments from developing countries compared to official foreign aid given to developing countries

Source: UNCTAD. 2010. Responding to the challenges posed by the global economic crisis. Retrieved from: www.unctad.org/en/docs/gdsddf20091_en.pdf.

poorest countries, where debt forgiveness has had some beneficial effects. In 2008, sub-Saharan countries paid US$15.4 billion in debt service payments and received just under US$40 billion in total aid. Even before the recent global financial crisis, it had become increasingly difficult for the poorest countries to pay just the minimum interest on their loans. Some had fallen so far behind that they would never have been able to rid themselves of debt. In the most heavily indebted countries, the debt was two or three times greater than the GDP, with repayment costs consuming more than 30 percent of the government's budget.

A complex picture finally boils down to this: In order for poor countries to pay the interest on what were frequently unjust loans, they have had to divert funds away from the poorest segments of their societies. The result is a direct link between debt, increasing poverty, and unnecessary illness and death. Estimates vary, but the cumulative result of the debt has undoubtedly adversely affected the lives of millions upon millions of blameless children. Fortunately (at least for the very poorest countries), debt relief mechanisms have produced clear improvements, but for the heavily indebted middle-income countries that hold the majority of the debt, their large and ever-increasing debt-servicing requirements are a constant drag on their economic development.

Developing World Debt Relief

It is important that the fundamental unfairness, even illegality, of the developing world debt is widely understood. Much of this debt should certainly be forgiven, not out of a sense of charity but simply because the debt had little to do with the people who are currently left holding the bill. The first phase of the debt is probably illegal under the doctrine of non-succession of state debts. Many of the debts formed in the second phase should also be unenforceable under the principle of odious debt. In addition, the subsequent years of economic and social changes forced on developing countries by the IMF and the World Bank have clearly been shown to be harmful. The developing world debt and its contribution to an increasing spiral of poverty and misery is, to a large extent, the fault of the richest nations. Again, there is plenty of precedent to support the concept of low-interest loans and limited-condition debt relief (Addison et al., 2004):

- Following World War II, the United States allowed Britain (a current G8 member) to repay loans at well below market rates in order to help the country recover from the effects of war.
- Britain's debt to the US following World War I was forgiven in the 1930s. Britain simply stopped paying!

- In 1953, European countries jointly agreed to grant Germany (a current G8 country) significant debt relief in order to help that country's struggling postwar economy. The process of international co-operation that resulted in that decision would serve as a useful model for a new approach to developing world debt.
- In 2000, major credit banks wiped out more than half of Russia's US$31.8 billion debt. They also awarded a seven-year grace period free from repayment. This process did not include the lengthy six-year Highly Indebted Poor Countries (HIPC) qualification process that is forced upon the poorest countries, even though Russia had defaulted on previous payments. Russia is a member of the G8 group that helps to dictate the HIPC Initiative conditions.

The move to forgive some part of the enormous developing world debt (rather than simply rescheduling it on better terms) has been a relatively recent development. It is a long story, but it can be briefly covered here. Not much more than 10 years ago, a feeling developed at many levels of society that developing world debt was a pressing problem that needed urgent attention. At a popular level, several large debt activist organizations were formed, the best known of which was probably the United Kingdom Jubilee Debt Campaign (Jubilee Debt Campaign, 2011). In response to worldwide campaigns, plus support from several high-profile public figures, politicians in developed countries soon got the message that their constituents expected action on this subject. It is important to understand that debt relief mechanisms depend on the type of debt. As touched on in the previous section, there are, broadly speaking, three groups of debt, and each has different relief mechanisms.

Multilateral debt: This is debt owed to large multilateral banks such as the IMF, the World Bank, the Inter-American Development Bank, and the African Development Bank. These institutions hold much of the debt of the poorest countries because they represent their only source of credit. They are also preferred creditors, so their repayments take precedence over all other creditors. Following the enhanced HIPC Initiative in 1999 and the Multilateral Debt Relief Initiative (MDRI) in 2005, significant progress has been made. So far 26 countries have met their obligations and have received substantial debt cancellation. Debt service ratios for the poorest African countries are now far better than those of any of the Western donor countries. Some European countries, such as Spain, Italy, Portugal, and Greece, are currently so indebted that they qualify for an IMF bailout. In 2007, the Inter-American Development Bank followed suit and cancelled debts held by five heavily indebted South American countries.

The HIPC process applies to countries meeting strict indebtedness conditions. Negotiations for indebted but slightly richer countries usually take place through the Paris Club.

Bilateral debt: These are debts resulting from bilateral country-to-country loans. They are frequently given to support trade deals through export credit agencies. The need for one agency to scrutinize and maintain the standards of export deals has been taken over by the European Network on Debt and Development (Eurodad, 2011). To support this work, Eurodad has developed a Charter on Responsible Financing, which European countries are expected to respect when developing bilateral export credit deals. Eurodad has also pressured governments not to inflate their development assistance claims by including cancelled commercial debts.

Private debt: These are debts held by private banks and bondholders. This form of debt is particularly common in middle-income countries that still have access to private credit sources. Some creditors have been aggressive in their pursuit of repayment. In some cases the debts have been sold at a discount to funds prepared to take the trouble to demand repayment at full value from the debtor. These have been called vulture funds. European countries have now agreed not to sell their debts to such funds in an attempt to stop the practice. A more benign resolution is often found through the London Club, which represents the interests of major commercial lenders.

SUMMARY

In practice, poverty is a complex issue with different presentations, different measurement techniques, and, of course, different solutions according to the underlying contributory causes. The health effects of poverty begin to operate from the moment of conception and continue throughout the child's life. No matter what statistical games can be played with the data, poverty is not the fault of the poor. Leaving aside the effects of acute disasters, most poverty cycles continue because of the effects of unfairness on a large scale perpetuated by poor governance. Poor people may well be unable to prevent injustice, but they certainly don't cause it. Also, there is a tight and complex relationship between poverty and education, much of it probably mediated by poverty's effects on nutrition. Poorly nourished children miss far more school time due to illness.

The Western concept of poverty (having little or no money) is not sufficient to deal with the broader reality of poverty in developing countries. Lack of money is obviously part of the picture, but as the World Bank's revolutionary study titled "Conversations with the Poor" revealed, poverty is also closely tied to social and cultural isolation, lack of education, marginalization, and the absence of power. There is no single measure or definition of poverty that reliably tracks the magnitude and extent of poverty under all circumstances around the world. The best approach is to use different scores and measures in order to get a general idea of the progress of poverty reduction, such as income analysis, consumption analysis, multidimensional analysis, sense of well-being, and so on. The first of the SDGs is on poverty: "End poverty in all its forms everywhere." Eradicating poverty in all its forms remains one of the greatest challenges of our times. One in five people in developing regions still live on less than US$1.25 a day. Malnutrition, discrimination, lack of clean drinking water and basic sanitation, limited access to education, and social discrimination are a few of the many manifestations of poverty.

A significant contributing factor to poverty is the enormous debt burden carried by developing countries. Developing world debt stems from the fact that developing countries of the world have been consistently held back by the need to service an ever-increasing financial debt owned by the richest countries in the world. Broadly, there are three classes of debt: multilateral debt, bilateral debt, and private debt. The Third World debt developed in three distinct stages. The first was the arbitrary imposition of debt onto newly independent countries by their previous colonial masters. The second was a decade of indiscriminate lending of vast amounts of money to poorly prepared dictatorships; money that was subsequently wasted and pillaged by corrupt governments, with little or no benefits for their people. The third was a period of financial collapse secondary to rising interest rates and falling commodity prices. If recent developments become sustainable, then we will hopefully enter a fourth stage: debt forgiveness. It is important that the fundamental unfairness of the developing world debt is widely understood so that it may be forgiven, not out of a sense of charity but simply because the debt had little to do with the people who are currently left holding the bill.

DISCUSSION QUESTIONS

1. What is poverty? How do you measure poverty?
2. In what ways can poverty be inherited? Is poverty the fault of the poor?
3. How is poverty related to geography?
4. How does low income affect health? What are the health risks associated with households in poverty?
5. What are the most cost-effective interventions to prevent poverty? How are these interventions reflected in the SDGs?
6. Why is it so difficult to measure poverty? How do the SDG targets reflect the various measurements of poverty?

7. How much progress has actually been made toward poverty eradication in the last 15 years?

8. What is multilateral debt? What are the arguments for cancelling developing world debt?

9. How does developing world debt undermine development? What can be done about it?

10. How can indiscriminate lending be stopped/checked by lenders?

RECOMMENDED READING

Bhalla, S. 2002. *Imagine there's no country: Poverty inequality and growth in the era of globalization.* Pub: Institute for International Economics.

Blustein, P. 2003. *The chastening: Inside the crisis that rocked the global financial system and humbled the IMF.* Pub: Public Affairs.

Easterly, W. 2002. *The elusive quest for growth: Economists' adventures and misadventures in the tropics.* Pub: MIT Press.

Feuerstein, M. 1997. *Poverty and health: Reaping a richer harvest.* Pub: Macmillan.

Perkins, J. 2004. *Confessions of an economic hit man.* Pub: Berrett-Koehler Inc.

Sachs, J. 2005. *The end of poverty: Economic possibilities for our time.* Pub: Penguin Press.

Sen, A. 1981. *Poverty and famines: An essay on entitlement and deprivation.* Pub: Clarendon Press.

Stiglitz, J. 2002. *Globalization and its discontents.* Pub: W. W. Norton.

World Bank & IMF. 2016. Development goals in an era of demographic change. Global monitoring report, 2015/2016. Retrieved from: http://pubdocs.worldbank.org/en/503001444058224597/Global-Monitoring-Report-2015.pdf.

REFERENCES

ABS. 2011. Australian Bureau of Statistics. Indigenous population, 2006. Retrieved from: www.abs.gov.au/ausstats/abs@.nsf/Lookup/4713.0Chapter82006.

Adams, P. 1991. Odious debts. Probe International. Retrieved from: http://journal.probeinternational.org/odious-debts/read-odious-debts-the-book/.

Addison, T., et al. 2004. *Debt relief for poor countries.* Pub: Palgrave MacMillan.

Alkire, S., et al. 2010. Acute multidimensional poverty: A new index for developing countries. Oxford Poverty and Human Development Initiative. Retrieved from: www.ophi.org.uk/wp-content/uploads/ophi-wp38.pdf.

Bhalla, S. 2000. Trends in world poverty—ideology and research. Retrieved from: http://www.oxusinvestments.com/files/pdf/em280600.pdf.

Bramley, D., et al. 2004. Indigenous disparities in disease-specific mortality, a cross-country comparison: New Zealand, Australia, Canada, and the United States. *New Zealand Medical Journal*, 117: 1215–1223.

Braun, K., et al. 1996. Life and death in Hawaii: Ethnic variations in life expectancy and mortality, 1980 and 1990. *Hawaii Medical Journal*, 55: 278–283.

Chen, S., et al. 2004. How have the world's poorest fared since the early 1980s? *The World Bank Research Observer*, 19: 141–169. Retrieved from: http://unstats.un.org/unsd/mdg/
Resources/Attach/Capacity/Chen%20&%20Ravallion%20(WBRO%202004).pdf.

Chen, S., et al. 2008. The developing world is poorer than we thought, but no less successful
in the fight against poverty. World Bank Development Research Group working paper no.
4703. Retrieved from: http://ideas.repec.org/p/wbk/wbrwps/4703.html.

CNN. 2011. Philippine nuclear plant to become tourist attraction. Retrieved from: http://news.
blogs.cnn.com/2011/05/11/philippine-nuclear-plant-to-become-tourist-attraction/.

Cow Politics. 2005. *New York Times* editorial. Retrieved from: www.nytimes.com/2005/10/27/
opinion/27thur1.html.

CPI. 2015. Transparency International's Corruption Perception Index. Retrieved from: http://
www.transparency.org/cpi2015.

Deaton, A. 2003. Measuring poverty in a growing world (or measuring growth in a poor world).
National Bureau of Economic Research working paper no. 9822. Retrieved from: www.
econ.yale.edu/seminars/develop/tdw03/deaton-030929.pdf.

EH Net. 2010. The English Poor Laws. Retrieved from: http://eh.net/encyclopedia/article/boy-
er.poor.laws.england.

Elo, I. 2009. Social class differentials in health and mortality. *Annual Review of Sociology*, 35:
553–572.

Eurodad. 2011. The European network on debt and development. Retrieved from: www.
eurodad.org/.

Friedman, M. 1997. John Maynard Keynes. Retrieved from: www.wissensnavigator.com/
documents/keynesfriedman.pdf.

Feuerstein, M. 1997. *Poverty and health: Reaping a richer harvest*. Pub: MacMillan.

Geremek, B. 1997. *Poverty: A history*. Pub: Basil Blackwell.

Hausler, S., et al. 2005. Causes of death in the Sami population of Sweden, 1961–2000.
International Journal of Epidemiology, 34: 623–629.

HDI. 2010. Human Development Index. Retrieved from: http://hdr.undp.org/en/statistics/hdi/.

HDI. 2016. Human Development Index. Retrieved from: http://hdr.undp.org/en/content/
human-development-index-hdi.

Health Canada. 2005. First Nations comparable health indicators. Retrieved from: www.
hc-sc.gc.ca/fniah-spnia/diseases-maladies/2005-01_health-sante_indicat-eng.
php#life_expect.

Hess, P. 1989. Force ratios, arms imports, and foreign aid receipts in the developing nations. *Journal of Peace Research*, 26: 399–412.

IBRD. 2005. The International Bank for Reconstruction and Development. Global development finance: Mobilizing finance and managing vulnerability. Retrieved from: http://siteresources.worldbank.org/GDFINT/Resources/334952-1257197866375/gdf05complete.pdf.

ICP. 2011. International Comparison Program. Retrieved from: http://siteresources.worldbank.org/ICPEXT/Resources/ICP_2011.html.

IFPRI. 2010. International Food Policy Research Institute. Global Hunger Index report. Retrieved from: www.ifpri.org/sites/default/files/publications/ghi10.pdf.

ILO. 2016. International Labour Organization. World employment and social outlook 2016: Transforming jobs to end poverty. Retrieved from: http://www.ilo.org/global/research/global-reports/weso/2016-transforming-jobs/lang--en/index.htm.

IMF. 2008. Heavily Indebted Poor Countries (HIPC) Initiative and Multilateral Debt Relief Initiative (MDRI)—status of implementation. Retrieved from: www.imf.org/external/np/pp/eng/2008/091208.pdf.

Jubilee Debt Campaign. 2011. Retrieved from: www.jubileedebtcampaign.org.uk.

Live 8. 2006. Retrieved from: www.live8live.com.

Michael, E., et al. 2003. Mixed signals from Kerala's improving health status. *Journal of the Royal Society of Health*, 123: 33–38.

Millet, D., et al. 2005. *Who owes who? Fifty questions about the world debt.* Pub: Zed Books.

Narayan, D., et al. 1999. Consultations with the poor: Global synthesis. World Bank Poverty Group. Retrieved from: http://siteresources.worldbank.org/INTPOVERTY/Resources/335642-1124115102975/1555199-1124138742310/synthes.pdf.

OPHI. 2010. Oxford Poverty and Human Development Initiative. Retrieved from: www.ophi.org.uk/policy/multidimensional-poverty-index/.

Panizza, U. 2008. Domestic and external public debt in developing countries. UNCTAD discussion paper no. 1882. Retrieved from: www.unctad.org/en/docs/osgdp20083_en.pdf.

Patterson, R. 1997. *Foreign aid after the Cold War: The dynamics of multipolar economic competition.* Pub: Africa World Press.

Perkins, J. 2004. *Confessions of an economic hit man.* Pub: Berrett-Koehler.

Pinkovskiy, M., et al. 2009. Parametric estimates of the world distribution of income. NBER working paper no. 15433. Retrieved from: www.voxeu.org/index.php?q=node/4508.

Ravallion, M. 2003. The debate on globalization, poverty, and inequality: Why measurement matters. *International Affairs*, 79: 739–754. Retrieved from: www-wds.worldbank.org/servlet/WDSContentServer/WDSP/IB/2003/05/30/000094946_03051604080285/Rendered/PDF/multi0page.pdf.

Ravallion, M., et al. 1991. Quantifying absolute poverty in the developing world. *Review of Income and Wealth*, 37: 345–361. Retrieved from: www.roiw.org/1991/345.pdf.

Reddy, S., et al. 2005. How not to count the poor. Retrieved from: www.columbia.edu/~sr793/count.pdf.

Reisen, H., et al. 2008. Prudent versus imprudent lending to Africa: From debt relief to emerging lenders. OECD Development Centre working paper no. 268. Retrieved from: www.oecd.org/dataoecd/62/12/40152567.pdf.

Rowntree, B. 1910. *Poverty: A study of town life.* Pub: MacMillan.

Sachs, J. 2005. *The end of poverty: Economic possibilities for our time.* Pub: Penguin Press.

Saith, A. 2005. Poverty lines versus the poor: Method versus meaning. *Economic and Political Weekly*, 40(43): 4601–4610. Retrieved from: http://repub.eur.nl/res/pub/19178/wp420.pdf.

Sen, A. 1981. *Poverty and famines: An essay on entitlement and deprivation.* Pub: Clarendon Press.

Sen, A. 1999. *Development as freedom.* Pub: Basil Blackwell.

Sillers, D. 2002. National and international poverty lines: An overview. Retrieved from: www.povertyfrontiers.org/ev_en.php?ID=1075_201&ID2=DO_TOPIC.

South Bulletin. 2004. Third world debt: A continuing legacy of colonization. *South Bulletin*, 85: 2–5.

Stambuli, P. 1998. Causes and consequences of the 1982 world debt crisis. University of Surrey. Retrieved from: http://129.3.20.41/eps/if/papers/0211/0211005.pdf.

StatCan. 2011. Statistics Canada, Aboriginal Peoples. Retrieved from: www12.statcan.ca/census-recensement/2006/rt-td/ap-pa-eng.cfm.

UN Millennium Development Goals. Retrieved from: www.un.org/millenniumgoals.

UN Resolution 1538. 2004. Independent inquiry into the Oil for Food Programme. Retrieved from: www.iic-offp.org.

UNCTAD. 2010. Responding to the challenges posed by the global economic crisis. Retrieved from: www.unctad.org/en/docs/gdsddf20091_en.pdf.

UNDP. 2015. Human development report. Retrieved from: http://hdr.undp.org/en/reports/global/hdr2015/.

UNICEF. 2010. Childinfo. Retrieved from: www.childinfo.org/index.html.

Wagstaff, A. 2000. Socioeconomic inequalities in child mortality: Comparisons across nine developing countries. *Bulletin of the WHO*, 78: 19–29.

Wall Street Journal. 2011. US prime rate history. Retrieved from: www.wsjprimerate.us/wall_street_journal_prime_rate_history.htm.

WGI. 2015. Worldwide governance indicators (government effectiveness). Retrieved from: http://info.worldbank.org/governance/wgi/index.aspx#home.

World Bank. 2006. Directions in development: Repositioning nutrition as central to development. Retrieved from: http://siteresources.worldbank.org/NUTRITION/Resources/281846-1131636806329/NutritionStrategy.pdf.

World Bank. 2010. Measuring inequality. Retrieved from: http://go.worldbank.org/3SLYUTVY00.

World Bank. 2011. Global economic prospects: Maintaining progress amid turmoil. Retrieved from: http://go.worldbank.org/PF6VWYXS10.

World Bank. 2016. Health expenditure per capita. Retrieved from: http://data.worldbank.org/indicator/SH.XPD.PCAP?locations=CU-US.

World Bank & IMF. 2016. Development goals in an era of demographic change. Global monitoring report, 2015/2016. Retrieved from: http://pubdocs.worldbank.org/en/503001444058224597/Global-Monitoring-Report-2015.pdf.

WTRG Economics. 2009. Oil price history and analysis. Retrieved from: www.wtrg.com/prices.htm.

CHAPTER 6

Malnutrition

Hunger is not an issue of charity. It is an issue of justice.

—*Jacques Diouf, director general, Food and Agriculture Organization, 1997*

OBJECTIVES

Malnutrition is not simply due to lack of food any more than poverty is simply due to lack of money. Both are the end result of numerous interlocking economic and social factors, such as poverty, lack of education, social inequity, and chronic recurrent infections. The effects of malnutrition are so widespread that estimating the mortality and morbidity directly attributable to malnutrition is very difficult—but both are horrifyingly high. A detailed examination of malnutrition is essential for any understanding of population health. After completing this chapter, you should be able to:

- understand the underlying causes, adverse effects, and prevalence of malnutrition in developing countries
- understand the different types of malnutrition (ranging from micronutrient to macronutrient deficiencies)
- understand the main methods used to measure and define malnutrition in population studies
- understand the common causes of inadequate food supply, and the complexities and problems associated with food aid to developing countries

INTRODUCTION

> You cannot achieve environmental security and human development without addressing the basic issues of health and nutrition.
>
> —*Gro Harlem Brundtland*

Malnutrition (and the more insidious effects of micronutrient deficiencies) stunts the development of affected children, and also reduces their ability to survive serious infections such as measles and gastroenteritis. Along with poverty, malnutrition traps populations in a never-ending cycle of ill health and poor productivity. As large famines have become less common, chronic moderate malnutrition has become much more important than acute severe starvation. Nowadays, one of the main consequences of malnutrition is the increased mortality from common childhood illnesses. Case mortality rates in measles, whooping cough, and bronchiolitis are many times higher among malnourished children.

The broad topic of nutrition is an essential subject for anyone studying global health. Along with poverty and human rights, malnutrition lies at the root of the health problems affecting developing world populations. Despite the importance of malnutrition, a sophisticated understanding of severe malnutrition has been slow to develop. Prior to Amartya Sen's study of famine 30 years ago, it was generally thought that Malthus's early 19th-century theory was correct—that malnutrition was an unavoidable feature of life in developing countries because there would always be far more people than food was available. The

Box 6.1 History Notes

Dr. Cicely Williams (1893–1992)

Dr. Cicely Williams was born in Jamaica. Despite the attitudes of her day, she was allowed to study medicine at Oxford because the war had left classes half empty. After graduating, she worked in the British Colonial Service, initially in Ghana. Her first major discovery was that sick children survived better if they were not separated from their mothers. Her early studies of malnutrition in West Africa led her to identify and name *kwashiorkor*. When working in Malaysia, she was the first to criticize the infant food companies for their advertising practices. Her paper, "Milk and Murder," was influential and ultimately helped the slow process of re-establishing breastfeeding. She is widely considered to be the founder of the study of maternal and child health (MCH). During World War II, she narrowly survived imprisonment in a Japanese camp. After the war, she became the first head of MCH in the newly formed WHO. After retiring, she continued to lecture past her 90th birthday. For more information, please follow the reference: Craddock (1984).

research stimulated by Sen's work subsequently showed that malnutrition is far more complex than that and is usually the result of numerous interrelated contributory factors.

The most important point to understand about malnutrition is that shortage of food is only one of many reasons behind its onset. A perfect example is the Ethiopian famine between 1983 and 1985, popularized by the Live Aid series of concerts. Drought and famine certainly caused enormous loss of life in the Sahel region, but there was always plenty of food in the country. The trouble was that none of it was sent to the famine-affected areas. Visiting journalists in Addis Ababa were not short of food, a point raised by a surprisingly small number of them (De Waal, 1997). The Soviet-backed government of the day was fighting US-backed rebels. They restricted food supplies to rebel-held regions and also resettled large numbers of the population to unproductive parts of the country. Starvation was inevitable, but it could easily have been avoided by a normally competent government. Whatever the scale, malnutrition is the end result of numerous social problems ranging from civil war to lack of maternal education. Even if local food shortages might originally have stemmed from drought and crop failure, the development of widespread starvation is ultimately a failure of food distribution from the rest of the country. The persistent starvation in Darfur, Sudan, was mainly due to lack of political will, even though the original shortage of food was agricultural in nature.

Not surprisingly, the adverse effects of malnutrition are as complicated as its causes. With time, the epidemiology of malnutrition has changed. Although it is still possible to die from lack of food in some parts of the world, severe starvation is becoming increasingly uncommon. Nowadays, mild and moderate degrees of malnutrition are the principal problem. Apart from reducing the growth and development potential of entire generations of children, lesser degrees of malnutrition

Box 6.2 Moment of Insight

Percentage of preschool children overweight or obese, average 1998 value for all Latin American and Caribbean countries:	Percentage of preschool children underweight, average 1998 value for all Latin American and Caribbean countries:
6.8% (and rising)	**6.8%** (and falling)
Source: de Onis, M., et al. 2010. Global prevalence and trends of overweight and obesity among preschool children. *American Journal of Clinical Nutrition*, 92: 1257–1264.	*Source:* de Onis, M., et al. 2004. Methodology for estimating regional and global trends of child malnutrition. *International Journal of Epidemiology*, 33: 1–11.

also reduce a child's immune function, which greatly increases mortality from common diseases such as measles, pneumonia, and gastroenteritis. The more insidious effects of micronutrient deficiencies can also have severe clinical effects, even in children who might otherwise appear well nourished. Examples include scurvy, hypothyroidism, and anemia.

Over the last 10–15 years, measurable improvements have been made in worldwide levels of childhood malnutrition. However, these average figures are heavily influenced by improvements in India and China. There are still areas of the world where progress has been very slow. Unfortunately, in the last few years, the effects of increased food prices, the global recession, and an increasing number of wars have combined to halt or even reverse the gains made before 2005. Many well-established interventions are available that have direct or indirect nutritional benefits. These include supplementary feeding programs, micronutrient fortification, maternal education, agricultural extension projects, and many others. Whatever approach is used, the project must be based on careful research so it can be tailored to meet the specific needs of the local population.

CAUSES AND EXTENT OF MALNUTRITION

> If a choice must be made, free school meals are more important for the health of poor children than immunization programmes, and both are more effective than hospital beds.
>
> —*T. McKeown, 1980*

Basic Nutrition

Humans are basically mobile chemical factories. Using simple ingredients available at any supermarket, our cellular mechanisms are able to construct and maintain an organism of staggering complexity. The fuel that keeps this process running is, of course, food. Since every cell in the body requires nutritional support, it is not surprising that a shortage of food can produce disease in every organ of the body. The adverse effects of malnutrition are particularly important during rapid growth periods such as childhood and pregnancy. Early malnutrition during the period of major organ development can have lifelong adverse effects.

After initial processing within the gut, food is absorbed into the bloodstream and lymphatic vessels before entering a huge variety of chemical pathways. Every organ has metabolic capacity, but the most important one is the liver. Larger molecules are slowly broken down in an oxidative process catalyzed by enzymes, which are often dependent on cofactors and minerals present in minute quantities in the diet. We capture the energy released during this chemical breakdown and use it to power our cellular processes. Small molecules are either stored for future use or used for immediate repair and growth. Apart from solid waste residues, the end results of all our efforts are heat, carbon dioxide, and water.

Along with water and oxygen, our principal nutritional components are protein, carbohydrate, and fat (USDA, 2011). These are the large items, or macronutrients, on which the system principally depends. Under normal circumstances, our energy is largely derived from carbohydrates and, to a lesser extent, from fats. The body usually uses protein for building purposes, but it can turn protein into energy if required. A diet deficient in all three macronutrients is often referred to as protein-energy malnutrition. The body can compensate for some dietary deficiencies by manufacturing chemicals that it needs. However, some types of fats and amino acids cannot be produced by our bodies, so they can only be obtained from our food. These essential fats and amino acids are constituents of a healthy diet.

In addition to the major nutritional components, a complete diet must also contain dozens of micronutrients (MNI, 2009). Most cannot be made in the body, so they must be present in the diet. Micronutrients include essential vitamins such as thiamin, vitamin C, and folic acid, plus minerals such as iron, calcium, and iodine. Deficiency of any one of these essential factors can result in serious disease even

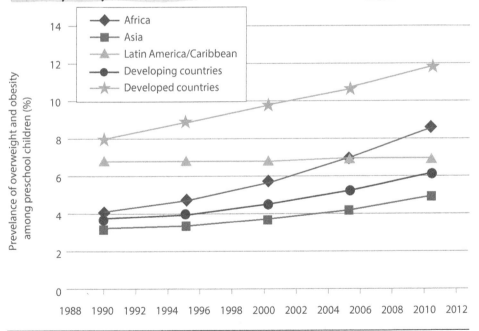

Figure 6.1: Prevalence of overweight and obesity among preschool children in different regions of the world

Source: de Onis, M., et al. 2010. Global prevalence and trends of overweight and obesity among preschool children. *American Journal of Clinical Nutrition, 92:* 1257–1264.

though the remainder of the diet is adequate. Examples include scurvy (vitamin C), anemia (iron), and hypothyroidism (iodine). Collectively, these are referred to as micronutrient deficiencies.

It is important to remember that "malnutrition" means "bad" nutrition—it is not just another word for starvation. The term refers to a wide range of diseases resulting from abnormalities in dietary intake. Children suffering from significant micronutrient diseases are not necessarily hungry and may appear relatively well fed from a macronutrient perspective. At the other end of the spectrum are the problems resulting from too much food intake. Obesity is the fastest-growing nutritional problem in the world (Figure 6.1). The rising number of obese people most likely exceeded the steadily falling numbers of starving people in the late 1990s (Popkin, 2007). The phenomenon of childhood obesity even applies to developing countries. As the "Moment of Insight" box shows, there are now more obese children in Latin America and the Caribbean than there are starving ones.

Causes of Malnutrition

> When I gave food to the poor, they called me a Saint. When I asked why the poor were hungry, they called me a communist.
>
> —*Dom Helder Camara*

The newcomer to malnutrition might have the initial impression that malnutrition is simply a case of not having enough food. Although this is certainly part of the problem, it is nowhere near the full story. It is important not to oversimplify the problem of malnutrition, because the underlying causes have to be understood fully before any practical sustainable treatment program can be implemented. Provision of food is indeed necessary for a starving population, but enabling that population to feed itself in a sustainable manner requires a complex program with multiple interventions based on a clear understanding of the local factors behind the malnutrition. A good example of the complex nature of malnutrition is demonstrated by plotting a composite measure of malnutrition (IFPRI, 2010) against income (Figure 6.2). Although there is a broad average relationship, levels of nutrition still differ widely between countries of similar income. Explanations include variations in agricultural performance, pro-poor government policies, civil unrest, and attitudes toward women. Ghana has only a quarter the income of Angola, but less than half the malnutrition.

Obtaining adequate nutrition for adults is hard enough in a developing country, but the problem is considerably more complicated where children are concerned. Their total dependence upon caregivers means that an endless list of problems at

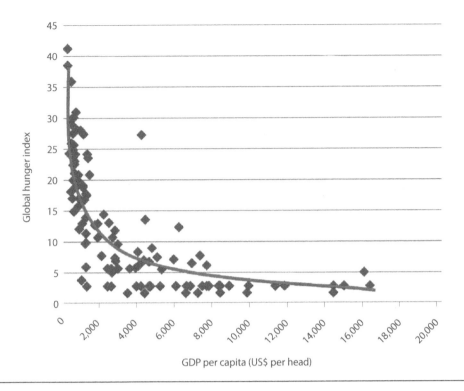

Figure 6.2: Plot of the composite Global Hunger Index against GDP per capita

Source: IFPRI. 2010. International Food Policy Research Institute. Global Hunger Index. Retrieved from: www.ifpri.org/publication/2010-global-hunger-index.

the level of family and society can, individually and collectively, reduce the chances that a spoonful of food will ultimately be put in that child's mouth (Smith et al., 2000). There are three broad groups of requirements that must be met before a population's children can have reliable nutrition (UNICEF, 1998):

- The first, of course, is that there must be adequate access to a reliable source of nutritious food (this is commonly referred to as household food security).
- There must be adequate care provided for children and women.
- There must be a safe and healthy society with adequate access to preventive care advice and basic health services.

Under each of these headings, there are numerous subheadings (Table 6.1). The possible range of complex interrelationships is almost endless. Each community will have its own set of contributory factors that underlines the absolute necessity for basing long-term intervention programs upon careful local research.

The following is only a short list of the possible variables that can ultimately affect the child's nutrition.

The child: Chronic intestinal parasites and infections (such as whooping cough, gastroenteritis, and measles) can all contribute to a worsening spiral of malnutrition and an increased susceptibility to further infection (Keusch, 2003). Recurrent attacks of gastroenteritis are a particularly common precipitating cause of malnutrition in a child with marginal nutrition. Unfortunately, HIV infection and tuberculosis are both becoming increasingly common secondary factors.

The mother: The combination of maternal poverty and lack of education leads to inadequate child-rearing practices. Two small meals a day given by an exhausted mother, with child care subsequently left in the hands of young siblings, is not a scenario that allows normal growth to occur. Lack of basic knowledge about breastfeeding, contraception, and nutritional requirements of children all contribute to the problem (Mishra et al., 2000).

The family: Traditional customs based on a stable extended family are not sufficient to meet the demands of life in an informal peri-urban settlement. Economic necessity that forces both parents to work, or the loss of a father due to migrant labour, HIV, or war, places severe strains on disrupted family structures and inevitably results in poor care for the children.

The society: Education for women, laws protecting children, and widespread provision of contraceptive and nutrition education often have low priorities in countries where money for social programs is limited. Traditional presence of gender

Table 6.1: Major factors determining the development of malnutrition in a child

Child:	• Recurrent illness (measles, gastroenteritis, whooping cough, TB, HIV)
	• Chronic intestinal parasites
Mother/family/ household:	• Poverty
	• Lack of hygiene (food and water handling and storage)
	• Poor child care (lack of stimulation, baby left in care of children)
	• Inadequate support for mother (overwork, poor access to medical care, education, family planning, and child care advice)
	• Family disruption (migrant labour, war, HIV, both parents working)
	• Inadequate housing (access to clean water, sanitation, waste disposal)
	• Inadequate food (lack of breastfeeding, poorly prepared infant formula feeds, poor-quality and irregular supply of food)
Society:	• Discrimination against women and girls (maldistribution of food within the household, unequal access to education and employment)
	• Lack of social support for the poor
	• Violence, social chaos, war

inequity can also have profound effects on nutrition ranging from the maldistribution of food within the family all the way to limited access to employment and education (Rousham, 1996).

As a further example of the complex contributing factors behind malnutrition, even the type of food in a child's diet may be a factor. The use of high-volume, low-caloric-density starch porridges can mean that the child may feel full even though he or she has still not obtained sufficient nutrition. The widespread dependence on a largely vegetarian diet can also be associated with nutritional problems. For example, high phytate levels in some cereal diets can inhibit absorption of calcium to the extent that it contributes to the development of rickets.

Prevalence of Malnutrition

During the last three decades, the epidemiology of malnutrition has changed considerably. Famines and deaths due solely to starvation have become increasingly rare events. Unfortunately, the world recently faced a new famine in Sudan that threatened millions of people, but this was the first large famine in 25 years. It is important to understand that the clinical presentation of malnutrition has changed greatly over this time period. Nowadays, acute severe starvation has largely been replaced by the more insidious effects of chronic malnutrition. While death due to absolute starvation is now less common, affected children suffer from lifelong physical and developmental impairments that trap them in an endless cycle of poverty, ill health, and poor expectations. Apart from its long-term adverse effects on the growth and development of affected children, malnutrition greatly increases the mortality of common diseases by reducing the child's immune response (Pelletier, 1995). Whether malnutrition acts as a chronic disease with a high morbidity and lower mortality or kills rapidly with a high mortality due to acute starvation (more rarely nowadays) does not change its importance. A detailed knowledge of all aspects of nutrition is vital for any serious study of global health.

The fundamental importance of nutritional health is reflected in its inclusion as one of the Millennium Development Goals. The aim was to halve the proportion of people suffering from undernutrition between 1990 and 2015. The proportion of undernourished people in the developing regions has fallen by almost half since 1990, though more than 90 million children under age five are still undernourished and underweight.

Measured end points vary from composite indicators such as the Global Hunger Index (IFPRI, 2010) to anthropometric surveys of height and weight (de Onis et al., 2004, 2010). The Food and Agriculture Organization is the monitoring agency for the nutrition goal. They chose to assess malnutrition by measuring daily caloric

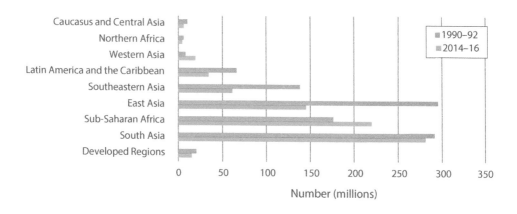

Figure 6.3: Numbers of undernourished people by region, 1990–1992 and 2014–2016

Source: FAO. 2015. The state of food insecurity in the world. Retrieved from: www.fao.org/hunger/en/.

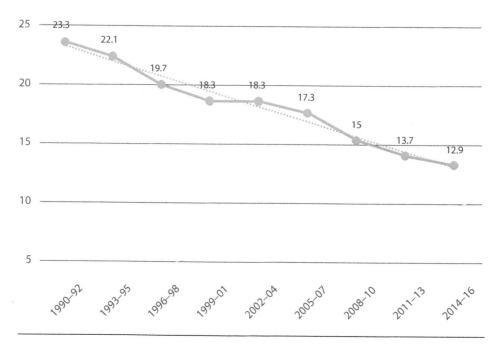

Figure 6.4: Proportion of undernourished people in the developing regions, 1990–2016

Source: United Nations. 2015. The Millennium Development Goals report. Retrieved from: www. un.org/millenniumgoals/reports.shtml.

intake derived from household surveys, the most common of which is the widely used household income/expenditure survey process. The fraction of the population with caloric intake below normal values is considered undernourished (FAO, 2003). The method is open to criticism—it does not assess food eaten outside the home and the results are often based on money spent on food rather than the exact type of food.

Today, 795 million people are undernourished globally, which is about one in nine individuals. The vast majority of them live in developing regions. However, the proportion of undernourished people in the developing regions has fallen by almost half since 1990, from 23.3 percent in 1990–1992 to 12.9 percent in 2014–2016 (Figure 6.4), which is close to the MDG hunger target of 11.6%. This reduction varies across regions. Two regions, South Asia and sub-Saharan Africa (Figure 6.3), now account for substantially larger shares of global undernourishment. The number of undernourished people in these regions has increased by 44 million since 1990, reflecting the regions' high population growth rate.

Global average levels of childhood stunting (low height for age, Figure 6.5) and childhood underweight (low weight for age, Figure 6.6) greatly vary by region, and progress has been slow. Sub-Saharan Africa and South Asia continually have a high prevalence of childhood stunting and childhood underweight. In 2014, 1 in 7 children were estimated to be underweight in less-developed regions. High prevalence combined with a large population means that most underweight children live in South Asia. It should be remembered that average levels are skewed by large improvements in China and India. While some African countries, such as Ethiopia, Ghana, and Mozambique, did well during this period, many others actually worsened. Setbacks in a small area can go unnoticed if there are large improvements in another region.

Undernutrition is not distributed evenly around the world (Figure 6.7). The greatest numbers of people affected by malnutrition are in Asia because of the population effects of India, China, and Bangladesh. However, the countries with the highest percentage of undernutrition are in Africa, particularly in sub-Saharan Africa. Some of the most affected African countries are Burundi, Chad, the Democratic Republic of Congo, and Eritrea. In Asia, badly affected countries include Bangladesh, Nepal, North Korea, and Cambodia. Once again, it is important to remember to study the local causes of malnutrition before rushing ahead with plans to cure it. What might work in one place may have much less relevance in another. For example, the principal contributory factors in Asia are poor education, gender inequity, and poverty, while the major factors in Africa are conflict, government ineffectiveness, and high rates of HIV/AIDS (IFPRI, 2010). The invariable finding in countries with the highest levels of malnutrition is a protracted humanitarian or natural disaster (sometimes both). Examples include North Korea, Afghanistan, Sudan, and Haiti.

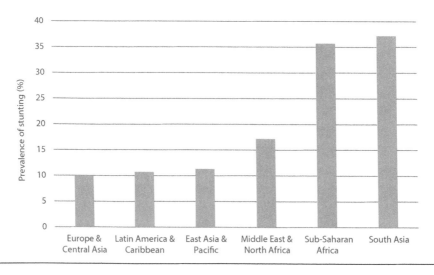

Figure 6.5: Recent trends in prevalence of stunting in preschool children by World Bank Region, 2014

Source: WHO. 2016. Data from Global Health Observatory visualizations: Joint child malnutrition estimates (UNICEF-WHO-WB). Retrieved from: www.who.int/nutgrowthdb/estimates/en/.

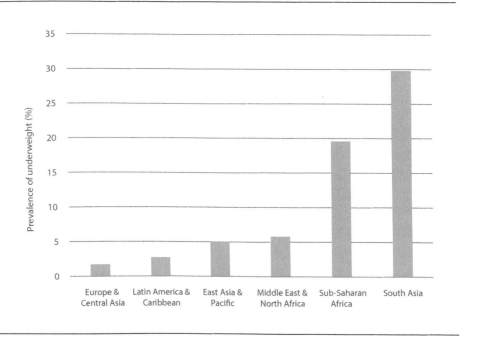

Figure 6.6: Recent trends in prevalence of underweight in preschool children by World Bank Region, 2014

Source: WHO. 2016. Data from Global Health Observatory visualizations: Joint child malnutrition estimates (UNICEF-WHO-WB). Retrieved from: www.who.int/nutgrowthdb/estimates/en/.

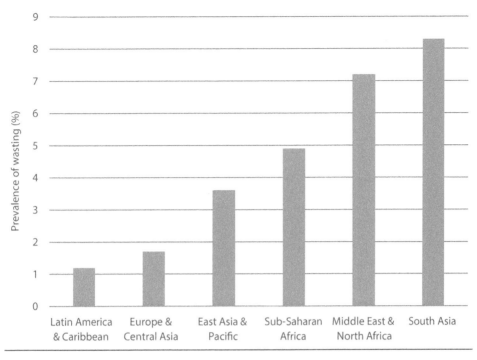

Figure 6.7: Prevalence of wasting in children under 5 years of age by World Bank Region, 2014

Source: WHO. 2016. Data from Global Health Observatory visualizations: Joint child malnutrition estimates (UNICEF-WHO-WB). Retrieved from: www.who.int/nutgrowthdb/estimates/en/.

Unfortunately, after 2005, nutritional standards worsened rapidly because of a combination of rising world food prices (Figure 6.8) and the global financial recession. By 2009, it was estimated that well over a billion people were suffering from undernutrition—a long way from the MDG goal to halve, between 1990 and 2015, the proportion of people who suffer from hunger. Since then, numbers have improved, but it should be remembered that vulnerable families live on the edge of disaster—they cannot just bounce back quickly. They must absorb the shocks of recession by selling their possessions and cutting back on health and education spending until there is finally nothing left to do but reduce their minimal food intake. Such actions weaken the family and leave them with financial and health problems from which they may take years to recover. As usual, the burden falls most heavily on women and small children. Globally, the MDG goal to cut hunger by half was almost reached. While some regions, such as Latin America and the Caribbean, met their nutrition goals by 2015, other regions, such as sub-Saharan Africa, did not meet their MDG target on hunger.

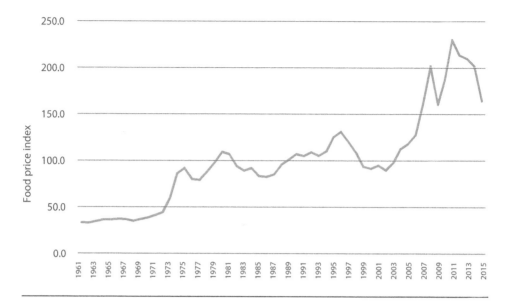

Figure 6.8: Recent trends in the FAO's Food Price Index, which is an average of 55 commodity prices in five groups (meat, dairy, cereal, oils, and sugar)

Source: FAO. 2015. World food price index. Retrieved from: www.fao.org/worldfoodsituation/wfs-home/foodpricesindex/en/.

The first two specific targets of the new SDG goal on hunger (Table 6.2) include:

1. By 2030, end hunger and ensure access by all people, in particular the poor and people in vulnerable situations, including infants, to safe, nutritious and sufficient food all year round, and
2. By 2030, end all forms of malnutrition, including achieving, by 2025, the internationally agreed targets on stunting and wasting in children under 5 years of age, and address the nutritional needs of adolescent girls, pregnant and lactating women and older persons.

No matter what criteria are used to define nutritional levels, it is estimated that about 795 million humans currently suffer from some form of malnutrition (FAO, 2015). Preschool children make up roughly 20–25 percent of that total. At a time when Western countries are facing an epidemic of childhood obesity, many tens of millions of children in developing countries go to bed hungry every night. (It should be added that obesity is an increasing problem in some middle-income developing countries.) The numbers are too large to comprehend adequately. While there have been improvements in rates of stunting and underweight in most areas of the world, huge numbers of children still have their ultimate potential limited by recurring cycles of illness and poor growth. A child who is moderately malnourished is two times more likely to die from infectious diseases than a well-nourished child, and the risk is five times as high for a severely malnourished child (Pelletier, 1994). The great majority of children who die from a combination of malnutrition and infection are either mildly or moderately undernourished (Pelletier et al., 1995) and often show no abnormal clinical signs other than their size. If height and weight are symmetrically reduced, they can look completely normal. In many

Table 6.2: Some targets of SDG 2: End hunger, achieve food security, improve nutrition, and promote sustainable agriculture

TARGETS	
2.1	By 2030, end hunger and ensure access by all people, in particular the poor and people in vulnerable situations, including infants, to safe, nutritious and sufficient food all year round
2.2	By 2030, end all forms of malnutrition, including achieving, by 2025, the internationally agreed targets on stunting and wasting in children under 5 years of age, and address the nutritional needs of adolescent girls, pregnant and lactating women and older persons
2.3	By 2030, double the agricultural productivity and incomes of small-scale food producers, in particular women, indigenous peoples, family farmers, pastoralists and fishers, including through secure and equal access to land, other productive resources and inputs, knowledge, financial services, markets and opportunities for value addition and non-farm employment
2.4	By 2030, ensure sustainable food production systems and implement resilient agricultural practices that increase productivity and production, that help maintain ecosystems, that strengthen capacity for adaptation to climate change, extreme weather, drought, flooding and other disasters and that progressively improve land and soil quality
2.5	By 2020, maintain the genetic diversity of seeds, cultivated plants and farmed and domesticated animals and their related wild species, including through soundly managed and diversified seed and plant banks at the national, regional and international levels, and promote access to and fair and equitable sharing of benefits arising from the utilization of genetic resources and associated traditional knowledge, as internationally agreed
2.a	Increase investment, including through enhanced international cooperation, in rural infrastructure, agricultural research and extension services, technology development and plant and livestock gene banks in order to enhance agricultural productive capacity in developing countries, in particular least developed countries
2.b	Correct and prevent trade restrictions and distortions in world agricultural markets, including through the parallel elimination of all forms of agricultural export subsidies and all export measures with equivalent effect, in accordance with the mandate of the Doha Development Round
2.c	Adopt measures to ensure the proper functioning of food commodity markets and their derivatives and facilitate timely access to market information, including on food reserves, in order to help limit extreme food price volatility

Source: UN. 2015. Transforming our world: The 2030 Agenda for Sustainable Development. Retrieved from https://sustainabledevelopment.un.org/post2015/transformingourworld/publication.

developing countries, a quarter or more of all children have some degree of malnutrition (de Onis et al., 2004). When working in such countries, it is easy to become habituated to the sight of thin children and to forget the social and health costs associated with their poor diets. "All the kids here are skinny—what does it matter?" It matters a lot.

TYPES OF MALNUTRITION

> Many of the things we need can wait. The child cannot. Right now is the time his bones are being formed, his blood is being made and his senses are being developed. To him we cannot answer "Tomorrow."
>
> —*Gabriela Mistral, 1948*

Macronutrient, or Protein-Energy, Malnutrition

When the intake of major nutrients (fat, carbohydrate, and protein) persistently falls 10–20 percent below minimal requirements, increasingly obvious changes occur. The final result depends on many other variables, including associated micronutrient deficiencies, individual variation, and infections, particularly pneumonia and intestinal parasites. Children and pregnant women are especially vulnerable. The case fatality rate of severe malnutrition is very high. Even with good-quality hospital care following the 10-step WHO treatment plan (Ashworth et al., 2003), at least one in four will likely die (Ashworth et al., 2004). Although every organ can be affected, the principal effects are covered under the following headings.

Growth

Without fuel, the body simply stops growing. The most obvious and easily measurable result of malnutrition is poor growth. The final result depends on the severity and extent of the malnutrition and also the age at onset of malnutrition. There are three common measurements used to assess growth: height for age, weight for age, and weight for height. Standardized charts allow a child's measurements to be compared to normal population values (WHO, 2011). The body mass index (BMI) is harder to calculate, so it is used less commonly in surveys.

Children affected by relatively short-term malnutrition will have a weight that falls well below the mean for their age (underweight), but their height for age may be reasonably well preserved. Consequently, the child will also be well below normal on a chart of weight plotted against height (wasting). Chronic malnutrition reduces all aspects of growth. Weight and height for age will both be well below the mean for age (underweight and stunted), but the child's weight for height may be fairly normal if both are reduced symmetrically.

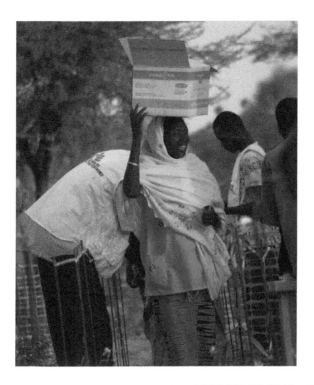

Photo 6.1: A woman in Niger collects a peanut-based nutritional supplement for her children.

Source: Photo courtesy of the European Community Humanitarian Office (ECHO: http://ec.europa.eu/echo).

The most extreme form of wasting and stunting results in two definable clinical conditions called "marasmus" (typically a very wasted but symmetrically small child without edema) and "kwashiorkor" (typically a child with less growth failure, but conspicuous poor skin and edema). Although both are becoming increasingly uncommon, they still gain a disproportionate amount of attention in the malnutrition literature. Some even use the terms as if they were synonymous with malnutrition (which, of course, they are not). There is a good deal of confusion surrounding both conditions. Some of the most common mistakes include the meanings of the names and their nutritional origins.

"Marasmus" is the simpler of the two and is derived from the Greek word for "wasted." "Kwashiokor" is a term from the Akan language of Ghana. It does not mean "abandoned child," "second child," or any number of similar fanciful expressions. In Ghana, "Kwashi" is the name given to a male child born on a Sunday (Kofi Annan gets his name from being born on a Friday). "Korkor" is the word for "red" and presumably refers to the reddish hair colour of children with severe malnutrition.

Claims that the differences between kwashiorkor and marasmus are due to different levels of protein intake are also incorrect. The problem is far more complex and is still incompletely understood (Krawinkel, 2003). Proposed theories include aflatoxins in the grain, abnormal hormonal or immune responses to the stress of starvation, and multiple associated micronutrient deficiencies. One thing is absolutely certain—if children get enough to eat, the problem disappears. It is best to categorize degrees of malnutrition as mild, moderate, and severe and leave these two diagnoses for medical texts. Hopefully, nutritional advances will one day consign both of them to the history books.

Development

Unfortunately, malnutrition can have a profound effect on neurological development and subsequent school performance (WHO, 2010b). The early growth and organization of brain cells are both dependent on adequate nutrition (before and after birth). The child's brain grows most rapidly during the period from conception to the second or third birthday. Severe undernutrition affecting the pregnant mother or the young child can have measurable and irreversible effects on subsequent brain development. Malnutrition in the early school years causes apathy, reduced activity, and lack of curiosity, which will inevitably reduce the child's ability to learn. Once again, the full picture depends on many other factors, particularly the effects of serious illness and associated iodine deficiency.

Table 6.3: Selected micronutrient deficiency by UN region

	PREVALENCE OF IODINE DEFICIENCY (%)	PREVALENCE OF ZINC DEFICIENCY (%)	PREVALENCE OF VITAMIN A DEFICIENCY (%)		PREVALENCE OF IRON DEFICIENCY (%)	
Region	Overall	Overall	Children <5	Pregnant women	Children <5	Pregnant women
Global	28.5	17.3	33.3	15.3	18.1	19.2
Africa	40.0	23.9	41.6	14.3	20.2	20.3
Americas & Caribbean	13.7	9.6	15.6	2.0	12.7	15.2
Asia	31.6	19.4	33.5	18.4	19.0	19.8
Europe	44.2	7.6	2.9	2.2	12.1	16.2
Oceania	17.3	5.7	9.2	17.3	15.4	17.2

Note: Iodine deficiency is defined as urine concentration <100 µg/L (2013); zinc deficiency is defined as inadequate zinc intake as determined from a weighted average of country means; vitamin A deficiency is based on serum retinol <0.7 µmol/L (1995–2005); iron-deficiency anemia is based on hemogloblin <110 g/L (2011).

Source: Black et al. 2013. Maternal and child undernutrition and overweight in low-income and middle-income countries. The Lancet, 382: 427–451.

Immune Response

It has been known for a long time that severe malnutrition has profound adverse effects on a child's immune system (Keusch, 2003). Relatively recent research has shown that mild and moderate malnutrition also poses significant risks to a child's health that are far greater than was previously appreciated. Such underweight or stunted children may, on first glance, look like rather skinny but otherwise fairly healthy youngsters. However, once they are stressed by infectious diseases, their mortality rate is greatly increased.

Of the approximately 10 million children a year who die from the major killers such as respiratory infections, diarrhea, malaria, and measles, it is estimated that the underlying effects of malnutrition were contributing causes to those deaths in 25–50 percent of the cases (Pelletier et al., 1995).

Micronutrient Malnutrition

Apart from the three major components of a normal diet, the body also requires dozens of other minerals and vitamins, often in very small amounts (MNI, 2009). Some of these chemicals are so commonly distributed that deficiency is almost unknown even among people suffering from poor nutrition. Others, such as iron, are often in marginal quantities even in a normal diet, so deficiency can be found in any population around the world. It is possible to have micronutrient deficiencies despite an apparently normal diet. Consequently, micronutrient deficiency is often referred to as "the hidden hunger." The return on investment on nutrition initiatives is very high. Regular provision of micronutrients returns that investment many times over in terms of improved growth, development, and survival. As a result, increasing amounts of aid are being spent on international efforts to eradicate micronutrient deficiencies, particularly in iodine, vitamin A, folate, zinc, and iron (MNI, 2011).

Iodine Deficiency

Roughly a third of the world's population live in areas where there is little or no iodine in the soil and consequently very little in the diet. Literally hundreds of millions of people are at risk of iodine deficiency disorder, particularly in large parts of China (ICCIDD, 2011). Iodine is an essential factor in thyroid hormone, which, in turn, is an essential factor needed for early brain development. Although some affected children suffer severe developmental delay, the problem is usually more subtle and manifests as poor school performance and lack of energy. Iodine deficiency is the single most common cause of preventable mental retardation and brain damage. The average IQ is 13 points higher in an iodine-supplemented population

compared to one that is iodine deficient. For decades, many countries have legislated the addition of iodine either to table salt or cooking oil. Food fortification is
effective and very cheap.

Vitamin A Deficiency

Vitamin A is part of a large family of chemicals called carotenoids, which contribute to the orange colour of foods such as carrots and mangos. Vitamin A is widely
distributed in a normal diet, but large parts of the developing world are at high risk
of deficiency, particularly their pediatric populations (UNICEF, 2007). Vitamin
A is a cofactor in many important chemical reactions; consequently, deficiency
causes a wide range of abnormalities, including severe eye disease (xerophthalmia),
which can ultimately lead to blindness and increased susceptibility to infections
(particularly to measles and diarrheal diseases). Prior to widespread vitamin A
supplementation and measles vaccination, it was estimated that 250,000 children
were blinded each year due to vitamin A deficiency and lack of measles vaccination.
The majority of those children lived lives of such deprivation that most died from
the combined effects of malnutrition and further infections.

It is almost unbelievable that this terrible toll on child health can now be
effectively treated and avoided for a few cents. Apart from its effects on vision,
the administration of vitamin A at regular immunization visits has been shown
to reduce all-cause mortality by about 25 percent. The mortality rate for measles
is almost halved with the addition of vitamin A. The cause of this reduction in
mortality is not known, but it is very real. Since 1997, the WHO has advocated
the routine administration of vitamin A at the same time the child is vaccinated—one of the major aid-funded health advances. Many countries now fortify
foods such as maize, wheat, and sugar with vitamin A. Fortification is effective
and also cheap.

Iron Deficiency

This is the most common micronutrient deficiency in the world, but appreciation
of the adverse effects of iron deficiency in children has been a relatively recent
development. Iodine and vitamin A fortification of foods were both widely introduced long before iron fortification was seriously discussed (Olivares et al., 1999).
Children born to iron-deficient mothers, whose breast milk is also low in iron, have
only marginal stores at birth to deal with a period of rapid physical and neurological
growth. It is estimated that at least half of the developing world's children between
six months and two years of age are iron deficient during this critical development
period. The worst affected are often found in countries where children are weaned
onto a rice porridge low in iron.

Apart from its effect on children, severe iron-deficiency anemia reduces the ability of adults to work and greatly increases risks during childbirth for women. Fortifying infant foods with iron is practised widely in developing countries, but these foods are expensive and may not reach the worst-affected populations. Supplementation with iron-containing tablets and syrups is another approach, but delivering the supplements to the huge numbers of at-risk families is a problem (as is compliance with treatment). Recent research has developed the concept of fortification using a vitamin and mineral preparation (Schauer et al., 2003) that can be easily added to the child's food (Sprinkles, 2011). There have also been innovations such as iron-fortified salt, tea, and even biscuits that are being developed and deployed in developing countries.

Zinc Deficiency

Zinc is analogous to vitamin A's actions. It has specific beneficial effects against gastroenteritis, but general use also reduces all-cause mortality by significant amounts, possibly due to its effects on the immune response. In keeping with iron deficiency, as many as a third of the world's population are at risk of marginal intake because they live in regions with low soil levels of zinc (IZINCG, 2011). Early studies in low-zinc areas of Turkey showed that zinc-supplemented fertilizers increased crop yields and also improved child health. Zinc is necessary for brain development and for normal labour. Zinc-deficient women have a higher rate of obstructed labour. Since 2004, zinc has been an essential part of gastroenteritis treatment along with oral rehydration solution (UNICEF, 2004). Acute use shortens the duration of the illness. Longer-term use reduces the risk of pneumonia, malaria, and recurrent gastroenteritis.

Folate Deficiency

Folic acid or folate is a water-soluble vitamin in the B group (vitamin B_9). It is an essential factor in fetal growth and development and also in the production of red blood cells. It is commonly found in leafy green vegetables. Deficiency is less common in areas where cereals and bread are fortified. Folate deficiency during pregnancy is associated with severe anemia in the mother and fetal defects (particularly forms of spina bifida) in the child. Early studies showed clear reductions in neural defects among babies of supplemented mothers (Lumley et al., 2007). Subsequent experiments have shown that folate given during pregnancy also seems to reduce other developmental abnormalities, particularly congenital heart defects. Combined folate-iron supplementation is an essential part of prenatal care for women in all parts of the globe. Ideally, folate should be started before the woman gets pregnant.

DEFINITION AND MEASUREMENT OF MALNUTRITION

True genius resides in the capacity for evaluation of uncertain, hazardous, and conflicting information.

—Winston Churchill, 1948

Measurement Systems

Several methods of assessing malnutrition have been proposed, each with its own techniques, measurement errors, and cut-off definitions. Over the last 15 years, there has been a much-needed move toward standardization. Although most research is now based on the WHO-recommended z-score methodology (WHO, 2009), this is still not universally used, so it is necessary to be familiar with some of the other measurement techniques found in the literature.

Small errors can make large differences in interpretation, particularly in small children. It is important to remember that any assessment of malnutrition must be based on simple, robust, and portable equipment that yields reproducible, statistically relevant results under what are often difficult conditions. The following methods are still used, or at least mentioned, in nutrition studies:

- *Road to health charts (de Onis, 1996):* Originally developed by David Morley in Nigeria in 1970, successors are found in clinics all over the world, often with space to record immunizations. Charts vary, so care is necessary before plotting a child's growth and making conclusions. These early growth charts can be confusing. They have only two lines: the upper represents the median weight for age for boys, while the lower represents the third percentile for girls.
- *Gomez system (Gomez et al., 1956):* This was widely used in the 1960s and 1970s and is still used by some countries. Malnutrition is graded using weight for height measurements.
- *Wellcome classification (Wellcome Trust Working Party, 1970):* This system includes marasmus and kwashiorkor as part of the classification. It is falling out of use as severe malnutrition is becoming less common. It is based on weight for age and the presence of edema.
- *Upper arm circumference (Collins, 1996):* The diameter of the upper arm remains relatively constant between one and five years of age, so this measurement can be used for rapid screening of large refugee populations, particularly when ages of children are unknown. It is of some value as a rough population screening tool, but is too inaccurate for clinical use.

- *Skin-fold thickness (Frisancho et al., 1982):* It is strongly depe ̄   ̄   ̄
  measurement technique. Small errors alter interpretation. It is ᴄ
  ally used in long-term nutritional studies, but more usually as a
  of obesity.
- *Body mass index (Ferro-Luzzi, 1994):* Weight is expressed as a ratio of surface area; calculation is needed; there is no cut-off value. BMI changes
  with age, so newly published WHO tables are required (WHO, 2006). It
  is more commonly used for obesity research.
- *Waterlow system (Waterlow et al., 1977):* Acute starvation (termed "wasting") is assessed using weight for height curves. Chronic starvation
  (termed "stunting") is assessed using height for age curves. Technique was
  adopted and developed by the WHO as its recommended method of nutrition assessment.
- *WHO Standard (Bern et al., 1997):* Addition of weight for age (underweight) to Waterlow; all are expressed as z-scores.

Standardized Reference Values

Since malnutrition is defined by comparing a child against standard values, the
choice of those universal reference values is very important. Since the late 1970s,
the WHO has used the widely available US growth charts developed by the
National Center for Health Statistics (NCHS). They combined two sets of data:
one for children under two years based largely on White Americans going back to
1929, and the other on older children from more recent surveys of schoolchildren.
The validity of the NCHS reference data has been criticized for various reasons,
including the age of the data, 24-month dysjunction (i.e., the curves don't meet!),
poor inclusion of breastfed infants, narrow racial base, and unrepresentative incidence of obesity (de Onis, 1997). The production of updated growth charts has
necessarily been a slow process. The WHO Multicentre Growth Reference Study
(MGRS) was proposed in 1994. After collecting growth data on several thousand
children from widely different backgrounds, the updated charts were released in
May 2006 (WHO, 2006).

Once a reference has been chosen, the child's measurement must be expressed
in relation to that standard. Inevitably, this has not been standardized either; three
different methods are used (Table 6.4) (Ge et al., 2001):

- *Percentiles:* The mid-position on any growth chart is referred to as the 50th
  percentile. It refers to the percentage of children who fall below this level.
  There is crowding of the lines at the 10th, 5th, and 3rd percentiles, so the

technique is of limited use for differentiating between varying degrees of childhood malnutrition.

- *Percent of the median:* The child's measured value is expressed as a percentage of the median reference value for his or her age—the most common method used in the past.
- *Z-score:* The term "z" is statistical notation for one standard deviation. The child's deviation from the reference mean value is expressed in numbers of standard deviations. Interpretation of a z-score is independent of the child's age or gender and can also be manipulated statistically. It is the method of choice recommended by WHO.

For example, using NCHS/WHO reference tables, the median weight for a 22-month-old girl is 11.55 kg with a standard deviation of 1.22 kg. A girl of this age weighing 8.89 kg can be plotted three ways:

1. *Percentiles:* Calculation—plots below 3rd percentile for age when plotted on standard weight for age NCHS growth chart. Interpretation is subjective.
2. *Percent of median:* Calculated by $(8.89 \div 11.55) \times 100 = 77$ percent. Classified as mild or grade I malnutrition by Gomez, but as moderate malnutrition using Road to Health and Wellcome criteria. It is unclassified by Waterlow criteria since there are no weight for age norms.
3. *Z-score or standard deviations below median:* Calculated by $(11.55 - 8.89) \div 1.22 = -2.18z$. Classified as moderate malnutrition (underweight) using WHO's definition. Does not apply to other systems.

This is not just statistical nitpicking—progress toward the targets of SDG 2.1 of ending all forms of malnutrition is monitored by nutritional surveys, which can be strongly skewed by careless measurements and choice of different methodology. The best solution is to standardize to the WHO growth charts and define a child's position on the chart by z-score.

Table 6.4: Approximate equivalence between the three methods used for defining a child's position on a growth chart.

MALNUTRITION	NORMAL	MILD	MODERATE	SEVERE	VERY SEVERE
Z-score	0	−1Z	−2Z	−3Z	−4Z
% of median	100%	90%	80%	70%	60%
Percentile	50	15.8	2.28	0.13	<0.1

FEEDING INFANTS

Artificial Feeding of Infants

> Formula feeding is the longest lasting uncontrolled experiment lacking informed consent in the history of medicine.
>
> —*Frank Oski, MD, retired editor, Journal of Pediatrics*

Babies have been successfully raised using formula feeds for many decades. In fact, the great majority of today's baby boomers (well over 50 percent) were fed solely on infant formula. At first glance, it is difficult to imagine what could be wrong with infant formulas or the vast industry that makes them, but as usual, a closer look reveals a more complex story.

In the 18th century, parents who could afford it would often choose a wet nurse. In some cases, the baby was lodged with the nurse and taken back only when the child was weaned. In the 19th century, the practice of using animal milk grew in popularity (called "dry nursing"). Milk from cows, goats, mares, and donkeys was used; donkey milk was considered to be the best option (Apple, 1987). Although there was no knowledge of nutritional science, it was already obvious to 19th-century observers that children who were not breastfed suffered a much higher mortality. Babies were fed by cup and spoon or with early versions of baby bottles. Until the introduction of the first rubber teat in 1845, nipples were made from soft leather or sponge.

Johann Simon published the first chemical analysis and comparison between cow and human milk in 1838, but this information was not used for development of artificial formulas until the 1860s. At that time, a German chemist, Von Leibig, and a Swiss inventor, Nestlé, both independently developed breast-milk substitutes based on cow's milk, wheat, malt, and sugar. Despite its expense, this new approach to infant feeding spread rapidly around the world (Schuman, 2003). By 1900, there were three available forms of infant feeding: breast milk, commercial breast-milk substitutes, and numerous recipes and recommendations (formulas), all of which were based on condensed milk. This product was developed during the American Civil War, when it was discovered that adding sugar to partially evaporated cow's milk extended its storage life. Cookbooks of the day usually included a recipe for evaporated milk formula. Typical additives included cow's milk, cod liver oil, orange juice, and sugar. By World War II, evaporated milk recipes had grown to become the most common form of infant nutrition.

The commercial baby food industry followed a similar course and introduced a variety of new formulas based on different fat sources. SMA (simulated milk adapted) was introduced in 1919. Lactogen was introduced in 1920, and the research of a milk chemist and a Boston pediatrician resulted in a formula called Similac (similar to lactation) in 1924. By the time Mead Johnson introduced Enfamil in 1959, commercial milk had become the most common form of infant nutrition. This rise continued to replace breastfeeding as the norm. By the 1970s, only 25 percent of two- to three-month-old children in the US were breastfed; this pattern was followed throughout most of the developed countries.

Legislation to establish minimum standards for infant formulas was surprisingly slow to arrive. It was not until the discovery of electrolyte abnormalities in some children fed commercial formulas that minimum legal standards for nutrients and testing were established in 1980. Formulas have continued to develop and a wide range of specialty products is now available, particularly for the complex nutritional requirements of preterm infants.

A major factor behind the popularity of commercial formulas was aggressive marketing by the baby food industries. Apart from direct advertising, formula was also provided in hospital to new mothers, a practice that was supported by many pediatricians as a move toward "scientific motherhood." As the baby boom market decreased, the industry looked to developing countries for new markets where they could use much of the same advertising practices (IBFAN, 2011).

So far so good. Current formula feeds are the result of many years of research and have a definite part to play in the nutrition of children in developed countries. However, the story is not so clear in developing countries where populations must raise small children without easy access to education, sanitation, or clean water. Under these circumstances, infant formulas may do far more harm than good. Apart from its socializing advantages, breast milk is sterile and nutritionally tailored for the baby. Its delivery is not complicated by malnutrition and infection resulting from incorrect mixing of the powder with dirty water by a mother who has not had any access to education. As early as 1939, one of the pioneers of maternal and child health, Dr. Cicely Williams, was warning about the increased mortality associated with the replacement of breastfeeding by bottle-feeding in developing countries. Unfortunately, these warnings had no effect. The industry continued to depict healthy-looking babies in its advertisements, dressed salespeople as nurses (mother craft nurses), and provided free supplies of baby formula to maternity wards.

These promotion methods produced the same effect in the developing world as they had elsewhere. By the 1960s, it was clear that this trend was associated with greatly increased mortality among bottle-fed children living in poverty. The term "commerciogenic malnutrition" was coined by Jelliffe (1972). He had already published a pamphlet, "Child Nutrition in Developing Countries," with the World Health Organization, which called attention to the dangers of bottle-feeding in poor populations. The fight now began in earnest with War on Want's publication in 1974 of a report on infant food promotion and its adverse effects called "The Baby Killer." Widespread interest in this campaign ultimately led to an international boycott of Nestlé products starting in 1977.

US Senate hearings in 1979 on the marketing of baby formula in developing countries and a subsequent joint WHO/UNICEF meeting on the same subject finally resulted in recommendations covering the international marketing of breast-milk substitutes, which resulted in a code of conduct endorsed by the WHO in 1981 and reaffirmed through the Innocenti Declaration in 1990. The code places restrictions on advertising of baby formulas and requires that salespeople do not provide milk, Pablum, or promotional gifts in hospitals (INFAC, 2011). The code has no legal power, but it has been adopted into law by many developing nations. The promotion of infant formulas in these countries is now well controlled, but in countries without legislation, there is still plenty of evidence to suggest that the infant food industry does not fully comply with the WHO International Code (Aguayo et al., 2003). Regular reviews of the situation are published by the International Baby Food Action Network (IBFAN, 2011).

Breastfeeding and the Impact of HIV/AIDS

> It is almost as if breastfeeding takes the infant out of poverty for those first few months in order to give the child a fairer start in life and compensate for the injustice of the world into which it was born.
>
> —*James P. Grant, former director, UNICEF, 1982*

The benefits of breastfeeding are so widely advertised that it is now easy to forget that only 30 years ago, there were real concerns that breastfeeding would almost die out as a cultural practice. Although breastfeeding has advantages for both the mother and child, it is important not to overstate the case; infants can grow and develop completely normally using properly prepared modern infant formulas. A mother who cannot breastfeed her child should not be made to feel that she has, in some way, failed her child. Breastfeeding is still the recommended form of infant feeding, but in a developed country, it is not a matter of life and death.

However, for a child born into poverty, the situation is very different. Exclusive breastfeeding in the first six months of life protects the child from a wide range of diseases, particularly malnutrition and gastroenteritis (Duijts et al., 2010). The infant of an overworked mother who has to leave the baby with older children each day cannot be nourished adequately. Poverty forces the family to dilute the expensive feed to make it last longer. It is then mixed with contaminated water that cannot be sterilized because the family has no cooking fuel. Numerous studies have confirmed this observation. A Mexican study showed that bottle-fed babies living in poverty are six to thirteen times more likely to die in the first two months of life compared to breastfed babies, and four to six times more likely to die between three and five months (Palloni et al., 1994).

Earlier reports by UNICEF estimated that the deaths of over a million children a year could be prevented with the exclusive breastfeeding of all children below the age of six months. Unfortunately, this was before research into HIV-infected mothers showed a significant cumulative risk of transmission of the virus in breast milk. This has been a major challenge to breastfeeding initiatives. The risk of early mortality associated with formula feeding has to be weighed against the risk of contracting HIV from breast milk. There have been heated debates on this topic, but a consensus has emerged (WHO, 2010a). Current recommendations are that an infected mother should remain on antiretroviral therapy for her lifetime and exclusively breastfeed her child for at least 6 months, and preferably for 12 months. A course of nevirapine (a medication to treat and prevent HIV/AIDS) for the child is also effective (Chasela et al., 2010). There is limited information on heat-treating expressed breast milk, but this is not a practical option in the social circumstances that surround many affected families. This is a very common problem in contemporary practical pediatrics. It is essential that people considering work in a developing country familiarize themselves with these recommendations.

Comparative studies have clearly shown that whether a new mother is HIV-positive or not, if she lives in poor socio-economic conditions, the risk of disease and death is higher for her child if she elects to bottle-feed (Bahl et al., 2005). It is very important that all mothers living in poverty are encouraged to breastfeed their children. Unfortunately, until relatively recently, hospitals did not encourage breastfeeding. In fact, practices such as mother and baby separation, rigid feeding regimes, and the convenience of formula food for staff all combined to reduce the emphasis on breastfeeding. Once widespread commercial formula advertising and provision of free milk in hospitals were added, it is easy to see why formula feeding was steadily supplanting breastfeeding in many parts of the world; the fault is not entirely to be laid at the door of the baby food industry.

The first large attempt to repopularize breastfeeding was taken at a joint WHO/UNICEF meeting in 1989. The result was a pamphlet titled "Protecting, Promoting, and Supporting Breastfeeding: The Special Role of Maternity Service." This contained several suggestions to improve the role of breastfeeding in maternity hospitals. The Baby-Friendly Hospital Initiative (UNICEF, 2011) that grew from this early report was launched as a joint UNICEF and WHO strategy in 1991. The criteria for designation as a "baby-friendly hospital" include extra training for health care staff, the promotion of breastfeeding both before and after pregnancy, and support for breastfeeding by trained lactation consultants. The baby is roomed in with the mother to encourage breastfeeding on demand and the child is not given any commercial milk or a pacifier. The program also restricts use of free formula or other products provided by the formula companies. The concept has been very popular and has spread widely throughout the developed and developing world (BFCC, 2011). Taken together, the international code of marketing of breast-milk substitutes and the Baby-Friendly Hospital Initiative have helped control the unregulated spread of formula foods and are slowly re-establishing breastfeeding as the nutrition of choice for young children.

FOOD SECURITY AND FOOD AID

Food Security

> Starvation is characteristic of some people not having enough to eat. It is not the characteristic of there not being enough to eat. While the latter can be a cause of the former, it is but one of many possible causes.
>
> —*Amartya Sen, 1983*

According to the Food and Agriculture Organization (FAO), food security exists when all people, at all times, have physical, social, and economic access to sufficient, safe, and nutritious food to meet their dietary needs and food preferences for an active and healthy life. The four pillars of food security are availability, access, utilization, and stability (FAO, 2009). Availability refers to supply of food; access reflects the demand side; utilization refers to food use and its metabolism by individuals; and stability refers to the capacity to obtain food over time (Barrett, 2010; FAO, 1997).

The Indian economist Amartya Sen (1983) was the first to publish a serious study of the causes of famines. He examined four famines, but concentrated on the 1943 famine in Bengal. Up to that point, it was generally believed that famines were simply caused by intermittent crop failures in developing countries, and were the inevitable consequence of too many people and not enough food. Some observers even blamed the victims themselves, either for having too many children or for not working hard enough. However, Sen pointed out that the Bengal harvest in 1943 was actually bigger than the harvest in 1941, which had not been a famine year. Clearly, there must have been many other factors involved—principally hoarding and redistribution to troops fighting World War II. There was plenty of food; it just was not given to the local poor.

The situation is no different from the great Irish potato famine of 1845. It is commonly believed that widespread crop failure and overpopulation resulted in the deaths of a million people and large-scale migration of the population to North

America. On closer examination, it was not quite that simple (Woodham-Smith, 1992). The only crop affected by blight was the potato, and the only people affected were the poor, who relied on potatoes. Throughout the famine period, Ireland was a net exporter of grain to Europe and Britain. Similar to the later Bengal famine, there was no total shortage of food, just a shortage of potatoes and a lack of political will to redistribute the available grain surplus. Indeed, every famine has its own unique features. Whether you look at food shortage from a family or a national point of view, there is always a great deal more to starvation than simple lack of food (Peng, 1987).

One beneficial result of Sen's early work has been the development of famine early warning systems. These can give enough advance notice to allow time to mobilize increased food supplies to a high-risk area. USAID's Famine Early Warning System is a good example (FEWS, 2011). At time of writing, its major area of interest is in south Somalia, where consecutive droughts and endemic civil war have produced the worst famine in over 25 years. Some of the most common variables that can produce famine by interrupting production and distribution of food are given in Table 6.5. The term "food security" has evolved to describe the degree to which a population has access to food.

The majority of the world's poor live in rural areas and depend on agriculture for both food and income. The direct and indirect benefits from agricultural improvement are numerous. Improved agricultural output raises nutritional levels and provides rural populations with income. Good farming practices also reduce ecological degradation and keep people on the land. Failure of agricultural programs is a disaster for the health and prosperity of rural communities. The final result is migration of the rural poor into destitute shantytowns surrounding the major towns. Unfortunately, many developing countries have neglected the rural sector, concentrating instead on urban areas and industrialization. Any attention paid to agriculture has been focused on cash crops for export rather than producing food for local consumption. Until recently, the aid industry had also given agriculture a

Table 6.5: Common causes of poor food security

POOR FOOD PRODUCTION	POOR FOOD DISTRIBUTION
• Poverty	• Poverty
• Crop failure, drought	• Corruption, hoarding, black market
• Lack of property rights, agricultural land, and pasture	• Lack of storage for surpluses
• Lack of credit for seeds, fertilizers, or tools	• Poor distribution infrastructure
• Lack of crop failure insurance	• Absence of social safety net
	• Religious or tribal discrimination
	• Powerlessness of the poor
	• War

steadily reducing priority (from over 15 percent in the 1980s to less than 5 percent by 2005). This trend has only recently been changed (FAO, 2009). Unfortunately, leadership in this vital area is lacking. The FAO has been under increasing criticism that culminated in a highly critical external review published in 2007. The organization is currently at the end of a three-year reform that cost over US$20 million, so it is hoped that improvements will be seen.

At the 1974 World Food Conference, delegates produced the declaration that "every man, woman, and child has the inalienable right to be free from hunger and malnutrition." The conference also predicted that this happy state would be achieved by 2000. Unfortunately, despite the gains of the Green Revolution, we are nowhere near achieving that goal. At the turn of the century, over 800 million people living in almost 90 nations were chronically malnourished. Delegates to the 1996 World Food Conference in Rome pragmatically accepted this failure of progress by setting a less ambitious goal of halving chronic malnutrition by the year 2015. This was subsequently adopted as one of the first targets of the MDGs set in 2000. As discussed above, progress has been made by many countries, but for parts of Asia and sub-Saharan Africa, meeting this goal was not possible.

Food Aid

Food aid was first provided to developing countries in the 1950s as a way for the United States and a few other countries (Canada, Japan, Australia, and the European Union) to dispose of grain surpluses. Aid money was used to buy the grain and transport it to developing countries suffering production shortfall. It was initially seen as a benefit for farmers and poor alike, but as usual, it turned out to be much more complicated than that. In humanitarian disasters, food aid has been of some value, but outside this narrow indication, it has generated enormous controversy and accusations that it produces more harm than good. The volume of food aid has fallen significantly since the 1960s and 1970s; the largest donors are the United States, at around 50 percent, the European Union at 15 percent, and Canada at 5 percent.

Food aid has always attracted considerable criticism (Oxfam, 2005a). It is blamed for creating disincentives, depressing food prices, distorting markets, and delaying the need for policy reforms. Powerful vested interests, including agricultural producers, truckers, and shippers, all tend to slow the rate of change. In response to widespread criticism, the major food donors agreed upon a Food Aid Convention in 1999, but the process lacked monitoring or enforcement. There is a strong move toward an effective Global Food Aid Compact (Barrett et al., 2005) that will hopefully produce a more accountable and efficient food aid process. Rather than being seen as altruism, some forms of food aid can be viewed as

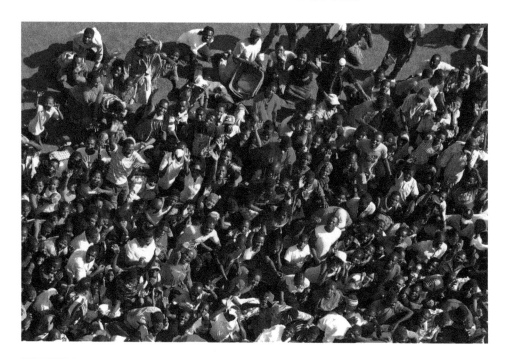

Photo 6.2: Mass food distribution following a disaster is a very difficult task. The image shows Haitians waving to a helicopter crew after they delivered water and food in the early period following the earthquake.

Source: UN Photo/Logan Abassi, with kind permission of the UN Photo Library (www. unmultimedia.org/photo).

subsidized dumping of agricultural surpluses (Oxfam, 2005a). This has led to its inclusion in the current Doha round of international trade talks, where it has been a topic of great irritation. Finally, the donation of genetically modified (GM) crops has added further complexity, particularly following Zambia's much-publicized refusal of GM crop donations. Taken altogether, food aid is a very complex issue.

It is important to remember that there are different types of food aid, each of which has its own advantages and disadvantages (Timmer, 2005):

- *Program food aid:* Food aid started in the 1950s with donations of agricultural surpluses from one government to another. The grains were usually sold in the recipient's local market and the money was then used for other development activities. This "monetized" form of food aid has been heavily criticized, particularly since the proceeds of sales are usually tied to purchases from the donor country. Apart from depressing local food markets, the practice can also be viewed as subsidized dumping and an unfair means to open up new markets. Program food aid now forms only a small proportion of total donated food.

- *Project food aid:* Starting in the 1970s, food aid was used to support specific projects such as school feeding programs, payment in kind for development work projects, and food support for vulnerable women and children. Donations are distributed through NGOs, local government agencies, or the World Food Program. Concerns about fostering dependency are minimized by targeting the donations to groups who have no other options. An apparent problem is the cost of shipping food. At least 50 percent of the aid grant is lost in shipping costs. It is more efficient to use the money to buy food locally or at least in neighbouring countries. The European Union has moved toward direct financing more quickly than the United States (Oxfam, 2005b).

- *Emergency food aid:* In the last 20 years, the distribution of free food to people suffering from natural disasters or political emergencies has become the major form of food aid. Even this seemingly simple process is open to criticism. The response to the recent Asian tsunami is a good example. Although inland food production and markets recovered quickly in Sri Lanka, the World Food Program made only small purchases within the country. Even if these markets had failed, purchases would have been easier from India or Thailand. Inevitable delays in bulk transport also run the risk of flooding the local market with donated food at a time when the next harvest is due, with inevitable results on the local economy. Again, direct donation of money would probably be more efficient in many cases.

SUMMARY

Food is an important social determinant of health and has a far-reaching impact on the overall well-being of populations. The fundamental importance of nutrition is reflected in its selection as one of the Millennium Development Goals. The aim was to halve the proportion of people suffering from undernutrition between 1990 and 2015. Today, 795 million people are undernourished globally, which is about one in nine individuals, with the vast majority living in the developing regions. However, the proportion of undernourished people in the developing regions has fallen by almost half since 1990. This reduction varies across regions. For example, South Asia and sub-Saharan Africa now account for substantially larger shares of global undernourishment. Furthermore, average levels of childhood stunting and underweight greatly vary by region, and progress to address these outcomes has been slow. Sub-Saharan Africa and South Asia continually have a high prevalence of childhood stunting and underweight. In 2014, 1 in 7 children were estimated to be underweight in less-developed regions.

High prevalence combined with a large population means that most underweight children live in South Asia. The new SDG goal on hunger, *End hunger, achieve food security and improved nutrition, and promote sustainable agriculture*, builds on prior MDGs. Achieving the SDG also requires tackling micronutrient deficiency, often referred to as "the hidden hunger." The return on investment for nutrition initiatives is very high. As a result, increasing amounts of aid are being spent on international efforts to eradicate micronutrient deficiencies, particularly in iodine, vitamin A, folate, zinc, and iron.

DISCUSSION QUESTIONS

1. What are the MDGs and SDGs related to food security? How do they differ from each other?
2. What is the prevalence of wasting in children under five years of age, by World Bank region? Are there specific treatments to improve the health of children suffering from stunting?
3. What are some of the links between nutrition and health?
4. What are some of the links among nutrition, education, and economic advancement?
5. What is the impact of micronutrient deficiency on health? How does this affect children and pregnant women?
6. Which parts of world have the worst nutrition problems and why?
7. What are the major micronutrient deficiencies facing developing countries?
8. What is food security? What are the pillars of food security?
9. What is food aid? What are the advantages and disadvantages of food aid?
10. Do you think hunger can be eliminated in our lifetime? Why or why not?

RECOMMENDED READING

De Waal, A. 1997. *Famine crimes: Politics and the disaster industry in Africa*. Pub: Indiana University Press.

Leathers, H., & Foster, P. 2004. *The world food problem: Tackling the causes of undernutrition in the Third World*. Pub: Lynne Rienner Publishers.

Savage-King, F., & Burgess, A. 2005. *Nutrition for developing countries*. Pub: Oxford University Press.

Semba, R., & Bloem, M. 2001. *Nutrition and health in developing countries*. Pub: Humana Press.

Sen, A. 1983. *Poverty and famines: An essay on entitlements*. Pub: Oxford University Press.

REFERENCES

Aguayo, V., et al. 2003. Monitoring compliance with the International Code of Marketing of Breast Milk Substitutes in West Africa. *British Medical Journal*, 326: 127–133.

Apple, R. 1987. *Mothers and medicine: A social history of infant feeding, 1890–1950*. Pub: University of Wisconsin Press.

Ashworth, A., et al. 2003. Guidelines for the inpatient treatment of severely malnourished children. WHO. Retrieved from: www.who.int/nutrition/publications/guide_inpatient_text.pdf.

Ashworth, A., et al. 2004. WHO guidelines for management of severe malnutrition in rural South African hospitals: Effect on case fatality and the influence of operational factors. *The Lancet*, 363: 1110–1115.

Bahl, R., et al. 2005. Infant feeding patterns and risks of death and hospitalization in the first half of infancy. *Bulletin of the World Health Organization*, 83: 418–426.

Barrett, C. B., 2010. Measuring food insecurity. *Science*, 327(5967; special issue on food security): 825–828. Retrieved from: www.jstor.org/stable/40509899 (Accessed: August 24, 2016).

Barrett, C. B., & Maxwell, D. G. 2006. Towards a global food aid compact. *Food Policy*, 31(2): 105–118. Retrieved from: http://papers.ssrn.com/sol3/papers.cfm?abstract_id=715002#%23.

Bern, C., et al. 1997. Assessment of potential indicators for protein-energy malnutrition in the algorithm for integrated management of childhood illness. *Bulletin of the World Health Organization*, 75: 87–96.

BFCC. 2011. Breastfeeding Committee for Canada. Retrieved from: http://breastfeedingcanada.ca/default.aspx.

Black, R. E., et al. 2013. Maternal and child undernutrition and overweight in low-income and middle-income countries. *The Lancet*, 382(9890): 427–451.

Chasela, C., et al. 2010. Maternal or infant antiretroviral drugs to reduce HIV-1 transmission. *New England Journal of Medicine*, 362: 2271–2281.

Cohen, D. 2005. Achieving food security in vulnerable populations. *British Medical Journal*, 331: 775–777.

Collins, S. 1996. Using middle upper arm circumference to assess severe adult malnutrition during famine. *Journal of the American Medical Association*, 276: 391–395.

Craddock, C. 1984. *Retired except on demand: The life of Dr. Cicely Williams*. Pub: Oxford University Press.

de Onis, M. 1997. Time for a new growth reference. *Pediatrics*, 100: 8–9.

de Onis, M., et al. 1996. The WHO growth chart: Historical considerations and current scientific issues. *Bibliotheca Nutritio et Dieta*, 53: 74–89.

de Onis, M., et al. 2004. Methodology for estimating regional and global trends of child malnutrition. *International Journal of Epidemiology*, 33: 1–11.

de Onis, M., et al. 2010. Global prevalence and trends of overweight and obesity among pre-school children. *American Journal of Clinical Nutrition*, 92: 1257–1264.

De Waal. 1997. *Famine crimes: Politics and the disaster industry in Africa*. Pub: Indiana University Press.

Duijts, L., et al. 2010. Prolonged and exclusive breastfeeding reduces the risk of infectious diseases in infancy. *Pediatrics*, 126: 18–25.

FAO. 1997. The food system and factors affecting household food security and nutrition. Agriculture, food and nutrition for Africa: A resource book for teachers of agriculture. Retrieved from: www.fao.org/docrep/W0078E/W0078E00.htm.

FAO. 2003. Measurement and assessment of food deprivation and undernutrition. Retrieved from: www.fao.org/docrep/005/Y4249E/y4249e00.htm.

FAO. 2006. FAO's Special Programme for Food Security. Retrieved from: www.fao.org/spfs/en/.

FAO. 2009a. Rapid assessment of aid flows for agricultural development in sub-Saharan Africa. Retrieved from: www.fao.org/docrep/012/al144e/al144e.pdf.

FAO.2009b. Declaration of the World Food Summit on Food Security. Retrieved from: www.fao.org/fileadmin/templates/wsfs/Summit/Docs/Final_Declaration/WSFS09_Declaration.pdf.

FAO. 2010. The state of food insecurity in the world. Retrieved from: www.fao.org/publications/sofi/en/.

FAO. 2015. The state of food insecurity in the world. Meeting the 2015 international hunger targets: Taking stock of uneven progress. Retrieved from: www.fao.org/3/a-i4646e.pdf.

Ferro-Luzzi, A. 1994. Body mass index defines the risk of seasonal energy stress in the Third World. *European Journal of Clinical Nutrition*, 48: 165–178.

FEWS. 2011. USAID Famine Early Warning System. Retrieved from: www.fews.net/Pages/default.aspx.

Frisancho, A., et al. 1982. Relative merits of old and new indices of body mass with reference to skin-fold thickness. *American Journal of Clinical Nutrition*, 36: 697–699.

Ge, K. Y., & Chang, S. Y. 2001. Definition and measurement of child malnutrition. *Biomedical and Environmental Sciences*, 14(4): 283–291.

Gomez, F., et al. 1956. Mortality in second- and third-degree malnutrition. *Journal of Tropical Pediatrics*, 2: 7783–7788.

IBFAN. 2011. International Baby Food Action Network. Retrieved from: www.ibfan.org.

ICCIDD. 2011. International Council for Control of Iodine Deficiency Disorders. Retrieved from: www.iccidd.org/index.php.

IFPRI. 2010. International Food Policy Research Institute. Global Hunger Index. Retrieved from: www.ifpri.org/publication/2010-global-hunger-index.

INFAC. 2011. Infant Feeding Action Coalition, Canada. Retrieved from: www.infactcanada.ca.

IZINCG. 2011. International Zinc Nutrition Consultative Group. Retrieved from: www.izincg. org/.

Jelliffe, D. 1972. Commerciogenic malnutrition? *Nutrition Review*, 30: 199–205.

Keusch, G. 2003. The history of nutrition: Malnutrition, infection, and immunity. *The Journal of Nutrition*, 133: 336S–340S.

Krawinkel, M. 2003. Kwashiorkoris still not fully understood. *Bulletin of the World Health Organization*, 81: 910–911.

Lumley, J., et al. 2007. Periconceptual supplementation with folate for preventing neural tube defects. *Cochrane Database of Systematic Reviews*, Issue 4. Retrieved from: http://apps. who.int/rhl/reviews/CD001056.pdf.

Mishra, V., et al. 2000. Women's education can improve child nutrition in India. *National Family Health Survey Bulletin*, 15: 1–4.

MNI. 2009. Micronutrient Initiative. A united call for action on vitamin and mineral deficiencies. Retrieved from: www.gainhealth.org/sites/default/files/report/investing_in_the_future_ pdf_11749.pdf.

MNI. 2011. Micronutrient Initiative. Retrieved from: www.micronutrient.org/English/view. asp?x=1.

Olivares M, et al. 1999. Anaemia and iron deficiency disease in children. *British Medical Bulletin*, 55: 534–543.

Oxfam. 2005a. Food aid or hidden dumping? Oxfam briefing paper no. 71. Retrieved from: www.intermonoxfam.org/UnidadesInformacion/anexos/2969/0_2969_310305_Food_ aid_or_dumping.pdf.

Oxfam. 2005b. Making the case for cash: Humanitarian food aid under scrutiny. Oxfam briefing note. Retrieved from: http://reliefweb.int/node/22059.

Palloni, A., et al. 1994. The effects of breastfeeding and the pace of childbearing on early childhood mortality in Mexico. *Pan American Health Organization Bulletin*, 28: 93–111.

Pelletier, D. 1994. The relationship between child anthropometry and mortality in developing countries: Implication for policy, programs, and future research. *Journal of Nutrition*, 124 (Suppl. 10): 2047–2081.

Pelletier, D., et al. 1995. The effects of malnutrition on child mortality in developing countries. *Bulletin of the World Health Organization*, 73: 443–448.

Peng, X. 1987. Demographic consequences of the great leap forward in China's provinces. *Population and Development Review*, 13: 639–670.

Popkin, B. 2007. The world is fat. *Scientific American*, 297: 88–95.

Rousham, E. 1996. Socio-economic influences on gender inequalities in child health in rural Bangladesh. *European Journal of Clinical Nutrition*, 50: 560–564.

Schauer, C., et al. 2003. Home fortification with micronutrient sprinkles—a new approach for the prevention and treatment of nutritional anemia. *Journal of Pediatrics and Child Health*, 8: 87–90.

Schuman, A. 2003. A concise history of infant formula. *Contemporary Pediatrics*, 2: 91–93.

Sen, A. 1983. *Poverty and famines: An essay on entitlements*. Pub: Oxford University Press.

Smith, L., et al. 2000. Explaining child malnutrition in developing countries: A cross-country analysis. International Food Policy Research Institute. Retrieved from: www.ifpri.org/publication/explaining-child-malnutrition-developing-countries-0.

Sprinkles. 2011. Sprinkles Global Health Initiative. Retrieved from: www.sghi.org/about_sprinkles/about_sprinkles.pdf.

Timmer, C. 2005. Food aid: Doing well by doing good. Center for Global Development working paper. Retrieved from: www.cgdev.org/content/publications/detail/5342.

UN. 2010. The Millennium Development Goals report. Retrieved from: www.un.org/millenniumgoals/pdf/MDG%20Report%202010%20En%20r15%20-low%20res%20 20100615%20-.pdf#page=13.

UN. 2015. Transforming our world: The 2030 Agenda for Sustainable Development. Retrieved from: https://sustainabledevelopment.un.org/post2015/transformingourworld/publication.

UNICEF. 1998. The state of the world's children 1998. Focus on nutrition. Retrieved from: www.unicef.org/sowc98.

UNICEF. 2004. Clinical management of acute diarrhoea. Retrieved from: www.childinfo.org/files/ENAcute_Diarrhoea_reprint.pdf.

UNICEF. 2007. Vitamin A supplementation: A decade of progress. Retrieved from: www.unicef.org/publications/files/Vitamin_A_Supplementation.pdf.

UNICEF. 2011. Baby-Friendly Hospital Initiative. Retrieved from: www.unicef.org/programme/breastfeeding/baby.htm.

USDA. 2011. United States Department of Agriculture: Food and Nutrition Information Center. Retrieved from: www.nal.usda.gov/fnic.

Waterlow, J., et al. 1977. The presentation and use of height and weight data for comparing the nutritional status of groups of children under the age of 10 years. *Bulletin of the World Health Organization*, 55: 489–498.

Wellcome Trust Working Party. 1970. Classification of infantile malnutrition. *The Lancet*, 2: 302–303.

WHO. 2006. Global database on child growth and malnutrition. Retrieved from: www.who.int/nutgrowthdb/en.

WHO. 2009. Child growth standards and the identification of severe acute malnutrition in infants. Retrieved from: www.who.int/nutrition/publications/severemalnutrition/9789241598163_eng.pdf.

WHO. 2010a. Guidelines on HIV and infant feeding. Retrieved from: www.who.int/child_adolescent_health/documents/9789241599535/en/index.html.

WHO. 2010b. Neurological disorders associated with malnutrition. Retrieved from: www.who.int/mental_health/neurology/chapter_3_b_neuro_disorders_public_h_challenges.pdf.

WHO. 2011. WHO global database on childhood growth and nutrition. Retrieved from: www. who.int/nutgrowthdb/en/.

WHO. 2016. Data from Global Health Observatory visualizations: Joint child malnutrition estimates (UNICEF-WHO-WB). Retrieved from: www.who.int/nutgrowthdb/estimates/en/.

Woodham-Smith, C. 1992. *The great hunger: Ireland, 1845–1849*. Pub: Penguin.

CHAPTER 7

Governance and Human Rights in Developing Countries

The aim of all political association is the preservation of the natural and imprescriptible rights of man. These rights are liberty, property, security, and resistance to oppression.

—Declaration of the Rights of Man and of the Citizen, 1789

OBJECTIVES

Lasting improvements in population health cannot simply be based on a combination of medical treatments and economic growth. The essential foundation for any lasting development work must be an improvement in that population's human rights and standards of governance. Rights (and the good governance that fosters them) are not a luxury given only to rich people; they are an indispensable component of any national development effort. It is important to appreciate that improvements in governance and human rights are just as important as poverty alleviation and they should be a central feature of any sustainable development work. This chapter will examine the basic features of governance and also the history and development of human rights (both for adults and children). After completing this chapter, you should be able to:

- appreciate the broad concept of human rights and the slow development of human rights legislation for both adults and children
- understand the essentials of good governance and the indivisible relationship between governance and human rights
- understand the need for improvements in governance and human rights as a foundation for any lasting development intervention
- understand the details of some of the most common human rights abuses

INTRODUCTION TO GOVERNANCE AND HUMAN RIGHTS

> I am not interested in picking up crumbs of compassion thrown from the table of someone who considers himself my master. I want the full menu of rights.
>
> *—Bishop Desmond Tutu, 1985*

At time of writing, governance and human rights are highly topical issues. The revolt against tyrannous authority that started in Tunisia has subsequently spread throughout the Arab world in a broad band of countries stretching from the Arab peninsula across North Africa (Photo 7.1). Apparently unassailable regimes in Egypt and Libya have fallen, and Syria has been engulfed in a civil war. There is nothing new about a move toward benign governance, but the Arab uprisings have certainly accelerated the usual snail's pace of progress. Freedom House is one of the oldest non-governmental organizations and recently celebrated its 75th anniversary. Over much of that time, it has acted as a monitor of political rights and freedoms (Freedom House, 2011). Using their classification system, only 29 percent of countries were classified as "free" in 1975. This has slowly risen to 44 percent by 2015 (Figure 7.1). During those decades, some terrifyingly bad dictators have been

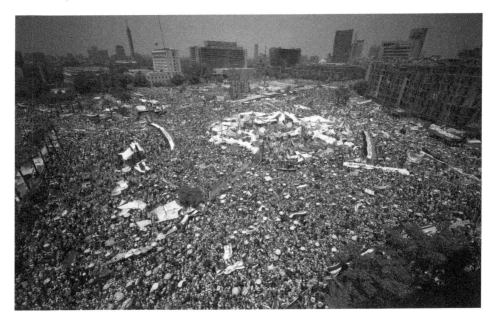

Photo 7.1: A shot of Tahrir Square in Cairo showing a vast crowd of Egyptian citizens demanding an end to their corrupt and oppressive regime.

Source: Photo by Ahmed Abd El-Fatah, courtesy of Wikimedia Commons.

removed—Idi Amin, Macias Nguema, Pol Pot, and Slobodan Milosevic are good examples. Unfortunately, there seems to be no shortage of others willing to take their place, such as Kim Jong-un of North Korea or al-Bashir of Sudan.

For those used to the peace and stability of a modern democratic country, it is difficult to imagine how badly many countries are still governed. It is hard to believe that there are still states—plenty of them, in fact—that torture and kill their own people. These governments don't care about national interest and they certainly don't care about their own people. Their actions are driven by one imperative—staying in power. If that requires a well-armed private militia rather than teachers, or tanks rather than schools, then those are the investments they'll make. Simply put, these countries would be much better off if their governments just agreed to do nothing. Even with the slow advances brought on by rebellion and, increasingly, outside intervention, roughly a quarter of the world's countries and over a quarter of the world's population live under tyrannous regimes. Collier's term "the bottom billion" (Collier, 2007) neatly sums up the lives of these unfortunate people, but it underestimates the total by half a billion.

The relationship between bad governance and population ill health is an obvious one. In fact it is so obvious and so clearly harmful to everyone involved that it is a mystery why these governments don't try some of the alternatives. The dictates of government self-interest produce terrible policies. At best, such

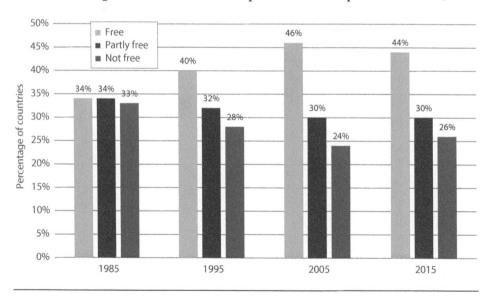

Figure 7.1: Trends in percentages of countries classified as free, partly free, or not free, 1985–2015

Source: Freedom House. 2016. Freedom in the world. Retrieved from: www.freedomhouse.org/template.cfm?page=1.

administrations simply don't care about the poor. For example, after cyclone Nargis, the Burmese government diverted food aid to the military rather than distributing it to affected survivors. At worst, once tribal or religious conflicts are added to the mix, governments can become positively dangerous to segments of their population, as happened in Darfur. The government of Sudan actively obstructed the delivery of food aid to the famine area and also used their oil profits to support military attacks against the local population. These actions were so blatant that the International Criminal Court issued an arrest warrant against al-Bashir, the president of the Sudanese government.

While it is true that the poor health of people living in such countries is largely due to the complicated end results of poverty, this is obviously not the full story. For a full understanding of the problem, it is necessary to ask the obvious question: Why are these people poor in the first place? Unfortunately, the answer is invariably a mixture of bad governance and lack of basic human rights—the two are just opposite sides of the same coin. They are absolutely central to population health and are also a fundamental requirement for any sustainable and effective interventions.

The problems of quantifying government efficiency will be discussed later, but no matter what measures are used, there are close relationships between governance

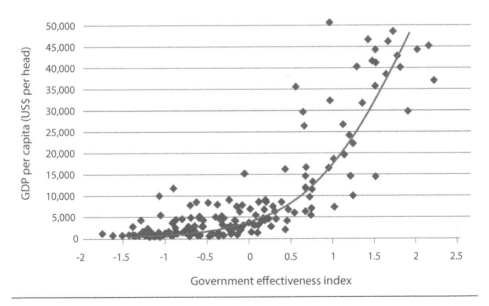

Figure 7.2: The relationship between government effectiveness and per capita income. The effectiveness index is based on the analysis of 17 national variables and ranges from −2.5 (very bad) to +2.5 (very good).

Sources: World Bank. 2011b. World development indicators. Retrieved from: http://databank.worldbank.org/ddp/home.do?Step=12&id=4&CNO=2; World Bank. 2010. World Bank governance indicators. Retrieved from: http://info.worldbank.org/governance/wgi/index.asp.

indicators and any conventional measures of health. A full analysis of the effects of bad governance would fill several books. Basically, bad governance is harmful for every level of society that requires coherent planning and management. Whether it is infrastructure development, economic policy, foreign relations, or investments in agriculture, health, and education, bad governments get bad outcomes. Predictably, as governance standards worsen, populations become poorer (Figure 7.2), they become hungrier (Figure 7.3), and they become sicker (Figure 7.4). As many Arab governments have now discovered, they also become increasingly desperate and angry.

Governance and human rights are tightly bound together. As a simple example, you don't get good government without the right to vote, but you aren't granted the right to vote without good government. Chicken or egg, it doesn't matter—you need them both for a healthy civil society. For the purposes of clarity, each is reviewed separately in this chapter, but in practice, they form an indistinguishable continuum. Whether they are called natural rights, universal rights, or human rights, the concept that humans are entitled to a range of freedoms, simply because they are human, has taken a very long time to develop. Although there have been brief periods of

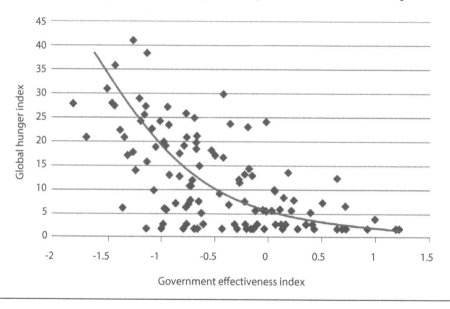

Figure 7.3: The relationship between government effectiveness and the adequacy of food supply. The Global Hunger Index is based on the analysis of three national variables. The higher the number, the worse the degree of hunger. Values below 5 are normal. Those above 30 represent countries with severe levels of hunger.

Sources: World Bank. 2010. World Bank governance indicators. Retrieved from: http://info.worldbank. org/governance/wgi/index.asp; IFPRI. 2010. International Food Policy Research Institute: Global Hunger Index. Retrieved from: www.ifpri.org/publication/2010-global-hunger-index.

enlightened rule in various countries, for much of human history average people have had little or no control over their own lives or over those who rule them. The theoretical ideas of human rights proposed by philosophers in the 17th and 18th centuries finally reached practical application during the late 18th century in the popular revolutions of America and France. It still took another 150 years and two world wars before the majority of the world's countries would come together in the mid-20th century to sign the first universal declaration of human rights.

It is worth remembering that the rights enjoyed by citizens of stable democracies did not appear overnight. They are the results of long struggles against unfair treatment and injustice. In Canada, the women's suffrage movement resulted in the granting of federal voting rights in 1920, but Aboriginal Canadians did not get the same privilege until 1960. It is also easy to forget just how recently international protocols against slavery, exploitation of children, and violence against women have been widely ratified. For example, universal agreement on the rights of children was not reached until the end of the 20th century. The rights, privileges, and, perhaps above all, the freedom from daily fear enjoyed by much of the world's population is just a dream for those unfortunate enough to live under the

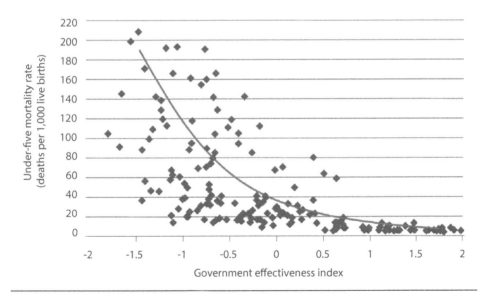

Figure 7.4: The relationship between government effectiveness and population health represented by the child mortality rate; similar graphs could be drawn using population life expectancy or maternal mortality as indicators.

Sources: World Bank. 2010. World Bank governance indicators. Retrieved from: http://info.worldbank.org/governance/wgi/index.asp; UNICEF. 2010. ChildInfo. Retrieved from: www.childinfo.org/mortality.html.

most oppressive regimes. Arbitrary arrest, state-sanctioned torture, religious or political persecution, and a host of other abuses are still daily realities for many people around the world.

In a society where abuse and repression are the norm, it is difficult for donor agencies and the local people to escape the dead hand of their government and participate as full partners in aid projects (Annan, 2005). There has been a growing realization that the absence of human rights acts as a very real barrier to successful development work. Sustainable improvements in population health require more than medical treatment and economic initiatives. Long-lasting gains have to be based on a foundation of social change and improved rights and freedoms for that population. Such changes are becoming an increasingly important part of large-scale population health initiatives.

GOVERNANCE IN DEVELOPING COUNTRIES

Little else is requisite to carry a state to the highest degree of opulence from the lowest barbarism but peace, easy taxes, and a tolerable administration of justice: all the rest being brought about by the natural course of things.

—Adam Smith, 1755

The Elements of Governance

The term "governance" refers to the total interplay of forces within a country that, taken together, determine how a country is run. It should not be confused with "government," which is only one part of the picture. The part played by government in the overall task of governance varies widely. In a few countries, such as Somalia, Chad, and Sudan, there is no effective government outside the major cities. As with Afghanistan, power in such failed states usually devolves to warlords and their armed militias. Some of the major contributors to governance are listed below.

Government Sector

In the Western model this is the country's legislative and administrative body. It is elected by a majority of the voting public. Systems vary, but the common factor in democracy is that voting rights are universal and principally restricted only by age. The country's judicial sector may be partly elected and partly appointed. Its task is generally to interpret and apply the law. It is the legislature's task to make new laws. There are, of course, many alternatives, including dictatorships (North Korea, Libya), theocracies (Yemen, Iran), and monarchies (Saudi Arabia, Swaziland). Democracy is not synonymous with good governance. Nigeria is nominally a democracy, but its economic and human rights histories are poor.

Box 7.1 History Notes

Nelson Rolihlahla Mandela (1918–2013)

Many leaders in history have paid a high price for their open support of human rights: Dr. Martin Luther King Jr. and Aung San Suu Kyi are good examples. Perhaps the most iconic is Nelson Mandela, of South Africa. Mandela was born in the Transkei in 1918. After mission school, he enrolled in college, but was suspended for joining a student protest. He studied law by correspondence and served his clerkship in Johannesburg. He first entered politics by joining the African National Congress (ANC) in 1942. Along with Sisulu, Tambo, and others, he began to change the ANC to a far more radical organization. The organization launched its Campaign for the Defiance of Unjust Laws in 1952. Its only weapons were boycotts, strikes, and civil disobedience.

Arrested for his part in the campaign, Mandela was given a suspended sentence. He opened a law practice with Oliver Tambo to represent the poorest people. Mandela was constantly harassed during the 1950s, including being banned from the Law Society, arrested, and imprisoned. After the Sharpeville massacre in 1960, where 69 protesters were shot dead, the ANC was outlawed. Mandela had to go underground, but was arrested in 1962. He was initially sentenced to five years, but when retried for other charges, he was sentenced to life in prison. He was finally released in 1990. He consistently refused earlier release in exchange for approval of apartheid, arguing, "Prisoners cannot enter into contracts. Only free men can negotiate." He was awarded the Nobel Peace Prize in 1993 and served as the first democratically elected president of South Africa from 1994 until he retired in 1999. He remained active through the work of three foundations that bear his name until his death in 2013. Follow the reference for more information: Nelson Mandela Biography (2017).

Public Sector (Civil Service)

Public sector institutions are responsible for the everyday administration of government services, such as the supply of electricity and water and the provision of education. Belgium's public sector is strong enough to run the country without any government intervention. In China, as far as outsiders can tell, the single ruling party and the powerful state bureaucracy appear to be almost on an equal footing. In Canada, there are public services at each level of government (federal, provincial/territorial, and local), which easily makes government the country's major employer.

This is the area of governance that is particularly important in terms of the administration of aid money going to government. For large interventions to stand any chance of success, the public service must be efficient, transparent, and accountable. Services are "transparent" when they are open to regular audits by an external body able to check administrative and financial procedures. An institution is "accountable" when it has to justify its expenditure and its decisions through the provision of regular financial and administrative reports. The strength of the public sector is the principal factor limiting the move toward "basket" aid funding for government ministries.

Civil Sector

An active and involved civil sector is an important aspect of good governance as it allows average people to be involved in the government process. The mechanism usually works through special interest groups that use the larger voice of the group to advance their interests with local government. The obvious example is a non-governmental organization such as Amnesty International. Others include citizen pressure groups, religious groups, and professional organizations. See Chapter 15 for more on this topic.

Other Elements—Developed Countries

Every country contains a complex mixture of influential groups. While developed countries certainly have problems with organized crime, gang warfare, and corruption, these usually don't become a threat to national stability. Mexico is, unfortunately, an example where, despite a stable democratic national government, corruption and a weak police force have resulted in a non-existent rule of law in the northern border regions. Other influential forces in developed countries include powerful political lobby groups, such as the US National Rifle Association, media moguls, and enormously wealthy transnational corporations.

Other Elements—Developing Countries

Malign influences in some developing areas that have lost central authority include warlords and their militias (Pakistan tribal areas), terrorist group Boko Haram (northeastern Nigeria), armed criminal gangs for hire (Kenya slums), predatory military (Burma), and a country's major export firms—often resource-extraction industries or external transnational companies.

MEASURING GOVERNANCE

I often say that when you measure what you are speaking about, and express it in numbers, you know something about it; but when you cannot express it in numbers, your knowledge is of a meagre and unsatisfactory kind.

—*Baron Kelvin, 1855*

Over the last 10 to 15 years, the topic of governance has become a central issue in the business of foreign aid. The professionalism of a developing country's public service, its ability to manage funds in a transparent manner, the levels of corruption and violence within the country, and the chances of the government's long-term survival are all of interest to many groups. Large agencies' allocation of foreign aid is increasingly dependent upon countries meeting acceptable levels of these and other variables. It should also be remembered that aid is only one part of the financial flows to developing countries. As will be discussed in Chapter 11, foreign investment in developing countries is now four to five times higher than aid, so governance indicators are of interest to a range of groups, including large investment firms, transnational corporations, government policy-makers, and academics. In response to this demand for information, there are now well over 100 governance indicators—so many, in fact, that there are now guides to governance indicators (UNDP, 2007).

The importance of governance indicators is such that anyone interested in the field of global health should have a good idea of their strengths and weaknesses. As with any other form of aggregated data collection, it is important to remember there are associated measurement errors—sometimes surprisingly large ones. Those errors increase rapidly every time a new variable is added to the mix. They are very definitely not to be viewed as flawless indicators that magically sum up the complexity of governance in a single number. It is important not to use them as a drunk uses a street lamp—more for support than illumination (Arndt, 2006). Some measures are based on quantifiable end points (debt levels, infant mortality rate, GDP per capita, etc.) but most rely more on subjective assessments of various questions scored by in-country representatives. Such measures are inevitably open to political or ideological observer bias. For example, central planning and closed markets might be viewed as very good or very bad governance, depending on the observer's point of view.

Before leaning too heavily on governance scores, it is important to look into their background. What are the affiliations and biases of the collecting agency? Do they have the funding to produce reliable reports for many countries over a long period?

Box 7.2 Moment of Insight

Total number of developing world women who died during pregnancy in 2008:	Total number of deaths if two fully loaded Boeing 747s crashed every day for a year:
343,000	**343,000**
Source: Hogan, M., et al. 2010. Maternal mortality in 181 countries, 1980–2008: A systematic analysis of progress towards MDG 5. *The Lancet*, 375: 1609–1623.	*Source:* Boeing. 2011. 747 family. Retrieved from: www.boeing.com/commercial/747family.

Do the scores measure government process, or do they ignore process and concentrate on measured outcomes? Are the end points quantifiable or based on subjective scores? Are the scored questions well designed or are they broad-based and open to many interpretations? Does the agency put in their own research or do they do nothing more than borrow scores from others and construct a weighted average? Do they publish the individual scores and do they make any estimate of error? These and other questions should be answered before using a score to help make decisions that may affect people's lives. The following are the most commonly used scores:

- *International Country Risk Guide (PRS, 2011):* The ICRG dates back to 1980, which makes it one of the oldest governance indicators. It is generated by a private company (PRS Group), which publishes regular updates on about 150 countries and territories in a monthly journal. This is the hard world of business, so you have to pay to get access to the scores. The score has three risk-assessment elements—financial, economic, and political. As a good example of the mixture of measures used in governance scores, the first two are based on quantifiable scores, while the third is based on expert subjective opinions about topics such as corruption, military influence, and potential for violence. No error estimates are given.

- *Freedom House (Freedom House, 2011):* This is another long-standing and much-quoted source of governance data. It was founded in 1941 as a voice for freedom and democracy. Its annual publication *Freedom in the World* rates over 200 countries and territories by their political rights and civil liberties. Each is based on expert opinion of a standardized list of questions and given a score from 1 (good) to 7 (bad). There are no objective measures used. The average of the two scores is used to classify countries as either free (score below 3) or not free (score above 5) (Figure 7.1). Answers for the individual questions and error estimates are not published.

- *Corruption Perception Index (CPI, 2011):* The CPI is not as old as the first two, but is certainly as influential. It was started in the mid-1990s when the end of the Cold War allowed the World Bank to start placing emphasis on corruption. The score ranges from 0 (most corrupt) to 10 (least corrupt). The final score is based on local questionnaire surveys, plus expert opinion. The component scores are not published, but the originating agency, Transparency International, does provide confidence limits covering the possible range of values for each country's score.

- *Country Policy and Institution Assessment (IEG, 2009):* The World Bank has been using some form of performance-based aid allocation since the 1970s. During that time the process has been refined and is now called the CPIA.

The final rating is based on scores for 16 variables grouped within four main categories (economic management, structural policies, equity, and public sector management). The four clusters are then used in a formula that calculates the final International Development Association (IDA) Resource Allocation Index (IRAI, 2010). In calculating the IRAI, 24 percent is given to the first three clusters, 68 percent is given to the fourth, and the remaining 8 percent is distributed between other variables, particularly the Portfolio Performance (World Bank, 2011a). The final score is calculated annually for about 80 IDA countries. It varies between 1 (poor) and 6 (high). Resources are generally allocated to countries above 3.5. The process was not transparent until the World Bank decided to publish CPIA and IRAI scores in 2006. Apart from its use by the World Bank, the score also influences the allocations of many other large agencies.

* *Worldwide governance indicators (WGI, 2010):* This group of six separate indicators has been published since 1996. They are often referred to as the KKZ indicators after the initials of the three originators of the project. Within the six different categories, scores are given for: voice and accountability, political stability, government effectiveness, regulatory quality, rule of law, and control of corruption. They are published annually by the World Bank Institute. A single unified average score is not used. They are complex indicators constructed using data from 31 different organizations. The WGI scores are as widely used as the CPIA. They form a large part of the selection criteria for the Millennium Challenge Account—particularly the Corruption score. The individual scores are not published, but, in common with the CPI, they do provide confidence intervals indicating the range of possible error for each score.

Governance and Aid Allocation

The problem of allocating aid—who gets what—is often lost in the noisier debate surrounding aid quantity, but it is a very important topic. Over the last two decades, there has been increasing attention paid to standards of governance as one of the major determinants of aid allocation, principally by multilateral organizations. Bilateral donors are slowly entering the debate, but as recently as 2008, Hoeffler showed that roughly half of bilateral aid was governed by donor-specific considerations (colonial ties, language), one-third was based on recipient need (poverty, disease), but only 2 percent was based on recipient merit (governance, corruption, human rights) (Hoeffler et al., 2008). Despite much talk of aid harmonization and efficiency, bilateral aid allocation lacks structure. To a

large extent, multilateral organizations are freed from individual past colonial associations and so are able to base their decisions on rather more objective criteria.
The World Bank has based allocations on a score balancing merit and need for
several decades (IEG, 2009). The newer Millennium Challenge Account selects
recipients using a number of scoring systems that are weighted toward merit,
particularly corruption control (WGI, 2010).

An egalitarian approach to funding is clearly too simple since India would do
rather better than the Solomon Islands using a per capita calculation (Utz, 2010).
In practice, some balance between merit and need is becoming the usual practice,
particularly since the study by Collier et al. (1999). While their methodology has
subsequently been criticized, the recommendation that aid should be used in countries with high needs (measured by poverty) and reasonable merit (defined as good
governance) has been highly influential. Unfortunately, there aren't many low-
income or lower-middle-income countries with good governance—Mali, Malawi,
Ghana, and Madagascar are examples. They are obviously attractive to donors,
giving rise to the term "donor darlings." At the other end of the spectrum are poor
countries with bad governance—Sudan, Somalia, and Zimbabwe are good examples. These "aid orphans" tend to be underfunded because of concerns by donors
about poor returns on investment.

Since the mid-1990s, governance has become such a central part of aid that it
is now both a major objective of aid projects and also a principal condition for aid
allocation. As usual, the reasons are complex and contentious:

- *Failure of economic reforms:* The economic reforms imposed on developing countries during the 1980s and 1990s were widely accepted as unsuccessful. Rightly or wrongly, these failures were principally attributed
  to government weakness and corruption. This led to a significant shift in
  policy at the World Bank toward good governance and the need to control
  corruption (World Bank, 1998).
- *End of the Cold War:* Before the fall of the Soviet Union, some truly terrible
  dictators were supported with aid because corruption and bad governance
  were ignored in favour of ideological allegiance. With the end of the Cold
  War, many tyrants were cut off from aid money and major institutions
  were now free to include governance in their allocation decisions.
- *Private foreign investment:* Direct foreign investment in developing countries has greatly outpaced increases in foreign aid. Large companies are
  not charities and want a clear return on their investments, which requires
  long-term government stability, low levels of corruption, and freedom
  from violence—all of which eventually come back to good governance.

- *Research opinion:* The governance–economic growth literature is large, but the predominant conclusion is that aid works best in an enabling environment of good governance, peace, and low corruption. While the paper by Roodman (2007) accepts this conclusion, it is critical of the methodology. It is also a very good review of the relevant literature.

While governance-based allocation is fine for average to well-governed countries, what is the long-term effect of this policy upon badly governed, poor countries (Rogerson et al., 2009)? Is there a risk that donor darlings will get a steadily larger slice of the aid pie, at the expense of the aid orphans, whose populations are in greatest need of assistance? Bearing in mind that not one of the fragile sub-Saharan African countries is on track to meet any of the Millennium Development Goals, it should be clear that learning how to assist badly managed fragile states remains the most difficult challenge facing the aid community today.

HUMAN RIGHTS IN DEVELOPING COUNTRIES

> No society can surely be flourishing and happy of which by far the greater part of the numbers are poor and miserable.
>
> —*Adam Smith, 1776*

Introduction to Human Rights

> Freedom, from which men are said to be free, is the natural power of doing what we each please, unless prevented by force or law.
>
> —*Justinian Codex, AD 529*

Human rights are discussed and analyzed in such detail by so many special interest groups that it is easy to lose sight of the big picture. Even those two simple words, "human" and "rights," are debated endlessly. What does it mean to be a "human"? Do human rights apply to unborn children, those with mental disabilities, or prisoners? What about "rights"? Are they different from needs or obligations? Who imposes them, who monitors them, and how are violations to be punished? Are all human rights equal or are some more important than others? As an example of the complex debate needed to establish widespread agreement on these issues, it took 1,400 rounds of voting on practically every word in every clause before the General Assembly adopted the Universal Declaration of Human Rights on December 10, 1948, in Paris (HRT, 2000). Such legal and philosophical debates are necessary when setting international conventions and laws, but in practice, it is not that difficult to tell when rights have been trampled. There are endless and unambiguous examples of human rights abuses: state-sanctioned torture and murder, imprisonment without trial, sexual exploitation of children, trafficking of humans, slavery, female genital mutilation, child labour, and many more. Whenever there is poverty and powerlessness, there will inevitably be discrimination or inequity very close behind.

Human rights should be differentiated from the social and legal obligations that any citizen has to follow in a civil society. Human rights are rather more abstract entities. They are independent of culture, race, class, age, or any other human subset; they consist of a set of rights one has simply through being a human (OHCHR, 2010). There is, of course, a debate about what constitutes the most basic rights, but most would agree that the steady growth of international legislation promoted by the UN over the last 50 years has shown that it is possible to establish a universally accepted set of basic human rights that are applicable to all countries and cultures in the world (Table 7.1).

There are many ways to categorize human rights (Donnelly, 2007). The simplest is to divide them into negative and positive rights. These are not judgmental terms; they simply describe the degree of government involvement. The concept of negative human rights emerges from the English (and subsequently American)

Table 7.1: Major milestones on the long road to universal human rights legislation

539 BC	The Cyrus Cylinder
250 BC	Ashok's Edicts
529	Justinian Codex
1100	King Henry I, Charter of Liberties
1215	King John I, Magna Carta
1689	English Bill of Rights
1776	US Declaration of Independence
1789	French Declaration of the Rights of Man
1791	US Bill of Rights
1893	Women's Vote, New Zealand
1945	United Nations formed
1948	Universal Declaration of Human Rights
1976	International Bill of Rights
1979	Convention on Elimination of All Forms of Discrimination against Women
1990	Convention on the Rights of the Child
2002	International Criminal Court formed
2006	Convention on the Rights of Persons with Disabilities
	International Convention for the Protection of All Persons from Enforced Disappearance

historical tradition of opposing government involvement in private life. Negative rights require nothing from government except that it should keep out of the way. These rights include freedom of speech, freedom of religion, and freedom of assembly (and freedom to carry arms in some countries). Positive rights tra~~ ~~~~~~ roots to the European (particularly French) tradition of expecting the gove to do something useful. These include the rights to an education, a liveliho~~ protection of equality for all citizens, and health.

Another common form of categorization was derived by Karel Vasak, a former head of the International Institute of Human Rights. He proposed three generations of human rights based loosely on the concepts of the French Revolution (liberty, equality, and fraternity). The first generation, based on liberty, consists of civil and political rights and is mostly negative (rights to life, liberty, free speech, movement, political and religious practice, fair trial, privacy, and voting). The second generation, based on equality, consists of social, economic, and cultural rights; they are mostly positive (rights to education, employment, and equality among citizens). The final group, based on fraternity, is less widely accepted and includes collective rights (rights to a clean environment, respect for cultural traditions, and peace). The recent recognition by the UN that water and sanitation are basic human rights is the first time that third-generation rights have been accepted (UN, 2010).

Other specific categories of human rights exist, including humanitarian rights (protection for those affected by armed conflict) and special rights claimed by particular groups (rights of workers, women, children, minority groups, refugees, Indigenous peoples, people with disabilities, etc.). Vasak's first- and second-generation rights can be seen in the two UN International Covenants adopted in 1966 (Covenant on Civil and Political Rights, and the Covenant on Economic, Social, and Cultural Rights). These became legally binding obligations for all signatories in 1976. Third-generation rights have not been codified by an international agreement.

Whatever classification is used, rights are interdependent, so attempting to place them into neat categories is, to some extent, artificial. For example, the rights to education and health cannot be entirely separated from the rights to life and liberty. The right to security may well conflict with the right to privacy (see the extensive debate surrounding the Patriot Act in the US). With all this complexity, it is easy to predict that some rights will conflict. The right to respect for cultural traditions, such as female circumcision, certainly conflicts with the right to self-determination and traditional practice. The right to a fair trial may conflict with the right to privacy, and the right to work may conflict with the right to a healthy environment. These should be viewed as challenges to be met by compromise; they are certainly not an excuse to abandon human rights.

Numerous controversies exist concerning human rights, but the most difficult is the challenge of setting universal human rights in a culturally diverse world (Ayton-Shenker, 1995). The imposition of universal rules was initially viewed as a form of cultural imperialism by which powerful countries dictated those rights they considered most important. With time, as more and more developing world countries sign on to international human rights treaties against slavery, torture, and other outrages against humanity, this argument has weakened. While the debate is not over, it is increasingly accepted that there is a fundamental set of universal rules that can be applied to all countries and cultures.

History of Human Rights Legislation

I have enabled all lands to live in peace.

—Cyrus the Great's Babylonian cylinder, 539 BC

The idea that human beings have rights simply because they are humans is largely a 20th-century concept. However, if history is examined closely, there were brief flashes of enlightened law-making before this period. The quote at the start of this

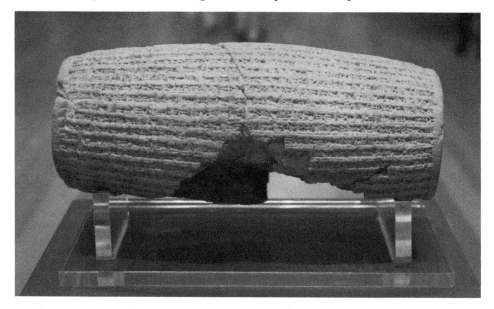

Photo 7.2: The original Cyrus cylinder in the British Museum; due to a widely circulated false translation, it has gained a reputation as an early declaration of human rights. A replica is displayed at the entrance of the United Nations headquarters.

Source: Photo by Mike Peel, courtesy of Wikipedia Commons.

section is from a small baked-clay cylinder uncovered in the 19th century at the site of Babylon. It is a 6th-century BC tablet, inscribed in cuneiform, describing the treatment of Babylonians after their conquest by Cyrus the Great (Photo 7.2). It is largely political propaganda, but due to a widely circulated false translation, it has gained a mistaken reputation as an early manifesto of human rights. As a result, a replica is displayed at the entrance to the United Nations headquarters. It should be added that after conquering Babylon, the inscription records that Cyrus didn't kill the population or destroy the city. By the standards of his day, that makes him an enlightened ruler worth remembering. The great 3rd-century BC Indian ruler, Ashoka the Cruel, later became Ashoka the Early Hippie after embracing Buddhism. Numerous inscribed rocks and pillars around his large kingdom can still be read and lay out enlightened rules, including religious tolerance and the abolition of slavery.

The great religions of the world all make extensive commentary on human nature, but the emphasis is usually on the duties and obligations of humans rather than their rights. This is typified by the ancient philosophical principle, often called the "golden rule" ("Do unto others as you would have them do unto you") (Wattles, 1996). This concept can be found throughout literature, ranging from the major religious texts to the popular character Mrs. Doasyouwouldbedoneby in the classical children's book *The Water Babies*. In the secular world, many ancient lawmakers collected lists of obligations and duties, but there was still very little emphasis on rights. The Code of Hammurabi from 1750 BC and the 6th-century Justinian Codex are good examples.

Throughout the Middle Ages, society was based on a hierarchical system, broadly separated into those who made war, those who prayed, and those who laboured (Bellatores, Oratores, et Laboratores). Very little time was wasted worrying about the rights of those at the bottom of the pile. The Magna Carta, signed by King John in 1215, is often thought to be the first crack in the structure of absolute power, but King Henry had already signed a charter of liberties limiting some of his powers 100 years earlier in 1100. By the 15th century, a small flicker of light had started to illuminate those dark European ages. Although various arbitrary names are given to the subsequent growth of humanism in Europe (Reformation, Enlightenment, Age of Reason), the rights we enjoy today can be traced back to the intellectual movement that started in Renaissance Italy (Rayner, 2006).

The Scottish philosopher John Locke (1632–1704) reflected the feeling of the times with his writing on human rights: "Every man has a property in his own person. This nobody has any right to but himself." Cromwell's revolution in 1640 did not do much for the rights of King Charles I, but the subsequent "Glorious Revolution" 40 years later, when the English swapped kings, led to the first European Bill of Rights in 1689. The desire for rights and freedoms developed further in the 18th century, ultimately leading to the Declaration of Independence by the American colonies in 1776. In common with many other attempts at human rights legislation, the words of the document ("We hold these truths to be self-evident, that all men are created equal") were more impressive than the subsequent deeds. Similarly, in 1789, the French Declaration of the Rights of Man and of the Citizen described human rights with equally impressive terms ("Men are born and remain free and equal in rights"), but that did not stop thousands of people from losing their heads during the subsequent Reign of Terror. Table 7.1 lists some of the main steps on the road to universal human rights.

The horrors of World War I and World War II managed to shock Western nations into realizing that human rights were not just an abstract debating point. In 1946, the newly formed United Nations established the Commission on Human Rights as the principal policy-making body for human rights legislation. Under the chairmanship of Eleanor Roosevelt, the commission started the difficult job of defining basic rights and freedoms. As noted above, after an exhaustive process, the General Assembly adopted the Universal Declaration of Human Rights on December 10, 1948, in Paris (UN, 2000).

The declaration did not have the legal force of a treaty, but widespread acceptance made it a cornerstone of the universal human rights movement. In 1966, the UN negotiated the International Covenant on Civil and Political Rights and another on Economic, Social, and Cultural Rights. Both came into force in 1976. Since they are legally binding, signatories are open to monitoring of their human

Table 7.2: Principal human rights legislation since World War II

1948	Universal Declaration of Human Rights
1965	International Convention on the Elimination of All Forms of Racial Discrimination
1966	International Covenant on Civil and Political Rights
	International Covenant on Economic, Social, and Cultural Rights
1979	Convention on the Elimination of All Forms of Discrimination against Women
1984	The Convention against Torture and Other Cruel, Inhuman, or Degrading Treatment or Punishment
1990	Convention on the Rights of the Child
	International Convention on the Protection of the Rights of Migrant Workers and Members of Their Families
2002	Rome Statute of the International Criminal Court
2006	United Nations Human Rights Council Formed
	International Convention for the Protection of All Persons from Enforced Disappearance
	Convention on the Rights of Persons with Disabilities
2007	United Nations Declaration on the Rights of Indigenous Peoples

rights practices. The two covenants, plus the universal declaration, are referred to as the International Bill of Rights (OHCHR, 2000); most modern countries are parties to both covenants. Six UN committees monitor compliance with various international treaties, including the Committee on the Rights of the Child, the Committee against Torture, and the Human Rights Committee. Table 7.2 summarizes the major human rights advances since World War II.

In the last decade, the UN has continued to make advances in this important area. A major achievement was the General Assembly's creation of the International Criminal Court (ICC, 2011). This developed from a variety of smaller, short-term courts established in the 1990s to prosecute war crimes in Rwanda and Yugoslavia. Around the same time, the existing UN Human Rights Commission had fallen into disrepute for allowing membership to countries with dreadful human rights records, such as Zimbabwe and Sudan. Finally, in a report in 2005, the UN secretary-general actually called for the abolition of the commission (Annan, 2005) and the establishment of a smaller council, which would meet throughout the year and restrict its membership to countries that meet accepted human rights standards. Despite opposition from the US, the new 47-member Human Rights Council held its first meeting in early 2006 (OHCHR, 2011).

Adult Human Rights

> Man's inhumanity to man makes countless thousands mourn.
>
> —*Robert Burns, 1786*

There seems no end to the abuses that cruel or greedy people can impose upon weak and powerless populations. The full range of those abuses of human rights is enormous; a complete review would fill a library. Many of these situations are virtually unknown to the general public. Some affect only a few thousand unfortunate people, so are too small to attract much attention. Examples include the abuse of child camel-racing jockeys in the Middle East (Caine et al., 2005) or the practice of child temple prostitution in southern India and Nepal (Mukhopadhyay, 1995). Others might affect millions and yet still be relatively unknown. For example, the rising price of gold has led to an enormous global gold rush. It is estimated that there are 15 million gold miners, working in 50 countries, mining under terrible working conditions (Spiegel, 2005). The 4 million women and 1 million children included in that total do not reach television screens, so the situation is virtually unknown, although the human and environmental costs are very real. In this section, we will examine a few of the most obvious and topical adult human rights abuses, including slavery, human trafficking, and violence against women.

Slavery

> Whenever I hear anyone arguing for slavery, I feel a strong impulse to see it tried on him personally.
>
> —*Abraham Lincoln, 1837*

Human nature being what it is, there have probably been slaves as long as there has been organized society—certainly as long as there has been war. Ancient Egyptian and Assyrian wall reliefs clearly show military captives. It seems unlikely that they would have wasted such a cheap source of labour. The Vikings traded and raided deep into Russia and eastern Europe; the term "slave" is derived from their word for Slavic "captive." The move to abolish slavery was a slow process; the major advances are summarized in Table 7.3. Although we are now at a point where all countries at least pay lip service to the concept of freedom, the widespread legal abolition of slavery has not brought the practice to an end. A recent review estimates there are 25–30 million people working as slaves today, probably more than there have ever been in history (Bales, 2004).

Slavery is common around the world, in both developed and developing countries. The Human Rights Center at the University of California, Berkeley, estimates that there are 10,000 slaves within the United States working in agriculture, factories,

Table 7.3: Major milestones in the slow progress against slavery

1787	Freed European slaves establish colony at Freetown, Sierra Leone
1794	France abolishes slavery
1804	Haiti, first republic of ex-slaves
1807	British abolish slave trading
1822	First Black American settlers land in Liberia (declared independent in 1847)
1833	Abolition of slavery in British colonies
1861–1865	American Civil War
1865	Emancipation of US slaves
1926	Slavery banned globally by the League of Nations
1948	Universal Declaration of Human Rights bans slavery
1956	UN Convention on the Abolition of Slavery
1966	UN Covenant on Civil and Political Rights becomes a legally binding agreement
2000	Protocol to Prevent Trafficking in Persons
2011	Charter of Fundamental Rights in the European Union, 2000, article 5, and Directive 2011/36/EU of the European Parliament and Council on preventing and combating trafficking in human beings and protecting its victims
2015	The Modern Slavery Act 2015 (an act of the Parliament of the United Kingdom)

restaurants, and hotels (UC, 2004). There is no reason to suppose that other developed countries are any different. Now that slavery is universally illegal, the movement of people to work in the various forms of slavery has become a criminal activity on an international scale. While it is important to appreciate the different forms of slavery, one should not lose sight of the larger picture by concentrating too much on definitions. Although there are obvious differences between a bonded labourer on a Central American farm and a West African child sold into the European sex trade, they share many common features that characterize the condition of slavery. These include the presence of force (mental or physical), physical restraint, absence of any individual power, and the ability to be sold or bought as a commodity. Modern examples of slavery include:

- *Bonded labour:* This is probably the most common form of slavery worldwide. Poverty forces people to sell themselves or their children as workers to repay a loan. The pay will never cover the repayments, so the debt never ends. The debt may also be passed on to the family's children.
- *Sex trade slavery:* This includes women and children forced into prostitution, pornography, or other forms of the sex trade. In some cases, debt or poverty is the motivation, while others may be tricked into working in another country with offers of domestic work.
- *Forced labour:* This term covers adults and children who are forcibly confined and made to work. Some are captured during war, as still happens in Sudan (Jok, 2001), while others are tricked into working and subsequently forced to endure harsh conditions with no pay through a variety of physical or mental threats. The category also includes involuntary domestic servitude. (Anti-Slavery International, 2011)

The average person can do little about the organized crime aspect of trafficking and slavery, but consumers can bring pressure to bear on unethical manufacturers through their choice of purchases. The fair trade labelling concept developed initially around coffee and cocoa production, but it has spread to a wide range of other products (Fairtrade Foundation, 2011). If manufacturers agree to introduce ethical codes of practice and follow international labour standards, their product is identified by a visible endorsement from one of a number of ethical trade organizations. As long as consumers subsequently buy those products, the pressure to change production practices is considerable.

Human Trafficking
The trafficking of humans, particularly women and children, is a rapidly growing global problem that is tied to international crime and slavery. The victim

profiles given in the US Department of State's annual report on human trafficking (USDS, 2011) provide human faces to this inhumane practice. Like slavery, trafficking is a problem in all countries, both developed (Kelly, 2002) and developing (Dottridge, 2002). Its illegal nature makes accurate numbers difficult to collect, but some estimates are available. The Department of State's report estimates that 600,000–800,000 men, women, and children are trafficked across international borders every year (USDS, 2011). Approximately 80 percent are women and up to 50 percent are minors. The principal reason for trafficking is commercial sexual exploitation. These estimates include only people trafficked across international borders and do not include the larger numbers trafficked within their own countries (Laczko et al., 2005). The International Labour Organization estimates that 200,000 women and children are internally trafficked in Southeast Asia alone (Derks, 2000) and that more than a million are moved globally every year. Reports from Bangladesh estimate that more than 13,000 children have been taken from the country over the past five years.

The US Federal Bureau of Investigation estimates that human trafficking generates US$9.5 billion in annual revenue; it is closely connected with large-scale international criminal organizations (Vayrynen, 2003). Profits are so high that there is a shift away from trafficking arms and drugs toward the movement of human beings. Drugs can only be sold once, but humans can be sold over and over again, providing a profit on each transaction. Forced transportation of humans through abduction, fraud, or some form of deception should be differentiated from human smuggling in which the participants are more or less willing.

The roots of trafficking are complex, but they include poverty, organized crime, violence, war, corruption, and discrimination against women. The most likely targets of traffickers are people from rural areas, children in large families, and ethnic minority groups (UNODOC, 2011). In some societies, there is a tradition of sending a young child to live with an extended family member in an urban centre. Traffickers can prey on such beliefs, promising the child's parents employment, training, or even marriage in town. In Africa, there is a large pool of street children who are particularly vulnerable to trafficking. They are the product of armed conflict, rural migration, poverty, and loss of parents to HIV/AIDS.

Such a profitable endeavour will not be stopped easily; eradication requires a combined approach. Improving educational and economical opportunities to vulnerable groups will give them better lives and reduce the likelihood that women and children will fall prey to human trafficking. Law enforcement has increasingly been helped by international treaties such as the United Nations Convention against Transnational Organized Crime and the Council of Europe's Convention on Action against Trafficking of Human Beings (Council of Europe, 2011). Reducing demand for the products of slave labour is also difficult. Ethical trade labelling can have an impact on a manufacturer's use of forced or slave labour, but the prosecution of those who travel to developing countries to use child prostitutes is still at a very early stage.

Violence against Women

The safest place for men is the home, the home is, by contrast, the least safe place for women.

—Susan Edwards, Policing "Domestic" Violence, 1989

Violence against women is a worldwide problem in developed and developing countries (Watts et al., 2002). The United Nations defines violence against women as "any act of gender-based violence that will likely result in physical, sexual, or psychological harm." Within this broad definition, a wide range of abuses can be included. These range from the insanity of so-called honour killings (Pope, 2005) to domestic violence, rape, forced child marriage, female genital mutilation, sex-selected abortion, and infanticide.

Exact statistics are not kept, but hundreds of millions of women around the world are affected. Even the single issue of domestic violence has been shown to be far more common than was accepted in past years. A review of various countries revealed the following rates of physical assault by a partner: Switzerland (21 percent lifetime, 7 percent in previous 12 months), Egypt (34 percent lifetime, 16 percent in previous 12 months), India (40 percent lifetime, 14 percent in previous 12 months), New Zealand (35 percent lifetime, 21 percent in previous 12 months), Nicaragua (28 percent lifetime, 12 percent in previous 12 months), Canada (29 percent lifetime, 3 percent in previous 12 months) (Watts et al., 2002). Research shows that almost all of the violence is perpetuated by men; women are at greatest risk from men they know, particularly male family members and intimate partners (Jeyaseelan et al., 2004). Physical abuse is usually also associated with long-standing psychological abuse. Experience has shown that social institutions have often blamed battered women or, at the very least, ignored them.

In countries where there are high rates of violence against women, there will inevitably be other gender-related abuses. For example, in areas of the world where females are not valued, the combination of early abortion of female fetuses and infanticide has seriously disturbed the gender ratio. In India, it has been estimated that there are 0.5 million missing female births annually (Jha et al., 2006). The health consequences of violence obviously include adverse physical and mental effects. Apart from the risks of physical injuries and in some cases death, abused women are more likely to suffer from depression, anxiety, psychosomatic symptoms, eating problems, and sexual dysfunction.

Although the UN passed a Convention on the Elimination of All Forms of Discrimination against Women in 1979, it was not until 1993 that abuse was explicitly targeted by the Declaration on the Elimination of Violence against Women. The very existence of violent acts against women is a manifestation of an unequal relationship between men and women within a society (WHO, 2003). Clearly, this has a long historical background. Apart from predisposing cultural attitudes toward women, some groups are at particular risk of abuse and violence. Examples include women in poverty, refugees, migrants, and minority groups.

As usual, the problem has to be dealt with at several levels. All countries should have strong laws prohibiting violent acts against women and, of course, those laws must be enforced. For example, the South African constitution is a model of gender equality, yet violence against women in that country's informal settlements is a serious endemic problem. Slow changes in societal attitudes toward domestic violence do occur with time as economy and education improve, but the process can be speeded up (WHO, 2011). Although it is a slow process, raising awareness of violence against women through educating boys and men is as important as passing laws protecting women's rights. It is also important to introduce education for the judicial services, such as judges and police officers who enforce the rules.

In Brazil, specific police stations have been introduced that deal only with women's issues such as domestic violence; they are staffed by women. The cycle of abuse will be broken only by collaboration among educators, health care authorities, the judiciary, the police, and mass information services. The state should also provide shelters, legal aid, and medical services for girls and women who have suffered violence. Apart from enforcing appropriate punishment, there should also be a system of treatment and counselling for the perpetrators.

The Rights of Children

> Please, sir, I want some more.
>
> —*Charles Dickens, Oliver Twist, 1837*

Development of Children's Rights

Prior to the 19th century, there were few supports for destitute children and little or no concept that a child might have rights. Abandoned children were collected by foundling hospitals, where they rapidly died. Children without homes either lived on the street or entered orphanages and workhouses. The idea of a long, happy childhood is a very recent development resulting from education and economic prosperity.

During the 19th century, there was a growing realization that children at least had the right to a roof over their heads. Dickens's work contributed to this sentiment. His books were accurate because he knew what he was writing about. By the age of 12, he had to work 10 hours a day, sticking labels on jars to support his family because his father was in debtors' prison. In the 1850s, it was estimated that 30,000 children were homeless in New York City alone. Charles Brace founded the Children's Aid Society in 1853 to help house these children. The approach of the day was to pick them off the streets and then send them west in trains to work on farms. This so-called "Orphan Train Movement" lasted into the 20th century and relocated over 120,000 children (CAS, 2011). A similar scheme was used in Britain. Between 1869 and the early 1930s, over 100,000 British "waifs and strays" were shipped off to Canada. Many suffered abuse and neglect while working as little more than bonded farm labourers (Snow, 2000).

The notion that children should be protected from the worst forms of child labour was reflected in the formation of the National Child Labour Committee in 1904 (NCLC, 2005). This organization still exists because there is still a need to protect children from exploitation in the workforce. The images of children working in early 20th-century America, captured by the American photographer Lewis Hine, became world famous. The first humanitarian agency specifically aimed at children (Save the Children) was started in 1919 by the Jebb sisters in England. It was initially planned as a short-term organization designed to help feed children affected by World War I. Unfortunately, the need continued and it has now grown to become a large international agency (ISCA, 2011).

Since World War II, all developed countries have established laws and societies aimed at protecting vulnerable children. However, until surprisingly recently, there was no international agreement specifically covering child rights. This was remedied in 1989 when a large meeting of world leaders accepted the Convention on the Rights of the Child (UNICEF, 2011). One year later, it became the first legally binding international agreement establishing the basic rights of the world's children. It has been ratified and accepted by every country in the world except Somalia and the United States. The Committee on the Rights of Children monitors implementation of the basic convention and also the implementation of two optional protocols introduced in 2000 (Protocol on the Involvement of Children in Conflict, and Protocol on the Sale of Children, Child Prostitution, and Child Pornography). Other relevant legislation includes the Protocol to Prevent Trafficking in Persons (especially women and children), adopted in 2000, and the International Labour Organization's Convention on the Worst Forms of Child Labour, adopted in 1999. These "worst forms" include trafficking, sale of a child, sexual exploitation, debt bondage, pornography, or excessively hazardous work.

Child Labour

> But they answer, "Are your cowslips of the meadows
> Like our weeds anear the mine?
> Leave us quiet in the dark of the coal-shadows,
> From your pleasures fair and fine!"

—*Elizabeth Barrett Browning, "The Cry of the Children," 1843*

The above poem was written in 1843 at a time when British society was waking up to the fact that living conditions for the poor were truly appalling—certainly, they were as bad as those in any developing country today. Although a bit sentimental for modern taste, it is impossible to read the poem without feeling a terrible sadness that such things were ever done to children (and are still done today). In 1833, the British Factory Commission Report revealed children were often employed from the age of six and made to work 14- to 16-hour days; they were kept awake by beating. The conditions in mines were even worse. The first legislation against child labour was passed in the same year that Barrett Browning wrote the above poem, but even then, it only raised the working age to 9 years in factories and 10 years in the mines!

The concept that childhood is an age of innocence is a very recent development. When Daniel Defoe visited Halifax in 1727, he thought it admirable that no child above the age of four was idle (Defoe, 1727). The liberal philosopher John Locke (1632–1704) recommended that poor children should be put to work at three years old, with a belly full of bread daily, supplemented, in cold weather, by a little warm gruel. In poor societies, children are viewed as small adults who have to work. Early in life, they are given jobs around the house and in the fields; this makes it very difficult to define acceptable and unacceptable forms of child labour.

Even the age limit of child labour is ambiguous. Most would agree that a 6-year-old is too young to work, but where is the line to be drawn—12 years, 14 years? Again, there is general agreement that what are termed the "worst forms" of child labour (prostitution, forced labour, child soldiers, etc.) are all clearly unacceptable, but part-time work in the family shop or piecework picking fruit in a local farm are not so clear-cut. The International Labour Organization keeps the best statistics on child labour (ILO, 2011). They tackle this problem by using four definitions of child labour:

- *Child employment:* Children getting pocket money for light work or helping in a family business; work does not interfere with school.
- *Child labour:* Children involved in excessively long or heavy work that either interferes with schooling or obliges them to leave school altogether.
- *Children in hazardous work:* Children involved in work that is hazardous to their physical and moral development; examples include the use of

dangerous equipment, excessively long hours, and exposure to physical and sexual abuse.

- *Worst forms of child labour:* This term is used to refer to the very worst ways in which children are used—prostitution (and the trafficking that goes with it), child soldiers, pornography, drug trade, and slavery. By the nature of the work, statistics are hard to gather.

These classifications have a large subjective element, but they provide the best available idea of the types and extent of child labour around the world.

In 2012, the ILO estimates that 264 million children, aged 5 to 17 years, were doing work of some form. For two-thirds of those children, the work was hard enough that it interfered with their schooling (child labour) and roughly a third of the labour was classified as hazardous to the child's safety (Figure 7.5). Although the world's population of children rose over that period, the numbers at work fell by many millions. Unfortunately, the economic crisis since those estimates were made has likely reversed that trend. Estimates of children in the worst forms of employment are hard to obtain. Based on the ILO's most recent figures, they form roughly 5 percent of the total, but this still represents millions of children living in utterly degrading and dangerous conditions (Table 7.4). The greatest numbers of working children are in Asian countries, but the highest percentages of children working are in sub-Saharan Africa (Figure 7.6).

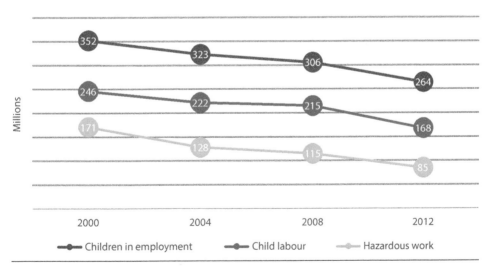

Figure 7.5: Trends in different forms of children's work between 2000 and 2012, age range 5–17 years

Source: ILO. 2013. Marking progress against child labour. Global estimates and trends 2000–2012. Retrieved from: www.ilo.org/ipec/Informationresources/WCMS_221513/lang--en/index.htm.

Table 7.4: Child labour distribution by level of national income, age range 5–17 years, 2012

NATIONAL INCOME CATEGORY	TOTAL CHILDREN ('000)	CHILD LABOUR ('000)	CHILD LABOUR (%)
Low income	330,257	74,394	22.5
Lower-middle income	902,174	81,306	9.0
Upper-middle income	197,977	12,256	6.2

Source: ILO. 2013. Marking progress against child labour. Global estimates and trends 2000–2012. Retrieved from: www.ilo.org/ipec/Informationresources/WCMS_221513/lang--en/index.htm.

Children work for a variety of reasons, the most important of which is poverty (Admassie, 2002). Although children are not well paid, they still serve as major contributors to family income in very poor developing countries. In places where education is inaccessible or of low quality, many children work simply because there is nothing else to do. Parents may find no value in sending their children to school when they could be home learning a skill such as agriculture and supplementing the family income. Traditional practices are also important. There is still a pervasive notion, in some areas, that educated females will not get married or have children. Young girls may be raised solely to take care of the household duties in order to release the mother for paid labour. Such practices restrict the education of females and

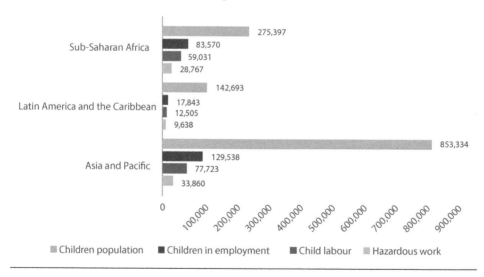

Figure 7.6: Children in employment, child labour, and hazardous work by region, age range 5–17 years, 2012

Source: ILO. 2013. Marking progress against child labour. Global estimates and trends 2000–2012. Retrieved from: www.ilo.org/ipec/Informationresources/WCMS_221513/lang--en/index.htm.

promote child labour. The acceptance of social class separation also perpetuates child employment. For example, people of India's lower castes are traditionally expected to perform manual labour; schooling may not even be considered.

There is a strong movement to abolish child labour in developing countries and require that children go to school (IPEC, 2011). This view is not as simple as it initially seems for a number of reasons. Although it is unfair that a young child should have to work every day, it is likely that many other factors in that child's life are also unfair. Simply banning work without putting in place other supportive social structures risks making a bad situation worse. This, of course, does not apply to the unconditional worst forms of child labour, but for the remainder, there are grey areas to consider.

Children will not attend school without an economic change in their condition. Schools must make it worthwhile for children to attend in order to make up for lost earnings. One necessary provision is that these schools should be free. Another possibility is that schools serve food supplements. If parents view schooling as having an advantage, then they will support attendance. The quality of education should also be improved so that schooling is considered an important factor in the future success of a child. Only after the introduction of such substitutes will school attendance increase. Another problem with complete abolition of child labour is that education and employment for children are not mutually exclusive. Many children go to school and also work in their spare time. In fact, many children have to work either to support their own tuition costs or those of their siblings.

Female Circumcision

Female circumcision (also known as "female genital cutting" or "female genital mutilation") is a term that covers a range of practices varying from a simple scratch of the clitoris to the partial or complete removal of the female genitalia (WHO, 2010). The procedure ranges from a mutilating excision of labia and clitoris (often with no hygiene) all the way to a ceremonial scratching or piercing of the labia. It is widely practised in central and northern Africa and is almost universal in some countries, such as Guinea, Egypt, Mali, and Eritrea (DHS, 2005). It is also practised in parts of the Middle East and in small areas of Asia. Some immigrant populations have imported the practice to European countries and North America. The practice is not condoned by any major religion, but it is sometimes given religious significance. In Egypt and Sudan, female circumcision certainly predates both Christianity and Islam by many centuries.

The justification for circumcision appears to be largely based on a belief that it will reduce sexual arousal in women (Kelly et al., 2005), making them less likely to engage in premarital intercourse or adultery. There are many other justifications for the practice, including a belief that contact with the clitoris is harmful to the husband or newborn baby. In countries where circumcision is commonly performed, uncircumcised women may have difficulty finding a marriage partner. The side effects of the more mutilating procedures include hemorrhage, painful scars, and chronic urinary and pelvic infections. Later in life, it can cause sexual dysfunction, depression, and a wide range of gynecological and obstetric complications (Lovel et al., 2000).

The UN Convention on the Rights of the Child is ambiguous about female circumcision. On one hand, Article 24 states that "parties shall take effective measures to abolish traditional practices prejudicial to the health of children," but Article 29 calls for "the development of respect for the child's parents and his/her own cultural identity and for the national values of the country in which the child is living." It is a question of personal rights, but whose rights? By making the eradication of female circumcision a human rights issue, it helps defuse accusations that this is just another example of cultural imperialism. Eradication of the worst forms of female circumcision is not aimed at cultures or religions; it is aimed at the most basic rights legally accorded to children.

The most mutilating forms of circumcision are found in areas of northeast Africa. In other parts of the world, particularly in Indonesia and Malaysia, the procedure has largely evolved into a symbolic ceremony with limited injury to the genitalia. Many would argue this is now a cultural tradition that is no worse than the widely accepted circumcision of males. The WHO estimates that 100–140 million women currently live with the effects of the procedure and over a million are performed every year (WHO, 2010a). Although it is important to pass laws making the practice illegal, legislation alone is not sufficient to reduce demand unless it is associated with interventions aimed at strategic points in society such as health professionals, health policy-makers, and the mass media. Programs based on community advocacy by religious and community leaders, plus the substitution of an alternative rite that does not involve any cutting, have been shown to be successful in Kenya, Senegal, and even Sudan (Diop et al., 2004).

SUMMARY

The term "governance" refers to the total interplay of forces within a country that, taken together, determine how a country is run. Lasting improvements in population health cannot simply be based on a combination of medical treatments and economic growth without good governance and human rights. Good governance and human rights are just as important as poverty alleviation and they should be a central feature of any sustainable development work. Good governance and human rights are mutually reinforcing elements. Without good governance, human rights cannot be respected and protected in a sustainable manner, and the implementation of human rights relies on a conducive and enabling environment. This includes appropriate legal frameworks and institutions as well as political, managerial, and administrative processes responsible for responding to the rights and needs of the population. The significance of good governance and human rights is reflected in its inclusion as one of the SDGs: "Promote peaceful and inclusive societies for sustainable development, provide access to justice for all and build effective, accountable and inclusive institutions at all levels." There has been a strong international focus on human rights starting with the General Assembly of the United Nations' adoption of the Universal Declaration of Human Rights in 1948, and then in the United Nations' Convention on the Rights of the Child in 1989. The issue of children's rights is particularly important as 168 million children worldwide are engaged in child labour, accounting for almost 11 percent of the child population as a whole. More than half of these children are also engaged in hazardous forms of work. Organizations like the International Labour Organization, and particularly the International Program for the Elimination of Child Labour, in the last few years have helped garner attention for the rights of children and have helped craft global and national frameworks, which has been a factor in the drop in the number of children in child labour in the last decade.

DISCUSSION QUESTIONS

1. What are the essential elements of good governance?
2. Why do improvements in governance and human rights lead to lasting developmental intervention?
3. What are human rights? What is the Universal Declaration of Human Rights?
4. Why has there been increasing attention paid to standards of governance as one of the major determinants of aid allocation?
5. What targets under SDG 16 relate to good governance and human rights?
6. What are the worst forms of child labour? How is the ILO helping child labourers around the world?
7. Why is the trafficking of humans, particularly women and children, a rapidly growing global problem?
8. What was the first legally binding international agreement establishing the basic rights of the world's children?
9. What is the "Orphan Train Movement"?
10. What are modern examples of slavery and how can they be addressed?

RECOMMENDED READING

Bales, K. 2004. *Disposable people: New slavery in the global economy*. Pub: University of California Press.

Donnelly, J. 2007. *International human rights*. Pub: Westview Press.

Malarek, V. 2004. *The Natashas: The new global sex trade*. Pub: Penguin Canada.

Shelley, L. 2010. *Human trafficking: A global perspective*. Pub: Cambridge University Press.

Skinner, E. 2008. *A crime so monstrous: Face to face with modern-day slavery*. Pub: Free Press.

United Nations. 2012. *The United Nations human rights treaty system*. Fact Sheet No. 30/Rev. 1. Available at: www.ohchr.org/Documents/Publications/FactSheet30Rev1.pdf.

REFERENCES

Admassie, A. 2002. Explaining the high incidence of child labour in Sub-Saharan Africa. *African Development Review*, 14: 251–275.

Annan, K. 2005. In large freedom: Towards development, security, and human rights for all. Retrieved from: www.un.org/largerfreedom/contents.htm.

Anti-Slavery International. 2011. What is modern slavery? Retrieved from: www.antislavery.org/english/slavery_today/default.aspx.

Arndt, C., et al. 2006. Uses and abuses of governance indicators. OECD Development Centre. Retrieved from: www.governance.unimaas.nl/training_activities/aau/download/Papers/Usesofabusesofgovernanceindicators%5B1%5D.pdf.

Ayton-Shenker, D. 1995. The challenge of human rights and cultural diversity. Retrieved from: www.un.org/rights/dpi1627e.htm.

Bales, K. 2004. *Disposable people: New slavery in the global economy*. Pub: University of California Press.

Basu, K., et al. 2003. The global child labour problem: What do we know and what can we do? *The World Bank Review*, 17: 147–173.

Boeing. 2011. 747 family. Retrieved from: www.boeing.com/commercial/747family.

Caine, D., et al. 2005. Child camel jockeys: A present-day tragedy involving children and sport. *Clinical Journal of Sports Medicine*, 15: 287–289.

CAS. 2011. Children's Aid Society. Orphan trains. Retrieved from: www.childrensaidsociety.org/about/history/orphan-trains.

Collier, P. 2007. *The bottom billion: Why the poorest countries are failing and what can be done about it*. Pub: Oxford University Press.

Collier, P., et al. 1999. Aid allocation and poverty reduction. World Bank Development Research Group. Retrieved from: http://go.worldbank.org/9ZRACQ2MT0.

Council of Europe. 2011. Action against trafficking in human beings. Retrieved from: www.coe.int/t/dghl/monitoring/trafficking/default_en.asp.

CPI. 2011. Transparency International's Corruption Perception Index. Retrieved from: www.transparency.org/policy_research/surveys_indices/cpi.

Defoe, D. 1727. *A tour through the whole island of Great Britain*. Pub: Everyman's.

Derks, A. 2000. Combating trafficking in South-East Asia. International Organization for Migration. Retrieved from: www.unesco.org/most/migration/ctsea.pdf.

DHS. 2005. Demographic health surveys: Female genital cutting 1990–2004. Retrieved from: www.measuredhs.com/topics/gender/FGC-CD.

Diop, N., et al. 2004. The TOSTAN program: Evaluation of a community-based education program in Senegal. Retrieved from: www.popcouncil.org/pdfs/frontiers/FR_FinalReports/Senegal_Tostan%20FGC.pdf.

Donnelly, J. 2007. *International Human Rights*. Pub: Westview Press.

Dottridge, M. 2002. Trafficking in children in West and Central Africa. *Gender and Development*, 10: 38–49.

Fairtrade Foundation. 2011. Retrieved from: www.fairtrade.org.uk.

Freedom House. 2011. Freedom in the world. Retrieved from: www.freedomhouse.org/template.cfm?page=1.

High Commission for Human Rights. 1989. Convention on the Rights of the Child. Retrieved from: www.unhchr.ch/html/menu3/b/k2crc.htm.

Hoeffler, A., et al. 2008. Need merit or self-interest—what determines the allocation of aid? Centre for Studies of African Economies. Retrieved from: www.csae.ox.ac.uk/working-papers/pdfs/2008-19text.pdf.

Hogan, M., et al. 2010. Maternal mortality in 181 countries, 1980–2008: A systematic analysis of progress towards MDG 5. *The Lancet*, 375: 1609–1623.

HRT. 2000. Human rights today: The Universal Declaration of Human Rights. Retrieved from: www.un.org/rights/HRToday/.

ICC. 2011. International criminal court. Retrieved from: www.icc-cpi.int/Menus/ICC?lan=en-GB.

IEG. 2009. The World Bank's country policy and institutional assessment. Retrieved from: http://siteresources.worldbank.org/EXTCPIA/Resources/cpia_full.pdf.

IFPRI. 2010. International Food Policy Research Institute. Global Hunger Index. Retrieved from: www.ifpri.org/publication/2010-global-hunger-index.

ILO. 2002. International Labour Organization. Every child counts: New global estimates on child labour. Retrieved from: www.ilo.org/public/english/standards/ipec/simpoc/others/globalest.pdf.

ILO. 2011. Global child labour developments: Measuring trends from 2004 to 2008. Retrieved from: www.ilo.org/ipec/ChildlabourstatisticsSIMPOC/lang--en/index.htm.

ILO. 2013. Marking progress against child labour: Global estimates and trends 2000-2012 Retrieved from: www.ilo.org/ipec/Informationresources/WCMS_221513/lang--en/index. htm.

IPEC. 2011. International programme on the elimination of child, action against child labor. Retrieved from: www.ilo.org/ipec/lang--en/index.htm.

IRAI. 2010. IDA resource allocation index. Retrieved from: http://go.worldbank.org/ S2THWI1X60.

ISCA. 2011. International Save the Children Alliance. Retrieved from: www.savethechildren. net/alliance/index.html.

Jeyaseelan, L., et al. 2004. World studies of abuse in the family environment: Risk factors for physical intimate partner violence. *Injury Control and Safety Promotion*, 11: 117–124.

Jha, P., et al. 2006. Low male-to-female sex ratio of children born in India: National survey of 1.1 million households. *The Lancet*, 367: 211–218.

Jok, J. 2001. *War and slavery in Sudan*. Pub: University of Pennsylvania Press.

Kelly, E. 2002. Journeys of jeopardy: A review of research on trafficking in women and children in Europe. International Organization for Migration, Research Series, no. 11. Retrieved from: www.evasp.eu/attachments/133_Journeys%20of%20Jeopardy.pdf.

Kelly, E., et al. 2005. Female genital mutilation. *Current Opinion in Obstetrics and Gynecology*, 17: 490–494.

Laczko, F., et al. (Eds.). 2005. Data and research on human trafficking: A global survey. International Organization for Migration. Retrieved: from:http://publications.iom.int/ bookstore/free/Global_Survey.pdf.

Lovel, H., et al. 2000. A systematic review of the health complications of female genital mutilation. Retrieved from: www.who.int/reproductivehealth/publications/fgm/who_ fch_wmh_00.2/en/index.html.

Mukhopadhyay, K. 1995. Girl prostitution in India. *Social Change*, 25: 143–153.

NCLC. 2005. National Child Labor Committee. Retrieved from: www.kapow.org/nclc.htm.

Nelson Mandela Biography. 2017. Retrieved from: www.nelsonmandela.org/content/page/ biography.

OHCHR. 2000. The International Bill of Human Rights. Retrieved from: www.ohchr.org/ Documents/Publications/FactSheet2Rev.1en.pdf.

OHCHR. 2010. What are human rights? Retrieved from: www.ohchr.org/en/issues/Pages/ WhatareHumanRights.aspx.

OHCHR. 2011. Office of the High Commissioner for Human Rights. Retrieved from: www. ohchr.org/EN/Pages/WelcomePage.aspx.

Pope, N. 2005. *Honor killings*. Pub: Palgrave Macmillan.

PRS. 2011. PRS Group's international country risk guide. Retrieved from: www.prsgroup.com/ICRG.aspx.

Rayner, M. 2006. History of universal human rights—up to WW2. Retrieved from: www.universalrights.net/main/histof.htm.

Rogerson, A., et al. 2009. Aid orphans: Whose responsibility? OECD Development Cooperation Directorate. Retrieved from: www.oecd.org/dataoecd/14/34/43853485.pdf.

Roodman, D. 2007. The anarchy of numbers: Aid development and cross-country empirics. Centre for Global Development. Retrieved from: www.cgdev.org/content/publications/detail/2745.

Snow, P. 2000. *Neither waif nor stray: The search for a stolen identity.* Pub: Universal Publishers.

Spiegel, S. 2005. Reducing mercury and responding to the global gold rush. *The Lancet,* 366: 2070–2072.

UC. 2004. Human Rights Center, University of California. Hidden slaves: Forced labour in the United States. Retrieved from: /digitalcommons.ilr.cornell.edu/forcedlabor/8/.

UN. 2000. Universal Declaration of Human Rights. Retrieved from: www.un.org/Overview/rights.html.

UN. 2010. UN resolution on the recognition of clean water and sanitation as basic human rights. Retrieved from: www.un.org/News/Press/docs/2010/ga10967.doc.htm.

UNDP. 2007. United Nations Development Programme. Governance indicators: A user's guide. Retrieved from: www.beta.undp.org/undp/en/home/librarypage/democratic-governance/oslo_governance_centre/governance_assessments/governance-indicators-2nd-edition.html.

UNICEF. 2010. ChildInfo. Retrieved from: www.childinfo.org/mortality.html.

UNICEF. 2011. Convention on the Rights of the Child. Retrieved from: www.unicef.org/crc/.

UNODOC. 2011. UN Office on Drugs and Crime. Human trafficking. Retrieved from: www.unodc.org/unodc/en/human-trafficking/index.html.

USDS. 2011. United States Digital Service. Trafficking in persons annual report. Retrieved from: www.state.gov/g/tip/rls/tiprpt/.

Utz, R. 2010. Will countries that receive insufficient aid please stand up? Concessional Finance and Global Partnership working paper no. 7. Retrieved from: http://go.worldbank.org/7Q74T3IXW0.

Vayrynen, R. 2003. Illegal immigration, human trafficking, and organized crime World Institute for Development Economics Research, discussion paper 2003/72. Retrieved from: www.wider.unu.edu/publications/working-papers/discussion-papers/2003/en_GB/dp2003-072/.

Wattles, J. 1996. *The golden rule.* Pub: Oxford University Press.

Watts, C., et al. 2002. Violence against women: Global scope and magnitude. *The Lancet,* 359: 1232–1237.

WGI. 2010. Worldwide governance indicators. Retrieved from: http://info.worldbank.org/governance/wgi/index.asp.

WHO. 2003. Multi-country study on women's health and domestic violence against women. Retrieved from: www.who.int/gender/violence/who_multicountry_study/en/index.html.

WHO. 2010. Female genital mutilation. Retrieved from: www.who.int/topics/female_genital_mutilation/en/.

WHO. 2011. Violence against women. Fact Sheet no. 239. Retrieved from: www.who.int/mediacentre/factsheets/fs239/en/.

World Bank. 1998. Development research group. Assessing aid: What works, what doesn't and why. Retrieved from: http://go.worldbank.org/2343YWFDQ0.

World Bank. 2010. World Bank governance indicators. Retrieved from: http://info.worldbank.org/governance/wgi/index.asp.

World Bank. 2011a. Annual report on portfolio performance. Retrieved from: http://go.worldbank.org/0500G3G5J0.

World Bank. 2011b. World Development Indicators. Retrieved from: http://databank.worldbank.org/ddp/home.do?Step=12&id=4&CNO=2.

CHAPTER 8

Water, Sanitation, and Infectious Diseases in Developing Countries

We shall not finally defeat AIDS, tuberculosis, malaria, or any of the other infectious diseases that plague the developing world, until we have also won the battle for safe drinking water, sanitation, and basic health care.

—UN Secretary-General Kofi Annan, 2001

OBJECTIVES

Much of the misery and ill health suffered by poor people on a daily basis is due to lack of the most basic provisions of a hygienic life. Apart from the discomfort and indignity caused by lack of sanitation, poor hygiene is the biggest single risk factor behind the high rates of infectious diseases in developing countries. Each year, roughly half a million children die from diarrhea simply because they don't have access to clean water. Another half a million die from pneumonia largely caused by the effects of overcrowding and terrible housing. Research has shown that diarrheal deaths can be halved simply by teaching caregivers to wash their hands! Water and sanitation initiatives are the most cost-effective aid initiatives, but this fact is greatly underappreciated. A knowledge of hygiene and its intimate connection with infectious diseases is absolutely vital for anyone interested in population health. After completing this chapter, you should be able to:

- understand the absolutely central place of water and sanitation in population health and the cost-effective nature of hygiene initiatives
- appreciate the extent of poor living standards around the world and the huge numbers of people who do not have access to clean water or sanitation
- understand the pathology and treatment of the three major infectious diseases—malaria, HIV/AIDS, and tuberculosis
- appreciate the range of less well-known but still important infectious diseases
- understand the pathology and treatment of the major infectious diseases of children

INTRODUCTION

> Public health is purchasable. Within a few natural and important limitations any community can determine its own health.
>
> *—Hermann Biggs, New York City's public health officer, 1899*

Children do not turn up at a medical clinic complaining of poor maternal education or lack of sanitation; they arrive with urgent medical problems—often infections—that demand immediate attention. It is easy to believe that treating those medical problems is the most important part of improving population health. Harsh experience with curative-based programs has shown clearly that long-term solutions must also be aimed at the underlying social problems that caused the infections. Once these are removed, measles, malnutrition, and dehydration slowly disappear (to be replaced by skateboard injuries). This does not, of course, mean that medical treatment has no value. Curative treatment is a vital part of the control of many diseases ranging from tuberculosis to gastroenteritis, but it is only a small part of a larger picture that has to include multiple interventions aimed at the underlying social inequities that produced those diseases in the first place.

Treating a severely dehydrated child with oral rehydration solution can produce dramatic temporary improvement, but if the baby is sent back to squalid,

Box 8.1 History Notes

James Grant (1922–1995)

Grant was born in China as a Canadian citizen; his father was a professor of public health at a medical college in what was then called Peking. He studied economics at the University of California and subsequently took law at Harvard. He became an American citizen after World War II. He started at the UN Relief Rehabilitation Administration in China and worked up through several international agencies until he founded and led the Overseas Development Council. He became head of UNICEF in 1980. In this position, he introduced the concept of the Child Survival Revolution. As a result of targeted programs for immunization, oral rehydration, and breastfeeding, an unimaginable number of children (perhaps as many as 25 million) cheated early death. Many millions more grew up stronger and healthier than they might otherwise have done. He also instituted the annual Progress of Nations Report and the State of the World's Children Report. He worked 12-hour days, six days a week, helped by assistants who worked in shifts. He was still dictating letters on the day of his death. His greatest achievement was to organize the UN Convention on the Basic Rights of the Child in 1989. He was awarded the Presidential Medal of Freedom in 1994. See the reference for further information: Jolly (2001).

overcrowded conditions with no access to clean water or sanitation, it will not be long before that child returns to hospital. Basic hygiene is and always has been important. With the possible exception of teenage boys, most humans have a natural tendency toward cleanliness. In Greek mythology, Asclepius's daughter Hygieia was the goddess of health and cleanliness 25 centuries ago. Despite this, it took a surprisingly long time before scientists such as Pasteur, Lister, and Koch established that micro-organisms were a common cause of disease (known as the germ theory). There was considerable resistance to the new ideas about germs and contagion—Florence Nightingale did not believe in it, and the famous obstetrician Ignaz Semmelweis was dismissed from his job and ridiculed because he made medical staff wash their hands between doing autopsies and examining patients (Thagard, 1997).

After discovering the causes of the problem, there was then another lengthy delay before anyone chose to do anything about it. London, in Queen Victoria's day, had sanitation standards no better than those of ancient Rome. They were forced to do something about their sanitation following the "Great Stink" of 1858, when the stench from the Thames was so bad that Parliament was not able to meet in the House of Commons. As a direct result, London was the first city to construct a system of closed sewers and pumping stations. The waste was pumped into the mouth of the Thames at high tide. Paris soon followed London's example, but Berlin didn't have anything similar to these cities until the very end of the 19th century. Even today, many of the world's growing "megacities" (population greater than 10 million people) have nothing approaching modern standards of universal clean water and sanitation. Examples include Delhi, Mumbai, Manila, Jakarta, and Karachi; each of these cities has over 15 million residents.

When standards of water and sanitation are poor, the importance of hygiene in personal health soon becomes apparent. When those standards fall rapidly, as happens following an acute disaster, the first results are water-borne diseases, such as gastroenteritis, plus their nastier cousins, cholera and typhoid. These are followed by skin infections and pneumonia. In chronic, long-standing areas of poor sanitation, hygiene becomes the principal determinant of ill health, particularly among the area's children. The resulting mortality is startlingly high and widely underappreciated. For example, 1.5 million children die annually from gastroenteritis secondary to contaminated water, and another 2 million die from chest infections largely caused by having to live in overcrowded, filthy shacks. At least another quarter of a million children die each year from accidents resulting from life in unregulated slums (Black et al., 2010). Improvements in hygiene can produce enormous benefits in reduced child mortality.

The general importance of hygiene and infectious diseases is reflected in their prominent place in the Sustainable Development Goals (SDGs). SDG 6, "Ensure availability and sustainable management of water and sanitation for all," has the following targets:

- By 2030, achieve universal and equitable access to safe and affordable drinking water for all.
- By 2030, achieve access to adequate and equitable sanitation and hygiene for all and end open defecation, paying special attention to the needs of women and girls and those in vulnerable situations.
- By 2030, improve water quality by reducing pollution, eliminating dumping and minimizing release of hazardous chemicals and materials, halving the proportion of untreated wastewater and substantially increasing recycling and safe reuse globally.
- By 2030, substantially increase water-use efficiency across all sectors and ensure sustainable withdrawals and supply of freshwater to address water scarcity and substantially reduce the number of people suffering from water scarcity.
- By 2030, implement integrated water resources management at all levels, including through transboundary cooperation as appropriate.
- By 2020, protect and restore water-related ecosystems, including mountains, forests, wetlands, rivers, aquifers and lakes.
- By 2030, expand international cooperation and capacity-building support to developing countries in water- and sanitation-related activities and programmes, including water harvesting, desalination, water efficiency, wastewater treatment, recycling and reuse technologies.
- Support and strengthen the participation of local communities in improving water and sanitation management.

In addition, the absolute importance of decent hygiene is reflected in the UN's decision to declare access to clean water and sanitation a basic human right (UN, 2010a).

It is not fair to load all the blame for this onto aid agencies. It should be remembered that contaminated water and lack of sanitation do not occur in isolation. They are simply a small part of a much larger problem of poverty and powerlessness that exists throughout many of the most fragile countries in the developing world. No significant improvement in hygiene, living standards, and their inevitable associated infectious diseases can be made without a comprehensive, multi-sectoral approach that addresses all levels of the problem. This is expensive, complicated,

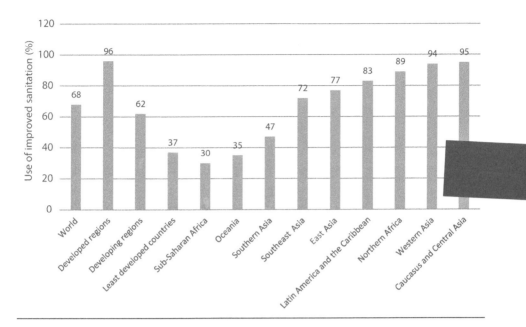

Figure 8.1: Use of improved sanitation for various world regions

Source: WHO/UNICEF. 2015. Progress on sanitation and drinking water: 2015 assessment and MDG update. Retrieved from: http://data.unicef.org/resources/progress-on-sanitation-and-drinking-water-2015-assessement-and-mdg-update.html.

and, above all else, requires enthusiastic and competent co-operation from all levels of government. There is a clear association between a country's development and the population's access to water and sanitation (Figure 8.1).

THE MAIN ELEMENTS OF HYGIENE

Clean Water

Thousands have lived without love, not one without water.

—*W. H. Auden, First Things First*

Easy access to a clean water supply is a fundamental requirement for a healthy life, and it has particular importance for the health of small children. The reduction of the numbers of people drinking dirty water on a daily basis is a major part of SDG 6. As usual, definitions are important. The monitoring agencies for the hygiene targets are WHO and UNICEF. They define three categories of water sources according to their level of safety (WHO/UNICEF, 2011):

- *Unimproved:* Surface water (stream, irrigation canal, lake, etc.), street vendor from carts, unprotected wells
- *"Other" improved:* Public taps, shared standpipes, protected and maintained wells and boreholes, rainwater collection
- *Improved:* Piped household water with the connection within the user's house or yard

At time of the last large survey in 2015, there had been steady improvements compared to the MDG starting point of 1990. Overall, 91 percent of the developing world's population has a safe drinking source. One of the targets of the MDGs was to halve, by 2015, the proportion of the population without sustainable access to safe drinking water and basic sanitation. The target for safe drinking water was surpassed in 2010, although Caucasus and Central Asia, Northern Africa, Oceania, and sub-Saharan Africa did not meet the target. Regardless, 2.6 billion people have gained access to an improved drinking water source since 1990, a number which represents 30% of the global population (Figure 8.2). However, there are still hundreds of millions of people drinking from unimproved sources.

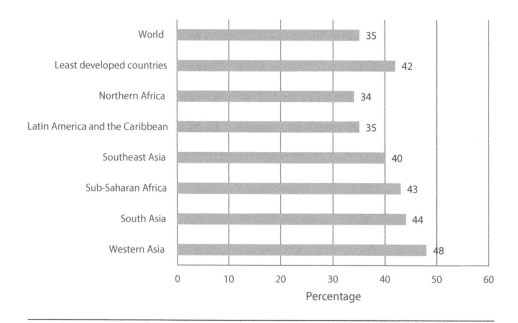

Figure 8.2: Proportion of 2015 population who gained access to an improved drinking water source since 1990 (%), by region

Source: WHO/UNICEF. 2015. Progress on sanitation and drinking water: 2015 assessment and MDG update. Retrieved from: http://data.unicef.org/resources/progress-on-sanitation-and-drinking-water-2015-assessement-and-mdg-update.html.

It is currently estimated that 663 million people worldwide do not have access to improved water sources; the majority of them now live in two developing regions: sub-Saharan Africa and South Asia (Figure 8.3).

The most obvious health risk associated with dirty water is the spread of water-borne infectious diseases. The most common agents in this group include bacteria (*E. coli*, salmonella), viruses (hepatitis A, rotavirus), helminths (schistosomiasis, Guinea worm), and protozoa (giardia, amebiasis) (WHO, 2016a). Mosquitoes also depend on stagnant untreated water for their larval stage. Apart from carrying numerous micro-organisms, water may also be dangerously contaminated by dissolved pollutants. Examples include arsenic and lead from industrial waste and high levels of nitrates from farming areas. While the portable water pumps used by many travellers are efficient at filtering infectious agents, it is important to remember that they cannot remove dissolved chemicals from a water source.

The United Nations responded to the importance of the clean water Millennium Development Goal by declaring an International Decade for Action on Clean Water. It started on March 22, 2005—World Water Day (UN, 2011). The main aim of the decade was to promote all aspects of the move

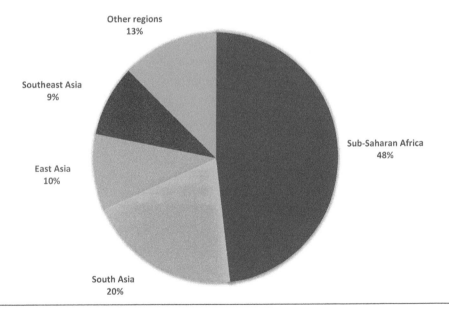

Figure 8.3: Proportion of population without access to improved sources of drinking water in 2015, by region; 663 million people lack access to improved drinking water sources in 2015.

Source: WHO/UNICEF. 2015. Progress on sanitation and drinking water: 2015 assessment and MDG update. Retrieved from: http://data.unicef.org/resources/progress-on-sanitation-and-drinking-water-2015-assessement-and-mdg-update.html.

Box 8.2 Moment of Insight

Total number of children who died from avoidable causes before their fifth birthday in 2010: **7,600,000**	Time taken, by the average person, to order a decaffeinated, double grande, triple macchiato with half and half, plus extra foam:
Number of seconds in a year: **31,536,000**	
One child dies of an avoidable cause every: **4.14 seconds**	**4.14 seconds**
Source: UNICEF. 2016. Child mortality. Retrieved from: www.childinfo.org/mortality.html.	*Source:* Independent research.

toward clean water. The sub-agency responsible is UN-Water (UN, 2016). There is no shortage of information for those interested. UN-Water runs two initiatives, including the UN Water Decade Programme for Capacity Development (UNW-DPC, 2011). The WHO Water, Sanitation, and Health website also provides information on the broader aspects of water safety, ranging from drinking water to waste-water treatment and water-borne infectious diseases (WSH, 2016). The WHO and UNICEF maintain a joint monitoring program for water supply and sanitation that provides updated estimates of drinking water and sanitation coverage based on household surveys (JMP, 2010).

It is estimated that the total volume of water on Earth is 1.4 billion km3, only 2.5 percent of which is fresh water. Since 70 percent of that water is locked in ice, that leaves less than 1 percent of the total for human use (UN, 2016). As a result of population growth and the associated increases in agriculture and industry, the world faces a very real crisis of water supply (UNESCO, 2003). Water's increasing scarcity has made it a more valuable commodity. Inevitably, private sector companies have grown to service this relatively new demand. The dominant companies are Thames Water, Vivendi, and Suez. Battle lines are drawn between those who believe clean water should be free and those who feel it should be paid for like any other service. The problem first became apparent in Bolivia when a private company obtained water rights for an area that included the town of Cochabamba (Shultz, 2000). Local activists organized widespread demonstrations that forced the government to reverse the privatization. Predictably, the poor were little better off after the reversal since they simply swapped privatized fees for local corruption.

Personal Hygiene

It must always be remembered that simply providing clean water is not sufficient on its own to make a significant impact on disease. Where populations have not had access to education, it is important to combine the provision of water with education on its use. This includes safe storage methods, care of pumps and wells, and personal hygiene. Apart from diarrheal diseases, lack of clean water is closely associated with a general lack of health, including skin and eye infections (particularly trachoma). It is estimated that over 5 million people worldwide are blinded by trachoma, and many times that number need treatment (Zhang et al., 2004). It is almost unbelievable that millions have lost their sight from a combination of dirty water and lack of soap to keep their hands and faces clean. The global alliance for the elimination of trachoma by the year 2020 relies on the SAFE strategy: Surgery, Antibiotic treatment, Facial cleanliness/handwashing, and Environmental changes (WHO, 2006a). Of all of these, regular cleanliness, based on a good supply of clean water, is the most important preventive factor.

Sanitation

> Again, our healthiest towns, such as Leamington, Cheltenham, Brighton, Hastings, and Scarbro', had little or no small-pox during the recent epidemic, whilst Birmingham, Leeds, Manchester, and similar large centres of industry suffered severely. Do not these facts confirm our previously expressed opinions that small-pox is a filth-disease, and like all filth-diseases, of the zymotic order, the only protection is in general and widespread cleanliness?
>
> *—John Pickering, 1876*

Good-quality housing and sanitation are as essential to health as access to clean water. Unfortunately, poor sanitation is at least three times more common than unsafe water supplies. Currently, roughly 50 percent of the developing world are without sanitation, as opposed to about 15 percent who lack clean water. As with clean water monitoring, the WHO and UNICEF define different categories of sanitation based on their degree of safety:

- *Open defecation:* Human feces disposed of or left in fields, bushes, or bodies of water
- *Unimproved facilities:* Facilities without safe separation from excreta, such as pit latrines without a slab, hanging latrines, or bucket latrines
- *Shared:* Acceptable facilities except that they are shared with other households or are open to public

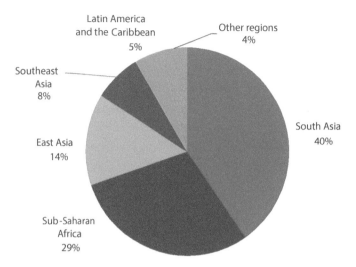

Figure 8.4: Proportion of population without improved sanitation in 2015, by region; 2.4 billion people do not use an improved sanitation facility.

Source: WHO/UNICEF. 2016. Progress on sanitation and drinking water: 2015 assessment and MDG update. Retrieved from: http://data.unicef.org/resources/progress-on-sanitation-and-drinking-water-2015-assessement-and-mdg-update.html.

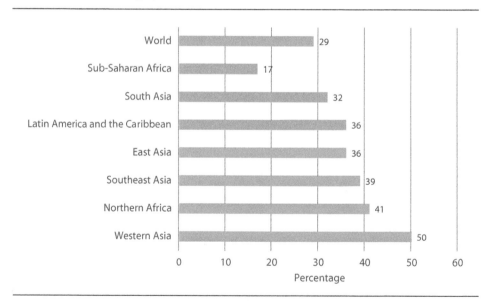

Figure 8.5: Proportion of the 2015 population who gained access to improved sanitation since 1990 (%), by region

Source: WHO/UNICEF. 2016. Progress on sanitation and drinking water: 2015 assessment and MDG update. Retrieved from: http://data.unicef.org/resources/progress-on-sanitation-and-drinking-water-2015-assessement-and-mdg-update.html.

- *Improved:* Flush toilet, composting toilet, pit latrine with ventilation and a covering slab

Nearly a third of the current global population has gained access to an improved sanitation facility since 1990, a total of 2.1 billion people (Figure 8.5). Western Asia and Northern Africa have provided access to 50 percent and 41 percent of the current population since 1990, while sub-Saharan Africa has provided access to less than 20 percent of the current population. In 2015, 2.4 billion people had no hygienic means of defecating (Figure 8.4), out of which 40 percent were in South Asia and 29 percent in sub-Saharan Africa (WHO/UNICEF, 2016).

Housing

Poor living conditions produce ill health through a number of mechanisms. Overcrowded, squalid huts provide breeding places for a number of disease vectors, including mosquitoes, fleas, and ticks. The mosquito is the worst of these vectors, spreading malaria, yellow fever, dengue, and filariasis. Poor handwashing, inadequate waste disposal, and absence of food and water storage inevitably lead to childhood diarrheal diseases. Poor air quality, particularly indoor smoke from cooking with wood or coal, predisposes children to a high rate of respiratory diseases. Respiratory infections now kill more children than diarrheal diseases each year (currently 2 million versus 1.5 million).

Polluted and overcrowded peri-urban slums are death traps for children. The World Health Organization estimates that 291,000 children were killed in 2003 from unintentional accidents such as traffic accidents, drowning, and poisoning; a further 14,000 were murdered (WHO, 2005). High levels of air pollution, open piles of household waste, low or absent standards for industrial waste disposal, chaotic traffic, and a host of other dangers lie in wait for careless children (Creel, 2002). An earlier study estimated 35 percent of the total burden of disease worldwide is due to environmental hazards (Kjellstrom, 1999). Finally, no restful or decent family life is possible when living under such circumstances. International studies have clearly shown that mental illness (particularly depression) is the most common cause of years lost to disability in the developing world (Stein et al., 2004). The daily grind of living under unbearable survival conditions is behind much of this morbidity. Poor living conditions are also closely associated with substance misuse, family violence, and child abuse. All are widespread (and often unacknowledged) problems in overcrowded settlements (Poznyak et al., 2005).

The importance of housing is reflected in the SDG to "make cities and human settlements inclusive, safe, resilient and sustainable of the targets" (SDG 11).

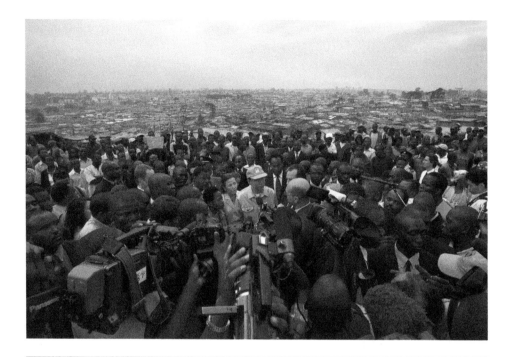

Photo 8.1: Former UN Secretary-General Ban Ki-moon briefs journalists about the UN-HABITAT project to resettle families living in the enormous Kibera slum, shown in the background. Kibera is only 5 km from the centre of Kenya's capital city, Nairobi. Its exact population is not known, but it is one of the largest slum settlements in the world.

Source: UN Photo/Eskinder Debebe, with kind permission of the UN Photo Library (www. unmultimedia.org/photo).

Specifically, target 11:1 states: "By 2030, ensure access for all to adequate, safe and affordable housing and basic services and upgrade slums." The continuing drift of people from the country into urban areas has now resulted in 3 billion people living in cities. A third of those, 1 billion people, live in slums without adequate sanitation, clean water, or any form of permanent shelter. The UN Human Settlements Programme (UN-HABITAT, 2005) and the World Bank formed the Cities Alliance and its "Cities without Slums" Action Plan (World Bank-UNCHS, 2005). Slum improvement schemes have had some claimed effects, with the proportion of slum dwellers falling in all regions (Figure 8.6). Total numbers are still rising because of population growth. Because of the past use of mass evictions to control slum populations, slum improvement remains a difficult and very contentious task (UN-HABITAT, 2006).

Although it takes many years to improve general living conditions in urban areas, disease control must work on a shorter time scale. Apart from improvements

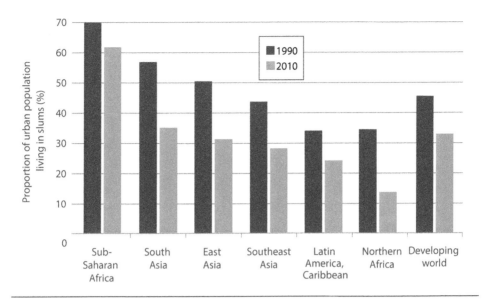

Figure 8.6: Trends in the proportion of urban populations living in slums for different regions of the world between 1990 and 2010

Source: UN. 2005. UN task force on improving the lives of slum dwellers. Retrieved from: www.unmillenniumproject.org/documents/Slumdwellers-complete.pdf.

in water and sanitation, one technique that can bring faster results is control aimed at the major disease-carrying biting insects. Vector control is no substitute for adequate standards of urban planning, but it does offer well-tested methods of interrupting some common diseases while longer-term urban solutions slowly develop (Townson et al., 2005). Vector-control techniques include treated bed nets (malaria), indoor residual spraying (Chagas disease), insect traps and screens (trypanosomiasis), and large-scale spraying (onchocerciasis).

THE RESULTS OF POOR HYGIENE

> To the people of poor nations, we pledge to work alongside you to make your farms flourish and let clean waters flow.
>
> —*President Barack Obama, inaugural speech, 2008*

The Disease Burden

Good hygiene is so central to human health that it should be no surprise to learn that lack of hygiene is responsible for a large share of the world's burden of disease. It is directly responsible for 10 percent of adult disease and as much as 20 percent of the

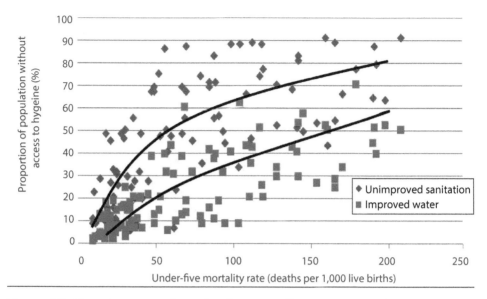

Figure 8.7: Plot of a country's under-five mortality rate against the proportion of its population that has no access to clean water or sanitation

Sources: WHO/UNICEF. 2011. Progress on sanitation and drinking water: 2010 update. Retrieved from: www.who.int/water_sanitation_health/publications/9789241563956/en/index.html; UNICEF, 2016, Child mortality, retrieved from: www.childinfo.org/mortality.html.

diseases of children (WHO, 2008). There is a clear relationship between a country's levels of hygiene and its child mortality rate. The relationship between mortality and clean water access is almost a completely straight line (Figure 8.7). This is an area where targeted aid spending can produce large benefits both in health and in economic improvement. The major diseases caused by the combination of polluted water, no sanitation, and a poor living environment are the following.

- *Diarrhea:* It is usually no more than a nuisance for adults, except during epidemics of severe water-borne infections such as cholera and typhoid. Among children, it is the second-most common cause of death. The introduction of oral rehydration solution has reduced the death rate, but current figures estimate that 1.5 million children still die from completely avoidable gastroenteritis every year.
- *Malnutrition:* Recurrent attacks of gastroenteritis result in worsening malnutrition. These days, a relatively small number die directly from starvation. The principal problem is that the weakened child suffers a far higher mortality rate from other common infections such as pneumonia. Overall, lack of hygiene causes an extra 800,000 deaths by this indirect mechanism (WHO, 2008).

- *Intestinal worms:* Roughly a third of the world's population is chronically infected with intestinal worms caused by fecal contamination of water. Examples include hookworm and ascariasis. Mortality is low, but economic and schooling costs associated with chronic illness are considerable.
- *Filariasis:* In both Asia and the Americas, filarial infections spread by mosquitoes from stagnant dirty water cause lymphatic filariasis in millions of people. At least 25 million are seriously incapacitated with swollen, immobile legs. Death rate is low, but economic cost is high.
- *Trachoma:* It is estimated that at least 5 million people are blind due to an eye infection spread through dirty water. When caught early, it can be easily treated with antibiotics. The best way to avoid it is to have schools teach regular hand and face washing. (S A.F. E)
- *Schistosomiasis:* This is a widespread parasitic infection caught from stagnant fecally infected water—commonly irrigation canals. Over 200 million people are infected worldwide. It causes significant economic costs from chronic ill health.
- *Malaria:* This is a parasitic disease spread by mosquitoes that breed in dirty water sources. Most adults in endemic areas have enough immunity to avoid death, but regular attacks have an enormous worldwide economic cost. Among children it is often lethal. Death rates have fallen recently, but malaria still kills at least 500,000 children every year.
- *Other mosquito-borne diseases:* Mosquitoes cause a lot more trouble than just spreading malaria. They are also the primary vector for a range of other serious illnesses, including various forms of viral encephalitis, dengue, and onchocerciasis.
- *Drowning:* Small children can get into trouble with surprisingly small amounts of water in bathtubs or sinks. Drowning is just one part of the broader picture of traumatic deaths among children living in slum conditions. Many of these deaths can be avoided through suitable legislation and education.

Taken together, the diseases associated with poor hygiene cause a large fraction of the world's disease burden. Among adults, lack of hygiene is responsible for 9.1 percent of all Disability-Adjusted Life Years (DALYs) lost and 6.3 percent of all deaths. Among children it causes 22 percent of all DALYs and 25 percent of all deaths (WHO, 2008). The contributions of the various causes to this disease burden are given in Figure 8.8.

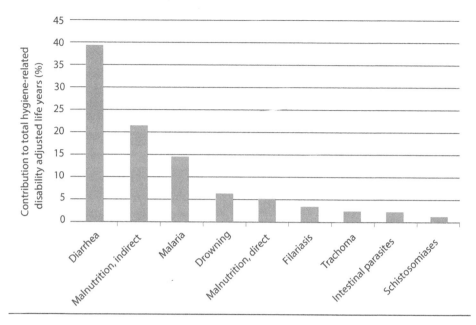

Figure 8.8: The contribution of various hygiene-related diseases to the overall total hygiene-related burden of disease

Source: Pruss-Ustun, A., et al. 2006. Preventing disease through healthy environments: Towards an estimate of the environmental burden of disease. WHO Report. Retrieved from: www.who.int/quantifying_ehimpacts/publications/preventingdisease.pdf.

The Economic Burden

Poor hygiene is obviously tightly bound up with poverty as both cause and effect. Poverty worsens hygiene because families and their local governments cannot afford the necessary investments in clean water, sanitation, and improved housing. In a horrible perpetuating cycle, lack of hygiene directly causes numerous health problems, which then worsen poverty because chronically ill adults cannot work and ill children do not go to school. Affected populations are trapped in an endless cycle of poverty, ill health, and terrible living conditions from which they cannot escape without assistance. There is a clear relationship between a country's hygiene standards and any measure of economic prosperity (Figure 8.9).

Economic estimates always contain a large subjective element, so they are to be used only as a guide. However, the WHO's numbers are still impressive (Hutton et al., 2004). The WHO estimates that if the sanitation goals were met, it would save 320 million productive days among adults each year, an extra 272 million school attendance days among older children, and 1.5 billion extra healthy days

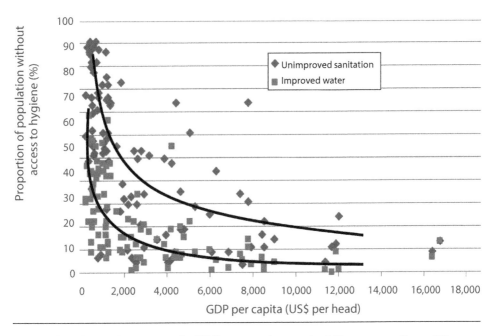

Figure 8.9: Plot of a country's GDP per capita against the proportion of its population that has no access to clean water or sanitation

Sources: WHO/UNICEF. 2011. Progress on sanitation and drinking water: 2010 update. Retrieved from: www.who.int/water_sanitation_health/publications/9789241563956/en/index.html; World Bank. 2011. GDP per capita. Retrieved from: http://data.worldbank.org/indicator/NY.GDP.PCAP.CD.

in children under five years! The total economic return, in terms of more working days, better health, and less time wasted on the simple tasks of keeping clean, is estimated to be US$84 billion per year.

INFECTIOUS DISEASES

> Infectious disease is one of the few genuine adventures left in the world. About the only sporting proposition that remains unimpaired by the relentless domestication of a once free-living human species is the war against those ferocious little fellow creatures, which lurk in dark corners and stalk us in the bodies of rats, mice, and all kinds of domestic animals; which fly and crawl with the insects, and waylay us in our food and drink and even in our love.
>
> —*Hans Zinsser, Rats, Lice, and History, 1935*

The Big Three

A combination of social change and scientific advances has produced huge advances against many infectious diseases. Previously common diseases such as measles, diphtheria, and pertussis have almost disappeared in developed countries. Progress against several others has been so good that they are now uncommon even in the poorest countries. Examples include polio, leprosy, onchocerciasis, Guinea worm, filariasis, and Chagas disease. Some members of that terrible group may even join smallpox one day as infectious agents that have been eradicated from the planet. It should be added that the cost of completely removing the last few cases is so high that strong arguments have been made to aim for "rare but still present" rather than complete eradication (Thompson, 2007). Unfortunately, there will always be infectious agents. Some will be old favourites, such as tuberculosis and malaria, which have parasitized humans as long as we have existed. Just when we deal with them, nature seems to create new ones, such as SARS and HIV, or old ones in a new form, such as avian influenza.

Obviously, there will never be an end to infectious diseases, but they can be kept under control. Currently, the greatest infectious threats to human health and productivity are HIV/AIDS, tuberculosis, and malaria; estimated total deaths from these diseases in 2009 were 1.8 million, 1.3 million, and 0.8 million, respectively. Doubtless that list will be completely different in 50 years, but right now those are the ones to deal with. Controlling the spread of these three agents consumes a lot of money either in direct targeted programs, such as Roll Back Malaria, or in indirect projects aimed at housing, sanitation, and nutrition. Anyone interested in the aid industry needs to have a good level of knowledge about these three infections.

Malaria

> Malaria defeated the international community 50 years ago. We cannot allow this to happen again.
>
> *—Margaret Chan, director-general, WHO, 2009*

Malaria has infected humans for thousands of years (CDC, 2010), likely for as long as there have been humans. Clear descriptions of the disease exist in early Chinese texts, such as the "Yellow Emperor's Medical Classic" (from about 200 BC). Hippocrates described typical cases in his writing and must have been familiar with the disease at least 25 centuries ago. Even though the exact cause of malaria was not discovered until the early days of the 20th century, it had long been associated with marshes and swamps. The enormous economic and social importance of the disease is reflected in the fact that three Nobel prizes have been awarded for research into malaria: Laveran for discovering the parasite, Ross for discovering the mode of transmission, and Müller for the introduction of DDT. The importance of reversing the increasing incidence of malaria is reflected in its selection as an SDG target (3.3).

Malaria is caused by a single-cell protozoan from the genus *Plasmodium*. Four members of the family cause disease in humans: *P. falciparum*, *P. vivax*, *P. ovale*, and *P. malariae*. Ancient names for the disease reflect its association with mosquito areas: *mal aria* means "bad air" in Italian. The parasite does not have an animal reservoir and is spread from human to human by the female anopheles mosquito (TDR, 2010). After entering the body through mosquito saliva, it multiplies in liver cells for a few days before rupturing into the bloodstream and invading red cells. *P. falciparum* does not have a liver cycle and, in general, produces the most severe form of disease. Waves of fever occur as merozoites subsequently burst out of infected red cells on a regular basis. The Romans noted differences in this periodicity and distinguished between tertian and quartan fevers. Destruction of red cells leads to anemia, jaundice, and fever. Some patients progressively slide into shock, renal failure, lung failure, involvement of the brain blood vessels (cerebral malaria), and death. Adults in endemic areas have sufficient immunity to keep the fatality rate low, but it remains a debilitating disease. Those with reduced immunity (children, travellers, and pregnant women) have a much higher mortality. Case fatality rates for travellers are roughly 5 percent, which is a good reason to take precautions when travelling.

Treatment relies on early use of effective anti-malarial drugs. This is a complex topic because of the extensive array of drugs (and drug combinations) and changing patterns of resistance (WHO, 2010d). The earliest effective anti-malarial was Qinghao, derived in China from *Artemesia annua*. Its use is described in the ancient manuscript "Fifty-Two Remedies," found in a 2,000-year-old tomb. Over the last decade, artemesinin drugs have been rediscovered. In combination forms, they are the mainstay of modern treatment. Jesuit missionaries in South America introduced quinine, another early drug, to Europe. Derived from the bark of the quina-quina tree, quinine remained the principal treatment until chloroquine was introduced in 1946. Chloroquine is still an effective drug against most strains of *P. vivax* and *P. malariae*, but *P. falciparum*'s almost universal resistance to chloroquine means other drugs must now be used. There is a growing trend to use combination therapy as standard treatment for malaria. Apart from combining the benefits of two individual therapies, it may also delay drug resistance (WHO, 2010d). Combinations such as sulphadoxine/pyrimethamine and atovaquone/proguanil are being replaced by Artemesinin-based Combination Therapy (ACT).

Unfortunately, the complexity of the malaria life cycle makes it very difficult to develop an effective vaccine (Targett, 2005). Several have been tested, but clinical efficacy has been low. Eradication efforts must be based on basic public health principles. In the early 1950s, the development of effective treatments (chloroquine) and effective long-lasting residual sprays (DDT) raised the hopes that malaria could be eradicated. The World Health Assembly proposed a worldwide eradication program in 1955 along the same line as the smallpox program. At the time, malaria had only just been eradicated from the United States and was still endemic in parts of Europe. The program was successful in many countries, but the emergence of drug resistance, insecticide resistance, wars, lack of funding, and poor involvement of affected communities ultimately led to abandonment of the project in 1969. The founding of Roll Back Malaria in 1998 (RBM, 2011), the MDGs in 2000, and RBM's subsequent Global Malaria Action Plan (RBM, 2008) have all combined to produce significant gains over the last decade. RBM has now grown into an enormous coalition of partners with the single aim of controlling malaria.

Malaria control is difficult, so the Global Action Plan is based on a combination of early diagnosis and treatment combined with methods aimed at preventing transmission. It consists of the following interventions (RBM, 2008):

- *Insecticide-treated mosquito nets:* Regular use of a treated net is effective and can reduce child deaths from malaria by over 20 percent (Eisele et al., 2010). Most are now treated with a long-lasting insecticide (LLIN), which lasts the life of a net—roughly three years. High rates of use produce benefits even for non-users because of the effective killing of local mosquitoes. Improved funding has allowed a rapid increase in bed net production.
- *Indoor residual spraying:* Spraying residual insecticide around living and sleeping areas is an effective barrier to malaria transmission. It must be done at least once a year, particularly before high-transmission times, by adequately trained personnel. DDT remains the most efficient long-acting insecticide. After much contentious debate, it has been reintroduced, only for malaria control, after a 30-year ban (WHO, 2009a).
- *Prompt diagnosis and treatment:* The tendency to delay seeking prompt attention and the habit of treating all fevers as "malaria" both reduce management effectiveness. Once effective treatment is known to help, those practices change. Diagnosis must be based on microscopy or modern rapid diagnostic tests, followed by effective treatment. Current therapy is based on artemesinin combination drugs for *P. falciparum*, plus chloroquine for other sensitive malaria forms (WHO, 2010a). The need for trained caregivers and sustainable supplies of drugs and testing reagents has large implications for organizational capacity and cost. Again, improved funding has greatly increased the supply of effective drugs.
- *Intermittent treatment during pregnancy:* Infection during pregnancy increases the risk of maternal anemia, low birth weight, and risk of premature birth. The final result is increased maternal and infant mortality

(Crawley et al., 2007). Management consists of two short treatment courses given in the second and third trimesters. Sulphadoxine-pyrimethamine is the usual choice of drug combination.

After a rocky start that resulted in a major organizational change in 2006, the RBM consortium has managed to achieve significant success in recent years. Measuring the exact numbers of cases and deaths is difficult because of the tendency to attribute all febrile illnesses to malaria. The best monitoring statistics are available for process rather than outcome. Examples include the numbers of pregnant women treated, children sleeping under nets, bed net production, and drug availability. Measured by these yardsticks, the RBM consortium has been busy and effective. Outcome statistics are not so detailed, but a clear picture of success does emerge (WHO, 2010b). In 2000, there were roughly 300 million cases and 1 million deaths, most of which were in children. By 2009, this had fallen to 225 million cases with 791,000 deaths. It is estimated that a million children's lives have been saved in that decade. While there are 106 countries where malaria remains endemic, three countries have recently been declared clear of the disease (Morocco, Turkmenistan, United Arab Emirates). In addition, 43 countries (11 in Africa) reported more than 50 percent reductions in malaria cases and deaths.

Tuberculosis

I saw pale kings and princes too,
Pale warriors, death-pale were they all;
They cried—"La Belle Dame sans merci
Hath thee in thrall!"

—John Keats, "La Belle Dame sans Merci," 1884

Tuberculosis has probably been a scourge of humanity as long as malaria. Definite evidence of infection has been found in mummified pharaohs and Neanderthal skeletons (Dormandy, 2001). The disease was called "Phthisis" by Hippocrates, who warned that the disease could be caught from infected patients. The name dates back to the 17th-century observation that infected lungs contain characteristic nodules (tubercles). Koch discovered the staining technique that enabled him to see the organism for the first time. Treatment relied upon nutrition and rest in sanitoria until the first tuberculosis drug (streptomycin) was developed in 1943. Waksman was awarded the Nobel Prize after searching for an active drug among 10,000 different soil microbes.

Tuberculosis is caused by a rod-shaped bacterium. Most disease is caused by *Mycobacterium* tuberculosis (CDC, 2011a). The principal source of infection is airborne droplets from infected patients, but intestinal infection still occurs in areas where milk from infected cattle is not pasteurized. What happens next depends on the host's resistance. The individual immune response is affected by individual susceptibility, nutritional level, age, and associated diseases (particularly HIV/AIDS)—social determinants of health are vitally important in the control of tuberculosis. Over 90 percent of well-nourished healthy people control the initial infection with no further disease beyond the small initial focus of lung infection. A large percentage of the world's population are infected with TB in this manner. The primary infection may remain latent for life or, under some circumstances, might reactivate years later. In susceptible patients, the bacterium spreads to other organs of the body, including the bones, kidneys, and brain. Overwhelming tuberculosis, often in children, leads to miliary tuberculosis.

In the early days of the 20th century, TB was the most common single cause of adult death throughout the world. Social change and medical treatments have greatly reduced that mortality, but TB still remains a serious threat to public health. The World Health Organization estimates there were 9.4 million new tuberculosis cases in 2009 and roughly 1.3 million deaths (WHO, 2010c). Ninety-eight percent of all deaths occurred in developing countries, particularly in sub-Saharan Africa. A particular concern has been the emergence—or at least the recognition—of resistant organisms. In 2008, over 400,000 cases (3–4 percent of total new cases) were resistant to at least two standard drugs (MDR-TB). Limited information suggests that 10 percent of these isolates were resistant to multiple drugs (XDR-TB). In that same year, 150,000 patients died from MDR-TB. Resistant TB is three times more lethal than sensitive TB, and is 10 times more expensive to treat (WHO, 2010d).

The diagnosis of TB is based on the clinical findings, chest X-ray, and examination of infected material (usually sputum). A skin test (Mantoux test) is available, but interpretation is difficult, particularly in the presence of HIV/AIDS. Treatment is, of course, based on combinations of antibiotics. After the introduction of streptomycin, it soon became obvious that single-drug treatment was associated with rapid development of drug resistance. Many variations of TB treatment courses exist, but all now rely on an initial period of three or four medications, which are cut back to two drugs as time progresses (CDC, 2011a). The *Mycobacterium* divides relatively slowly, so intermittent treatment schedules can be used. More complex (and far more expensive) multi-drug regimes are necessary to control resistant TB (Mitnick et al., 2008).

The importance of TB is reflected in the fact that major efforts were made to control it years before the Millennium Development Goals were established. In 1991, the World Health Assembly recognized TB as a major threat to world health. The initial aims were to detect 70 percent of all new cases using sputum staining and successfully treat 85 percent of those detected cases. The DOTS (Directly Observed Therapy, Short course) strategy (see below) was widely introduced in 1994, and the Stop Tuberculosis Initiative (Stop TB) was established in 1998 (StopTB, 2011). When it came to TB goals, the MDGs took a back seat to the Stop TB partnership. MDG 6 simply aimed to halt and reverse the increase in newly infected people, whereas, in addition to its earlier detection and treatment aims, Stop TB aims included to halve the 1990 mortality and prevalence rates by 2015, and to eliminate TB as a public health problem by 2015.

There was a 47% decrease in TB mortality between 1990 and 2015, with an estimated 43 million lives saved between 2000 and 2015 (WHO, 2015). The MDG target to reverse the spread of the disease by 2015 has been achieved on a worldwide basis, as the number of new cases of tuberculosis has been slowly falling by an average of 1.5 percent per year since 2000. It is important to note that the WHO includes HIV co-infection when it measures prevalence of TB, but its mortality figures refer to patients who died from single infection. They do not include mortality from HIV co-infection. The elements of the Stop TB Strategy were (WHO, 2006b):

- *Vaccines:* The BCG (*Bacillus Calmette Guerin*) vaccine was introduced in 1921 and has been shown to reduce mortality from tuberculosis in children. It appears to be less effective against reactivated pulmonary tuberculosis in adults. Several vaccines are under development around the world; it is hoped that a more effective vaccine will be available within a decade (Doherty et al., 2006).
- *DOTS strategy:* Patient compliance is an important factor in any form of drug treatment from hypertension to diabetes. Tuberculosis compliance is particularly important because open, untreated cases represent a threat to the greater population. Consequently, considerable effort has been put into ensuring that TB patients actually take their drugs. Whether in developed or developing countries, it has been shown that "Directly Observed Therapy, Short course" by a health worker or supervisor (DOTS strategy) is a vital element in TB treatment (CDC, 2011a).
- *Case detection:* New cases used to be detected by mobile population X-ray screening. Case detection now relies on sputum microscopy of symptomatic people seeking care (WHO, 2006b). This obviously requires investment in TB centres and trained technicians. Since HIV infection is closely related to an increased risk of tuberculosis, TB control centres should be closely linked with HIV/AIDS-control programs.
- *Treatment standardization:* Standardization of treatment is essential for optimum care and also to avoid development of drug resistance. The TB

Coalition for Technical Assistance has taken a lead in this area (TBCTA, 2006). Malaria treatment lags behind TB in this regard. Diagnosis, treatment, monitoring, and response to resistant organisms are best managed and controlled by internationally accepted standard protocols. A clear protocol for managing drug-resistant TB must be in place.

- *Drug access:* Treatment requires a supply of affordable and effective drugs, which, ideally, should be free of charge. Use of fixed drug combinations improves adherence to treatment. The Global Drug Facility (GDF) has been established to improve the global supply of effective anti-tuberculosis medication (GDF, 2011).

The WHO's End TB Strategy was launched in 2015 as a succession to the Stop TB initiative. It aims to end the global TB epidemic, to cut new cases by 90 percent between 2015 and 2035, and to ensure that no family is burdened with catastrophic expenses due to TB. The End TB Strategy includes a vision, a goal, and three high-level indicators with corresponding targets for 2030 and 2035. The 2035 targets are:

1. To reduce the absolute number of TB deaths by 95 percent compared with a baseline of 2015.
2. To reduce the TB incidence rate by 90 percent to ≤10 cases per 100,000 population per year, and
3. To eliminate the catastrophic costs faced by TB-affected families. This target is set to be achieved by 2020 (WHO, 2015b).

HIV/AIDS

> I asked about the cabbages. I assumed it supplemented their diet? Yes, they chorused. And you sell the surplus at market? An energetic nodding of heads. And I take it you make a profit? Yes again. What do you do with the profit? And this time there was an almost quizzical response as if to say what kind of ridiculous question is that.... "We buy coffins of course; we never have enough coffins."
>
> —*Stephen Lewis, former deputy director of UNICEF*

The first reports of a new acquired form of immune deficiency, predominantly among homosexual men, appeared in the Western medical literature in early 1981 (Gottlieb, 1981). Many initially believed that it was due to immune damage from recreational drug use, but epidemiological studies subsequently indicated an infectious etiology. By 1983, the Pasteur Institute had isolated what subsequently proved to be the causative virus. There was much subsequent argument about the naming and discovery of the virus (and rights to the lucrative HIV test) between French and American

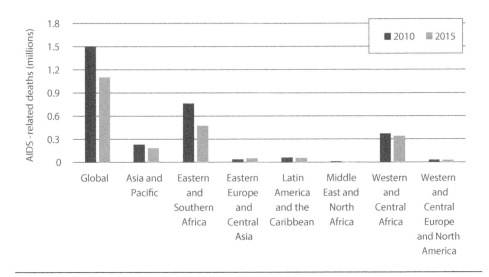

Figure 8.10: AIDS-related deaths, global and by region, 2010 and 2015

Source: UNAIDS. 2016. Global AIDS update. Retrieved from: http://www.unaids.org/en/resources/documents/2016/Global-AIDS-update-2016.

laboratories (Gallo, 2003). The final agreed name was "human immunodeficiency virus" (HIV). HIV is a single-strand RNA virus from the genus *Lentivirus*. Of the two forms, HIV1 is by far the most common; HIV2 is mostly found in West Africa. HIV is transmitted between humans by close contact with bodily fluids (blood, semen, breast milk), contaminated blood (needle exchange, transfusions), and mother-to-infant transmission (pregnancy, childbirth, breastfeeding).

Only a decade after the first reports, the virus was already established as a global epidemic affecting all parts of the world. While it certainly affects rich populations, as with any other infectious disease, its burden falls most heavily on the poorest people and the poorest countries, particularly those in sub-Saharan Africa (Figure 8.10). The size of the epidemic is hard to comprehend. Based on the most recent published estimates (UNAIDS, 2016), roughly 36.7 million people worldwide are living with HIV infection (Figure 8.11). During the total course of the epidemic, over 30 million people have died. As a result of an extraordinary international effort, some degree of control has been obtained. The number of new cases peaked in the late 1990s and annual deaths have slowly declined each year since 2005. The number of people living with the disease is still increasing because of greatly improved case survival rates.

The full clinical picture of HIV infection is enormous (CDC, 2011b). Its principal mechanism of action is to infect components of the immune system, particularly a subgroup of white cells called CD4+ T cells. Progressive damage

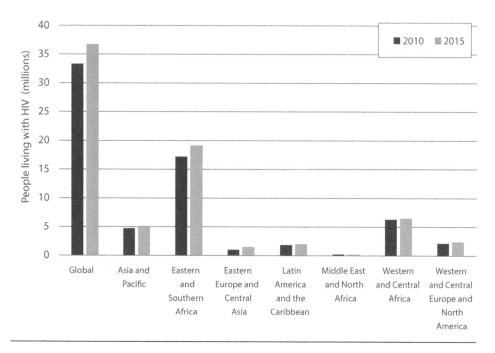

Figure 8.11: HIV epidemic estimates, global and by region, 2010 and 2015

Source: UNAIDS. 2016. Global AIDS update. Retrieved from: http://www.unaids.org/en/resources/
documents/2016/Global-AIDS-update-2016.

to the cellular immune system leads to a growing risk of opportunistic infections (pneumocystis pneumonia, tuberculosis, and cytomegalovirus) and also malignancies (Kaposi sarcoma, B-cell lymphomas, and cervical cancer in women). In late-stage disease, direct viral infection of other body organs such as the brain, kidneys, or liver can also cause significant disease. Progression of the disease is very variable, ranging from months to years. Subsequent development of the infection is influenced by age of onset, nutrition, other infections, and effective viral treatment. During the early stages, the patient may be completely asymptomatic except for an initial fever and lymphadenopathy. As the disease progresses, weight loss and various skin infections such as candida and herpes appear. Later stages are characterized by bacterial infections, tuberculosis, spread to the brain, and severe wasting.

The case fatality rate is ultimately very high. Roughly 5 percent of infected patients appear to remain stable over many years, but the majority slowly progress to fully expressed late-stage AIDS. Median interval from initial infection to severe immune deficiency is eight to nine years, but it is generally accepted to be shorter in most developing countries (Dorling et al., 2006). Survival time after onset of severe AIDS is also variable. In the absence of supportive care and antiviral treatment, the progression from full-blown AIDS to death usually occurs in less than a year, but this can be dramatically altered by provision of effective antiretroviral therapy. The classification of HIV cases is beyond the scope of this chapter, but two methods exist. The CDC's is based largely on CD4 counts and so requires laboratory services, while the WHO's system relies only on clinical criteria (AETC, 2011). In the early stages of disease, patients do not need antiretroviral drugs. Cut-off points for treatment are constantly updated, but the latest recommendations include a CD4 count less than 350 cells/mm^3, WHO clinical stage 3 or 4 (irrespective of CD4 count), and any patient with TB co-infection (WHO, 2009b). At any one time, roughly half of all cases meet criteria for treatment.

Before the introduction of Highly Active Anti-Retroviral Therapy (HAART), there were no treatments available other than supportive care, good nutrition, and treatment of common infections, such as candidiasis and pneumonia. At the time, feelings of frustration and resignation were a serious problem among developing world health workers. The first anti-HIV drug (AZT, zidovudine) was introduced in1987, followed by the steady introduction of many others in four different classes during the 1990s (WHO, 2016b). Their early use in combination therapy has dramatically changed the outlook for HIV-infected patients. Apart from improving health, HAART regimes also reduce transmission risks because of the very low viral loads in many treated patients.

Mother-to-child transmission is the most important source of HIV infection in children—about 150,000 children were newly infected in 2009 (UNAIDS, 2010). In developed countries, triple-combination regimes used before and after delivery (for both mother and child) can reduce transmission to close to zero (from an untreated average of about 25 percent) (WHO, 2004). Even under poor resource conditions, short courses of effective drugs can reduce transmission significantly. Several regimes have been tested, including zidovudine alone or in combination with lamivudine and nevirapine (WHO, 2004). This offers the promise of saving a generation of children in developing countries. The widespread introduction of trans-natal antiretroviral (ARV) treatment has been very slow considering the possible benefits. Depending on duration, viral load, and the mother's health, breastfeeding by an untreated mother increases the risk of transmission by a further 10–15 percent. Management is a contentious issue (WHO, 2007). Ideally, every child should be fed well-prepared formula, but in large parts of the world, formula feeding is associated with significant diarrhea-associated risks of its own. Treatment of mother and child with ARVs for the duration of feeding has been shown to be effective.

The growth of the fight against AIDS has been extraordinary. In 25 years, it has gone from a medical curiosity to a multi-billion-dollar industry employing tens of thousands of people, which doesn't mean it has always been effective, but it is certainly large. The UN agency responsible for coordinating the HIV response is UNAIDS. It was established in 1996 as part of the UN Development Group (UNAIDS, 2011). Many other organizations are involved in capacities ranging from funding to advocacy. Major groups include the Global Fund to Fight AIDS, TB, and Malaria; the William Clinton Foundation; and the President's Emergency Plan for AIDS Relief. After a slow start in the 1990s, funding picked up following the impetus of the MDGs. On World AIDS Day in 2003, the WHO and UNAIDS announced a plan to have 3 million patients on antiretroviral treatment by the end of 2005 (the "3 by 5 target"). At the time, WHO estimated that more than 4 million people living with AIDS in sub-Saharan Africa needed antiretroviral therapy, but only 315,000 had access to affordable treatment.

That early goal wasn't met, but progress has been made. Of the 14.6 million people who needed treatment in 2009, 5.25 million were receiving ARVs. Coverage varies between countries, but on average, about 35–40 percent of those needing treatment are now being reached (UNAIDS, 2010). There is a long way to go before universal coverage is attained, but there are already signs of measurable improvements in controlling the epidemic. The most recent global report shows that prevalence appears to have reached a plateau (UNAIDS, 2016). The Millennium Development Goal for HIV was to halt and reverse the spread of infection. This modest aim has been reached almost everywhere, including most of Africa. New HIV infections fell by approximately 40 percent between 2000 and 2013, from an estimated 3.5 million cases to 2.1 million (UN, 2016). The principal elements of the response to the epidemic are as follows:

- *HIV vaccine:* When the viral cause of AIDS was discovered in the early 1980s, there was initial enthusiasm that a vaccine would soon be discovered; unfortunately, this hope has not been met. There are two problems confronting HIV vaccine research. Firstly, the virus expresses a surprisingly complex antigenic variation for such a seemingly simple organism. Secondly, the body's ability to respond to a vaccine is reduced by the fact that HIV infects some of the cells that mediate that response. Several vaccines have been tested, but, unfortunately, none has shown any significant results so far. Since a small percentage of people appear to have innate immunity to HIV and a few infected patients appear to live for many years with normal health, hopes still remain high that a vaccine will ultimately be found (IAVI, 2011).
- *Routine testing:* Despite considerable debate about universal testing, contact tracing, and even quarantine, the issue of HIV testing remains a contentious one. The WHO took an early lead against the stigmatization of

HIV-positive people. Cuba was the only country to carry this policy to its conclusion. Between 1988 and 1993, all Cubans who tested HIV-positive were quarantined and allowed out only with a chaperone (Hansen et al., 2003). The country has subsequently adopted more enlightened policies; its provision of free antiretroviral therapy now makes it a leader in HIV control among developing countries. In the single area of mother-to-infant transmission, there is nearly universal support for routine prenatal testing because of the existence of highly effective treatment regimes that reduce the risk to the fetus (UNAIDS, 2004).

- *Behavioural change:* Changing human behaviour is not easy, as the failure rates of weight-loss and anti-smoking programs show. The steps needed to alter behaviour must start with changing knowledge and beliefs about HIV. Building on this base leads to changes in attitude and, finally, personal practice. Peer influence is an important factor in social change, whether dealing with teenage sexual practices or recreational drug use (Diaz et al., 2005). Unfortunately, the discussion of safe sex and provision of needles, syringes, and safe injection sites is still only slowly being accepted by some donor agencies and also by conservative governments. In developed countries, education programs have caused significant changes in behaviour with measurable reductions in the incidence of HIV infections among heterosexuals, homosexuals, and drug users. There have been concerns that improved survival produces a degree of complacency, which in turn may again increase high-risk behaviour.

- *Condoms:* The use of condoms is only one issue within the broad topic of behavioural change, but it attracts a disproportionate amount of attention and a great deal of heated argument. While regular condom use is clearly beneficial in reducing the spread of HIV and a number of other sexually transmitted diseases, its impact will always be limited by inconsistent use. At present, the supply of condoms through the UN Population Fund (UNFPA) and other agencies falls far below the many billions that are needed annually. Until condoms are readily and freely available, their impact will not justify the energy put into arguing about them (UNFPA, 2007). Condom use should be viewed as only one part of a broad coordinated strategy against HIV infection.

- *Partnerships:* In the developing world, Uganda has shown a lead in HIV/AIDS interventions. High-level aid partnerships, backed by widespread community involvement, have produced real changes in the population's attitude toward safe sexual practices and measurable reductions in the infection rate (Bunnell et al., 2006).

- *Drug treatment:* Brazil was the first developing country to provide universal antiretroviral therapy for infected patients. Brazil's AIDS program is estimated to have halved the country's predicted mortality and infection rates (Berkman et al., 2005). Success is due to a program that integrates prevention and treatment approaches. HIV treatment recommendations need to be regularly updated as knowledge and circumstances evolve. Research results, improved funding, access to medication, and clinical experience all improve, so treatment protocols must change to reflect those advances. Current decision levels for treatment, plus recommended protocols, are contained in the most recent WHO treatment report (WHO, 2009b).

Important but Neglected Infectious Diseases

The three main infections we have just covered are all associated with huge social and economic costs. They deserve all the attention they get, but it's important to remember that there are plenty of other infectious agents that cause chronic ill health in developing countries. The importance of these lesser-known diseases is not widely appreciated, so they do not attract research attention or medical funding. Because of this, they are called "orphan" or "neglected" tropical diseases. The lack of funding is not an accurate reflection of their importance. Table 8.1 lists the 14 main diseases included within the neglected category and shows the huge

Table 8.1: The prevalence of neglected tropical diseases in sub-Saharan Africa

Hookworm	198 million
Schistosomiasis	192 million
Ascariasis	173 million
Trichuriasis	162 million
Lymphatic filariasis	46–51 million
Onchocerciasis	37 million
Trachoma	30 million
Loiasis	13 million
Yellow fever	180,000
Trypanosomiasis	50,000–70,000
Leprosy	30,000
Visceral leishmaniasis	19,000–24,000
Dracunculiasis	10,000
Buruli ulcer	4,000

Source: Hotez, P., et al. 2009. Neglected tropical diseases in sub-Saharan Africa. Retrieved from: www.plosntds.org/article/info%3Adoi%2F10.1371%2Fjournal.pntd.0000412.

numbers of people they infect in sub-Saharan Africa alone. Many of those diseases are also represented in other poor areas of the world, so their cumulative effect is enormous. Attention is slowly being paid to research (NTD, 2011) and drug treatment (DNDi, 2011) in this area. This book is not intended to be a medical text, but the following two examples will hopefully give some insight into the importance of these long-neglected conditions.

Visceral Leishmaniasis (Kala Azar)

Different species of the protozoal parasite *Leishmania* can cause a spectrum of diseases ranging from superficial skin ulcers to invasive, slowly lethal multi-organ disease. The organism is spread by the bite of a sandfly. In its most severe form (visceral leishmaniasis, or kala azar), the parasite causes invasive disease with fever, weight loss, and steady deterioration to death over a few months. Exact numbers are not known because asymptomatic infection is common. In endemic areas, the disease has become an increasingly common opportunistic infection associated with HIV infection and is a developing pathogen in southern Europe. It is thought that 50,000 new cases occur each year, principally in Bangladesh, Brazil, and Sudan. The less severe, but still disfiguring, cutaneous form probably affects millions of people; exact data are not available.

The most common form of treatment is a drug called pentavalent antimony, which has been available for over 50 years. It is a toxic drug with, in some cases, severe side effects, including death. Newer drug alternatives, such as ambisome, miltefosine, and paromomycin, have not been widely used in treatment because of the familiar story of expense and limited research targeted at neglected diseases. However, now that large numbers of Western soldiers are at risk of catching the parasite while serving in high-prevalence areas, research has been given higher priority (Zapar et al., 2005). So far, research in India has shown that miltefosine shows considerable promise as a safe oral alternative for invasive disease (Olliaro et al., 2005).

African Trypanosomiasis (Sleeping Sickness)

There are two closely related forms of sleeping sickness caused by different types of the protozoan parasite *Trypanosoma brucei*. The disease is spread by tsetse flies and is distributed widely throughout Central Africa. After infection, the first symptoms are relatively mild, so patients often remain undiagnosed. As the parasite spreads and invades the central nervous system, the patient's mental state undergoes a change that includes intense pain, confusion, somnolence, and ultimately death. The disease was well controlled in the 1960s by a combination of medical treatment and tsetse fly control. Unfortunately, war and social upheaval have interrupted control measures and the disease is returning. Disease surveillance is poor, so exact numbers are not available, but it is estimated that in some high-risk areas of Central Africa, sleeping sickness has become the most common cause of death, ahead of TB and AIDS.

Sleeping sickness is very difficult to treat (Jannin et al., 2004). In its early stages, pentamidine and suramin are used for patients who have not progressed to the neurological stage. The drugs are expensive and associated with side effects. The treatment of late-stage, neurologically affected patients requires melarsoprol, which is toxic enough to kill about 5 percent of treated patients; drug resistance is also becoming increasingly common. Eflornithine is a safer and more effective alternative for the West African disease, but as an example of the low priority given to these diseases, it was withdrawn from manufacture in 1995. Political pressure persuaded the producer to restart production (Wickware, 2002). A new oral drug (so far called DB 289) has entered clinical trials (Jannin et al., 2004).

SUMMARY

Water and sanitation are fundamental to human development and overall health. The importance of safe water and sanitation in population health and global development is reflected in SDG 6: "By 2030, achieve universal and equitable access to safe and affordable drinking water for all; By 2030, achieve access to adequate and equitable sanitation and hygiene for all and end open defecation, paying special attention to the needs of women and girls and those in vulnerable situations." These are not just goals in their own right, they are also critical to the achievement of other global health initiatives such as adequate nutrition, food security, and the eradication of poverty. Much of the misery and ill health suffered by poor people on a daily basis is due to lack of the most basic provisions of a hygienic life. Apart from the discomfort and indignity caused by lack of sanitation, poor hygiene is the biggest single risk factor behind the high rates of infectious diseases in developing countries and plays an adverse central role in population health. Unfortunately, 663 million people still lack access to safe water and 2.4 billion people still lack access to sanitation. The lack of sanitation, lack of safe water, and otherwise poor living environments lead to major health conditions such as diarrhea, malnutrition, intestinal worms, filariasis, trachoma, Schistosomiasis, malaria, and a host of others. Taken together, the diseases associated with poor hygiene make up a large fraction of the world's disease burden. Obviously, there will never be an end to infectious diseases, but they can be kept under control. Currently, the greatest infectious threats to human health productivity are HIV/AIDS, tuberculosis, and malaria. These major global public health threats undermine development in many resource-poor countries and have huge social and economic costs. Controlling the spread of these three agents consumes a lot of money both directly through targeted programs such as Roll Back Malaria and the Global Fund to Fight AIDS, Tuberculosis and Malaria, and indirectly through projects aimed at improving housing, sanitation, and nutrition.

DISCUSSION QUESTIONS

1. What are the SDGs related to clean water and sanitation?
2. What are the SDG targets related to water and sanitation? Do you think these targets will be met by 2030?
3. Why is sanitation linked to high childhood mortality?
4. What are the most prevalent infectious diseases in developing countries?
5. Why is malaria control very difficult?
6. What are neglected tropical diseases (NTDs)?
7. What groups are especially at risk of NTDs? What steps would you take to reduce the burden of NTDs?
8. What is DOTS? What are the key elements of this approach?
9. What is the most prevalent source of HIV infection in children?
10. What steps would you take to continually reduce the burden of HIV/AIDS?

RECOMMENDED READING

Gandy, M., et al. (Eds.). 2003. *The return of the white plague: Global poverty and the new tuberculosis*. Pub: Verso.

Ghosh, J., et al. (Eds.). 2003. *HIV and AIDS in Africa: Beyond epidemiology*. Pub: Blackwell Publications.

Hotez, P. 2008. *Forgotten people, forgotten diseases: The neglected tropical diseases and their impact on global health and development*. Pub: American Society of Microbiology.

Liu. L., et al. 2015. Global, regional, and national causes of child mortality in 2000–13, with projections to inform post-2015 priorities: An updated systematic analysis. *The Lancet*, 385: 430–440.

Seear, M. 2000. *Manual of tropical pediatrics*. Pub: Cambridge University Press.

Shah, S. 2011. *The fever: How malaria has ruled humankind for 500,000 years*. Pub: Picador.

REFERENCES

AETC. 2011. AIDS education and training centers: HIV classification. Retrieved from: www. aids-ed.org/aidsetc?page=cg-205_hiv_classification.

Berkman, A., et al. 2005. A critical analysis of the Brazilian response to HIV/AIDS: Lessons learned for controlling and initiating the epidemic in developing countries. *American Journal of Public Health*, 95: 1162–1172.

Black, R., et al. 2010. Global, regional, and national causes of child mortality in 2008: A systematic analysis. *The Lancet*, 375: 1969–1987.

Bunnell, R., et al. 2006. Changes in sexual behaviour and risk of HIV transmission after antiretroviral therapy and prevention interventions in rural Uganda. *AIDS*, 20: 85–92.

CDC. 2010. Centers for Disease Control and Prevention. The history of malaria, an ancient disease. Retrieved from: www.cdc.gov/malaria/history/index.htm.

CDC. 2011a. Tuberculosis. Retrieved from: www.cdc.gov/tb/.

CDC. 2011b. HIV/AIDS. Retrieved from: www.cdc.gov/hiv/default.htm.

Crawley, J., et al. 2007. From evidence to action? Challenges to policy change and programme delivery for malaria in pregnancy. *Lancet Infectious Diseases*, 7: 145–155.

Creel, L. 2002. Children's environmental health: Risks and remedies. Population Reference Bureau. Retrieved from: www.prb.org/pdf/ChildrensEnvironHlth_Eng.pdf.

Diaz, S., et al. 2005. Preventing HIV transmission in adolescents: An analysis of the Portuguese data from the health behaviour of school-aged children study and focus groups. *European Journal of Public Health*, 15: 300–304.

DNDi. 2011. Drugs for Neglected Diseases initiative. Retrieved from: www.dndi.org/index.php/ overview-dndi.html?ids=1.

Doherty, T., et al. 2006. Progress and hindrances in tuberculosis vaccine development. *The Lancet*, 367: 947–949.

Dorling, D., et al. 2006. Global inequality of life expectancy due to AIDS. *British Medical Journal*, 332: 662–664.

Dormandy, T. 2001. *The white death: A history of tuberculosis*. Pub: Hambledon.

Eisele, T., et al. 2010. Protective efficacy of interventions for preventing malaria mortality in children in *Plasmodium falciparum* endemic areas. *International Journal of Epidemiology*, 39 (Suppl. 1): 81–101.

Gallo, R. 2003. The discovery of HIV as the cause of AIDS. *New England Journal of Medicine*, 349: 2287–2285.

GDF. 2011. The Global Drug Facility. Retrieved from: www.stoptb.org/gdf.

Gottlieb, M. 1981. Pneumocystis carinii pneumonia and mucosal candidiasis in previously healthy homosexual men: Evidence of a new acquired cellular immunodeficiency. *New England Journal of Medicine*, 305: 1425–1431.

Hansen, H., et al. 2003. Human immunodeficiency virus and quarantine in Cuba. *Journal of the American Medical Association*, 290: 2875–2878.

Hotez, P., et al. 2009. Neglected tropical diseases in sub-Saharan Africa. Retrieved from: www.plosntds.org/article/info%3Adoi%2F10.1371%2Fjournal.pntd.0000412.

Hutton, G., et al. 2004. Evaluation of the costs and benefits of water and sanitation improvements at the global level. WHO report. Retrieved from: www.who.int/water_sanitation_health/wsh0404/en/.

IAVI. 2011. International AIDS Vaccine Initiative. Retrieved from: www.iavi.org/Pages/home.aspx.

Jannin, J., et al. 2004. Treatment and control of human African trypanosomiasis. *Current Opinion in Infectious Diseases*, 17: 565–571.

JMP. 2010. WHO-UNICEF Joint Monitoring Programme. Retrieved from: www.wssinfo.org/.

Jolly, R. 2001. Jim Grant: UNICEF visionary. Retrieved from: www.unicef.org/publications/files/Jim-Grant-LR.pdf.

Kjellstrom, T. 1999. How much global ill health is attributable to environmental factors? *Epidemiology*, 10: 573–584.

MDG. 2010. Millennium Development Goals. Retrieved from: www.un.org/millenniumgoals/.

Mitnick, C., et al. 2008. Comprehensive treatment of extensively drug-resistant tuberculosis. *New England Journal of Medicine*, 359: 563–574.

NTD. 2011. Neglected Tropical Disease Program. Retrieved from: http://ntd.rti.org/.

Olliaro, P., et al. 2005. Treatment options for visceral leishmaniasis: A systematic review of clinical studies done in India, 1980–2004. *Lancet Infectious Diseases*, 5: 763–774.

Poznyak, V., et al. 2005. Breaking the vicious circle of determinants and consequences of harmful alcohol use. *Bulletin of the World Health Organization*, 83: 803–805.

Pruss-Ustun, A., et al. 2006. Preventing disease through healthy environments: Towards an estimate of the environmental burden of disease. WHO report. Retrieved from: www.who.int/quantifying_ehimpacts/publications/preventingdisease.pdf.

RBM. 2008. Roll Back Malaria. Global malaria action plan. Retrieved from: www.rbm.who.int/gmap/gmap.pdf.

RBM. 2011. A decade of partnership results. Retrieved from: www.rbm.who.int/ProgressImpactSeries/docs/report8-en.pdf.

Shultz, J. 2000. Bolivians win anti-privatization battle. *NACLA Report on the Americas*, 33: 44–45.

Stein, D., et al. 2004. Depression and anxiety in the developing world: Is it time to medicalize the suffering? *The Lancet*, 364: 233–234.

StopTB. 2011. The Stop TB Partnership. Retrieved from: www.stoptb.org/.

Targett, G. 2005. Malaria vaccines 1985–2005: A full circle? *Trends in Parasitology*, 21: 499–503.

TBCTA. 2006. Tuberculosis Coalition for Technical Assistance. International standards for tuberculosis care. Retrieved from: www.who.int/tb/publications/2006/istc_report.pdf.

TDR. 2010. Tropical Disease Research. Malaria. Retrieved from: apps.who.int/tdr/svc/diseases/malaria;jsessionid=8981050596F1EC9CD92D96AB9811E8D8.

Thagard, P. 1997. Retrieved from: http://cogsci.uwaterloo.ca/Articles/Pages/Concept.html.

Thompson, K., et al. 2007. Eradication versus control for poliomyelitis: An economic analysis. *The Lancet*, 369: 1363–1371.

Townson, M., et al. 2005. Exploiting the potential of vector control for disease prevention. *Bulletin of the World Health Organization*, 83: 942–947.

UN. 2005. UN task force on improving the lives of slum dwellers. Retrieved from: www.unmillenniumproject.org/documents/Slumdwellers-complete.pdf.

UN. 2010a. UN resolution on the recognition of clean water and sanitation as basic human rights. Retrieved from: www.un.org/News/Press/docs/2010/ga10967.doc.htm.

UN. 2010b. Millennium Development Goals report. Retrieved from: www.un.org/millenniumgoals/pdf/MDG%20Report%202010%20En%20r15%20-low%20res%2020100615%20-.pdf.

UN. 2011. Water for life, 2005–2015. Retrieved from: www.un.org/waterforlifedecade/background.shtml.

UN. 2015. The Millennium Development Goals report 2015. Retrieved from: www.undp.org/content/dam/undp/library/MDG/english/UNDP_MDG_Report_2015.pdf.

UN. 2016. UN-Water. Retrieved from: www.unwater.org/index.html.

UNAIDS. 2004. UNAIDS/WHO policy statement on HIV testing. Retrieved from: www.who.int/rpc/research_ethics/hivtestingpolicy_en_pdf.pdf.

UNAIDS. 2010. UNAIDS report on the global AIDS epidemic. Retrieved from: www.unaids.org/globalreport/global_report.htm.

UNAIDS. 2011. Joint United Nations Programme on HIV/AIDS. Retrieved from: www.unaids.org/en/aboutunaids/unaidsleadership/.

UNAIDS. 2016. Global AIDS update. Retrieved from: www.unaids.org/en/resources/documents/2016/Global-AIDS-update-2016.

UNESCO. 2003. Water for people, water for life: The world's water crisis. Retrieved from: www.unesco.org/water/wwap/wwdr/wwdr1/pdf/chap1.pdf.

UNFPA. 2007. Comprehensive condom programming: A strategic response to HIV and AIDS. Retrieved from: www.unfpa.org/hiv/programming.htm.

UN-HABITAT. 2005. UN-HABITAT's strategy for implementation of the Millennium Development Goal 7, target 11. Retrieved from: www.unhabitat.org/pmss/listItemDetails.aspx?publicationID=1805.

UN-HABITAT. 2006. Focus area 3: Access to land and housing for all. Retrieved from: www.unhabitat.org/content.asp?typeid=19&catid=10&cid=9525&activeid=929.

UNICEF. 2016. Child mortality. Retrieved from: www.childinfo.org/mortality.html.

UNW-DPC. 2011. UN-Water Decade Programme on Capacity Development. Retrieved from: www.unwater.unu.edu/.

WHO. 2004. Antiretroviral drugs for treating pregnant women and preventing HIV infection in women. Retrieved from: www.who.int/hiv/pub/mtct/en/arvdrugswomenguidelinesfinal. pdf.

WHO. 2005. World health report: Statistical annex. Retrieved from: www.who.int/whr/2005/ annex/en/index.html.

WHO. 2006a. A guide: Trachoma prevention through school health curriculum development. Retrieved from: www.who.int/blindness/CHF%20GUIDE%20FINAL%20EN.pdf.

WHO. 2006b. The Stop TB strategy. Retrieved from: www.who.int/tb/strategy/en/.

WHO. 2007. HIV transmission through breastfeeding. Retrieved from: whqlibdoc.who.int/ publications/2008/9789241596596_eng.pdf.

WHO. 2008. Safe water, better health: Costs, benefits, and sustainability of interventions to protect and promote health. Retrieved from: www.who.int/water_sanitation_health/ publications/safer_water/en/.

WHO. 2009a. WHO and DDT for malaria control. Retrieved from: www.who.int/malaria/ publications/who_ddt_malaria_control-june.pdf.

WHO. 2009b. Rapid advice: Antiretroviral therapy for HIV infection in adults and adolescents. Retrieved from: www.who.int/hiv/pub/arv/rapid_advice_art.pdf.

WHO. 2010a. Guidelines for the treatment of malaria, 2nd ed. Retrieved from: whqlibdoc.who. int/publications/2010/9789241547925_eng.pdf.

WHO. 2010b. World malaria report. Retrieved from: www.who.int/malaria/world_malaria_ report_2010/worldmalariareport2010.pdf.

WHO. 2010c. Global tuberculosis control. WHO report. Retrieved from: www.who.int/tb/ publications/global_report/en/.

WHO. 2010d. Multidrug and extensively drug-resistant TB (M/XDR-TB). Retrieved from: whqlibdoc.who.int/publications/2010/9789241599191_eng.pdf.

WHO. 2016a. Water and sanitation-related diseases. Retrieved from: www.who.int/ water_sanitation_health/diseases/diseasefact/en/.

WHO. 2016b. Antiretroviral therapy. Retrieved from: www.who.int/hiv/topics/treatment/en/.

WHO/UNICEF. 2011. Progress on sanitation and drinking water: 2010 update. Retrieved from: www.who.int/water_sanitation_health/publications/9789241563956/en/index.html.

WHO/UNICEF. 2016. Progress on sanitation and drinking water: 2015 assessment and MDG update. Retrieved from: http://data.unicef.org/resources/progress-on-sanitation-and-drinking-water-2015-assessement-and-mdg-update.html.

Wickware, P. 2002. Resurrecting the resurrection drug. *Nature Medicine*, 8: 908–909.

World Bank. 2010. World Bank governance indicators. Retrieved from: http://info.worldbank. org/governance/wgi/index.asp.

World Bank. 2011. GDP per capita. Retrieved from: http://data.worldbank.org/indicator/NY.GDP.PCAP.CD.

World Bank-UNCHS. 2005. Cities alliance for cities without slums. Retrieved from: web.mit.edu/urbanupgrading/sponsor/ActionPlan.pdf.

WSH. 2016. WHO's water, sanitation and health. Retrieved from: www.who.int/water_sanitation_health/en/.

Zapar, M., et al. 2005. Infectious diseases during war time. *Current Opinion in Infectious Diseases*, 18: 395–399.

Zhang, H., et al. 2004. Risk factors for recurrence of trichiasis: Implications for trachoma blindness prevention. *Archives of Ophthalmology*, 122: 511–516.

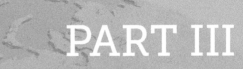

PART III

WHAT ARE THE TYPES AND EXTENT OF ILL HEALTH IN DEVELOPING COUNTRIES?

CHAPTER 9

How to Define and Measure Health

Whenever you can, count.

—Sir Francis Galton, 1865

OBJECTIVES

Health research has moved away from simple mortality data and increasingly adopted more sophisticated measures of the social burden that diseases produce. In
addition to the shorter-term pain and suffering caused by disease or death, chronic
health problems also impose a longer-term burden both on the affected individual
and on the broader society. Using a variety of techniques adapted from the world of
insurance, it is now possible to estimate the "cost" of different diseases in terms of
years of life lost. It should always be remembered that although these newer measurement techniques offer a greater insight into population health, they do bring
their own problems, including the increased expense of complex data gathering
and greater chances of measurement and calculation error. After completing this
chapter, you should be able to:

- understand the central importance of defining and measuring health outcomes in improving the effectiveness of aid projects
- appreciate the difference between simply counting the extent of disease and
  measuring the societal burden of disease
- know the definitions of the commonly used health variables
- understand how data is collected and appreciate the range of errors involved

INTRODUCTION

If you want to inspire confidence, give plenty of statistics. It does not matter that they should be accurate, or even intelligible, as long there is enough of them.

—Lewis Carroll

Ill health and poverty are intimately related. They run as two intertwined strands throughout the subject of global health; you will never find one without the other. Neither can be understood until they can be measured, so several agencies spend a great deal of time and money trying to collect accurate data about both of them. There is, of course, some overlap, but the World Bank tends to concentrate on poverty research, while the World Health Organization, the UN Population Division, and UNICEF collect vast amounts of information about population health. As we saw in Chapter 5, the measurement of poverty is a contentious subject, open to a great deal of criticism and potential error. The measurement of ill health is, if anything, even worse because there is not even a fully agreed-upon definition of health to act as a reference point. While there will always be arguments about the subjective elements involved within their calculation, these new methods of assessing health are here to stay and should be understood by anyone interested in this field.

Prior to the introduction of disease impact measures, developing world health research was dominated by studies of child mortality. It was generally thought that infectious diseases were the main health problem, while other important diseases, such as the dreadful annual mortality of women during childbirth, received very

Box 9.1 History Notes

John Graunt (1620–1674)

John Graunt was born in London into a middle-class 17th-century family. He received a basic education and was then apprenticed in his family shop. His business grew and he became quite a wealthy man. He mixed with the well-known people of his day, including Samuel Pepys.

Charles II had earlier introduced a system of weekly death registration (Bills of Mortality), which were intended to act as an early warning system of plague outbreaks. For unknown reasons, Graunt made a detailed study of these documents and published his findings, "Observations on the Bills of Mortality," in 1662. This is generally accepted as the earliest study of population health in the English language. He was the first person to calculate a life table, giving the probabilities of survival at each age. Despite his low social status as a merchant, he was elected as a fellow of the newly formed Royal Society, but it took a bit of pushing from the king. He later lost considerable property in the fire of London and also suffered for his conversion to Catholicism. He ultimately died in poverty. Follow the reference for more details: Rothman (1996).

little attention. Time has changed all those attitudes. An emphasis on children is obviously important, but a healthy society requires healthy adults, and research now reflects that view. For a variety of reasons—particularly the need to monitor large-scale projects such as the Sustainable Development Goals (SDGs) and the outcome measurements needed for cost-effective health planning—it has been necessary to introduce better measures of population health to meet those new demands.

These new techniques are not actually all that new. They have attracted more attention in the last decade, but their development goes back over 40 years (Sassi, 2006). Research that began in the 1960s led to the development of the Quality-Adjusted Life Year (QALY) in 1976. The concept is simple: time spent suffering from ill health or disability is discounted by a subjective factor. For example, a woman who lived with a lifetime debilitating disease with a subjective factor of 0.8 (only 80 percent of a healthy active life), and then died at 40 years, has clearly lived less than a completely healthy life. QALYs assess the amount of healthy life lived by multiplying years with the ill health or disability by the subjective factor ($0.8 \times 40 = 32$ QALYs). Treatments may lessen the degree of disability, therefore increasing the health factor, or they may increase life expectancy. Either way, effective treatments are assessed by their ability to *increase* QALYs.

The concept of the Disability-Adjusted Life Year (DALY) was introduced in 1994 and is a more complex calculation (Sassi, 2006). DALYs are, to some extent, the reverse of QALYs—they estimate the amount of life lost by ill health, disability, or early death rather than the quality of life achieved. The patient just mentioned has lost years of useful life in two ways—firstly by dying too early (sooner than the life expectancy of 82.5 years for women, and therefore a loss of years is represented by 42.5 [82.5 − 40]), and secondly by living with the disease (loss is years lived with disease x [1 − disease factor; the disease factor in this case is 0.8]). The total is the sum of these two: (42.5 + 40[1 − 0.8]). Therefore, the patient lost 50.5 DALYs from lifetime illness. Treatments may reduce life lost by increasing the health factor (disease factor gets smaller) or by reducing years of life lost from premature death (years lived gets larger). Either way, effective treatments *decrease* DALYs. The full calculation is more complex because it discounts total life lost by various factors, which are open to considerable debate, but the general method is unchanged (see more on DALY calculations later in this chapter).

Despite these problems, measurement techniques such as QALYs and DALYs now have an established place in the measurement of population health. The principal insight gained from their use has been an understanding that non-lethal diseases, such as mental ill health, and traffic accidents actually produce a greater burden of disease for society than the more intuitively obvious common causes of mortality. Apart from being useful in the monitoring of large-scale health projects,

Box 9.2 Moment of Insight		
Canada	**Angola**	**Pakistan**
Proportion of children who die before their fifth birthday:	Proportion of children who die before their fifth birthday:	Proportion of children who die before their fifth birthday:
1 in 200	**1 in 20**	**1 in 6**

UNICEF. 2015b. Levels & trends in child mortality report 2015. Estimates developed by the UN Inter-agency Group for Child Mortality Estimation. Retrieved from: www.who.int/maternal_child_adolescent/documents/levels_trends_child_mortality_2015/en/.

these newer measurement tools also allow health planners to target their limited budgets toward those diseases that cause the greatest burden in their local population. This might seem a cold-hearted way of allocating health finances, but when cash is limited, it must be used in the most effective way to improve public health.

Quite apart from straightforward measurement error, the conclusions derived from health or poverty studies can both be significantly altered simply by changing the basic definitions of the study variables. Whether you are using US$1 per day figures to assess poverty or Disability-Adjusted Life Years to assess health burden, it is very important to have a good working knowledge of the definitions and potential problems associated with the measurement of population health. It is important to understand that this is not a minor issue of interest simply to statisticians. Whether the topic is the best allocation of limited resources or the management of complex health initiatives, health assessment is an important subject and everyone involved in the broad aid industry should be very familiar with measurement techniques and their errors—particularly the errors. This chapter will examine the techniques used to measure population health in detail.

THE DEVELOPMENT OF HEALTH MEASUREMENT

History of Health Measurement

> Go number Israel from Beersheba even to Dan; and bring the number of them to me, that I may know it.
>
> —*1 Chronicles 21:2*

As far as it is possible to tell, the only measure of health recorded through most of human history was a simple head count. For many centuries, various administrations kept some record of the population depending on whether they wanted to tax them or recruit them to the army. As the quote at the start of this section shows, King David of Israel ordered a population census over 3,000 years ago. At least 2,000 years before David, the Babylonians had been keeping population tax records pressed into squares of mud. As far as governments were concerned, you were either dead or alive. Ill health and early death were probably so much a part of daily life that no one even thought to quantify them. Census-taking was an established part of Roman and Greek city administration. The first known census of the Roman Empire occurred in 28 BC under Augustus (it was 4,603,000). As a good example of the problems generated by imprecise statistics, no one knows if this referred only to males or whether women, children, and slaves were included. Although plenty of observers described the effects of plague as it swept through 14th- and 15th-century Europe (particularly the Arab historian and philosopher Ibn Khaldun), it was still some time before anyone studied the broad causes of death.

As early as 1523, the earl of Essex ordered that parish clerks should submit a record of deaths each week to act as an early warning system for plague epidemics. Data collection was only intermittent until Charles II put it on a more formal basis in the mid-17th century (Greenberg, 1997). These "Bills of Mortality" were published for the public to read. With steady improvements, they were continued until the middle of the 19th century. The table of diagnoses from 300 years ago (Table 9.1) again demonstrates the need for clear standard definitions in medical research. For unknown reasons, a wealthy London shop owner, John Graunt, became interested in the accumulated information held within these bills. His book, *Observations on the Bills of Mortality*, published in 1662, is widely accepted as the first attempt to measure population health (Rothman, 1996). Consequently, Graunt is variously described as one of the earliest demographers and epidemiologists. This work and similar studies by William Petty and Edmund Halley (of comet fame) gained wide recognition, not so much because of an interest in improving the lives

Table 9.1: The meaning of common diagnoses used in early bills of mortality

Chrisoms	(death before baptism)
Headmouldshot	(inflamed brain)
Planet struck	(paralyzed)
Rising of the lights	(lung disease)
Imposthume	(abscess)
Purples	(spotted fever)
Looseness	(dysentery)

Source: Slought Museum. 2011. Bills of mortality, London. Retrieved from: slought.org/content/410265/.

of the poor but because life insurance had just been introduced. The earliest insurers wanted actuarial data to predict how long people might live at different ages.

Eighteenth-century medicine's tendency to respect ancient authority without question meant that progress over the next two centuries was embarrassingly slow. If you don't measure things, you don't learn anything. Although gifted observers like John Snow (UCLA, 2007) and Ignaz Semmelweis (Dodd Library, 2011) were able to make valuable advances based on their own clinical observations, it took a long time before population health was measured in a scientific manner. The absence of hard data meant that, even in the mid-19th century, doctors still believed infection was spread by dirty air and that most diseases were the result of unbalanced humours. When Semmelweis suggested that child-bed fever could be avoided by handwashing rather than purging, he was laughed at. The lack of reliable health information (and the prevailing notion that it wasn't even necessary) greatly slowed medical progress. Apart from the discovery of anaesthesia, there had been few medical advances between the time of Hippocrates and the reign of Queen Victoria.

It was not until the 1860s that William Farr, of the British General Registry Office, applied statistical techniques to the observations of Snow and others to prove that infected water was the cause of disease (Bingham et al., 2004). The subsequent move by European cities to build sewage management systems was a direct result of this basic public health study. The enormous health benefits of improved hygiene were the first measurable results of the new science of epidemiology, and they were far more recent than is commonly appreciated. Berlin and Paris did not develop modern city sewage systems until the very end of the 19th century. Later, Ross and McKendrick placed the study of disease on a formal mathematical basis and provided powerful epidemiological tools to examine the causes of disease, tools that were soon widely adopted for medical research. One of the best-known early uses of medical epidemiology was the famous 1950 study by Doll and Hill, which finally proved that smoking was the main cause of lung cancer, rather than fumes from diesel trucks.

During the 1960s and 1970s, cost-effectiveness studies, developed in the business world, began to be applied to large-scale medical projects. Most of the current tools for measuring burden of disease were developed around this time. In 1990, these new epidemiological methods were used in a joint project between Harvard University, WHO, and the World Bank during their first study of global health. They used the Disability-Adjusted Life Year methodology to study the burden of more than 100 diseases in eight different world regions (WHO, 2016a). That early Global Burden of Disease (GBD) report was the first time the importance of chronic diseases, such as mental illness, became apparent.

Why Measure Health?

> We find no sense in talking about something unless we specify how we measure it; a defi-
> nition based on measurement is the one sure way of avoiding talking nonsense.
>
> —*Sir Hermann Bondi, 1964*

Information is vital to the advancement of any science. Without carefully collected data, treatments can be based only on the unreliable foundation of personal
bias and traditional dogmas; neither is an effective source of new information.
One of the greatest doctors of the 19th century, Rudolph Virchow, made himself very unpopular by ridiculing the theory of disease based on humours, which
dated back to before Hippocrates. However, even he did not believe in the germ
theory of disease and thought that infections emerged spontaneously out of dirt.
Clearly, Hermann Bondi's advice is correct. The best reason for doing accurate
health studies is to avoid talking nonsense. Some of the other reasons for measuring health are listed below.

Early Warning of Major Diseases
The first Bills of Mortality were intended to act as an early warning of plague epidemics. The 2003 epidemic of Severe Acute Respiratory Syndrome (SARS) and
concerns about the spread of avian influenza show that regular surveillance is still
very important (CDC, 2005). The World Health Organization's Global Alert and
Response section has the responsibility of coordinating a number of disease-sur-
veillance initiatives (WHO, 2016b). These include networks for surveillance of
influenza, cholera, yellow fever, and plague. Improvements in travel now make it
possible for a severe infectious agent to travel around the globe in 24 hours. The
principal lesson from SARS is that disease surveillance is now more important
than it has ever been.

Project Monitoring and Evaluation
Population health measurement is a vital part of outcome assessment in any
large-scale health initiative, particularly disease eradication programs. Modern
disease-tracking techniques were refined during the smallpox eradication program.
The Millennium Development Goals (MDGs) also included several defined and
measured health outcomes that have greatly improved general standards of health
measurement. Each of the eight main goals and 21 targets had a separate monitoring agency; examples include UNAIDS and UNICEF. Targeted programs against
tuberculosis, HIV/AIDS, polio, leprosy, and malaria all also need accurate data
monitoring to assess progress.

Health Planning

In the past, diseases that killed most people were assumed to be the greatest public health threats, so they attracted the bulk of health spending. However, once the broader burden of disease was measured, unexpected conditions such as accidents and mental illness became more obvious public health threats. This information can significantly affect decisions made about the distribution of available health money. Health measurement is also necessary to guide cost containment measures and the reorganization of existing health systems (WHO, 2016c).

Population Health Surveillance

States have a responsibility to monitor the health of their populations; in Canada this is the responsibility of the Public Health Agency of Canada (PHAC, 2016). Basic measurements include registration of birth, death, and marital status, plus derived variables such as infant and maternal mortality rates. Most developed countries also have some form of disease control and surveillance structure that can investigate newly identified health problems. Snow's early identification of cholera or James Lind's study of scurvy have their modern counterparts in the early identification of HIV/AIDS by the US Centers for Disease Control during the 1980s and the early warning of the SARS epidemic by Canada's Global Public Health Intelligence Network in November 2002.

MEASURING THE AMOUNT OF DISEASE

It was a great step in science when men became convinced that, in order to understand the nature of things, they must begin by asking, not whether a thing is good or bad, noxious or beneficial, but of what kind it is? And how much is there of it? Quality and Quantity were then first recognized as the primary features to be observed in scientific inquiry.

—*James Maxwell, 1890*

In these next two sections, we'll follow Maxwell's advice by looking at ways to measure first the quantity and then the quality of disease. Once a country advances to the point where births, deaths, and population are recorded, the first step in accurate health measurement has been made. Using this basic data, a large number of health-related statistics can be calculated. The obvious starting point is to measure deaths and their causes. Deaths may be expressed in raw numbers as fractions of the population or as numbers in a given time. Major diseases are often defined by their associated mortality rates, while less lethal conditions are quantified by their incidence and prevalence. As time passes and mortality rates fall, more subtle measures of health are needed. People are no longer looked on as being either alive or dead—the quality of their lives and the burden imposed by non-lethal diseases become increasingly important.

The measurement of population health in developing countries has followed that basic pattern. Thirty years ago, the principal topic of research interest was mortality and its causes, principally the mortality of children. Standards of data collection were in their infancy and the estimates produced were not at all accurate. Increasingly reliable methods of obtaining population health data were developed during the same period that childhood mortality steadily dropped. By the 1990s, the field of epidemiology was ready for a change. The WHO responded to the monitoring requirements of the rapidly growing global middle class by introducing measures of disease burden. They selected the DALY as their principal measuring tool and used it to study the effects of common diseases in over 100 countries. The first Global Burden of Disease study was published in 1999 (WHO, 2016a). It provided major insights into the diseases that cause the heaviest burden for a population and was the first to show that targeting high-mortality diseases is not necessarily the best way to reduce disease burden.

In epidemiological studies, it is often easier to identify and count diseases (numerator) than it is to count the total number of people at risk (denominator). This makes it difficult to determine accurate values for a wide range of indicators. Inaccuracies due to poorly defined denominators can significantly affect the conclusions of a health study. A few basic definitions are necessary for this chapter and are provided below. Further epidemiological information can be found in several good texts (Norman et al., 2008).

- *Rates:* A rate indicates the number of times an event happens in a particular population over a given time span. Its calculation requires a defined period of time, a defined population, and the number of defined events. For example, a birth rate requires the number of live births (in a year) and the population size to turn it into a rate (births per 1,000 population per year). Errors and uncertainties will affect both the numerator and denominator. When rates are calculated for particular sections of society, such as infants, newborns, or under-fives, they are referred to as specific rates. Commonly used examples include the maternal mortality rate and the infant mortality rate (Figure 9.1)

- *Incidence:* Incidence measures the number of new cases of a given disease that develop in a specific time (usually a year). If 12 people catch tuberculosis each year in a population of 1,000, then the annual incidence is 1.2 percent. For very small numbers, the incidence is sometimes expressed per 100,000 people. For infectious diseases, the local incidence is a rough indication of your risk of catching it. If you move into that community and live like the average person, then your chance of catching tuberculosis that year is roughly 1.2 percent.

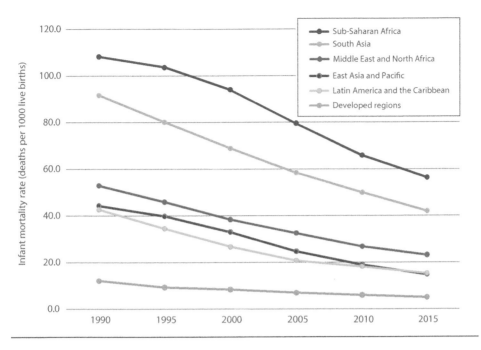

Figure 9.1: Trends in infant mortality rates for different world regions over the last 25 years; IMR is defined as deaths before the first birthday per 1,000 live births.

Source: UNICEF. 2015a. Estimates generated by the UN Inter-agency Group for Child Mortality Estimation (IGME) in 2015. Retrieved from: http://www.data.unicef.org/child-mortality/under-five.html.

- *Prevalence:* The prevalence is a measure of how much disease there is in a population at a given point in time and is used to guide provision of health services. Prevalence is calculated by dividing the number of people with the disease at any particular time point by the population at risk. Diseases of low incidence, such as cystic fibrosis, may have a high prevalence on the hospital ward simply because some will require frequent long-term admissions. Consequently, the need for health services for cystic fibrosis is higher than its simple calculated incidence would suggest.

Collecting Vital Statistics

To understand God's thoughts one must study statistics … the measure of His purpose.

—*Florence Nightingale, 1860*

Most countries at least pay lip service to the concept of collecting a basic package of health information on their citizens. The need for extensive infrastructure and a large budget means that this collection is often incomplete or, in many developing countries, almost non-existent. These so-called vital statistics usually include registration of birth, death, marital status, migration, and population.

Population Count

It seems likely that the very first population measure was a head count—it was certainly common practice in the Roman Empire. The foundation of all health measurements is the size of the population—every rate requires a denominator based on an accurate estimate of population or one of its subgroups. Examples include numbers of pregnant women or children under five years. The data are obtained by a regular national census count, often performed about every decade. Between census years, a fair estimate of the population and its subdivisions can be gained from regular analysis of the demographic data contained in the vital statistics. Obviously, accurate growth forecasts are important for planning future public services such as health and education.

Mortality Registration

Once the information gained from accurate death registration is added to the basic population data, a wide range of health indicators can be calculated. The simplest is a crude mortality rate (number of deaths in a given time divided by the total population in that period), but, as mentioned above, a wide range of specific rates can also be calculated. Breaking the basic data into subdivisions based on age, gender, or disease allows the calculation of specific indicators such as age-specific, gender-specific, or cause-specific mortality rates. Mortality rates are also used to calculate two other commonly quoted variables: standardized mortality ratio (SMR) and life expectancy at birth. Collecting accurate data in poor countries is a challenge. It is estimated that 70 percent of deaths worldwide are not certified (Sibai, 2004), so data collection must often rely on question-based surveys such as the sisterhood method (information is obtained by interviewing family members about survival of their adult sisters) developed to estimate maternal mortality (WHO, 1997).

Birth Registration

In many countries, a child is denied even the most basic registration of its existence at birth. Many children die of early neonatal causes before there has been time to register the child's birth. They are mourned by their families, but remain unknown to the state. UNICEF estimates that 30 percent of all births worldwide are unregistered, ranging from 22 percent in East Asia and the Pacific to 70 percent in sub-Saharan Africa (UNICEF, 2016a). Apart from introducing errors into health estimates, lack of a birth certificate can adversely affect a child throughout life. In some countries, a birth certificate is required for attendance at school, treatment in a clinic, immunization, obtaining credit, opening a bank account, or getting a passport. In some cases, there may be deliberate lack of birth registration intended to minimize the size of a particular ethnic minority, such as the Roma in central and eastern Europe.

Global Systems for Monitoring Health

It has always been important to monitor population health, but the establishment of the MDGs in 2000 brought the need for accurate health monitoring into focus. The MDGs set specific targets for a range of improvements in education, the status of women, the environment, poverty, and, of course, health. Four of the goals required the measurement of specific health outcomes. When the goals were established, it was well understood that monitoring information would often be incomplete and much of the data would require mathematical modelling rather than hard measurement. The MDGs acted as a catalyst for much-needed improvements in the gathering and measurement of health information—rather late in the day, it must be said. Four initiatives have been introduced that greatly improve the accessibility and quality of health information:

- *MDG Monitoring:* The monitoring requirements for the various MDGs and targets involved enormous amounts of work by many separate agencies. Beginning in early 2004, the World Bank and the IMF committed joint staff and funds toward an annual review of all these data sources that acted as an overview of progress toward the MDGs. The first Global Monitoring Report appeared in 2004 (GMR, 2011). It is published annually and provides a good review of the policies and actions of both developed and developing countries toward achieving the accepted targets.
- *SDG Monitoring:* The mechanics of SDG monitoring are still being worked out, but an emerging consensus suggests that the focus of SDG monitoring will be at the national level. As you saw in Chapter 1, the 17 SDGs come with 179 targets and 304 indicators. Indicators will be the backbone of monitoring progress toward the SDGs at the local, national, regional, and global levels. The goal is to use the indicators as a framework to help countries develop implementation strategies and allocate resources accordingly. The framework would also act as a report card to measure progress toward the SDG targets (SDSN, 2015).
- *Health Metrics Network:* A large alliance of countries, international partners, plus far-sighted funding from the Bill and Melinda Gates Foundation, came together in 2005 to form the Health Metrics Network. It

took 50 years and external private funding before the aid industry made serious efforts to collect accurate health statistics, but better late than never (HMN, 2011). It was originally an initiative of the World Health Organization. Their main strategy is termed MOVE-IT (Monitoring of Vital Events with Information Technology). The aim is to create a harmonized framework for the collection of health information that can then be shared on a global basis. The network also intends to provide technical and financial support for the establishment of these networks. Since a large part of the world does not even collect details of birth and death, this is a very ambitious undertaking, but also one that is long overdue.

- *Global Burden of Disease Project:* The GBD Project was started by the World Health Organization in response to the need for more precise insights into global disease. This represented a true revolution in health metrics. They moved away from traditional disease measures and used two newly developed tools—Disability-Adjusted Life Years (DALYs) to assess the burden of disease, and the Population Attributable Fraction (PAF) to quantify the contribution of various risk factors (WHO, 2016a). While there is controversy surrounding some of the subjective elements within the measures, they have provided unique insights into the burden and causes of disease around the world.

Measurement Error

Every careful measurement in science is always given with the probable error ... every observer admits that he is likely wrong, and knows about how much wrong he is likely to be.

—*Bertrand Russell, 1914*

In many developing countries, neither births, nor deaths, nor population are routinely recorded. Consequently, a calculated rate that depends on death registration for the numerator and accurate population information for the denominator is likely to suffer from a few errors. Research has shown wide variations between official government health statistics and the results of independent surveillance studies (Arudo et al., 2003). Note that a difference doesn't mean that either side is correct; it just means there's an appreciable error somewhere. In some cases, the final numbers are little more than informed guesses. This is not a criticism of the agencies that spend a great deal of time and effort on collecting data; it is simply the reality facing data gatherers in countries with poor administrative structures. Before basing a decision upon published health data, it is vital that some thought is given to the accuracy of that data.

An earlier comment in a paper by Cooper illustrates how recently data collection standards have improved (Cooper et al., 1998): "The statistics which appear in national ministries and international agencies are mainly guestimates formed from models, extrapolations, and common sense, constrained largely by the need to avoid deviating too far from previous estimates." It must be remembered that the data in the population health reports represent the best efforts given the current standards of health collection. The WHO data-gathering agencies try as much as possible to base their estimates on more than one source of information in order to improve accuracy, but the results should still be considered as the best available data rather than a reference gold standard.

A fairly recent report showed that even using loose criteria, death registration was complete for only 64 out of 115 countries studied (Mathers et al., 2005). Coverage ranged from close to 100 percent in Europe to less than 10 percent in sub-Saharan Africa. Using more stringent definitions, only 23 countries had data that were considered more than 90 percent complete and where poorly defined causes of death accounted for less than 10 percent of the total. It should be remembered that even when deaths are properly registered, the process is still not a completely reliable source of information. The widespread diagnosis of "malaria" for unexplained death with fever, or imprecise terms such as "heart failure," provide little information for the medical researcher. Similarly, compound causes of death are very difficult to classify properly. For example, a malnourished, unimmunized child who catches measles and dies from the subsequent pneumonia may be classified under several headings. Considering the numbers of children who die from multiple pathologies, there is surprisingly little research quantifying cumulative contributory causes of death (Pelletier et al., 1995).

Apart from errors involved in the raw mortality rates, the broader field of health measurement includes many other derived variables, each of which has its own particular errors. For example, poverty-associated inequalities in health are a popular topic of research. Unfortunately, different researchers rely on different means of measuring economic status. It has been clearly shown that varying the choice of economic measure will influence the final conclusion of the study of health and equality (Houweling et al., 2003). These effects can be so large that published differences in health and inequality between countries may be more of an artifact than a reality.

MEASURING THE BURDEN OF DISEASE

Let not your conception of disease come from words heard in the lecture room or read from a book. See, and then reason and compare and control. But see first.

—*William Osler, 1892*

Measurements of mortality are relatively easy to compile, but they are very crude indicators of the overall effects of disease, whether on individuals or on society. If a person dies, those potential years of lost life, production, and earnings have a profound effect that is not captured by a simple mortality statistic. Even if someone survives a disease, he or she may be left with disability for varying periods. That again is not adequately assessed if patients are simply classified as dead or alive. For over 30 years, increasingly sophisticated measurement tools have been devised to provide information on both the frequency of disease as well as the burden of disease carried by those who bear some form of disability. This requires a large amount of extra effort compared to simple mortality calculations, but the results have profound effects on the debate concerning health care. Once burden of disease is measured, a range of unexpected diseases (particularly mental illness and accidents) become much more obvious causes of potential lost life. This has important implications for the cost-effective allocation of health care budgets.

Two broad classes of measurement have emerged over time: health expectancy and health gaps; Figure 9.2 expresses these concepts graphically. Curve 1 represents a mythical population that lives in perfect health for 80 years and then suddenly dies. Curve 2 is a life expectancy curve for an average country. The difference between the two (Area C) is the health gap or lives lost due to various premature diseases. Curve 3 represents the expectancy curve for healthy life—people who are alive, but suffer some degree of illness. Area A is that population's expectancy of a disease-free life, while Area B represents the further life lived with some degree of limitation. Many attempts have been made to express the burden of disease by

Table 9.2: Life expectancy for UN groups (including high- and low-income countries) for 2014

REGION	LIFE EXPECTANCY
Sub-Saharan Africa	58.6
Latin America & Caribbean	74.9
Middle East & North Africa	72.9
South Asia	68.1
East Asia & Pacific	74.9
Europe & Central Asia	76.9
High-income countries	80.6
Low-income countries	61.3

Source: World Bank. 2016. Data from World Bank. World Development Indicators, Data Query. Available at: http://databank.worldbank.org/data/reports.aspx?source=2&series=SP.DYN. LE00.IN&country=.

combining the effects of lost life years (Area C in Figure 9.2) with a measure of the burden caused by living with a disease (Area B in Figure 9.2).

The concept of years of potential life lost was used in the early 1980s by the Ghana Health Assessment Team (GHAT, 1981) in order to improve their ability to measure the results of health spending in that country. Their shift from mortality data to burden of disease assessment produced unexpected results. They found that diseases with the highest health burden were not being targeted; money was principally going to a high-cost referral hospital that contributed very little to the health of the rural population. Based on these results, the government placed greater emphasis on community-based health care strategies that provided many times greater savings in life years per dollar spent. Subsequent research has produced a wide range of population health measures designed to integrate both mortality and morbidity into a single number. The best-known examples include the Disability-Adjusted Life Expectancy (DALE), published for 190 countries in 1999 (Mathers et al., 2001), and the Disability-Adjusted Life Year (DALY), used as a basis for the 1990 and 2000 Global Burden of Disease studies (WHO, 2016a).

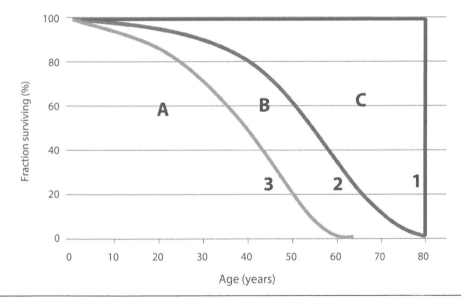

Figure 9.2: Idealized life expectancy curves

Curve 1: population with perfect health, then sudden death at 80; **Curve 2:** typical life expectancy curve for an average population; **Curve 3:** life expectancy curve for perfect health.

Area A: alive in good health; **Area B:** alive with some disability; **Area C:** premature death.

Measuring Health Expectancies

The conventional calculation of life expectancy considers people as either alive and healthy or dead. Obviously, this is unrealistic; every population includes people who are alive and yet limited in some degree by a persistent health disability. This brings up the concept of the two different life expectancy curves shown in Figure 9.2—one for total life and the other for disease-free life. The gap between the two is a measure of the extent of disease in the population. In order to measure the total life expectancy and the life expectancy in good health, it is necessary to weight different disabilities with regard to their severity, duration, and age of onset. Several indices have been developed for this purpose, including the Disability-Free Life Expectancy (DFLE) and Disability-Adjusted Life Expectancy (DALE) (Murray et al., 1997).

Early estimates of Disability-Free Life Expectancy (Sullivan, 1971) were dichotomous—that is, all disabilities were considered equal. People were considered "alive and well" or "alive and unwell," no matter what the disease. An international research network, Réseau Espérance de Vie en Santé (REVES, 2011), was established in 1989 with the objective of using this tool to assess and compare the health of populations. The more recently developed DALE (WHOSIS, 2011a) has superceded the DFLE. To add to the confusion, it is now more commonly called Health-Adjusted Life Expectancy (HALE). HALE adjusts for the degree of severity of a disability using self-reported health status and subjective allocation of weighted disease scores. The weighted years of ill health are subtracted from total life expectancy to produce an estimate of total years of healthy life expected at birth. Since personal opinions about degree of disability differ between cultures, care is required when adjusted life expectancies are compared between populations.

As shown in Figure 9.2, no matter what method is used to define good health, the result is two life expectancy curves: a disability-free life expectancy (curve 3) and a higher number representing total life expectancy (curve 2). Obviously, the difference between the two is the increasing burden of disability as the population ages. One use of this method has been to study the health of increasingly aging populations in developed countries. Has this simply been an extension of poor health, or do rich people actually live longer and healthier lives? Studies have shown that the slope of the increase in total life expectancy with time is the same as that for healthy life expectancy. This suggests that the observed increase in lifespan is not just an extension of ill health but is a real improvement in healthy years lived. The gender difference between healthy life expectancy is much smaller than it is for total life expectancy.

Table 9.3: Leading causes of death and DALYs globally

	DEATHS		DALYS
1	Ischemic heart disease	1	Ischemic heart disease
2	Cerebrovascular disease	2	Cerebrovascular disease
3	Chronic obstructive pulmonary disease	3	Lower respiratory infections
4	Lower respiratory infections	4	Low back and neck pain
5	Alzheimer's disease and other dementias	5	Preterm birth complications
6	Tracheal, bronchus, and lung cancer	6	Diarrheal diseases
7	Diabetes mellitus	7	Sense organ diseases
8	Road injuries	8	Neonatal encephalopathy
9	Diarrheal diseases	9	Road injuries
10	Chronic kidney disease	10	HIV/AIDS

Source: IHME. 2016a. Institute for Health Metrics and Evaluation. Rethinking development and health: Findings from the Global Burden of Disease study. Pub: IHME.

Table 9.4: Countries with the highest and lowest life expectancy at birth (in years), by sex, 2015

MALE		FEMALE	
Highest		**Highest**	
Switzerland	81.3	Japan	86.8
Iceland	81.2	Singapore	86.1
Australia	80.9	Spain	85.5
Sweden	80.7	Republic of Korea	85.5
Israel	80.6	France	85.4
Japan	80.5	Switzerland	85.3
Italy	80.5	Australia	84.4
Canada	80.2	Italy	84.4
Spain	80.1	Israel	84.3
Singapore	80.0	Iceland	84.1

Lowest		**Lowest**	
Lesotho	51.7	Chad	54.4
Chad	51.7	Cote d'Ivoire	54.4
Central African Republic	50.9	Central African Republic	54.1
Angola	50.9	Angola	54.0
Sierra Leone	49.3	Sierra Leone	50.8

Source: WHO. 2016e. World Health Statistics 2016: Monitoring health for the SDGs. Retrieved from: www.who.int/gho/publications/world_health_statistics/2016/en/.

The differences in life expectancies for different regions of the world are startling (Table 9.4). The average person in a developed country can expect to live 30 years longer than his or her counterpart in sub-Saharan Africa. When countries are examined individually, the differences are even more shocking. Revised data by Mathers et al., calculated for 191 countries, produced some interesting findings. Compared to developed countries, life in sub-Saharan Africa is significantly shorter and the time lived with disability is twice as long. People in Japan or Australia can expect to have over 40 more years of *healthy* life than the average person living in Sierra Leone (Mathers et al., 2001)!

Measuring Health Gaps

On two occasions, I have been asked, "Pray Mr. Babbage, if you put into the machine wrong figures, will the right answers come out?" I am not able rightly to apprehend the kind of confusion of ideas that could provoke such a question.

—*Charles Babbage (1791–1871), inventor of the first programmable calculating machine*

The Disability-Adjusted Life Year (DALY) has been adopted by the World Bank and the WHO as the standard method for measuring total disease burden, so it is important to have some idea about its calculation. The equations look impressive when written out in full and can give a misleading impression of scientific precision. However, the old computing adage should always be remembered: If you feed those equations bad basic data, you'll get garbage out no matter how complex the calculations might appear. By the time incomplete raw data have been manipulated and weighted, the final result can be open to several questions.

Summing up the full range of diseases in a single number is an ambitious undertaking. How can the death of a malnourished 9-month-old be compared to an HIV-positive 25-year-old woman who is well controlled on treatment? The DALY is one of a number of health measures designed to answer this question by estimating the total burden of disease (Gold et al., 2002). The final result is expressed in units of years of life lost, hence the term "health gap" rather than "health expectancy." The method is based on measuring two components of ill health: years lost due to premature death (YLL) and years lost due to disability (YLD) (WHO, 2016a):

DALY = YLL + YLD

A wide range of data is needed to feed this seemingly simple equation, including mortality statistics (numbers and causes of death) and disability statistics (age of onset and average duration of disability, plus average distribution of disability severity). Apart from the poor standard of data collection in many countries, the use of subjective weighting for age and disease is also a source of criticism (Rushby et al., 2001).

YLL (years lost from premature death): The basic calculation is simple:

YLL = expected years of life − age at death

It is assumed that men live an average of 80 years and women live 82.5 years. This is the only gender inequity allowed in DALY calculations. Unfortunately, it gets more complex once age at death is weighted by its "value." The extremes of age are counted less than early adulthood, and the final figure is also discounted at 3 percent per year. Once the weights and discounts are applied, an infant death corresponds to 33 DALYs.

YLD (years lost to disability): Again, the basic equation is simple:

YLD = duration of disability × disability weight

Complications occur with the choice of disability adjustment. The disability weighting score varies from 0 (perfect health) to 1 (dead); blindness is scored at 0.6 and loss of a limb at 0.3. For example, a five-year-old girl who loses a leg to cancer is expected to live a further 77.5 years with her disability. Once this is adjusted by disability weight, non-uniform age adjustment, and annual discount, it results in 10.5 YLDs. A previously healthy young man who suffers paraplegia at 20 years and dies of a heart attack at 60 years has lost years of life due to disability and also to premature death. The final DALY takes into account both those separate factors.

The DALY methodology provides a way to assess which diseases cause the heaviest burden within a country, allows comparisons to be made by country income (Table 9.5), and also helps assess the cost effectiveness of targeted initiatives—DALYs saved for dollars spent. DALYs have certainly allowed greater insights into the burden of less lethal diseases, such as psychiatric illnesses. However, as always, errors must be considered before placing too much faith in a single number that contains a significant subjective factor. It should be viewed as a practical tool that has errors, not as a universal gold standard. Apart from the problem of calculating standard disease weights for different countries, the DALY is calculated differently by different agencies—some do not weight productive age over old age, while others discount age. Other problems include the quantification of co-morbidities and non–health-related social effects of interventions.

Table 9.5: Leading causes of DALYs

DEVELOPING COUNTRIES	DEVELOPED COUNTRIES
1. Ischemic heart disease	1. Ischemic heart disease
2. Lower respiratory infections	2. Low back and neck pain
3. Cerebrovascular disease	3. Cerebrovascular disease
4. Low back and neck pain	4. Tracheal, bronchus, and lung cancer
5. Diarrheal diseases	5. Depressive disorders
6. Preterm birth complications	6. Chronic obstructive pulmonary disease
7. HIV/AIDS	7. Sense organ diseases
8. Road injuries	8. Diabetes mellitus
9. Malaria	9. Alzheimer's disease and other dementias
10. Chronic obstructive pulmonary disease	10. Self-harm

Source: IHME. 2016b. Institute for Health Metrics and Evaluation. GBD Compare Data Visualization. Pub: IHME, University of Washington. Available from: http://vizhub.healthdata.org/gbd-compare.

SOURCES OF POPULATION HEALTH INFORMATION

To study the phenomena of disease without books is to sail an uncharted sea, while to study books without patients is not to go to sea at all.

—*William Osler*

It has become very clear over the last 10–15 years that mortality statistics offer only a very restricted view of population health. In order to gain a deeper understanding of the complex variables underlying population health, it is necessary to find information on growth, nutrition, education, immunization, and many others. For those who plan large-scale health interventions, it is necessary to have access to much broader information, including economic data, population statistics, and even measured deficiencies of the existing health system. Although there are a great many sources of information, the following section gives information on the largest, easily accessible health information databases and reports for children and adults.

Child Health Data

Basic Mortality Rates

The most commonly used indicators of child mortality are neonatal mortality, the number of children who die before reaching 28 days of age per 1,000 live births in a given year, and the under-five mortality rate (U5MR), the number of children who die before their fifth birthday per 1,000 live births. In many parts of the world, 5 percent of live births are dead by one month of age, 10 percent by one year, and 15 percent by five years. Both neonatal mortality and U5MR have been chosen as targets for the SDGs, so updated information on the number and causes of child deaths is available in the World Health Statistics series—WHO's annual compilation of health statistics for its 194 Member States (WHO, 2016e). Both are also included in UNICEF's State of the World's Children annual report (UNICEF, 2016b).

Causes of Mortality

Although burden of disease measures, such as the DALY, are increasingly replacing simple mortality data in adults, this methodology can be questioned for very small children. Trying to calculate the years of life lost in a six-month-old child who dies from a combination of malnutrition and dehydration requires the use of a number of adjustment factors. Consequently, most observers still use mortality figures to assess the major diseases of children. A good source is the annual Global Burden of Disease study (GBD, 2016) and the Global Health Data repository. There are also a number of publications from the UN Inter-agency Group for Child Mortality Estimation (UN IGME).

Child Growth

As discussed in Chapter 6, the principal measures of child growth are underweight, stunting, and wasting. The prevalence of underweight children below five years of age is an SDG indicator; updated information for this variable can be found in "World Health Statistics 2016: Monitoring Health for the SDGs" (WHO, 2016e). A larger and more organized source of information is the Child Nutrition Database at the UNICEF website (UNICEF, 2016c). The WHO also maintains a Database on Child Growth and Malnutrition (WHO, 2016d).

Nutrition

The United Nations Food and Agricultural Organization (FAO) is the principal source of statistics about agricultural production. The statistical database, at its main website (FAO, 2016), deals with global data ranging from forestry to fish production. However, the organization also produces an annual summary of nutrition called the "State of Food Insecurity" (FAO, 2015), which is an excellent source for information on food supply, the prevalence of malnutrition, and progress toward the MDGs for nutrition.

Education

The vital place of education in overall population health and development is reflected in SDG 4 on education, "Ensure inclusive and equitable quality education and promote lifelong learning opportunities for all," and has seven targets and three means of implementation. Education is also included in goals on health, growth and employment, sustainable consumption and production, and climate change. Most education-monitoring research is done by the UN Educational, Scientific, and Cultural Organization (UNESCO). A great deal of educational data can be found at the UNESCO Institute for Statistics (UNESCO, 2016).

Immunization

Immunization is a basic foundation for child health, so global statistics, collected from a range of organizations, are updated on a regular basis by WHO (2016f) and UNICEF (2016d). Both these organizations produce a joint "Immunization Summary" every few years. The most recent summary covers data up to 2014 (UNICEF, 2016e). It provides a wide range of immunization data, by country and region, for the six major childhood vaccines (pertussis, tetanus, measles, polio, diphtheria, and BCG [*Bacillus Calmette Guerin*]).

Adult Health Data

General Mortality Statistics

Although the UN publishes a regular report on world mortality (UN, 2006), there has been a move away from mortality statistics toward the use of summary measures of health, such as the DALY. This concept was first introduced on a large scale during the 1990 Global Burden of Disease study. The GBD study generated an enormous amount of information, which was gradually published in the years following the initial study. The latest Global Burden of Disease study was carried out in 2010. Summaries of the most recently updated 2010 report can be found at the Global Burden of Disease website (GBD, 2016). The entire time series of GBD estimates are being updated annually to provide policy-makers, donors, and other decision-makers with the most timely and useful picture of population health. Many other research articles analyzing various aspects of the original data are available in the medical literature and also in the WHO's annual publication, the World Health Statistics Report (WHOSIS, 2011b).

Maternal Mortality and Morbidity

Improvement in maternal health is an important target of the SDG on health. Updated information can be found in the regular MDG reports (GMR, 2011). The primary information is held on UNICEF's Maternal Health Database (UNICEF, 2011f). The usual problems of incomplete birth and death registration complicate the collection of accurate data. The average world figure for maternal mortality ratio is 400, but it is over 800 in sub-Saharan Africa. Lifetime risk of maternal death varies from 1 in 2,800 in developed countries to less than 1 in 20 in parts of sub-Saharan Africa. The UNICEF Maternal Health Database also includes information on female morbidity, particularly statistics on female genital mutilation, antenatal care, contraceptive use, and fertility.

Population Statistics

Population numbers are a vital part of health measurement, so there are plenty of sources of current information. The UN Population Information Network is a good starting point (DESA, 2016a). The Population Reference Bureau is another good source of information concerning global population (PRB, 2016).

Contraception

Condom use is included within MDG 6 as part of the strategy to reduce the spread of HIV/AIDS. Clearly, information on the broader subject of contraceptive use is also of importance. The UN publication "World Contraceptive Use 2015" can be downloaded from the UN Population Division website (DESA, 2016a). Current information on contraceptive use and fertility rates is also available at the WHO Maternal Health Database (WHO, 2016g).

Clean Water and Sanitation Access

SDG 6 is related to safe drinking water and sanitation. Monitoring progress is a joint responsibility of WHO and UNICEF. Updated statistics are available at the UNICEF database (UNICEF, 2016g). The two organizations also produce a regular joint report on water and sanitation (WHO/UNICEF, 2015). The WHO also devotes an entire website to the topic of water, sanitation, and health (WHO, 2016h).

Other Useful Sources

The UN Common Database has a seemingly endless list of information grouped under different headings (UN, 2016). You can study everything from cement production to fertility rates. If you are looking for obscure information, this is a good place to start. The World Bank's annual publication, World Development Indicators (WDI, 2016), and its associated databank (World Bank, 2016) both provide access to an enormous range of development data—another good place to start if you are looking for obscure numbers. The CIA's World Factbook website provides easily digestible information for foreign travellers (CIA, 2016).

Apart from giving details of just about every country in the world, it also gives some data on the major demographic indicators, such as mortality, population, and economic indicators. It is an excellent first source for those travelling to exotic countries.

SUMMARY

The measurement of ill health can be challenging because there is no agreed-upon definition of health to act as a reference point. The World Health Organization defined health in its 1948 constitution as "a state of complete physical, mental, and social well-being and not merely the absence of disease or infirmity." The last three decades have witnessed a transformation in the way health is measured, moving from simple mortality data to more sophisticated measures that go beyond morbidity, mortality, and disability, such as DALYs or QALYs. While there will always be arguments about the subjective elements involved within their calculation, these new methods of assessing health provide a critical piece to the myopic outlook of life expectancy without taking into account additional years that are healthy, productive, and enjoyable. These new measures make it possible to estimate the "cost" of different diseases in terms of years of life lost. They are used internationally for assessing health care interventions and treatments. Their application also enables policy-makers to make informed decisions regarding various health interventions, and countries to choose vital, cost-effective health solutions.

DISCUSSION QUESTIONS

1. Why is it important to have composite indicators like DALYs and QALYs to measure the burden of disease?
2. How do newer measurement tools also allow health planners to target their limited budgets toward those diseases that cause the greatest burden in their local population?
3. Which report finally proved that smoking was the main cause of lung cancer rather than fumes from diesel trucks? How was this done?
4. What are the leading causes of DALYs globally? How do the leading causes of DALYs compare between high-income and low-income countries?
5. Which health measures do you consider to be most effective and why?
6. Why was the Global Burden of Disease Project started?
7. What measures could one use to measure life expectancy in good health?
8. Define DALY. How is it calculated?

9. What are some of the benefits of effective health measurements?

10. What are some of the major shortcomings of new health measures such as DALYs?

RECOMMENDED READING

Murray, C. J. L., et al. 2013. Disability-adjusted life years (DALYs) for 291 diseases and injuries in 21 regions, 1990–2010: A systematic analysis for the Global Burden of Disease study 2010. *The Lancet* 380(9859): 2197–2223. doi:10.1016/S0140-6736(12)61689-4.

Murray, C. J. L., et al. 2015. Global, regional, and national disability-adjusted life years (DALYs) for 306 diseases and injuries and healthy life expectancy (HALE) for 188 countries, 1990–2013: Quantifying the epidemiological transition. *The Lancet* 386(10009): 2145–2191. doi:10.1016/S0140-6736(15)61340-X.

Norman, G., et al. 2003. *PDQ Statistics*. Pub: McGraw-Hill.

WHO. 2016. World health statistics annual report: Monitoring health for the SDGs. Retrieved from: www.who.int/gho/publications/world_health_statistics/2016/en/.

REFERENCES

Arudo, J., et al. 2003. Comparison of government statistics and demographic surveillance to monitor mortality in children less than five years old in rural western Kenya. *American Journal of Tropical Medicine and Hygiene*, 68: 30–37.

Bingham, P., et al. 2004. John Snow, William Farr, and the 1849 outbreak of cholera that affected London. *Public Health*, 118: 387–394.

CDC. 2005. Centers for Disease Control and Prevention. Severe Acute Respiratory Syndrome. Retrieved from: www.cdc.gov/ncidod/sars.

Childinfo. 2011. Health statistics for women and children. Retrieved from: www.childinfo.org.

CIA. 2016. *The world factbook 2016–17.* Pub: Central Intelligence Agency. Retrieved from: www.cia.gov/library/publications/the-world-factbook/index.html.

Cooper, R., et al. 1998. Disease burden in sub-Saharan Africa: What should we conclude in the absence of data? *The Lancet*, 351: 208–210.

DESA. 2016a. UN Department of Economic and Social Affairs, Population Division. Retrieved from: www.un.org/en/development/desa/population/.

DESA. 2016b. World contraceptive use 2015. Retrieved from: www.un.org/en/development/desa/population/publications/dataset/contraception/wcu2015.shtml.

Dodd Library. 2011. Semmelweis. Retrieved from: http://dodd.cmcvellore.ac.in/hom/26%20-%20Semmelweis.html.

FAO. 2015. The state of food insecurity in the world. Retrieved from: www.fao.org/hunger/en/.

FAO. 2016. The UN Food and Agriculture Organization. Retrieved from: www.fao.org/.

GBD. 2015. Global, regional, and national age–sex specific all-cause and cause-specific mortality for 240 causes of death, 1990–2013: A systematic analysis for the Global Burden of Disease study 2013. *The Lancet*, 385(9963): 117–171.

GBD. 2016. Global burden of disease. Institute of Health Metrics and Evaluation: Retrieved from: www.healthdata.org/gbd.

GHAT. 1981. Ghana Health Assessment Team. A quantitative method of assessing the health impact of different diseases in less developed countries. *International Journal of Epidemiology*, 10: 1075–1089.

GMR. 2011. Global Monitoring Report. Retrieved from: http://go.worldbank.org/SUEMHZMEW0.

Gold, M., et al. 2002. HALYS and QALYS and DALYS, oh my: Similarities and differences in summary measures of population health. *Annual Review of Public Health*, 23: 115–134.

Greenberg, S. 1997. The "Dreadful Visitation": Public health and public awareness in 17th-century London. *Bulletin of the Medical Library Association*, 85, 391–401.

HMN. 2011. Health Metrics Network. Retrieved from: www.who.int/healthmetrics/en/.

Houweling, T., et al. 2003. Measuring health inequality among children in developing countries: Does the choice of indicator matter? *International Journal for Equity in Health*, 2: 8–20.

IHME. 2016a. Institute for Health Metrics and Evaluation. Rethinking development and health: Findings from the Global Burden of Disease study. Pub: IHME.

IHME. 2016b. Institute for Health Metrics and Evaluation. GBD Compare Data Visualization. Pub: IHME, University of Washington. Available from: http:// vizhub.healthdata.org/gbd-compare (Accessed January 01, 2016).

Mathers, C., et al. 2001. Healthy life expectancies in 191 countries, 1999. *The Lancet*, 357: 1685–1691.

Mathers, C., et al. 2004. Global patterns of healthy life expectancy in the year 2002. *BMC Public Health*, 4: 66–78.

Mathers, C., et al. 2005. Counting the dead and what they died from: An assessment of the global cause of death data. *Bulletin of the World Health Organization*, 83: 171–177.

Murray, C. J. L., et al. 1997. Regional patterns of disability-free life expectancy and disability-adjusted life expectancy: Global Burden of Disease study. *The Lancet*, 349: 1347–1352.

Norman, G., et al. 2008. *Biostatistics: The bare essentials*. Pub: McGraw-Hill.

Pelletier, D., et al. 1995. The effects of malnutrition on child mortality in developing countries. *Bulletin of the World Health Organization*, 73: 443–448.

PHAC. 2016. Public Health Agency of Canada, Surveillance Systems. Retrieved from: www.phac-aspc.gc.ca/surveillance-eng.php.

PRB. 2011. Population Reference Bureau. About PRB. Retrieved from: www.prb.org/About.aspx.

REVES. 2011. What are health expectancies? Retrieved from: http://reves.site.ined.fr/en/DFLE/definition/.

Rothman, K. 1996. Lessons from John Graunt. *The Lancet*, 347: 37–39.

Rushby, J., et al. 2001. Calculating and presenting disability adjusted life years (DALYs) in cost-effectiveness analysis. *Health Policy Planning*, 16: 326–331.

Sassi, F. 2006. Calculating QALYs, comparing QALY and DALY calculations. *Health Policy Planning*, 21: 402–408.

SDSN. 2015. Indicators and a Monitoring Framework for the Sustainable Development Goals: Launching a data revolution for the SDGs: A report to the Secretary-General of the United Nations by the Leadership Council of the Sustainable Development Solutions Network. Retrieved from: http://unsdsn.org/resources/publications/indicators/ (Accessed June 22, 2016).

Sibai, A. 2004. Mortality certification and cause of death reporting in developing countries. *Bulletin of the World Health Organization*, 82: 83–88.

Slought Museum. 2011. Bills of Mortality, London. Retrieved from: slought.org/content/410265/.

Sullivan, D. 1971. A single index of mortality and morbidity. *HSMHA Health Report*, 86: 347–354.

UCLA. 2007. John Snow. Retrieved from: www.ph.ucla.edu/epi/snow.html.

UN. 2006. Department of Economic and Social Affairs. World Mortality Report. Retrieved from: www.un.org/esa/population/publications/worldmortality/WMR2005.pdf.

UN. 2016a. Millennium Development Goals. Retrieved from: www.un.org/millenniumgoals.

UN. 2016b. UN Statistical Division. Retrieved from: http://data.un.org/.

UNESCO. 2016. UNESCO Institute for Statistics. Retrieved from: www.uis.unesco.org/Pages/default.aspx

UNICEF. 2015a. Estimates generated by the UN Inter-agency Group for Child Mortality Estimation (IGME) in 2015. Retrieved from: www.data.unicef.org/child-mortality/under-five.html.

UNICEF. 2015b. Levels & Trends in Child Mortality Report 2015. Estimates Developed by the UN Inter-agency Group for Child Mortality Estimation. Retrieved from: www.who.int/maternal_child_adolescent/documents/levels_trends_child_mortality_2015/en/

UNICEF. 2016a. Birth registration: Statistical tables. Retrieved from: www.unicef.org/protection/57929_58010.html

UNICEF. 2016b. The state of the world's children. Retrieved from: www.unicef.org/sowc/

UNICEF. 2016c. Childinfo: Child nutrition statistics. Retrieved from: www.childinfo.org/nutrition.html.

UNICEF. 2016d. Childinfo: Child immunization statistics. Retrieved from: www.childinfo.org/immunization.html.

UNICEF. 2016e. Maternal health statistics by region. Retrieved from: https://data.unicef.org/.

United Nations Population Division. n.d. United Nations population information network: Data. Retrieved from: www.un.org/popin/data.html.

UNICEF. 2016f. Joint UNICEF/WHO immunization summary. Retrieved from: www.who.int/
    immunization/monitoring_surveillance/routine/reporting/en/.

UNICEF. 2016g. Water and sanitation statistics by region. Retrieved from: www.childinfo.org/
    wes.html.

UNICEF. 2016h. Childinfo: Child health statistics. Retrieved from: www.childinfo.org/
    mortality_imrcountrydata.php.

WDI. 2016. World Development Indicators. Retrieved from: http://data.worldbank.org/
    data-catalog/world-development-indicators.

WHO. 1997. The sisterhood method for estimating maternal mortality. Retrieved from:
    whqlibdoc.who.int/hq/1997/WHO_RHT_97.28.pdf.

WHO. 2001. National burden of disease studies: A practical guide. Retrieved from: www.who.
    int/healthinfo/nationalburdenofdiseasemanual.pdf.

WHO. 2008. Global Burden of Disease: 2004 update. Retrieved from: www.who.int/healthinfo/
    global_burden_disease/2004_report_update/en/.

WHO. 2015a. Global tuberculosis report. Retrieved from: http://apps.who.int/iris/bitstre
    am/10665/191102/1/9789241565059_eng.pdf.

WHO. 2015b. Implementing the End TB Strategy: The essentials. Retrieved from: www.who.
    int/tb/publications/2015/end_tb_essential.pdf?ua=1.

WHO. 2016a. The Global Burden of Disease project. Retrieved from: www.who.int/healthinfo/
    global_burden_disease/about/en/.

WHO. 2016b. Global alert and response. Retrieved from: www.who.int/csr/en.

WHO. 2016c. Burden of disease and cost-effectiveness estimates. Retrieved from: www.
    who.int/immunization/monitoring_surveillance/burden/estimates/en/; www.who.int/
    water_sanitation_health/diseases/burden/en/.

WHO. 2016d. Global database on childhood growth and nutrition. Retrieved from: www.who.
    int/nutgrowthdb/en/.

WHO. 2016e. World Health Statistics 2016: Monitoring health for the SDGs. Retrieved from:
    www.who.int/gho/publications/world_health_statistics/2016/en/.

WHO. 2016f. Immunization in WHO regions. Retrieved from: www.who.int/topics/
    immunization/en/.

WHO. 2016g. Maternal and reproductive health database. Retrieved from: www.who.int/gho/
    maternal_health/en/index.html.

WHO. 2016h. Water sanitation and health. Retrieved from: www.who.int/
    water_sanitation_health.

WHO/UNICEF. 2015. Progress on sanitation and drinking water: 201555c update. Retrieved
    from: www.who.int/water_sanitation_health/monitoring/en/.

WHOSIS. 2011a. WHO statistical information system. Healthy life expectancy (HALE) at birth.
    Retrieved from: www.who.int/whosis/indicators/2007HALE0/en/.

WHOSIS. 2011b. The world health statistics report. Retrieved from: www.who.int/whosis/
    whostat/en/.

World Bank. 2011. World databank. Retrieved from: http://databank.worldbank.org/ddp/home.
    do?Step=12&id=4&CNO=2.

World Bank. 2016. Data from World Bank. World Development Indicators, Data Query.
    Available at: http://databank.worldbank.org/data/reports.aspx?source=2&series=SP.DYN.
    LE00.IN&country (Accessed December 20, 2016).

CHAPTER 10

The Diseases of Adults and Children in Developing Countries

Disease is not of the body but of the place.

—Lucius Seneca, 4 BC to AD 65

OBJECTIVES

The previous chapter examined the difficulties of defining and measuring disease accurately. In this chapter, we will examine the results of that research in order to answer the questions: What is the magnitude of morbidity and mortality in different regions of the world? What are the major underlying causes of that ill health? This is not a sterile academic topic—high-quality health data is an absolutely essential foundation for good health care. When combined with modern methods of risk analysis, it allows planners to adjust their programs to meet local requirements in the most cost-effective way. Because of the unique problems associated with pregnancy-related diseases, maternal mortality will be reviewed as a separate adult category. After completing this chapter, you should be able to:

- understand the major causes of adult morbidity and mortality in the developing world and their trends with time
- understand the magnitude and causes of avoidable child mortality in developing countries
- appreciate the central role of the mother in the safe growth and development of children
- understand the magnitude and underlying causes of maternal mortality

INTRODUCTION

The social environment in childhood affects achieved adult height, life chances, and ulti-mately even mortality rates in adult life.

—Sir Michael Marmot, 1987

Over the last two or three decades, population health research has provided an increasingly sophisticated understanding of ill health in developing countries. The World Bank and the WHO led the way by combining injury weighting meth-ods from the insurance industry with cost-effectiveness approaches developed for business. The combination of these two strands of research has resulted in a rev-olution in health epidemiology. Not surprisingly, the cost-effectiveness approach was championed by the World Bank. Beginning in 1993 with the first edition of Disease Control Priorities in Developing Countries, its Disease Control Priorities project (DCPP, 2011) has continued to help health planners develop policies based on measured evidence. The second edition was published in 2006 (DCP2, 2006) and as of April 2016, part of the third edition has been published (DCP3, 2016). Obviously, there can be no useful analysis without accurate data. The challenge of improving basic health information was taken on by the WHO's Global Burden of Disease project (WHO, 2011). Apart from improving basic mortality data, they also pioneered the use of the DALY to measure the burden of different diseases around the world. Their first Global Burden of Disease report, in 1993, was highly

Box 10.1 History Notes

Lillian Wald (1867–1940)

As with Virchow, it is difficult to imagine how someone managed to achieve so much in one lifetime. Wald was born to a wealthy middle-class American family and studied to be a nurse. She rebelled against strict hospital practice and took further training to join the newly formed visiting nurses who worked in the poorest areas of New York. She later coined the term "pub-lic health nurse" and, as an educator and administrator, advanced nursing as a respected professional organization. Based on her experiences of the squalor of the Lower East Side, she devoted the rest of her life to improving the conditions of the poor. The centre she started for the poor, the Henry Street Project, is still running today, as is the Public Health Nursing Organization. Her advocacy led to school nurses, school meals, the Women's Trade Union League, and respect for the rights of immigrants. Not surprisingly, she was also instrumental in the New York State women's suffrage movement. It is impossible to list all the health initia-tives started by this dynamo. After her funeral, the US president, New York governor, and New York mayor each talked about her life's work to a packed Carnegie Hall audience. For more information, follow the reference: Henry Street (2011).

influential and helped to broaden health analysis by including important but less lethal conditions, such as psychiatric disorders. The most recent update was in 2013 and led by the Institute of Health Metrics and Evaluation (IHME). The study produced estimates for 323 diseases and injuries, 67 risk factors, and 1,500 sequelae for 188 countries (GBD, 2013).

The first Global Burden of Disease study had a profound effect on the subsequent measurement of population health. Traditional mortality data have increasingly been replaced by broader measures of the total burden of ill health imposed by common diseases. Morbidity measurements became just as important as mortality measurements once it was shown that non-communicable diseases (alcohol abuse, road traffic accidents, tobacco-related diseases) caused a greater disease burden than HIV, tuberculosis, and malaria combined. The growing emphasis on health promotion and disease prevention has also stimulated research into the risk factors behind the major diseases (WHO, 2009). More recently, the need to monitor the SDGs has added further emphasis to the need for accurate population health data and has also placed a much-needed emphasis on the need for accurate data on maternal mortality and the risks associated with pregnancy. The trend toward measurement and analysis is a good one, but it must always be remembered that these new methods rely on complex calculations that are open to sampling error, measurement error, and problems of inaccurate data sources. Furthermore, these measurements may convey only limited dimensions of more complex issues.

In the past, the health industry has sometimes had a history of investing in expensive treatments without first checking to see if they were the most efficient way of improving population health. A good example was the early assumption that exporting Western-style hospital-based medical care to developing countries was the best way to improve their widespread health problems. It took 20 years and an international meeting at Alma Ata before it became widely accepted that expensive urban hospitals had actually done very little to improve the lives or health of the developing world's rural majority. The money spent maintaining what subsequently became dubbed "disease palaces" meant there was less money for rural health care. When examined carefully, the exported hospital likely made health worse for the poorest people.

The best way (in fact, the only way) to avoid wasting money on initiatives that are unlikely to work is to base health planning on the best available epidemiological health research. The methods first pioneered by the Ghana Health Assessment Team 40 years ago (GHAT, 1981) are increasingly being adopted by the developing world health industry. The Ghanaian team's response to a limited health budget was to fund initiatives that had the best predictable benefits for the lowest costs. They were the first to adopt the business techniques of risk analysis and cost-benefit analysis, which allowed them to modify their own plans so they could meet the most important needs of their local population. Modern developments of those earlier techniques have plenty of applications in terms of population health initiatives. Knowledge of trends in morbidity and mortality, combined with an understanding of the underlying behavioural, social, economic, and political causes, allows health projects to be planned in the most effective manner possible. This is an essential topic for anyone who plans to work in the field of developing world health care.

CAUSES OF DEATH AND CHRONIC DISEASE IN DEVELOPING COUNTRIES

Never use abstract nouns when concrete ones will do. If you mean "More people died" don't say "Mortality rose."

—C. S. Lewis, Letters to Children

In 1955, the world's population was 2.8 billion and the average global life expectancy was 48 years. At time of writing, in 2016, the population has just passed through 7 billion and life expectancy is just above 70 years. These improvements in mortality and morbidity are extraordinary and are surprisingly underappreciated. In many developing countries, life expectancy has increased by 25 years during that 50-year period—in each successive year, a newborn can expect to live another six months. A child born 10 years after an older sibling can expect to live 5 years longer! Some, but not all, of this progress can be explained—the topic was discussed at length in Chapter 3 under the determinants of disease. The contribution of the aid industry to this trend is a cause of heated debate, but a good deal of credit can certainly be claimed for the improvements in child health. No matter what the cause, the progress itself is undeniable.

The pattern of health improvement follows a predictable course. With the exception of HIV in the 1980s, basic improvements in sanitation, health care, and immunization have steadily reduced the burden of infectious diseases. Their place is taken by a completely new set of problems closely related to increasing affluence, including obesity, diabetes, tobacco-related diseases, ischemic heart disease, and strokes. The 1993 Burden of Disease report separated countries into rich and poor, but rapid progress in large countries such as India, China, Brazil, and Indonesia meant that by the 2000 update, a third category for middle-income countries had to be added. China and India are both good examples of the contrasts and paradoxes that can be seen in these transition countries. While they still have areas of great poverty, they also have growing numbers of billionaires. While both countries still receive aid, they are also becoming significant donors of aid. Their major causes of mortality and morbidity are rapidly resembling those of the richest countries, with reducing levels of major infections and rising levels of obesity and ischemic heart disease. This section will examine the causes of mortality and morbidity among adults living at these three income levels.

Common Causes of Mortality

> Twenty-five years ago, the world's leading experts in cardiovascular diseases warned of an impending epidemic of heart disease in developing countries. This warning was largely ignored.
>
> —*Gro Brundtland, former director-general of the WHO, 1999*

According to the first Global Burden of Disease study, 50 million people died in 1990, 12.7 million of whom were children below the age of five. The great burden of this mortality fell on developing countries; 98 percent of all childhood deaths and 83 percent of deaths in people 15–59 years occurred in developing countries (Murray et al., 1994). At the time of the first global study, the world was more clearly split between developed and developing countries. There was, of course, a global middle class, but their growth had not yet had a big impact on mortality rate statistics. With the exception of pneumonia, developed countries had almost eradicated infectious diseases as a major cause of mortality. The dominant causes of mortality were non-infectious diseases, such as atherosclerotic vascular disease and cancer. In contrast, five of the leading causes of mortality in developing countries were infectious (pneumonia, diarrheal diseases, tuberculosis, measles, and malaria). However, the effect of a growing affluent class was evident by the appearance of

---

Box 10.2 Moment of Insight

Average life expectancy of one Japanese woman:	Average life expectancies of women living in:
	Afghanistan: 43.8 years
	Mozambique: 42.4 years
	Total years lived by two women living in very poor countries:
86.2 years	**86.2 years**

Source: UN. 2006. Economic and social affairs, world population prospects. Retrieved from: www.un.org/esa/population/publications/wpp2006/WPP2006_Highlights_rev.pdf.

heart attacks and strokes as significant problems, even in developing countries. At that stage, the HIV/AIDS epidemic had not yet reached the top 10.

The ongoing development of China, Brazil, India, and other reduced-mortality areas of the developing world has effectively formed a global middle class that has greatly altered the distribution of mortality, shifting it away from infectious diseases in children and toward non-communicable diseases in people over 60 years old. In this area of research, the WHO classifies cause of death under only three headings:

Group 1: communicable, maternal, perinatal, and nutritional conditions

Group 2: non-communicable diseases

Group 3: injuries

Much of the world is currently going through an epidemiological transition from high pediatric mortality due to Group 1 causes, toward increasing death rates from Group 2 diseases in an increasingly older population. This trend has reached the point that three times as many people now die from non-communicable diseases as from Group 1 causes (Figure 10.1). Overall, 18 percent of all deaths occur in children, while 51 percent are in adults 60 years and older.

When the leading causes of global deaths are plotted, the mixture of Group 1 and Group 2 causes becomes obvious (Figure 10.2). Over the last few decades, the burden of disease has shifted toward non-communicable diseases globally. The most common cause of death worldwide is vascular disease—heart attacks and

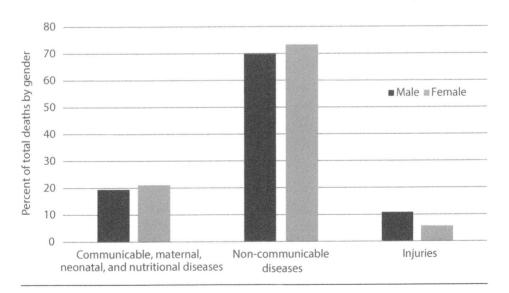

Figure 10.1: Distribution of deaths by cause and gender, 2015

Source: IHME. 2016. Data from Institute of Health Metrics and Evaluation. GBD heat map. Pub: IHME, University of Washington. Retrieved from: http://vizhub.healthdata.org/gbd-compare/.

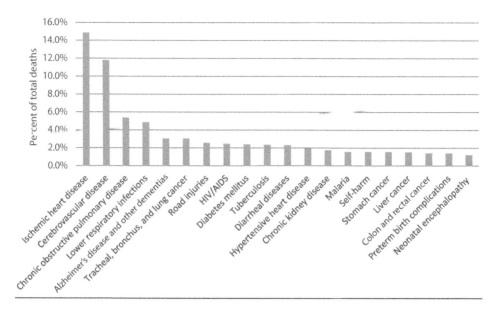

Figure 10.2: The leading causes of death in 2013 for all ages; frequency of deaths is expressed as a percentage of that year's total deaths.

Source: IHME. 2016. Data from Institute of Health Metrics and Evaluation. GBD heat map. Pub: IHME, University of Washington. Retrieved from: http://vizhub.healthdata.org/gbd-compare/.

strokes. Mixed in with these diseases of increasing affluence are the major killers of children in poor countries (diarrhea, HIV/AIDS, prematurity, and birth asphyxia). Apart from the fact that vascular diseases hold the top two mortality spots, the additional presence of lung cancer and chronic bronchitis highlights the burgeoning epidemic of tobacco-related disease, which will remain a major cause of death worldwide for several decades with current smoking patterns (Islami et al., 2015). Gender differences are significant in a few categories, particularly in cardiovascular disease, which now causes almost a third of all female deaths. Intentional and accidental injuries are far more common in men than women. Almost one in eight male deaths are due to injuries.

When causes of mortality are broken down by income group (Table 10.1), there are clear differences between rich and poor. Among high-income countries, diseases associated with affluence (heart attacks, strokes, diabetes), plus diseases of an aging population (dementias, cancer), dominate the picture. In the poorest countries, infectious diseases (diarrheal diseases, HIV, TB, malaria) and diseases of infancy (prematurity and neonatal diseases) are still the dominant causes of death, although even in the poorest countries, heart attacks and strokes are beginning to climb up the mortality table. The rapidly growing global middle class has made great progress in its transition from Group 1 diseases to those of Group 2—its top

Table 10.1: Leading causes of death for all ages for low- and middle-income countries and high-income countries, 2015. Disease frequency is expressed as percentage of total deaths.

LOW- AND MIDDLE-INCOME COUNTRIES			HIGH-INCOME COUNTRIES		
Rank	Cause	% Total	Rank	Cause	% Total
1	Ischemic heart disease	12.7	1	Ischemic heart disease	21.5
2	Cerebrovascular disease	11.6	2	Cerebrovascular disease	12.2
3	Chronic obstructive pulmonary disease	5.7	3	Alzheimer's disease and other dementias	7.0
4	Lower respiratory infections	5.2	4	Tracheal, bronchus, and lung cancer	5.3
5	HIV/AIDS	3.1	5	Chronic obstructive pulmonary disease	4.2
6	Tuberculosis	3.0	6	Lower respiratory infections	3.7
7	Road injuries	3.0	7	Colon and rectal cancer	3.1
8	Diarrheal diseases	3.0	8	Diabetes mellitus	1.9
9	Diabetes mellitus	2.5	9	Stomach cancer	1.8
10	Tracheal, bronchus, and lung cancer	2.3	10	Self-harm	1.8

Source: IHME. 2016. Data from Institute of Health Metrics and Evaluation. GBD heat map. Pub: IHME, University of Washington. Retrieved from: http://vizhub.healthdata.org/gbd-compare/.

five causes of mortality are identical to those in high-income countries. Only the presence of tuberculosis and road injuries on the list gives a clue to the presence of poverty and urban chaos.

Common Causes of Morbidity and the Burden of Chronic Diseases

Health is my expected heaven.

—John Keats, 1820

In the fairly recent past, death and its major causes dominated health research; this was particularly true for children. Even 20 years ago, child mortality was so high that little time was spent analyzing causes of chronic illness. As people clambered out of extreme poverty, they gradually achieved the time and money to worry about being alive and well rather than simply being alive. Epidemiologic research responded to this trend by starting to study morbidity along with mortality. The WHO selected the Disability-Adjusted Life Year (DALY) as its principal indicator and first used it in a landmark 1990 study of the burden of diseases around the world. As discussed in the last chapter, the total burden of disease is calculated by adding the years lost to disability (YLD) to the years of life lost from early mortality (YLL). Apart from the errors involved in collecting the necessary basic data, there is also a significant subjective element in the calculation of DALYs. The method has provided useful insights into the daily burden of disease, but it should still be interpreted with some caution.

At the time of the 1990 study, almost a quarter of all deaths were in children. This enormous burden of potential years lost to avoidable diseases meant that pediatric conditions dominated the list of diseases with the greatest burden. The presence of pneumonia, diarrheal diseases, perinatal conditions, and measles reflected the prevailing high rates of childhood disease in the developing world. The HIV/AIDS epidemic had not yet grown sufficiently to enter the top 10 list. The most surprising finding of the first 1990 study was the unexpectedly high burden caused by neuropsychiatric disorders (Chisholm et al., 2005). Four of the top 10 causes of years lost to disability in 1990 were psychiatric diseases (obsessive-compulsive disorder, schizophrenia, bipolar disorder, and depression). It should be remembered that this was the first attempt at assessing global disability. Direct comparisons between the leading causes of years lost due to disability between 1990 and 2004 should be made with great care because of the changes and improvements made to measurement techniques with time.

Before using complex methods to measure the burden of illness, the first place to start is simply to look at prevalence—how many people are sick in the world at any one time? There are also cases of common low-mortality conditions, which lack the drama of malaria or tuberculosis and so tend to be discounted, but they still cause a great deal of misery, reduced activity, and economic loss. By far the most common single cause of illness around the world is iron-deficiency anemia. This is followed by depression, arthritis, poor vision and hearing, and severe infestations with intestinal parasites. These are not minor issues—with access to good-quality medical care, much of this disease load can be improved, with great benefits in terms of population health and productivity.

After counting diseases, the next step is to quantify the cumulative burden they impose on a population, which is done by measuring DALYs. The method allows the cost of a medical intervention to be compared against effective gains in health and also helps health planners to target the most serious diseases within a community. It is important to remember that mortality statistics and DALYs measure different aspects of disease, so they do not always agree about which disease is the most important. The 10 leading causes of death DALYS for low- and

Table 10.2: Leading causes of DALYs for low- and middle-income countries, 2015

LOW- AND MIDDLE-INCOME COUNTRIES			HIGH-INCOME COUNTRIES		
Rank	Cause	% Total	Rank	Cause	% Total
1	Ischemic heart disease	5.3	1	Ischemic heart disease	10.4
2	Lower respiratory infections	5.2	2	Low back and neck pain	7.6
3	Cerebrovascular disease	4.4	3	Cerebrovascular disease	5.6
4	Low back and neck pain	3.7	4	Tracheal, bronchus, and lung cancer	3.4
5	Diarrheal diseases	3.5	5	Depressive disorders	3.2
6	Preterm birth complications	3.3	6	Chronic obstructive pulmonary disease	3.1
7	HIV/AIDS	3.3	7	Sense organ diseases	
8	Road injuries	3.2	8	Diabetes mellitus	
9	Malaria	3.2	9	Alzheimer's disease and other dementias	
10	Chronic obstructive pulmonary disease	2.9	10	Self-harm	2.2

Source: IHME. 2016. Data from Institute of Health Metrics and Evaluation. GBD heat map. Pub: IHME, University of Washington. Retrieved from: http://vizhub.healthdata.org/gbd-compare/.

middle-income countries and for high-income countries in 2015 are highlighted in Table 10.2. Clearly, diseases with the highest DALY scores don't always match up with those that have the highest mortality. The leading individual causes of DALYs in low- and middle-income countries are ischemic heart disease, lower respiratory infractions, cerebrovascular disease, etc. This differs substantially from the 10 leading causes of DALYs in high-income countries and reflects the high burden of conditions related to birth in low-resource settings.

Table 10.2 lists the most common causes of DALYs by income group. There are, of course, many similarities with the equivalent mortality table (Table 10.1), but there are also significant differences. Important diseases in richer countries that are missed by a crude mortality analysis include alcohol abuse, vision loss, hearing loss, and the long-term effects of road traffic accidents. DALY scores are heavily influenced by chronic severe infections and early child deaths. Consequently, in poor countries, there is little difference between the causes of mortality and the largest sources of DALYs. However, illnesses such as lower back and neck pain and malaria that are missed in the crude mortality analysis represent significant causes of DALYs in low- and middle-income countries.

The Major Disease Risk Factors

If one is forever cautious, can one remain a human being?

—Aleksandr Solzhenitsyn, 1968

When it comes to major diseases, prevention is a lot better than a cure. It took the aid industry many years to learn this simple lesson. The failure of Western-style hospital-based medical care to improve population health in poor countries was finally accepted at the Alma Ata meeting in 1978 (see Chapter 3). The subsequent adoption of primary health care (PHC), with its greater emphasis on research and prevention, represented a revolution in the approach to disease. Diseases aren't magical—they are caused by risk factors that can usually be identified, quantified, and, in many cases, avoided. You can't prevent a disease until the underlying causes are known, so the shift to PHC was associated with greater emphasis on the study of diseases and their underlying causes. Once major risk factors have been identified, several attempts are made to concentrate limited financial resources on those identifiable problems.

The first package of treatments aimed at identified proximal risk factors was proposed as part of the UNICEF-sponsored Child Survival Revolution in the 1980s (UNICEF, 1984). It included immunization, breastfeeding, and oral rehydration solution. The World Bank proposed its own essential services package in the 1993 World Development Report (World Bank, 1993). It was aimed at major risk factors for adult and child disease; the interventions ranged from school deworming programs to alcohol and tobacco control. The World Health Organization's Integrated Management of Childhood Illnesses program is also designed around major pediatric risks (Lambrechts et al., 1999). The subject of essential health packages is examined further in Chapter 13. It is also important to note the limited paradigm of risk in these approaches, which tend to focus on biomedical risk factors and not on the broader forces of poverty and social, economic, political determinants of health. As discussed in Chapter 3, these broader forces play important roles in the health of populations.

CHILD HEALTH IN DEVELOPING COUNTRIES

The child was diseased at birth, stricken with a hereditary ill that only the most vital men shake off.... I mean poverty; the most deadly and prevalent of all diseases.

—Eugene O'Neill, Fog, early one-act play, 1914

Before starting this next section on child health, it is important to begin by addressing the widespread misconception that treating sick children in developing countries is a pointless exercise: "High child mortality is just nature's way of keeping the population down." Although this notion is commonly held, it is completely false. In developing areas of the world, children represent a form of security that will provide support to the parents when they are too old to earn a living. Consequently, families will continue to have children until they can be sure that at least a few will survive to adulthood. The American demographer W. Thompson (Hirschman, 1994) described a four-stage process (demographic or fertility transition) that is followed by most countries as they emerge from poverty. It is characterized by large families during periods of poverty and poor social development, followed by a steady decrease in family size once living standards and health care start to improve (see "Family Planning" in Chapter 12 for more details). There is no unified fertility theory that fully explains this observation (rather, there are several that raise furious debate), but its existence has been repeatedly demonstrated, including in the recent histories of the currently industrialized countries.

Child Mortality Rates

Time and fevers burn away
Individual beauty from
Thoughtful children, and the grave
Proves the child ephemeral

—*W. H. Auden, "Lullaby," 1937*

Child deaths have been monitored since the 1950s, but there was no clearly organized methodology and data distribution system until surprisingly recently. The 1990 World Summit for Children in New York generated an ambitious plan of action for child health, which acted as a catalyst for broad improvements in data collection. The UN Population Division and UNICEF started the large task of organizing the available data from 1960 onwards (Hill et al., 1999). They also placed great emphasis on making the results available to researchers through publications and the UNICEF website (UNICEF, 2011). In order to meet the monitoring demands of the MDGs, the next step was the formation of the Child Health Epidemiology Reference Group (CHERG, 2016) in 2001, followed by the Interagency Group for Child Mortality Estimation in 2004 (IGME, 2011a). The aim of both organizations is to share data and standardize estimates within the UN group. Their most recently published mortality estimates were in 2015 (IGME, 2015).

Significant progress has been made in reducing child deaths since 1990. The number of under-five deaths worldwide has declined from 12.7 million in 1990 to 5.9 million in 2015. Progress against childhood mortality has been one of the success stories of international aid. In many countries, death rates have fallen by 50 percent since 1990. This has not always been enough to meet the rather ambitious MDG

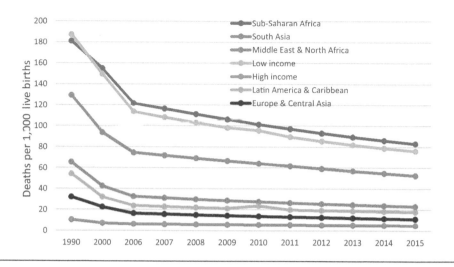

Figure 10.3: Trends in under-five mortality rates for different world regions over the last 25 years

Source: World Bank. 2016a. Data from the World Bank. World Development Indicators: Mortality. Retrieved from: http://data.worldbank.org/indicator/SP.DYN.IMRT.IN?display=graph.

4 target of two-thirds reduction in the under-five mortality rate by 2015 (i.e., 30 deaths per 1,000 live births), but it is still a huge step forward (Figure 10.3). The region with the highest under-five mortality rate in the world (sub-Saharan Africa) has also registered a substantive acceleration. Its annual rate of reduction increased from 1.6 percent in 1990s to 4.1 percent in 2000–2015 (IGME, 2015). Since 1990, the global under-five mortality rate has dropped 53 percent, from 91 deaths per 1,000 live births in 1990 to 43 in 2015. According to the latest estimates by WHO and the Maternal and Child Epidemiology Estimation Group, of the 5.9 million deaths in children under five that occurred in 2015, about half were caused by infectious diseases and conditions such as pneumonia, diarrhea, malaria, meningitis, tetanus, HIV, and measles (Figure 10.5). The main killers of children under age five in 2015 include preterm birth complications (18 percent), pneumonia (16 percent), intrapartum-related complications (12 percent), diarrhea (9 percent) and sepsis/meningitis (9 percent). Importantly, almost half of all under-five deaths are attributable to under-nutrition, as discussed in Chapter 6. There is also a change in trends in infant mortality shifting to greater percentage accounted for by neonatal deaths in the first month of life. Most child deaths are caused by diseases that are readily preventable or treatable with proven, cost-effective interventions. Although we can measure the numbers and causes, and even estimate the tens of millions of potential years of life lost, how do we measure the accumulated grief produced by these tragedies? Some will believe that developing world families are hardened to the death of children—that the loss of

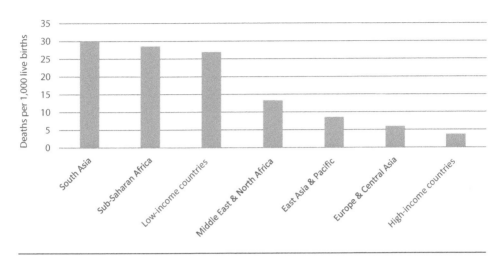

Figure 10.4: Neonatal mortality (NMR) in 2015 for different world regions

Source: World Bank. 2016b. Data from the World Bank. World Development Indicators. Retrieved from: http://data.worldbank.org/indicator/SH.DYN.NMRT?display=graph.

one from eight is much easier to bear than the loss of one from two. This is not true. Perhaps a new measure of sadness is required—a grief-adjusted life year. Maybe this would help to put a human face on these otherwise unimaginable numbers.

The three measurements of mortality commonly used are:

- *Under-five mortality rate:* The number of deaths before the fifth birthday per 1,000 live births is the most widely used indicator of a country's child health status because it is the final result of all adverse factors averaged over a five-year period.
- *Infant mortality rate:* The number of deaths before the first birthday per 1,000 live births. Children are particularly vulnerable to poor social and economic factors during the first year. The infant mortality rate correlates well with social standards, so it is used as an indicator of state competence as well as an indicator of child health.
- *Neonatal mortality rate:* The number of deaths before 28 days of life per 1,000 live births. Neonatal mortality is a measure of the adequacy of delivery and newborn standards in a country. It is closely correlated with maternal mortality because both are affected by a similar set of variables.

In high-mortality areas like sub-Saharan Africa, neonatal causes account for less than 30 percent of total under-five deaths. In lower mortality areas, where social improvements have allowed more older children to survive, neonatal causes make up 40 percent or more of the total. Controlling neonatal and maternal deaths requires significant investments in delivery and newborn services, so these two rates are the last to show significant improvement.

Common Causes of Childhood Mortality

Figure 10.5 illustrates the most common causes of childhood death up to five years of age. Improvements in vaccination coverage, increasing emphasis on sanitation, and use of oral rehydration solution have greatly reduced deaths from a wide range of pediatric illnesses. As a reflection of improved sanitation and better treatment for dehydration, pneumonia overtook diarrhea as the leading cause of death some years ago. At present, diarrhea is slightly ahead as a killer of older children, but a high rate of pneumonia among infants has allowed pneumonia to keep its place as the most common overall infectious cause of death. Progress against HIV infection in children has meant that deaths due to AIDS seem to have reached a plateau.

Figure 10.6 gives the most common causes of death for those children who die within the first four weeks of life. While the under-five mortality rate reflects average health standards of a society averaged over a period of years, neonatal

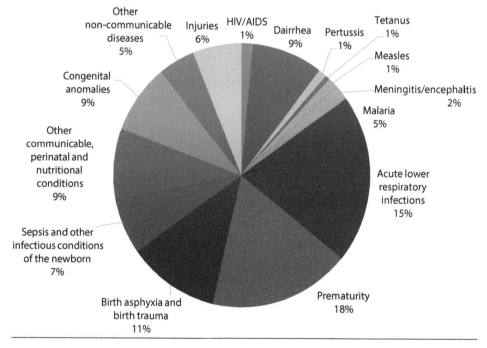

Figure 10.5: Causes of under-five child death, globally, by percentage, 2015

Source: WHO. 2016. Global Health Observatory Data Repository: Mortality and global health estimates. Retrieved from: http://apps.who.int/gho/data/node.main.CM3002015REGWORLD?lang=en

mortality is more an indicator of pregnancy and early child care standards. Causes of neonatal death are split fairly evenly between infectious diseases (neonatal sepsis and pneumonia) and the complications of pregnancy and delivery (birth asphyxia and prematurity). These causes do not respond to the provision of basic primary health care and public health provisions, such as clean water and immunization. They are medical emergencies and require medical treatment in properly equipped and staffed health centres. This comprehensive approach requires money, planning, and sustainable long-term investment. Prior to the impetus of the MDGs, all three were lacking, inhibiting improvements in infant and maternal mortalities.

Ninety-eight percent of all under-five deaths occur in developing countries—the poorer the country, the higher the rate; the correlation is not difficult to detect. Many of the major causes can be avoided by immunization, and most of the remainder can be treated effectively. Whatever the exact survival figures might be, given access to good health care, it is fair to say that millions of children die unnecessarily every year. Effective treatments exist for pneumonia, malaria, diarrhea, and neonatal infections. Reliable vaccines have almost abolished polio and can do the same for measles and neonatal tetanus. HIV transmission from mother to child can be efficiently inhibited by the use of antiretroviral therapy, and neonatal causes

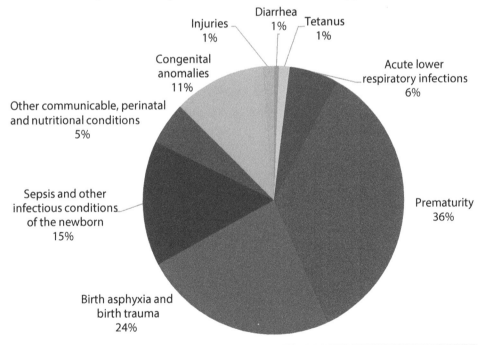

Figure 10.6: Causes of neonatal deaths, globally, by percentage, 2015

Source: WHO. 2016. Global Health Observatory Data Repository: Mortality and global health estimates. Retrieved from: http://apps.who.int/gho/data/node.main.CM3002015REGWORLD?lang=en.

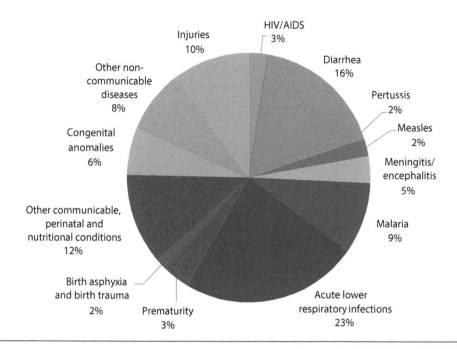

Figure 10.7: Causes of post-neonatal under-five deaths, globally by percentage, 2015

Source: WHO. 2016. Global Health Observatory Data Repository: Mortality and global health estimates. Retrieved from: http://apps.who.int/gho/data/node.main.CM3002015REGWORLD?lang=en.

of death can also be significantly reduced by the presence of well-trained attendants during pregnancy and delivery. The problem of global child mortality is not due to lack of treatment options—it is due to lack of political will.

Maternal and Child Health Approach

> There is no such thing as a baby.
>
> —*Dr. Donald Winnicott, pediatrician, psychoanalyst*

Dr. Winnicott's famous saying, quoted above, sums up the complete reliance of a child on his or her mother. Clearly, whatever harms a mother will also harm her child. Child care given by a healthy, educated woman, who has access to postnatal care and advice, can protect the infant against a range of infectious and environmental dangers. As the 2005 World Health Report pointed out, no serious advances in child mortality can be made until equivalent attention is paid to female health, particularly education, gender equality, and pregnancy-related medical care (WHO, 2005a). The bond between mother and child is so close that there is a natural tendency to view the health concerns of women and children as a single issue. The original term used to describe this combined approach (maternal-child health, or MCH) was certainly in common use a century ago—there was already a US Bureau of Maternal and Child Health by 1935. In recognition of the combined medical approaches used for mothers and newborns, the more commonly used terms are now "maternal and newborn health" (MNH) (UNICEF, 2009) or "maternal, newborn, and child health."

The delivery of a child is a risky time for a woman in a poor country. Nearly half of all maternal deaths occur within a day of delivery, and most of the remainder are spread out over the next month. A quarter of all newborn deaths also happen on the first day of life and another half occur within the first week. Women die mostly from blood loss, sepsis, obstructed labour, and eclampsia. Newborns die most commonly from prematurity, birth asphyxia, and infections. Once the causes of death are listed, the necessary interventions are quite obvious—good-quality, accessible health care. To some extent, we need to relearn the lessons of Alma Ata from 1978. There needs to be a continuum of competent care for women and their children with at least part of the follow-up centred on the home. All interventions should be supported by relevant clinical research and data collection. The total package requires investment in buildings, logistic support, trained staff, non-medical infrastructure and transportation, and research, so it is considerably more expensive than selective therapies such as vaccination. However, the results, in terms of a healthy population, are worth the investment.

The main features of a comprehensive MNH continuum of care consist of the following minimum standards (UNICEF, 2009):

- *Prenatal care:* Regular clinic visits to assess for risk factors; monitor growth; provide iron and folate supplements, deworming, preventive malarial treatment, HIV/syphilis screening, tetanus toxoid to protect the infant, treated bed nets, and counselling to use a trained birth attendant. (Newer versions of MNH are now including a focus on reproductive health of women before pregnancy, including access to contraception, their own nutrition, etc.)
- *Basic delivery care:* Basic monitoring by a skilled birth attendant, good standards of hygiene, active management of third stage to prevent post-partum hemorrhage, and basic care of the newborn, as well as application of an HIV protocol for mothers testing positive.
- *Emergency provisions:* Birth attendants should be trained to recognize and refer developing emergencies. A referral centre should be accessible by local ambulance. The centre should be able to provide antibiotics, oxytocin,

magnesium sulfate, intravenous fluid, and blood transfusion, as well as have surgical staff, facilities, and anaesthesia for Caesarean section.

- *Postnatal care for the mother:* The birth attendant should be trained to recognize complications such as bleeding and infection. The mother should be given counselling about breastfeeding, child care, and family spacing. A nurse's first follow-up visit to the woman's home should be within three days.
- *Care for the newborn:* Dry and wrap the newborn, exclusive breastfeeding, and clean umbilical cord care. The child and mother should be reviewed together at home three days after discharge. The attendant should be trained to detect key problems, such as infection and poor weight gain.

MATERNAL HEALTH IN DEVELOPING COUNTRIES

There is a crying need for an international agency for women. Every stitch of evidence we have, right across the entire spectrum of gender inequality, suggests the urgent need for a multilateral agency. The great dreams of the international conferences in Vienna, Cairo, and Beijing have never come to pass. It matters not the issue: whether it's levels of sexual violence, or HIV/AIDS, or maternal mortality, or armed conflict, or economic empowerment, or parliamentary representation, women are in terrible trouble. And things are getting no better.

—*Stephen Lewis, addressing a high-level panel on UN reform, 2006*

If resolutions could sort out maternal deaths, the problem would have been solved long ago. The first large-scale conference on maternal deaths was held in 1987 by the Inter-agency Group for Safe Motherhood. After mergers and name changes, they are currently called the Partnership for Maternal, Newborn, and Child Health (PMNCH, 2011). The goal for reducing deaths, set at that early meeting, has been long forgotten. There were many more meetings on this subject, including the International Conference on Population and Development in 1994, the Fourth World Conference on Women in 1995 (plus their regular follow-up evaluations), and the MDGs in 2000. The pattern of rather more talk than action is demonstrated by the slow progress in reducing maternal deaths (Table 10.3) and increasing the prevalence of skilled birth attendants, neither of which changed significantly throughout the 1990s (Adegoke et al., 2009).

It must be remembered that pregnancy-related ill health is only one of many examples in which the lives of women receive insufficient attention. It doesn't matter what aspect of a woman's life in the developing world is examined—the effects of war, economic indicators, the levels of personal violence, human rights, access to education, or HIV/AIDS—women always do worse than men. As Stephen Lewis has pointed out, there is an urgent need to improve the historical second-class status of women in many parts of the world. He has suggested the establishment of a new international agency that will basically have the same mandate for women that UNICEF currently has for children.

The Extent of Maternal Mortality

The importance of women's health was reflected in the targets of SDG 3:

- *Target 3.1: By 2030, reduce the global maternal mortality ratio to less than 70 per 100,000 live births.* Measurements are not accurate, but world estimates for the maternal mortality ratio (MMR) in 2015 were 216 deaths per 100,000 live births, which means that the 2030 MMR goal would have to be reduced to 70 (Table 10.3).
- *Target 3.7: By 2030, ensure universal access to sexual and reproductive health-care services, including for family planning, information and education, and the integration of reproductive health into national strategies and programmes.* This is a very optimistic goal for large parts of the developing world. The term "reproductive health-care services" includes: access to family planning advice, access to contraceptives, adequate antenatal care, presence of a trained birth attendant, provision of emergency obstetric services, and reduction of teen pregnancy rates.

Maternal mortality is defined as the death of a woman while pregnant or within 42 days of termination of that pregnancy. In some jurisdictions, the definition includes deaths within one year after the end of a pregnancy. Deaths are defined as being due either to direct causes (complications of pregnancy and delivery) or indirect causes (death from pre-existing disease such as heart failure). Three separate indicators are calculated using the basic mortality data: (1) maternal mortality ratio, or MMR (maternal deaths per 100,000 live births), (2) maternal mortality rate (maternal deaths per 100,000 women of reproductive age), and (3) lifetime risk of pregnancy-associated death. The maternal mortality ratio is the most commonly used variable. Apart from the practical problems of measurement, MMR gives no indication of associated birth injuries or lifetime risk of death.

Unfortunately, making accurate estimates of maternal mortality (and any variables derived from that basic data) is notoriously difficult. It requires knowledge of a range of variables, including accurate information about deaths of women at reproductive age, the cause of death, and whether or not the woman was pregnant

Table 10.3: Comparison of maternal mortality ratio and number of maternal deaths, 1990 and 2015

MDG REGION	1990		2015		
	MMR	Maternal deaths	MMR	Maternal deaths	Lifetime risk of maternal death: 1 in
World	385	532,000	216	303,000	180
Developed regions	23	3,500	12	1,700	4,900
Developing regions	430	529,000	239	302,000	150
Northern Africa	171	6,400	70	3,100	450
Sub-Saharan Africa	987	223,000	546	201,000	36
Eastern Asia	95	26 000	27	4,800	2,300
Eastern Asia excluding China	51	590	43	380	1,500
Southern Asia	538	210,000	176	66,000	210
Southern Asia excluding India	495	57,800	180	21,000	190
Southeastern Asia	320	39,000	110	13,000	380
Western Asia	160	6,700	91	4,700	360
Caucasus and Central Asia	69	1,300	33	610	1,100
Latin America and the Caribbean	135	16,000	67	7,300	670
Latin America	124	14,000	60	6,000	760
Caribbean	276	2,300	175	1,300	250
Oceania	391	780	187	500	150

Source: WHO. 2015. Trends in Maternal Mortality: 1990 to 2015 Estimates by WHO, UNICEF, UNFPA, World Bank Group, and the United Nations Population Division. Retrieved from: www.who.int/reproductivehealth/publications/monitoring/maternal-mortality-2015/en/.

or had been recently pregnant (WHO, 2006). Unfortunately, only a few developing countries register births and deaths, fewer still record the cause of death, and hardly any note pregnancy status on the death certificate. In the absence of accurate registration data, various approaches are used to obtain accurate mortality estimates. These include direct household surveys, the sisterhood method, and reproductive age mortality studies (MMM-R, 2009).

In response to the need for better information, in 1990 the WHO, UNICEF, and UNFPA agreed to co-operate in order to improve standards of data collection and dissemination. They subsequently published updated summaries of maternal mortality statistics, the most recent of which was in 2015 (WHO, 2015). The UNICEF website also publishes accessible statistics on maternal health (Childinfo,

2011). While there have been measurable improvements in women's health around the world, progress toward the various parts of MDG 5 has been slow, particularly in South Asia and sub-Saharan Africa. Estimates of maternal mortality vary with the estimating agency, but some progress can be seen no matter which figures are used (Table 10.3). The worsening HIV epidemic slowed progress during the 1990s, but the annual death rate does seem to be dropping (WHO, 2015). Improvements in maternal mortality ratio have been seen everywhere, but South Asia and sub-Saharan African countries lag far behind world averages. The MMR in some African countries is still well above 500, with a 1 in 36 lifetime risk of death during delivery.

The biggest single determinant of maternal safety during delivery is the presence of a well-trained attendant. Although this has been common knowledge for decades, little more than 40 percent of the deliveries in the poorest countries have access to a skilled assistant. Roughly 75 percent of women in developing countries have at least one antenatal visit, but less than half those in South Asia or sub-Saharan Africa get the recommended four visits. Again, in the poorest countries, access to family planning information and easily available contraceptives is poor—coverage is barely 25 percent in sub-Saharan Africa. Not surprisingly, teen birth rates are very high in these poorly served areas. This exposes the mother and child to significantly higher medical risks. Overall, health care is slowly improving for women. However, many poor countries in Africa and Asia will not be included within that average estimate.

Causes of Maternal Mortality

There are inevitable similarities between maternal deaths and childhood deaths. The vast majority of both are treatable and/or avoidable. Figure 10.8 shows that in nearly one-third of cases, the mother simply bled to death—an almost completely avoidable and treatable problem. Most of those women would have lived if they had delivered in a developed country. Not surprisingly, most maternal deaths occur in developing countries, principally in sub-Saharan Africa and India (WHO, 2010). Less than 1 percent of maternal deaths occur in developed countries. If women do not die in developed countries, then there is no good reason why they should be dying anywhere else. Women and children differ in one important respect—childhood mortality is decreasing after two decades of interventions, but progress in maternal mortality has been very slow. Despite a lot of fine words, women's health still appears to be a scandalously low priority.

It should always be remembered that for every woman who dies, there are millions more who suffer chronic disabling complications of pregnancy. It has been estimated that of the nearly 140 million women who give birth each year, roughly

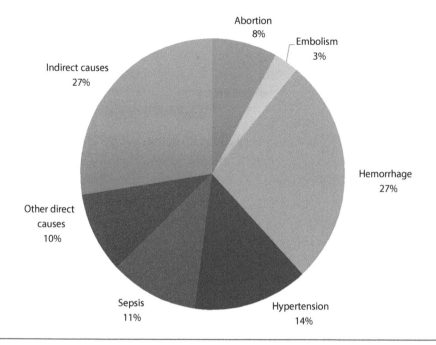

Figure 10.8: Distribution of causes of maternal death in low- and middle-income countries

Source: Say, L., et. al. 2014. Global causes of maternal death: A WHO systematic analysis. *The Lancet Global Health 2014*, 2: e323–333.

half experience some form of complication during pregnancy (Ashford, 2002). Ten to 15 percent of these women subsequently develop chronic disabilities, such as severe anemia, incontinence, fistulae from the uterus to the bladder or colon, depression, chronic pain, and infertility. As another example of the low priority placed on women's health, there is little accurate information about this huge burden of disease. The WHO's Department of Reproductive Health and Research has only recently started to formalize the collection of data concerning maternal morbidity (DRHR, 2009). Clearly, better data concerning the broad subject of reproductive health is an urgent priority.

Practical Solutions

The statistics concerning poorly managed pregnancy and delivery are staggering. As we have discussed above, roughly 1,000 women die every day from pregnancy-related causes. Complications of delivery leave millions more women with disabilities and contribute to the deaths of the 3.5 million children who die within the first 28 days of life. What makes it worse is that most of this mortality and morbidity is completely

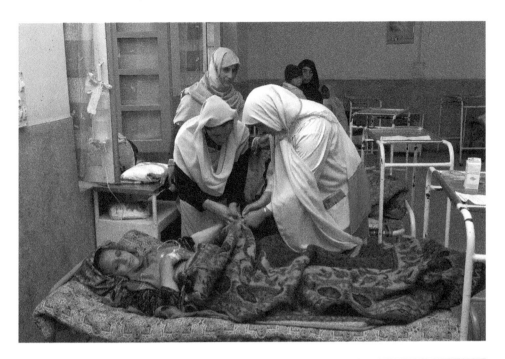

Photo 10.1: A woman who has just delivered her baby is cared for by trained birth attendants. She is being treated in the Mansehra District Hospital in Pakistan. Although this is a very poor region, her chances of a successful birth are greatly increased by the presence of properly trained midwives.

Source: UN Photo/Evan Schneider, with kind permission of the UN Photo Library (www. unmultimedia.org/photo).

avoidable with access to basic medical care. Although primary health care has produced great improvements in the health of children, it has had less effect on maternal mortality. Sanitation and immunizations are fine for a population, but they do not scratch the surface of pregnancy-associated diseases. Pregnancy and delivery are associated with sudden and unpredictable complications that can only be treated by having rapid access to trained attendants and basic medical care (WHO, 2005a). Numerous studies have shown that the major determinants of outcome in pregnancy are access to competent antenatal care and delivery by a trained attendant (Photo 10.1).

History provides plenty of support for the need for midwives. Sweden adopted a national policy favouring the presence of a midwife for all births in the 19th century. By 1900, the maternal mortality ratio in Sweden had fallen to 230 per 100,000 live births (Högberg, 2004). In contrast, the United States focused on hospital delivery by doctors and paid little attention to midwives. The maternal mortality ratio in the United States was still 700 per 100,000 live births in 1930 and did not fall until increasing emphasis was placed on the need for trained birth attendants. Despite all the technological gadgets associated with modern medicine, the place of the midwife has not changed. The central factor in any attempt to reduce pregnancy-related deaths must be the provision of skilled attendants during birth (UNFPA, 2006).

Obviously, the presence of a well-trained midwife needs to be backed up by access to a wide range of services. Even routine obstetric procedures, such as Caesarean section or blood transfusion, will require relatively expensive staff and equipment. By the time the associated costs of a district obstetric referral centre are added up, the cost of a comprehensive obstetric care program is significant. This is one reason why maternal care has lagged behind. However, it is worth it. Whether looked at from the point of view of child health, maternal health, or the general standard of living in a community, serious investments in maternal health are highly cost effective and long, long overdue (Adam, 2005). Medical treatments will be covered in more detail in Chapter 13, but briefly, a comprehensive intervention plan aimed at reducing neonatal maternal death would consist broadly of the following (WHO, 2005a):

- *Prenatal care:* During pregnancy, women should have access to regular monitoring (including testing for HIV and syphilis), intermittent preventive treatment for malaria, supplementation of micronutrients (particularly iron, vitamin A, and calcium), and macronutrient supplementation for the poorest women.
- *Care during delivery:* Every delivery should be attended by a trained midwife, with easy access to higher-level care when necessary, which includes the need for safe transportation. Minimum facilities in the referral centre should include safe blood transfusion, drugs for treatment of basic complications (infections, hypertension, and seizures), and access to Caesarean section. There should also be basic resuscitation equipment for treating unstable children (suction, incubator, oxygen). For HIV-positive women, there should be a national protocol for labour management, backed by regular supplies of antiretroviral drugs.
- *Postnatal care:* The new mother should have access to breastfeeding advice, post-delivery medical care, family-planning advice, and follow-up for her child (such as immunizations).

In an attempt to catalyze funding, focus on the plight of women and children, the United Nations' eighth secretary-general, Ban Ki-moon, launched the Global Strategy for Women's and Children's Health in September 2010 (UN, 2010). This strategy galvanized political leadership, strengthened commitment, attracted billions of dollars in financial commitments, and created

Every Woman Every Child, a powerful multi-stakeholder movement for health. The new Strategy puts women, children, and adolescents at the heart of the new UN SDGs and provides a roadmap to achieving the highest attainable standard of health for all women, children, and adolescents. The Strategy was updated in 2015 (Every Woman Every Child, 2015a). According to the latest progress report, more than 300 organizations (including governments, civil society, foundations, academia, businesses, and international organizations) have made over 400 specific commitments ranging from service delivery to advocacy and financial commitments. The Global Strategy has played an essential role in bringing new attention and action to areas where progress has lagged the most, such as newborn survival, still births, family planning, adolescent health, and access to life-saving commodities (Every Woman Every Child, 2015b). It is a lot of work, but it is worth it.

SUMMARY

The leading cause of death and DALYs globally is ischemic heart disease, followed by stroke. Most of the other leading causes of death, with the exception of lower respiratory infection, HIV/AIDS, and TB, are non-communicable. The burden of disease globally is largely non-communicable in all regions except sub-Saharan Africa and South Asia. There has been progress in all regions of the world in increasing life expectancy over the last several decades.

Although remarkable progress has been made in reducing child deaths in the last three decades, child mortality is still a significant global health challenge. Approximately 5.9 million children around the world died in 2015 before they reached their fifth birthday. Since 1990, the global under-five mortality has dropped by 53 percent. The largest cause of deaths of under-five children globally is prematurity, which killed 18 percent of all children who died before reaching age five in 2015. The main killers of children under age five in 2015 include preterm birth complications (18 percent), pneumonia (acute lower respiratory infections)(15 percent), birth asphyxia and trauma (11 percent), and diarrhea (9 percent). Also, almost half of all under-five deaths are attributable to undernutrition.

Maternal mortality has continued to be a challenge globally. In 2015, there were 303,000 deaths. Developing regions account for approximately 99% (302,000) of the global maternal deaths in 2015, with sub-Saharan Africa alone accounting for roughly 66% (201,000), followed by South Asia (66,000). Achieving the SDG target of a global maternal mortality ratio below 70 under SDG 3.1 would require intensifying the efforts and progress catalyzed by

MDG 5. The new Global Strategy for Women's, Children's and Adolescents' Health launched in 2015 is spearheading an enhanced global collaborative response aimed at ending all preventable maternal deaths. Improving health outcomes of women requires health systems that provide cost-effective services in relation to nutrition prenatal care, family planning, and, most importantly, deliveries attended by skilled health care providers.

DISCUSSION QUESTIONS

1. What are the leading causes of death globally? How has that changed in the last three decades?
2. How do you think the burden of disease will evolve by 2030?
3. What are the critical factors that determine a person's health in a low-income country?
4. Why is it important to use composite indicators like DALYs to measure burden of disease?
5. Which regions of the world have the highest maternal mortality and why?
6. What would be your key recommendations for reduction of maternal mortality?
7. What are the SDG targets for maternal mortality? Are these targets achievable?
8. Why does life expectancy differ significantly between high-income and low-income countries?
9. What are the major causes of death for neonates, infants, and children younger than five years?
10. What are the most effective interventions to improve the health of women in low-income countries?

RECOMMENDED READING

Bale, J., et al. 2004. *Improving birth outcomes: Meeting the challenges in the developing world*. Pub: National Academic Press.

Koblinsky, M. (Ed.). *Reducing maternal mortality: Learning from Bolivia, China, Egypt, Honduras, Indonesia, Jamaica, and Zimbabwe*. Pub: World Bank Publications.

Liu, L., et al. 2015. Global, regional, and national causes of child mortality in 2000–13, with projections to inform post-2015 priorities: An updated systematic analysis. *The Lancet*, 385: 430–440.

WHO. 2015. *Trends in Maternal Mortality: 1990 to 2015: Estimates by WHO, UNICEF, UNFPA, World Bank Group and the United Nations Population Division*. Retrieved from: www.who.int/reproductivehealth/publications/monitoring/maternal-mortality-2015/en/.

REFERENCES

Adam, T. 2005. Cost-effectiveness analysis of strategies for maternal and neonatal health in developing countries. *British Medical Journal*, 331: 1107–1114.

Adegoke, A., et al. 2009. Skilled birth attendants—lessons learnt. *British Journal of Obstetrics and Gynaecology*, 116 (1; Suppl.): 33–40.

Ashford, L. 2002. Hidden suffering: Disabilities from pregnancy and childbirth in less developed countries. Population Reference Bureau. Retrieved from: www.prb.org/pdf/HiddenSufferingEng.pdf.

Black, R., et al. 2010. Global, regional, and national causes of child mortality in 2008: A systematic analysis. *The Lancet*, 375: 1969–1987.

CHERG. 2016. Child Health Epidemiology Reference Group. Retrieved from: http://cherg.org/main.html.

Childinfo. 2011. Maternal health statistics. Retrieved from: www.childinfo.org/health.html.

Chisholm, D., et al. 2005. Cost effectiveness of clinical interventions for reducing the global burden of bipolar disorder. *British Journal of Psychiatry*, 187: 559–567.

DCP2. 2006. Disease control priorities in developing countries, 2nd ed. Retrieved from: www.dcp2.org/page/main/About.html.

DCP3. 2016. Disease control priorities in developing countries, 3rd ed. Retrieved from: www.dcp-3.org/disease-control-priorities-third-edition.

DCPP. 2011. World Bank's Disease Control Priorities project. Retrieved from: www.dcp2.org/page/main/About.html.

DRHR. 2009. Department of Reproductive Health and Research. Retrieved from: whqlibdoc.who.int/hq/2009/WHO_RHR_09.02_eng.pdf.

Every Woman Every Child. 2015a. The global strategy for women's, children's and adolescent health (2016–2030). Retrieved from: www.who.int/life-course/publications/global-strategy-2016-2030/en/.

Every Woman Every Child. 2015b. Saving lives, protecting futures: Progress report on the global strategy for women's and children's health. Retrieved from: http://everywomaneverychild.org/images/EWEC_Progress_Report_FINAL_3.pdf.

GBD. 2013. Global, regional, and national age–sex specific all-cause and cause-specific mortality for 240 causes of death, 1990–2013: A systematic analysis for the Global Burden of Disease study 2013. *The Lancet*, 385(9963): 117–171.

GHAT. 1981. The Ghana Health Assessment Team. A quantitative method of assessing the health impact of different diseases in less developed countries. *International Journal of Epidemiology*, 10: 1075–1089.

Henry Street. 2011. Lillian Wald. Retrieved from: www.henrystreet.org/about/history/lillian-wald.html.

Hill, K., et al. 1999. Trends in child mortality in the developing world, 1960–1996. Retrieved from: www.childinfo.org/mortality_methodology.html.

Hirschman, C. 1994. Why fertility changes. *Annual Review of Sociology*, 20: 203–233.

Högberg, U. 2004. The decline in maternal mortality in Sweden: The role of community mid-wifery. *American Public Health Association*, 94: 1312–1320.

IGME. 2011a. Inter-agency Group for Child Mortality Estimation. Retrieved from: www.childinfo.org/mortality_igme.html.

IGME. 2015. Levels and trends in child mortality. Retrieved from: www.unicef.org/media/files/IGME_report_2015_child_mortality_final.pdf.

IHME. 2010. Institute for Health Metrics and Evaluation. Building momentum: Global progress toward reducing maternal and child mortality. Retrieved from: www.healthmetricsandevaluation.org/publications/policy-report/building-momentum-global-progress-toward-reducing-maternal-and-child-mor.

IHME. 2016. Data from Institute of Health Metrics and Evaluation. GBD heat map. Pub: IHME, University of Washington. Retrieved from: http://vizhub.healthdata.org/gbd-compare/.

Islami, F. et al. 2015. Global trends of lung cancer mortality and smoking prevalence *Transl Lung Cancer Res.*, 4(4): 327–338.

Lambrechts, T., et al. 1999. Integrated management of childhood illnesses: A summary of first experiences. *Bulletin of the World Health Organization*, 77: 582–594.

MMM-R. 2009. Maternal Mortality Measurement Resources. Retrieved from: www.maternal-mortality-measurement.org/index.html.

Murray, C. J. L., et al. 1994. The global burden of disease in 1990: Summary results, sensitivity analysis, and future directions. *Bulletin of the World Health Organization*, 72: 495–509.

PMNCH. 2011. Partnership for Maternal, Newborn, and Child Health. Retrieved from: www.who.int/pmnch/en/.

Say, L., et al. 2014. Global causes of maternal death: A WHO systematic analysis. *Lancet Global Health 2014*, 2: e323–333.

UN. 2006. Economic and social affairs, world population prospects. Retrieved from: www.un.org/esa/population/publications/wpp2006/WPP2006_Highlights_rev.pdf.

UN. 2010. The global strategy for women's and children's health 2010–2015. Retrieved from: http://www.who.int/pmnch/activities/advocacy/globalstrategy/2010_2015/en/.

UN. 2011. Department of Economic and Social Affairs: Fertility and Family Planning section. Retrieved from: www.un.org/esa/population/publications/wcu2010/Main.html.

UNFPA. 2006. Towards MDG5: Scaling up the capacity of midwives to reduce maternal mortality and morbidity. Retrieved from: www.unfpa.org/public/publications/pid/1279.

UNICEF. 1984. The state of the world's children. Retrieved from: www.unicef.org/sowc/archive/ENGLISH/The%20State%20of%20the%20World's%20Children%201984.pdf.

UNICEF. 2008. Progress for children: A report card on maternal mortality. Retrieved from: www.childinfo.org/files/progress_for_children_maternalmortality.pdf.

UNICEF. 2009. The state of the world's children: Maternal and newborn health. Retrieved from:

www.unicef.org/protection/SOWC09-FullReport-EN.pdf.

UNICEF. 2010. Countdown to 2015: Maternal, newborn, and child survival. Retrieved from: www.unicef.org/media/media_53814.html.

UNICEF. 2011. Childinfo. Child mortality statistics. Retrieved from: www.childinfo.org/.

WHO. 2005a. World health report 2005: Make every mother and child count. Retrieved from: www.who.int/whr/2005/en.

WHO. 2005b. Pregnancy, childbirth, postpartum, and newborn care: A guide for essential practice. Retrieved from: whqlibdoc.who.int/publications/2006/924159084X_eng.pdf.

WHO. 2006. Reproductive health indicators: Guidelines for their generation, inter- pretation, and analysis for global monitoring. Retrieved from: whqlibdoc.who.int/ publications/2006/924156315X_eng.pdf.

WHO. 2008. Global Burden of Disease: 2004 update. Retrieved from: www.who.int/healthinfo/ global_burden_disease/2004_report_update/en/.

WHO. 2009. Global health risks. Mortality and burden of disease attributable to selected major risks. Retrieved from: www.who.int/healthinfo/global_burden_disease/global_health_ risks/en/index.html.

WHO. 2011. Global Burden of Disease project. Retrieved from: www.who.int/healthinfo/ global_burden_disease/about/en/index.html.

WHO. 2015. *Trends in Maternal Mortality: 1990 to 2015: Estimates by WHO, UNICEF, UNFPA, World Bank Group and the United Nations Population Division*. Retrieved from: www. who.int/reproductivehealth/publications/monitoring/maternal-mortality-2015/en/.

WHO. 2016. Global Health Observatory Data Repository: Mortality and glob- al health estimates. Retrieved from: http://apps.who.int/gho/data/node.main. CM3002015REGWORLD?lang=en.

World Bank. 1993. World development report. Investing in health. Retrieved from: http://files. dcp2.org/pdf/WorldDevelopmentReport1993.pdf.

World Bank. 2011. World Bank indicators. Retrieved from: http://data.worldbank.org/indicator.

World Bank. 2016a. Data from the World Bank. World Development Indicators: Mortality. Retrieved from: http://data.worldbank.org/indicator/SP.DYN.IMRT.IN?display=graph.

World Bank. 2016b. Data from the World Bank. World Development Indicators. Retrived from: http://data.worldbank.org/indicator/SH.DYN.NMRT?display=graph.

PART IV

WHAT CAN BE DONE TO HELP?

CHAPTER 11

The Structure of the Foreign Aid Industry

No one would remember the Good Samaritan if he'd only had good intentions. He had money as well.

—Margaret Thatcher, 1980

OBJECTIVES

In an ideal world, aid would be given, without strings attached, to benevolent governments that would then use it solely for the benefit of its citizens. Unfortunately, reality isn't that simple. Once aid money leaves an external donor's hand, it follows a complicated path before it reaches the intended recipient. This chapter follows that course in some detail. After completing it, you should have an understanding of the following elements of international aid:

- the major external funding sources available to developing countries
- the full range of aid agencies from large to small
- the types of aid on which the money is spent
- the various implementation methods used to improve service delivery
- aid effectiveness—measuring it and improving it
- the future of the aid industry

INTRODUCTION

> If the international aid regime were a national economy, one thing is clear: the World Bank and the International Monetary Fund (IMF) would be after it to reform.
>
> —*Dennis Whittle and Mari Kuraishi, 2005*

As we discussed in Chapter 2, the pattern for the modern aid industry was established by the Marshall Plan in 1948. In those early days the United States was the only significant donor. The money was managed by the first bilateral agency (Economic Cooperation Administration, ECA) and distributed to 15 European countries through a single agency, the Organisation for European Economic Co-operation (OEEC) (Photo 11.1). Since then, times have changed; aid has become very big business, and those first two agencies have grown out of all recognition. The ECA became the US Agency for International Development (USAID), while the OEEC grew into the Organisation for Economic Co-operation and Development (OECD)—both are major players in the current aid industry.

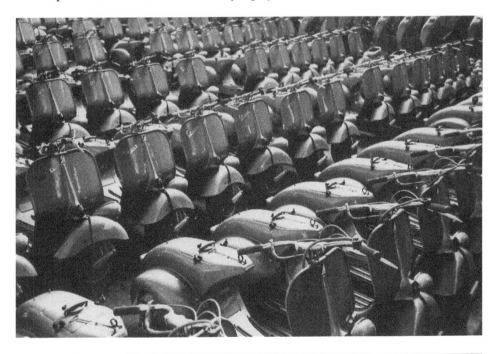

Photo 11.1: The Marshall Plan helped to rebuild Europe's economy after the devastation of World War II. It remains a model for effective economic assistance. This 1951 photograph shows new Vespas rolling out of the Piaggio plant, which was rebuilt with Marshall Plan funds.

Source: US National Archives, courtesy of Wikimedia Commons.

Since the early development of foreign aid was led by governments, an expanding bureaucracy was inevitably close behind. It is often stated that no aid agency has ever been closed. With the exception of some Soviet-era co-operation agencies, this is likely true (Burall et al., 2006). Aid agencies have continued to increase at a faster rate than the increase in financial flows they are supposed to manage. Now that roughly 40 countries donate foreign aid, the resulting administrative support structure has become unmanageably complex. Bilateral agencies, multilateral agencies, and the countless non-governmental organizations have grown far beyond the point where any unified attempt at reform or control is possible (Hewitt et al., 2004).

The system is not without any guidance—some large organizations, such as WHO, UN Development Programme, World Bank, UNICEF, and a few others, carry particular weight in their areas of expertise. While their policies and recommendations are influential, there is no structure that functions as a governing body. Donor countries are free to design, administer, and implement their own aid policies, each influenced by a varying mixture of altruism, self-interest, and past history. Multilateral agencies even out some of these biases, but in the absence of leadership and common goals, the development of foreign aid over the last 60 years (particularly direct state-to-state aid) has been influenced by a variety of external events and changing theories. The results have been policies that have, at times, had very little to do with helping the poor.

Although aid from most Development Assistance Committee (DAC) countries falls well below the original target of 0.7 percent of gross national income (GNI) (Figure 11.1), it still represents a great deal of money, at least on paper. Annual

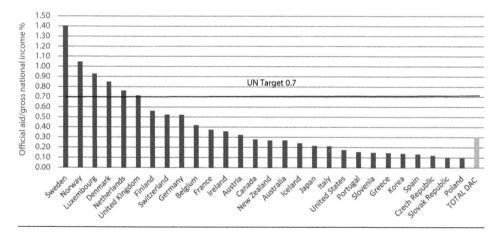

Figure 11.1: Official aid as a percentage of gross national income for Development Assistance Committee members in 2015

Source: OECD. 2016a. Organisation for Economic Co-operation and Development, International Development Statistics (database). Retrieved from: https://data.oecd.org/.

aid flows have been above US$100 billion since 2005 (Figure 11.2). In 2015, net official development assistance (ODA) flows from member countries of the DAC rose by 6.9% in real terms from 2014 to reach US$131.6 billion, representing 0.30% of GNI (Figure 11.2) (World Bank, 2016a). It is encouraging that ODA continues to remain high and stable. However, it would be naive to imagine that countries donate such large sums of money without expecting some commercial or political return. Apart from the practice of tying aid to purchases from the donor, aid is further diluted by using it for highly paid technical consultants, the transaction costs of multiple visiting missions, double-counting debt relief, and even including the costs of caring for refugees within the donor's borders (Greenhill, 2006). Estimates vary, but it is likely that at least a quarter of quoted aid is lost in these ways. The terms "real aid," "core aid," or "country programmable aid" (CPA) have been coined to describe the portion of aid that finally filters through to the recipient countries. OECD's estimates of programmable aid over the last decade are also plotted in Figure 11.2. To their credit, donor countries have taken this problem seriously through the Paris and Accra meetings on aid effectiveness (OECD, 2008a). The OECD now publishes annual estimates of CPA.

Unfortunately, apart from lack of leadership, the aid system also has no organizational response to feedback from the poor who are, of course, the aim of the whole exercise. It was only in the late 1990s that the Poverty Reduction Strategy process first gave the poor some nominal voice in their own development plans. Prior to that time, they had no say at all in the growth and development of the system intended to serve them. True to form, aid agencies don't listen to the source

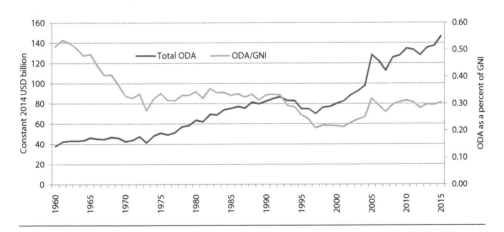

Figure 11.2: Net official development assistance, 1960–2015

Source: OECD. 2016b. Development co-operation report 2016: The Sustainable Development Goals as business opportunities. Pub: OECD Publishing, Paris. Retrieved from: http://dx.doi.org/10.1787/dcr-2016-14-en.

of their money either—the taxpayers in individual countries. Large-scale public influence in foreign aid distribution began with the HIV epidemic, but reached extraordinary levels in response to the issue of developing world debt. Politicians' realization that many of their constituents are passionately interested in aid has had a beneficial effect on the priority given to aid in many countries.

The continued proliferation of aid sources means that many countries have more projects than they can manage. The aid allotted to some countries becomes fragmented into many small projects whose administrative burden outweighs any likely value (Acharya et al., 2004). Such countries are deluged with agencies—it is not difficult to find examples. An OECD survey (OECD, 2006) found that the average developing country must host 200 donor missions each year. Quite apart from the endless rounds of meetings, there are also reports, budgets, and outcome measurements to be completed for each of these projects. Administrators in both Cambodia and Vietnam have to find time and staff to host more than one visiting mission every day of the year.

The problems associated with the organization of aid are no secret. As early as 1969, a large-scale review of aid, chaired by Lester Pearson, produced recommendations that would still be perfectly relevant today—more money, less tied aid, better harmonization, and fewer agencies. Despite a great deal of talk in the subsequent 40 years, it is only within the last decade that substantive efforts have been made to improve the quantity and quality of aid. As shown in Figure 11.2, dissatisfaction with the system was such that the average percentage of GDP given as aid in OECD countries fell to its lowest level ever as recently as 1997. The organizational and financial demands of the MDGs were likely the main catalysts for change. These led to significant agreements on development funding prompted by the Monterrey round of meetings. These, in turn, prompted equally significant declarations on aid effectiveness following international meetings in Rome, Paris, and Accra.

There is a sense that the new millennium is a time of great promise for foreign aid. The days of donor and recipient are to be replaced by serious partnerships with responsibilities and obligations applying to both sides of the relationship—all backed by significant cash flows. Like it or not, the old order will have to adapt or become increasingly irrelevant; everything about the world of aid is simply changing too fast. The presence of large non-OECD donors like China and India is introducing external competition into what used to be a DAC monopoly. In addition, increases in alternative funds, such as remittance income, foreign direct investment, and private philanthropy, all allow developing countries more choice and fewer conditions when looking for sources of external funding. Even the traditional disease patterns are changing, moving away from high childhood mortality and toward the health problems associated with increasing affluence.

EXTERNAL FUNDING SOURCES FOR DEVELOPING COUNTRIES

> Each economically advanced country will progressively increase its official development assistance ... to reach a minimum net amount of 0.7 percent of its GDP by the middle of the decade.
>
> —*UN resolution 2626, October 1970*

When commentators analyze and measure aid, the term is usually used to mean the money donated by the 24 members of the Development Assistance Committee (DAC) of the OECD. The term "official development assistance" (ODA) is also commonly used. Although the DAC is still a major source of funds, it is no longer the only (or even the largest) source of money available to developing countries. The alternatives are certainly not linked by a common definition of what constitutes aid—they are grouped together by nothing more than their availability as external supplies of money. Each has its own idiosyncrasies that should be clearly understood. For example, the origins, uses, and magnitude of direct foreign investment are very different from those for remittance earnings. As mentioned in the introduction, times are changing; aid is no longer synonymous with ODA, and a much broader view of funding alternatives is now necessary.

The OECD's Development Assistance Committee

The DAC started as a special interest group of 11 members within the OECD's predecessor (Organisation for European Economic Co-operation). The DAC was formally established as a major subcommittee of the OECD in 1961, acting within the Development Co-operation Directorate (DCD-DAC, 2011). Since then, the OECD has grown to include 34 members, 24 of whom are united as major aid donors within the DAC. This group includes 23 states, plus the European Commission, which acts as a bilateral donor even though it has multilateral sources of funds. Apart from acting as a forum for the world's major donor countries, the DAC has several subsections that deal with important aspects of aid, such as effectiveness, evaluation, and particularly the statistical monitoring of cash flows.

Although there is no universally agreed-upon definition of aid, the DAC's version is widely used (OECD, 2008b). Official development aid (ODA) is defined as government funding for development or humanitarian purposes—military funding is excluded. There is no agreement on debt relief. It is currently included, but there are moves to make it separate from ODA. It is important to remember that donated money may be a mixture of grants and loans. It qualifies as ODA as long as the grant element is greater than 25 percent of the total and the loan is

Box 11.1 History Notes

George Marshall (1880–1959)

Marshall was born in the United States and trained as a career soldier. He served in World War I, rising to colonel. He was the chief planner of the final offensive that broke through the Hindenburg line at the end of the war. He subsequently rose to become chief of staff in charge of all American troops during World War II. In 1947, he was appointed secretary of state under Truman. In this position, he devised the European Recovery Program (subsequently called the Marshall Plan), which played a major role in the reconstruction of Europe. It is generally accepted as the start of modern large-scale aid projects. Its organizational framework remains a model for current development assistance. He received the Nobel Peace Prize for his humanitarian contribution in 1953. Despite this, he was publicly criticized during the McCarthy era as being soft on communism and subsequently resigned, disillusioned by politics.

For further information, follow the reference: George C. Marshall Foundation (2009).

given at concessional rates of interest. In recent years the grant fraction has been close to 100 percent for most DAC donors, so loans now form only a very small part of total ODA.

Donor countries understandably wish to retain some control over their own decisions, so the majority of the donations are made directly from state to state (bilateral aid). The remainder is given to large agencies such as the World Health Organization, the World Bank, or agencies of the United Nations (multilateral aid). The distinction between multilateral and bilateral aid is not completely clear-cut because some countries give aid to large institutions as long as it is used for a given purpose. The fraction of bilateral aid is roughly 70 percent, but individual countries vary widely. The pros and cons of the two forms of aid are discussed in the next section.

Early attempts were made to define the obligation of aid. The World Council of Churches called for countries to donate 1 percent of their GDP in 1958. The UN resolution quoted at the start of this section was adopted in 1970 and was based on the recommendation of a committee led by Lester Pearson. The mathematical justification for the 0.7 percent GDP figure is not clear, but the target is widely accepted. Currently, only five DAC members exceed that figure (Figure 11.1), while the DAC average is below half of that target (Figure 11.3). The term "gross national income" (GNI) has now replaced "gross domestic product" (GDP). GNI is the GDP plus receipts from international companies (minus their international taxes).

The variables affecting an individual country's aid allocation are a complex mixture of altruism and strategic and commercial interests. Some countries, such as France, Belgium, and Portugal, favour their old colonies. Others may use some

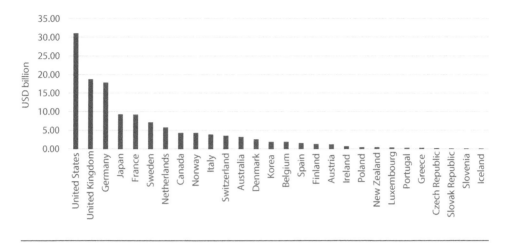

Figure 11.3: Net official development assistance from DAC donors in 2015

Source: OECD. 2016a. Organisation for Economic Co-operation and Development, International Development Statistics (database). Retrieved from: https://data.oecd.org/.

of their aid for commercial advantage by insisting that the money must be spent on services from the donor country (usually called "tied" aid). Political motives did not end with the Cold War, but were simply replaced by others, such as the war against drugs and, more recently, the war against terrorism. For example, the two top recipients of US aid in 2010 were Afghanistan and Iraq. While there are many poor people in those regions, it is likely that there are other considerations behind the allocation of this aid.

Over the last 60 years, many external factors have influenced the degree of donor generosity; the struggle to influence various countries by those on either side of the Cold War was the biggest of these. The quantity and reliability of aid flows have both varied over the years. When expressed as a percentage of GDP, aid spending fell steadily from the early 1980s. Aid measured as cash flow fell sharply in the 1990s after the end of the Cold War. It is important to remember that this is not ancient history. As recently as 1997, ODA had fallen to a low point of US$67.9 billion. In the same year, the average fraction of GDP donated by DAC countries was only 0.22 percent. At the time, there were concerns that traditional forms of aid might become increasingly irrelevant and replaced by rising levels of foreign investment and remittance incomes.

Although there had been signs of increasing aid flows in the late 1990s, the High-Level Forum on development funding in 2001, under Ernesta Zedillo, followed by the UN Conference on Financing for Development at Monterrey in 2002 (United Nations, 2003), acted as significant stimuli. Funding levels in

2010 were nearly double those of the low point in 1997. The level of generosity of DAC members still varies widely. The largest individual donor is the United States (Figure 11.3), but when expressed as a percentage of GNI, the US lags far behind Norway, Luxembourg, Sweden, and others (Figure 11.1). Despite the long list of past problems with DAC development aid, there does now seem to be a window of opportunity to repair those mistakes. Substantive efforts at improving the quantity, reliability, and also quality of DAC-sourced aid are now being made. The future of ODA looks a lot brighter than it did only a dozen years ago.

Non-DAC Donors

The steady spread of global prosperity has meant that many smaller countries have now become aid donors. A few, such as South Korea, have gone from being a major aid recipient 50 years ago to being a significant donor. In fact, South Korea is the most recent country to join the DAC. Some countries, such as India and China, are in the strange position of being aid donors and aid recipients at the same time. The non-DAC donors are usually studied as three separate groups:

- OECD countries that are not in the DAC (Czech Republic, Hungary, Iceland, Israel, Poland, Slovak Republic, Slovenia, Turkey)
- Arab countries (Kuwait, Saudi Arabia, United Arab Emirates)
- Non-OECD countries (Taipei, Thailand, China, India)

The OECD tracks donations by all these countries, with the exception of China and India (OECD, 2010). Estimated development co-operation flows by 29 providers beyond the DAC reached US$33 billion in 2014, compared to US$24 billion in 2013 (OECD, 2016b).

Two of the most influential non-OECD donors are India and China. Unfortunately, neither country publishes regular reviews of its aid policies. China has recently produced a government white paper on its aid policy, but it contains rather more rhetoric than hard statistics (Chinese Aid, 2011). While there is no information on annual aid flows, the paper states that China has donated a total of US$38.83 billion since its program started. This money was given in the form of grants and concessional loans. If anything, India gives even less information (Chanana, 2009). India's foreign aid program has slowly increased since its start in the 1960s. It is estimated that it currently donates US$150 million to $200 million each year.

Remittance Income

The first question that many newcomers to very poor countries ask is, "How do local people manage to pay for their daily needs?" In many cases the answer is that families are supported by members working overseas who send cash back to their country of origin. This money is termed "remittance income" and its magnitude is large—nearly three times larger than ODA flows (Figure 11.4). The World Bank's Remittance and Migration site contains detailed statistics (World Bank, 2011). Their best estimates show that over 160 million people work outside their country of origin for economic reasons (Table 11.1). Despite the financial recession, they currently repatriate far in excess of US$300 billion per year! The problems of tracking cash sent by small private firms rather than large electronic transfer companies, and the presence of large numbers of unregistered illegal workers throughout OECD countries, make accurate data collection difficult.

In 2015, worldwide remittance flows are estimated to have exceeded US$601 billion. Of that amount, developing countries are estimated to receive about US$441 billion, nearly three times the amount of official development assistance. The top recipient countries of recorded remittances were India, China, the Philippines, Mexico, and France (Figure 11.5). High-income countries are the main source of remittances. The United States is by far the largest, with an

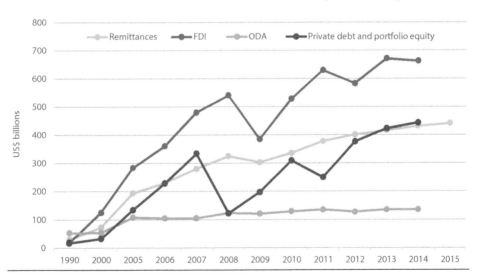

Figure 11.4: Three forms of cash flow from the developed to the developing world; annual flows of remittance income, foreign direct investment, and official development aid over the last 25 years

Source: World Bank. 2016a. Migration and remittances factbook 2016 (3rd ed.). Retrieved from: https://openknowledge.worldbank.org/handle/10986/23743.

Table 11.1: Regional estimates of remittance incomes (US$ billions)

	2010	2013	2014	2015E	2016F	2017F	2018F
Developing countries	331.7	416.6	429.9	431.6	447.9	465.7	484.7
East Asia and Pacific	94.1	113.4	121.8	127.0	131.0	135.5	140.3
Europe and Central Asia	31.4	47.7	43.4	34.6	36.3	38.3	40.3
Latin America and Caribbean	55.7	61.1	63.6	66.7	69.3	71.9	74.6
Middle East and North Africa	38.9	48.8	50.8	50.3	51.6	53.0	54.5
South Asia	82.0	110.8	115.5	117.9	123.3	129.3	135.8
Sub-Saharan Africa	29.7	34.7	34.8	35.2	36.4	37.7	39.1
World	460.5	573.0	592.0	581.6	603.2	626.4	651.3

Source: World Bank. 2016b. Migration and remittances, recent developments and outlook. Migration and Development brief 26.

estimated US$56.3 billion in recorded outflows in 2014. Saudi Arabia ranks as the second largest, followed by the Russia, Switzerland, Germany, United Arab Emirates, and Kuwait (World Bank, 2016b).

There is nothing new about economic migrants. Several developed European countries, such as Italy and Ireland, have relied heavily on this source of money in the past. Greece and Spain still receive substantial remittance income. Most of the work is manual labour, so returns are affected by economic swings. Returns sent from Russia are closely tied to the oil price, while those from the US are principally related to the strength of the new housing market. Despite this, remittances appear to have survived the recent global financial crisis.

Apart from the separation of family members, the biggest drawback of migrant labour is that better-trained workers tend not to go home, so the investment in their education is lost. The brain drain of locally trained nurses and other health care workers from developing countries to rich countries is a particular example of this problem. Assessing the final impact of remittances is difficult because their social and economic effects are so varied. Finding a balance between the loss of a young worker and the new source of income is hard enough at a family level. When this is scaled up to a national level, the effects will vary widely between countries (Sharma, 2009).

Remittances certainly seem to have been beneficial to countries struggling after natural or humanitarian crises, such as Somalia in the 1990s or Haiti after the earthquake. Their long-term economic benefits depend strongly on a supportive national policy toward this source of cash. Examples include easy access to bank accounts, remittance-linked loans, and income tax exemptions. Some countries are even issuing investment bonds to raise money from migrant labourers. Greece is currently

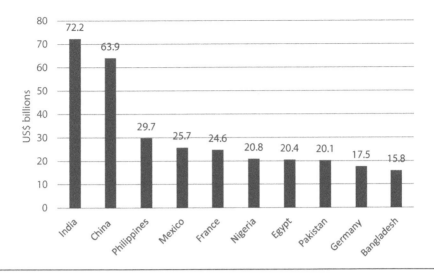

Figure 11.5: The largest recipients of remittance income for 2015

Source: World Bank. 2016a. Migration and remittances factbook 2016 (3rd ed.). Retrieved from: https://openknowledge.worldbank.org/handle/10986/23743.

following Israel's past example by offering diaspora bonds to help deal with its current debt crisis. Whatever their benefits might be, it should be remembered that remittances are private flows to individual families. They are influential and deserve careful study, but they should not be viewed as an alternative to foreign aid.

Foreign Direct Investment

Increasingly liberal attitudes toward global trade over the last decade have been associated with rapid increases in foreign direct investment (FDI) in developing countries (Figure 11.6). Subsidiaries of transnational corporations contribute the great majority of FDI. With a rising global middle class, an increasing proportion of this sum comes from large companies in developing countries such as China and India. The sums involved are larger than ODA and remittances combined (Figure 11.5). Total global FDI was US$1.12 trillion in 2010—developing countries attracted US$524 billion of that total, or just over half. The best source of information is the Statistics Division of the UN Conference on Trade and Development (UNCTAD, 2011). Its data show how rapidly FDI in developing countries has grown since 1995. It should be remembered that this is the harsh world of business. The principal aim of FDI is to make money, not help the poor. That investment is expected to make money, so there are FDI outflows to consider as well.

Such enormous sums of money can have beneficial effects, but they can also cause a great deal of harm. For example, there are valid concerns that countries might relax environmental and labour laws in order to be more attractive to foreign mining companies. Analyzing the final domestic advantage is not easy (OECD, 2002). Apart from regulatory concerns, the repatriation of profits and interest repayments lead to substantial FDI outflows. The results will depend largely on the conditions of the host economy, the degree of corruption, and the strength of local industry regulations. A good start was made in 2002 with the establishment of the Extractive Industries Transparency Initiative (EITI, 2011). Fifty of the world's biggest mining companies have already joined, but this is still a long way from applying modern standards of labour and environmental protection to companies working in developing areas.

Private Philanthropy

As the response to the Asian tsunami and other natural disasters has shown, the generosity of individual citizens appears to be greater than that of their governments. As an example, less than five months after the Haitian earthquake, private and voluntary organizations had donated US$1.1 billion to the relief effort. Private funding differs from traditional ODA in many ways, including the use of innovation and technology. Following the same disaster, the Red Cross was able to raise US$32 million in separate $10 donations by text message (Hudson Institute, 2011). The sources of philanthropical donations are so varied that tracking accurate statistics is difficult. The annual Index of Global Philanthropy, produced by the Hudson Institute, provides some estimates, but they are based mostly on OECD data that are incomplete (OECD, 2010). France and Norway, for example, are both listed as having zero private donations. Both these sources suggest that total private charity may be roughly the same magnitude as governmental ODA. The estimated range of private donations from DAC countries for 2009 was US$22.7 billion to $52.5 billion (Hudson Institute, 2011).

Traditionally, privately funded NGOs have raised money from their own countries. Advertisements for Oxfam or World Vision are common examples. Some larger NGOs are now raising part of their support from the population of the host country. This follows a trend among many aid organizations to decentralize their decision-making to missions and community-based groups within the target country. Apart from the very large range of traditional philanthropic foundations, ranging from CARE to the Aga Khan Foundation, the establishment of new agencies by major figures in the business world has been another obvious trend in recent years. The Soros Foundation, the Turner Foundation, and particularly the Bill and Melinda Gates Foundation all give substantial sums of money for aid work. Warren Buffett's donation of US$31 billion to the Gates Foundation in 2006 has allowed that organization to grow into a very influential agency (Bill and Melinda Gates Foundation, 2011). At present, the Bill and Melinda Gates Foundation is the only private entity reporting to the OECD on its activities with developing countries, with a reported disbursement of US$2.9 billion in 2014 (OECD).

Innovative Funding Mechanisms

Prior to the MDGs, the only alternative funding sources outside traditional ODA were based on private charity. As Figure 11.2 shows, the DAC countries have greatly increased their donations, but there is still a need for alternative or innovative funding sources. The term was first used at the Monterrey Conference on Development Funding in 2002. The fortuitous arrival of successful business entrepreneurs into the world of aid has likely helped this process. All of the mechanisms described below have been introduced within the last few years, but given the problems associated with traditional ODA, this list will probably grow rapidly in the near future. They provide an idea of the exciting possibilities for the future direction of development aid.

UNITAID

This organization was established in 2006; it now has 34 member countries. Its aim is to provide sustainable flows of funding to support the purchase of drugs and diagnostics for use against the major infectious diseases, particularly HIV/AIDS, TB, and malaria. Apart from its innovative approach to organization, it was established from the outset to rely on new forms of funding. Some countries, such as the UK and Spain, provide direct funds, but the remainder raise money through the levy of a few dollars on airline tickets. By 2009, it had raised nearly US$1 billion (UNITAID, 2009). It reduces bureaucracy by running its secretariat through the WHO and directs the sustainable flows of cash through implementing agencies, such as the Clinton Foundation and the Global Fund to Fight Aids, Tuberculosis, and Malaria.

GAVI

The Global Alliance for Vaccines and Immunisations (GAVI) was proposed at the World Economic Forum in 2000. It is a very broad-based group consisting of governments, philanthropists, financial organizations, multilateral agencies, and vaccine manufacturers. Its governance was overhauled in 2008. Its aim is to improve access to immunizations, to strengthen local vaccine delivery capacity, and also to support development of new vaccines. Apart from government grants and private donations, it receives much of its financing through two innovative mechanisms: the International Finance Facility (IFF) and a binding business contract for vaccine development called the Advance Market Commitment (AMC). Over 10 years, the alliance has provided US$2.8 billion to more than 70 countries (GAVI, 2010). The concept of an IFF was devised by the UK government. It raises short-term money through bond issues against the promise of long-term confirmed funding from donors. The first test of the idea was an IFF for immunizations, started in 2004 (IFFim, 2011). The UK government estimates that this funding method is capable of generating up to US$50 billion per year.

GFATM

The Global Fund to Fight Aids, Tuberculosis, and Malaria (GFATM) is another broad coalition of government and public agencies that has tried new ideas to attract money. It was founded in 2002 and initially relied on the WHO for administrative services. Since 2008 the Global Fund has been an autonomous agency. Its aim is to improve funding for the prevention and treatment of the three major infectious diseases, AIDS, TB, and malaria. Although the bulk of its funds come from multilateral aid agencies, it also receives alternate funds from private foundations and UNITAID. Other innovative sources of funding include the Product Red initiative (companies are allowed to display the Product Red logo in exchange for a percentage of sales) and various debt conversion arrangements where creditors agree to accept less debt repayment as long as the forgiven amount is used for local health initiatives within the debtor country (Debt2Health, 2007).

AID AGENCIES

The sources of funding represent only the first step in the path of money from donor to final recipient. The next level of complexity is made up of the aid agencies that administer the cash, and it is every bit as confusing as the number of funding sources. The most obvious question is: Why are all these agencies necessary? With the move toward directing funding to government budgets rather than individual programs, one possible future for aid would be the one-cheque-a-year model. The Millennium Challenge Account has made moves in that direction, but until that simple day arrives, spending has to be planned and administered and that needs agencies, probably not nearly as many as currently exist, but that is their general justification. For the purposes of discussion, agencies fall into the following three groups.

Bilateral Agencies

Bilateral aid refers to the donation of money directly from one government to another. The model was established by the Marshall Plan at the end of World War II. DAC countries are no longer the only donors, but they are still the largest; the US, the UK, France, Germany, and Japan lead the way. With the steady proliferation of multilateral agencies, the fraction of bilateral aid has fallen with time, but it remains the dominant donation method. The DAC average is 70 percent bilateral, but individual countries vary from the US (over 80 percent bilateral) to Italy and Austria (less than 50 percent). This presumably reflects a desire for countries to retain control of such large sums of money. Each donor country has at least one national agency, so there are now well over 50 bilateral agencies. Examples include the US Agency for International Development (USAID), Global Affairs Canada, and the UK's Department for International Development (DFID).

Altruism is not the only motivating factor behind bilateral aid decisions. Donors understandably look for other advantages from their generosity, so aid allocation is sometimes influenced by political interests (the Cold War, the war on terror) and also by economic interests (tied aid, opening new markets). In countries where there is a level of public suspicion toward large multilateral agencies,

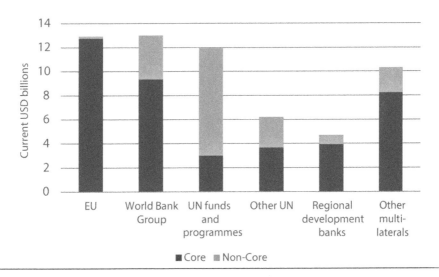

Figure 11.6: Division of multilateral funding between core and non-core programs in 2013; the major UN programs in order of funding are: WFP, UNDP, UNICEF, UNHCR, UNRWA, and UNFPA. The major regional banks are the African and Asian Development Banks.

Source: OECD. 2015. Multilateral aid 2015: Better partnerships for a post-2015 world. Pub: OECD Publishing, Paris. Retrieved from: http://dx.doi.org/10.1787/9789264235212-en.

bilateral aid is an easier sell to the electorate because it is seen as more efficient, less bureaucratic, and better able to serve national interests.

Multilateral Agencies

Multilateral aid is given by large agencies made up of varying numbers of donor states; allocation decisions are made by a governing body. Their origin can also be traced back to World War II, when the first multilateral agencies (IMF and the precursor to the World Bank) were established at Bretton Woods. From large to small, there are now over 200 multilateral agencies (DAC, 2010). In total they receive about 30 percent of ODA. Roughly 80 percent goes to the main five groups, with only 20 percent left for the remainder (Figure 11.6). Apart from the long-standing major groups—the UN group, EU institutions, the World Bank group, and international development banks, there has been the recent addition of targeted, or vertical, funds. Some of these special interest organizations have become a major part of the aid scene. Examples include the Global Fund, GAVI, Education for All—Fast Track Initiative, and the President's Emergency Plan for AIDS Relief (EURODAD, 2008).

Since the recent financial crisis, many donors are taking a hard look at the value received from their multilateral funding choices (DFID, 2011). With Britain's practice as an example, the recent trend has been to increase funding for efficient agencies, but reduce or stop funding for those perceived as giving poor returns on investment. The fraction of multilateral aid has fallen below 30 percent in the last few years. Donors also try to maintain control of their money by earmarking part of their donation to multilateral agencies rather than throwing it into the general pot and trusting the agency to use it efficiently. This non-core, or multi-bi, funding has increased to about 30 percent of the total. It is higher among UN programs and lower among EU institutions (Figure 11.6).

Compared to bilateral aid, multilateral funding is seen as less political but more bureaucratic. The advantages of scale and the concentration of expertise under one agency must be balanced against the extra bureaucracy and more inflexible decision-making process. Neither funding method is able to avoid conditionality. While the strategic and economic conditions associated with bilateral aid are avoided, they are simply replaced by other forms of conditionality applied by the multilateral lending agencies.

Non-Governmental Organizations (NGOs)

In terms of numbers, the private, non-profit groups generally known as NGOs greatly outnumber the traditional large agencies. The widespread use of the term

"NGO" gives the incorrect idea that there are unifying features common to all these thousands of groups. That is not true. There is no widely accepted definition for NGOs, there is no guiding body, no regulatory framework, and no one even knows how many there are (likely in the tens of thousands). Consequently, any attempt at generalization is impossible. Some, like Save the Children or Oxfam, are large, highly competent organizations with respected international reputations. At the other end of the spectrum are small groups with very variable levels of training, preparation, or even basic understanding of local problems. Rules vary between developing countries, but it is still possible for a group of enthusiasts to work within remote rural communities, handing out medications or advice without any controls or limitations on their actions. The International Committee of the Red Cross sits in a category of its own since it has an international mandate to support the Geneva Convention.

Not surprisingly, NGOs as a group face the same broad criticisms as the large official agencies—lack of regulation, poor or absent outcome analysis, variable training and qualifications of their members, inadequate sustainability, and lack of transparency concerning costs. The arrival of Médecins sans Frontières (Doctors without Borders) in the 1970s brought a much-needed sense of professionalism to the area of aid work, but amateurism is far from over—either among workers or their agencies. McCall et al.'s (1999) study of large private agencies showed extraordinarily poor standards of training and field support, even for workers going to potentially dangerous regions. The rise of national NGOs within developing countries has been a relatively new development. Again, their sizes and standards vary widely, but some, such as the Bangladesh Rehabilitation Assistance Committee (BRAC, 2012), are now large enough that they run projects in other developing countries.

TYPES OF AID

> Clean water and health care and school and food and tin roofs and cement floors, all of these things should constitute a set of basics that people must have as birthrights.
>
> —*Paul Farmer*

This section concentrates on the *what* of foreign aid, not the *why*, but it is still worth making a few comments about the reasons why rich countries decide to invest money to help poorer countries. Since the end of the Cold War, altruism has risen to the top of the list, but on occasion, it is still followed by economic advantage, political and security considerations, and historical ties of language and colonialism. In a world shrunken by modern travel and communications, poverty—with all its health and social consequences—sits right next door to great wealth. Under those circumstances, most would agree that helping those living in the poorest countries does not need much justification. Whether it is a moral imperative or simple common sense, foreign aid is a good idea. The fact that the aid industry is easily criticized or that foreign aid has often been done badly in the past is not a valid argument against the concept of aid; it is an argument in favour of doing it properly.

Assuming benign intentions, a source of cash, and a selection of professional agencies, what types of aid are available? For the purposes of review, aid can be placed into four very broad groups, plus one extra that will likely become more important in the future:

- *Economic aid:* From micro credit to free trade zones, the main aims are poverty reduction and economic growth.
- *Health aid:* From oral rehydration to large vertical funds, the main aim is improved population health.
- *Civil society aid:* From rehabilitating child soldiers to drafting a national constitution, the main aims are peace, good governance, and the rule of law.
- *Disaster relief:* From refugee camps to disaster preparedness training, the main aim is to help those affected by natural and humanitarian disasters.
- *Climate aid:* From low-emission power generation to large-scale water conservation projects, the aid industry gets set to face climate change in developing countries.

There is, of course, overlap between the four main aid groups. However, for the purposes of analysis, they can be viewed as separate entities, each with its own history of trial and error. Although the development of international aid was covered in detail in Chapter 2, it is worth emphasizing some of the main points using these separate headings.

Economic Aid

Economic aid was the first form of foreign aid. Economic theories of the day, based on the Marshall Plan, suggested that aid-supported infrastructure led to growth, which led to prosperity. While this had worked in postwar Europe, it did not work in developing countries (Easterly, 2002). By the 1970s, this approach had left the developing world littered with expensive dams, railways, and hospitals, but with little sign of economic growth. Failure of the accumulationist theory of aid was overshadowed by the increasing debt crisis, which reached a critical point in the early 1980s with Mexico's first default. The subsequent imposition of stringent conditions for further loans was widely unpopular and ultimately led to the IMF developing the current Heavily Indebted Poor Countries (HIPC) Initiative in the mid-1990s. The Poverty Reduction Strategy process within the HIPC program, combined with the emphasis on poverty reduction within the MDGs, reflects a profound change of attitude. Economic aid is now focused directly on the poor rather than on trying to help countries pay their debts at the expense of the poor.

Health Aid

Health aid was the second major form of aid. Early projects were based on scientific discoveries made during World War II, particularly penicillin, chloroquine, and DDT. The optimistic hope was that science would soon allow us to have a world free from several diseases, including malaria and tuberculosis. Those top-down imposed programs did not succeed, except for two examples—the near eradication of yaws from Africa, and the total eradication of smallpox. Implementation lessons learned from those early days have allowed subsequent teams to make huge advances against a range of diseases, including polio, leprosy, river blindness, Guinea worm, and filariasis. Despite those successes, malaria and tuberculosis remain major causes of human disease. Since the early 1980s, those two ancient diseases have, of course, been joined by the human immunodeficiency virus. A large portion of health aid is now directed toward controlling these three infections using recently developed vertical programs such as the Global Fund.

From a health systems perspective, the first approach was to export Western medicine in the form of hospitals and expensive technical equipment. Widespread dissatisfaction with technological solutions for social problems led to the Alma Ata meeting in 1978 and a switch in emphasis toward primary health care (PHC). Enthusiasm for PHC was such that optimists talked of "health for all by 2000." Unfortunately, these high hopes weren't reached (at least in part because of arguments about interpretation and implementation). However, the PHC era still produced some of the most easily recognizable and measurable benefits of foreign aid, such as widespread immunization and oral rehydration. While PHC has passed out of fashion, it has not been replaced by a widely accepted alternative model for funding and delivering health care to developing world populations. The current importance of health aid is reflected in the fact that three of the eight MDGs are directly related to health.

Civil Society Aid

Civil society aid, with its emphasis on good governance, peace, and human rights, has been a growing ideological feature of foreign aid in recent times. It didn't start with the end of the Cold War, but it certainly gained more attention once the political allegiances of foreign leaders were seen as less important than their human rights record. A civil society is increasingly viewed as an essential foundation for effective aid. Without it, aid projects stand a higher chance of failure. In the past, conditions have been attached to aid in a usually unsuccessful attempt to induce beneficial changes. Rather than trying to change governments, donors are now switching to performance-based allocation, which tends to reward countries with good human rights records. For example, IDA grants are allocated on the basis of a scoring system—at least part of which includes measures of civil society. While this might be good for aid outcomes, it means that the poor in these increasingly forgotten, difficult partnership countries are excluded.

Disaster Relief

Disaster relief efforts predate the modern aid industry. The US Congress first donated food surpluses to aid Venezuela as early as 1812, and the International Committee of the Red Cross was founded in 1863. Delivering and coordinating services as different as housing, health care, food delivery, and security are major challenges in the chaos of an acute crisis. The biggest review of a major disaster was organized by the Tsunami Evaluation Coalition (TEC, 2007). Multiple needs-assessment teams, poor coordination (even competition) among agencies, arbitrary funding decisions, multiple groups of enthusiastic but untrained relief workers, and insufficient reliance on local capacities were major problems. The major donors spent US$11 billion on disaster relief in 2010, so it is important to learn from this experience. With the establishment of large coordinating agencies such as the UN's Office for the Coordination of Humanitarian Affairs and the European Commission Humanitarian Office, uniform standards will slowly be accepted. However, the recent responses to earthquakes in Pakistan and Haiti, Hurricane Katrina, and the Japanese tsunami show there is still plenty of room for improvement in the international responses to disasters.

Climate Aid

Climate aid is the newest form of aid, an inevitable development given the size of the global movement to combat climate change. The first moves toward assisting developing countries to deal with climate change were made by the 1992 UN Framework Convention on Climate Change. Despite widespread ratification of the UNFCCC's recommendations, developed countries gave only a trickle of climate aid. The more recent 2010 UN climate conference in Cancun agreed to provide US$10 billion for climate aid over the next two years. This was optimistically scheduled to rise to US$100 billion by 2020. The money will be channelled through a newly developed Green Climate Fund whose interim trustee is the World Bank. This will be in addition to several climate funds that already exist (Climate Funds, 2011).

Since many of the climate initiatives will overlap with conventional aid projects (agriculture improvements, water conservation, etc.), developing countries have expressed concerns that donors may try to double-count aid under two headings. Efforts to raise climate funding to 0.5 percent of GDP, in addition to the target of 0.7 percent GDP for ODA, are not meeting with enthusiasm. A recent report by the UN's Advisory Group on Climate Change Finance pragmatically accepts that, in common with trends in foreign direct investment, the private sector contribution might ultimately turn out to be the largest source of climate funding for developing countries (AGCCF, 2011).

TYPES OF IMPLEMENTATION

> Aid agencies have a long history of trying to "cocoon" their projects using free-standing technical assistance, independent project implementation units, and foreign experts—rather than trying to improve the institutional environment for service provision.... They have neither improved services in the short run nor led to institutional changes in the long run.
>
> —*World Bank, 1998*

So far, we have looked at the different funding sources, the types of aid on which the money can be spent, and the broad range of agencies that administer the funds. There's one last step—someone finally has to do something useful with all that cash. This is obviously the most important part of the process, but it gets surprisingly little attention. Will you achieve your goals, or will the money disappear like water poured on sand? We're not talking about the endless practical problems that confront any project—that's all part of the fun of development work—we're looking at the bigger picture in this section. Basically, what is the best way to implement projects so that money ends up going where it is intended?

At one end of the implementation spectrum, you can cut out the middlemen and simply give the money directly to poor people as a form of welfare (or as budget support for their government) and trust that they will know best how to spend it. At the other end, money can be used for projects that are completely separate from local authority. Import the necessary equipment (all purchased from the donor country), use only expatriate staff, complete the project, and then go home. In the middle, there are varying degrees of involvement with local authorities, ranging from a town council, through specific ministries, and finally up to government or even regional organizations. The principal consideration behind the choice of methodology is the degree of trust in local administrative abilities. When there is a high degree of trust (a good example would be the Marshall Plan), direct grants are used. When local administrative capacity is less reliable (or non-existent in humanitarian disasters), programs shift toward greater degrees of independence. While there are degrees of overlap, the following broad approaches can be defined.

Project-Based Aid

The traditional form of project aid refers to stand-alone programs such as building schools, clinics, or clean-water systems that are largely funded, staffed, and planned by outside agencies. In a world of program-based aid and the widely accepted Paris Declarations on aid effectiveness, old-fashioned project aid has been getting a bad name. In practice, projects can be very large and involve varying degrees of local and governmental input, so definitions are not clear-cut. Good examples are vertical programs targeted against specific diseases, which may work outside the local country's health system. They are not strictly project aid, but they do carry some of the risks and problems associated with projects.

Project aid tends to be more common in environments where local administrative capacity is weak. It also tends to be the method used in the early chaotic days following an acute disaster—not necessarily a good thing, since that is one of the major criticisms of many disaster responses. Project aid has several advantages when viewed strictly from the donor's perspective. Funding and administration are more easily controlled and specific outcomes are easier to measure compared to large, sector-wide undertakings. Projects are also easier to visualize, which can help raise further funds from home.

There are also, of course, significant problems, which have prompted moves away from project funding. Strictly autonomous projects are open to a range of criticisms, principally due to lack of local input in the planning stages and poor sustainability when the expatriates go home. Even if outside agencies decide to work with local governments, it can make matters even worse because of the responsibilities generated by multiple uncoordinated and often overlapping projects. There are numerous stories of developing countries that have to host a new visiting delegation every single day and generate dozens of budget reports to different agencies. Duplication, fragmentation, and overlap are the principal reasons behind the current emphasis on donor coordination and aid harmonization (OECD, 2011).

Program-Based Aid

In an attempt to get around the problems of multiple uncoordinated projects, donors started experimenting with combined funding of an entire sector in the mid-1990s. They began in the areas of education, agriculture, and health. These new initiatives were initially called sector-wide approaches (SWAps), but the broader term "program-based aid" (PBA) is now more commonly used (Cabral, 2010). The Paris Declaration proposes that 66 percent of a donor's bilateral aid should be used for program-based funding. There is no convenient definition, but basically, program aid is used to coordinate budget support for a unified program. "Program" is an expandable term that includes support for a single sector, such as health; multisectoral support for broad aims, such as poverty alleviation; or even for multinational programs, such as the Nile Basin Initiative. The key factors are a common budget, local leadership, coordination of donor practices, and harmonization of the donors with local policy aims.

The anticipated advantages are improved local ownership of the program, better donor alignment with the recipient country's aims, reduction of administrative costs through donor coordination, and a results-based monitoring and evaluation methodology. It is important to understand that PBAs are intended to be a new way of doing business. They are not "the same old thing" dressed up to satisfy the Paris Declaration (Lavergne, 2003). Without substantive changes in organization and management, programs will simply swap the top-down approach of project aid for the top-down approach of the local ministry of health, with no real benefit (Cabral, 2010). The essential features needed for a functioning PBA are:

- a clearly defined program
- a common budget and financial monitoring framework
- guaranteed aid flows for the duration of the project
- use of local administrative structures for program planning and management
- in the absence of strong administration, investment in local systems to allow them to take full control with time

This looks good on paper and meets the main requirements of the Paris Declaration, but in a weak administrative environment, it isn't easy to make changes. A Swedish study of 11 health sector SWAps showed that donors must enter these arrangements with a long-term view that may involve several years of preparation before the country's administrative capacity is able to take on the management of large projects (SIDA, 2003).

Direct Budget Support

Direct budget support (DBS) is becoming an increasingly common form of foreign aid—the British government is a particular supporter of the concept (Warrener, 2004). This is not, of course, simply a one-cheque-a-year model for aid. The other necessary elements include policy dialogue, support for local capacity to manage the funds, and a detailed accountability mechanism—it is not just a matter of handing over the cash (UNCTAD, 2008). The money is either given into the country's general budget, or it may be earmarked for a particular sector. This form of support has obvious advantages in terms of simplicity, low administration costs, and local ownership. Concerns include the possibility that DBS can lead to corruption, difficulty in determining whether funds were used to support agreed-upon aims, difficulties in monitoring outcomes when money is placed into a general fund, and the preferential support of government over the private sector and NGOs.

Some examples will help illustrate the increasing emphasis placed on different forms of direct cash transfer. At one end of the spectrum are cash transfers, in-kind food donations, or various forms of redeemable vouchers given directly to poor people. Aid-funded work schemes for unemployed youth fit under the same general heading. On the surface, these seem to be a good idea—simply a form of unemployment insurance for the poorest. They may be particularly applicable in countries recovering from war or other disasters, such as Sierra Leone (Holmes et al., 2008). Examples include several cash- or voucher-transfer programs in Latin America that are conditional on school attendance, and the child grant system in South Africa (Barrientos et al., 2006). The advantages are that poor families have cash to meet their immediate needs, and spending then also improves the local economy—similar in many ways to remittance income. The potential disadvantages include fostering a sense of aid dependence, increasing local inflation, producing unknown effects on the broader economic aims of the country, and creating a risk that targeting the money to particular groups might exacerbate underlying tensions in the area.

On a larger scale, the best example of direct financial transfer is the Millennium Challenge Corporation (MCC), established in 2004 by the Bush administration. Money is granted in a three-step process (MCC, 2011). The country must first pass a selection process based on measures of governance, economic policies, and willingness to support the poor. MCC staff then work with the country to establish a development plan. Once that is complete, funding is channelled through a locally managed Millennium Challenge account. Wherever possible, financial monitoring is maintained by an independent auditing company. Concerns include the choice of conservative selection criteria, slow release of available funds, and diversion of money to the government and away from the intended local non-governmental organizations.

AID EFFECTIVENESS

> If amid the scattered hopes of a failed development project, there was a little black box to record what had gone wrong, it would always turn out to be the case that, somewhere on the way, the people for whose benefit the project was intended had found better things to do with their time.
>
> —*James Grant, director, UNICEF, 1982*

What Has Aid Achieved?

For reasons that are unclear, development economists dominate the literature on aid effectiveness. Much-quoted books by Collier, Moyo, Easterly, and Sachs, listed in the Recommended Reading section, are all written by economists. This is unfortunate for several reasons. Firstly, economic aid is only a small part of the broad picture of aid. Of the four forms of aid listed earlier (economic, health, civil society, and disaster), economic aid is the only one that might be expected to produce measurable economic growth, so the use of economic growth as a proxy for the success of all other forms of aid is misleading (Clemens et al., 2004). Secondly, far too much faith is placed in the statistical abilities of economists. Those technical papers might look impressive, but their foundations are soft. Economic growth studies are frequently based on pooled measurements from many developing countries. The most basic comparison compares the amount of aid a country receives with its annual growth. This has been plotted many times in many papers and there appears to be no clear linear relationship between aid and growth (Rajan et al., 2005). This does not mean there is no relationship; it means the relationship (if one exists) is more complex than a simple straight line.

In an attempt to bring out more subtle relationships, the effects of multiple related variables can be tested by statistical methods. Unfortunately, there are a lot of potential variables that might explain some of the poor economic results of aid—dozens of them. Examples include standards of governance; distance from a port; annual rainfall; levels of poverty, health, or education in the recipient population; professional standards of the donor; strength of local currency; level of corruption—even the average annual temperature or murders per capita. It isn't difficult to find as many variables as there are measured points, which makes the final conclusions of such statistical fishing trips of questionable value. In statistical terms, this methodological problem makes the results fragile. This is not a minor problem. The claim that aid works only in countries with good governance (Burnside et al., 2004) has had an influential effect on the IDA's allocation of aid, but the methodology has been shown to be open to just this statistical error (Murphy et al., 2006).

This all brings up the long-standing question: Does aid work? Aid projects are complex undertakings—their results usually do not resolve themselves into simple yes/no answers. Examining the outcomes of a single large aid project will illustrate this problem. In 1960, the Kariba Dam and power station project was completed at a gorge on the Zambezi River between what were then northern and southern Rhodesia. The project was largely funded by the World Bank, and at that time, the dam was one of the biggest in the world. Money was given and a dam was built; clearly, on that level, it was a successful aid project (WCD, 2000).

However, if you look closely, the conclusions are not quite so simple. The 100 people who were killed building the dam are not usually discussed, and neither are the 57,000 Batonga who were forcibly displaced from their traditional home. Their displacement was poorly planned and was often associated with violence. To this day, the displaced Batongas live in absolute rural poverty, which is well documented by Dr. Sekai Nzenza-Shand (1997). They certainly did not benefit from this project—and neither did the thousands of animals who were stranded and drowned. The much-publicized animal rescue operation (Operation Noah) meant that the animals gained far more attention than the Batongas.

On the other side, the Zambian copper industry gained a source of cheap electricity—surely that was a clear benefit? Unfortunately, drought during the 1990s meant that the turbines did not turn, so the old coal-powered station had to be restarted. Environmentally, the huge lake increased the spread of malaria and schistosomiasis. Conversely, the hydroelectricity was certainly ecologically friendlier than the old coal-powered station. The lake provides a modest kapenta fishing industry, but the water was of only limited value for agricultural development because of the absence of irrigation pumping equipment. When everything is balanced out, was this project a success or a failure? By picking the facts that fit your biases, it can be made into an ecological disaster or an economic triumph. Now multiply this by the total number of aid projects and then decide if aid is of any value!

Although there is still a great deal of poverty and ill health in the world, the rapid rise of India and China over the last 20 years has been such that average global figures for poverty and malnutrition have halved over this time period. The dominance of these two developing countries is so great that their progress will likely allow most of the MDGs to be met in 2015 even though there are regions that do not share in their prosperity. How much, if any, of this progress (uneven as it is) can be attributed to aid? There are, of course, strong opinions on each side of this debate. Whatever else might be said of aid, it is certain that nothing lasting can be achieved quickly. The best reviews of aid are those that take a long look at a coherent policy over time. Two in particular are worth reviewing: the outcome of Australian aid investment in Papua New Guinea over

25 years (AusAID, 2003), and a similar review of US aid investment in Costa Rica over 50 years (USAID, 1998). The only conclusions that can be made are that well-designed projects, run by well-trained people acting in partnership with well-intentioned recipients, can—as long as there is sustainable funding and careful monitoring—improve the lives of poor people. If one or more of these essential elements is missing, aid money will be wasted.

Examples of Aid Outcomes

To get a broader view of the value of aid, it is useful to look at some of the successes and failures under the four separate types of aid.

The Results of Economic Aid

As noted above, this is a difficult question to answer because of the number of confounding variables. A slightly exaggerated example would be an attempt to explain differences in the growth of children in 50 countries by measuring the height of a few children in each one. You now have 50 sets of measurements (facts) and many ways of explaining why they vary (theories). Is it due to cross-country variation in poverty, rainfall, standards of agriculture, education of their parents, etc.? Fairly soon, you can have 50 theories and 50 measurement sets. In statistical terms, you have insufficient degrees of freedom. In commonsense terms, public policy should not be based on regression studies without extensive corroborating evidence.

Based on cross-country regression analyses, economists have claimed that aid produces measurable economic growth in an enabling environment (Burnside et al., 2004); aid works, but the relationship with growth is non-linear (Hansen et al., 2001); aid works after a civil war, with good governance (Collier et al., 2004); and aid works, but only outside the tropics (Dalgaard et al., 2003). Based on conclusions from many similar studies, aid allocation is currently influenced by claims that aid should be directed to countries with extensive poverty and signs of policy reform (Collier et al., 2001). In reality, the factors that combine to produce rapid economic growth are not known. In China, the catalyst might have been relaxation of government controls (Rusheng, 2006). In India, it might have been the reduction in bureaucratic red tape (Rodrick et al., 2004).

The correct combination of educated workers, suitable infrastructure, and government regulations will vary from country to country. The best that aid can expect is to target economic initiatives using the best available evidence in the hope that it will help a country develop whatever elements are needed for growth in that region. Successful examples can be found in the areas of agriculture and technology. Aid money and technical assistance led to the agricultural advances collectively

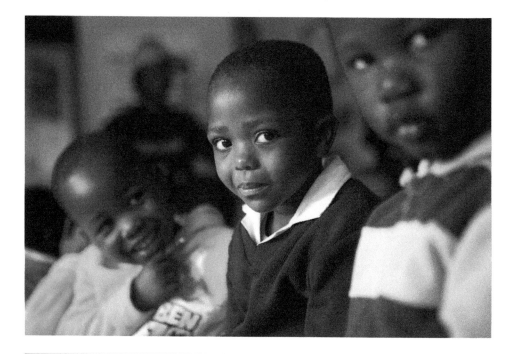

Photo 11.2: Arguments about the effects of aid on economic growth will likely never end, but there is no doubt about the benefits of aid directed toward child and maternal health. Although the families of these South African schoolchildren are not wealthy, their children are growing up healthy and strong. A large part of this is due to the combined effects of maternal education, vaccination, and basic hygiene.

Source: David Gough/Integrated Regional Information Network photo library (www.irinnews.org/photo).

known as the Green Revolution. This has lifted millions of people out of hunger and poverty in India and other Asian countries. Again, aid and technical assistance helped the Indian government establish what have now become the highly respected Indian Institutes of Technology.

The Results of Health Aid

Here we are on firmer ground. While health aid has had its own share of waste and mismanagement, it does not require exotic statistical tests to prove that health aid's best results have been of enormous benefit to poor people (Photo 11.2). The WHO's program against smallpox was the first time that a major infectious disease had been eradicated (the severe acute respiratory syndrome, SARS, can possibly be added to that list). Since then, single-focus programs have had huge successes against polio (reduced to less than 100 cases a year), measles, onchocerciasis, filariasis, and others, including leprosy. The current trend toward vertical programs aimed at malaria, tuberculosis, and HIV have all shown signs of success, but all three are very difficult diseases to control.

The move toward primary health care following the Alma Ata meeting in 1978 also resulted in major aid-funded health advances. These include the reduction in deaths from dehydration using oral rehydration solution (ORS), the marked reduction in vaccine-preventable deaths through widespread immunization, and a reversal of the trend away from breastfeeding. There is no doubt that money spent on health initiatives has been of benefit.

The Results of Civil Society Aid

Although one of the earliest actions of the new United Nations was to produce a declaration of human rights, it has taken quite a long time before significant aid funding has been directed to this area. However, there are now many clear examples of success stories. One early success was the conditional tying of US aid to land ownership reform in Taiwan. Breaking the hold of elite families allowed the country's economy to take off. Aid also supported the struggle for democracy in South Africa and has supported election monitoring around the world. The most recent advance has been the establishment of the International Criminal Court in 2002. Hopefully, the risk of future prosecution will make tyrants think twice before victimizing their own population. The use of aid to encourage and develop the elements of civil society has undoubtedly been beneficial.

The Results of Disaster Relief

Although the responses to the Asian tsunami and earthquakes in Pakistan and Haiti were inevitably chaotic, there is no doubt that humanitarian aid contributed to saving lives and speeding up the post-disaster recovery process. In all these cases, the responses were far from perfect, but the circumstances and working conditions were very difficult. Now that serious attention is being paid to the problems of organization and coordination, humanitarian aid has a significant and justifiable place in the broad field of foreign aid.

Improving Aid Effectiveness

> Because things are the way they are, things will not stay the way they are.
>
> —*Bertolt Brecht*

The 17 SDGs were agreed upon and adopted by every single one of the 193 member states of the United Nations on September 25, 2015. These goals, officially known as "Transforming Our World: The 2030 Agenda for Sustainable Development," are a successor to the MDGs. Such a widespread and unprecedented level of agreement among states in adopting the SDGs should definitely have a major influence on the current aid industry. Apart from the prior catalytic effect of the MDGs and now hopefully the new SDGs, the last decade has seen a convergence of other events that promise to help shake up the old order. The arrival of significant new donors, such as China, India, and Brazil, has introduced competition into the DAC monopoly, while the growing influence of successful business leaders (now termed "philanthrocapitalists") has brought innovative methods for raising money and administering aid. Finally, the analysis of past policies, such as the support of tyrants during the Cold War or the era of structural adjustments, has perhaps even brought a sense of humility that the poor could have been better served by all that aid money. Whatever the reason, change is certainly in the air.

The simplest sign that donor countries are serious about change is the steady growth of aid funding. Since the low point of 1997, aid funding has now doubled (Figure 11.2). The current emphasis on aid effectiveness dates to the 2002 Monterrey meeting on aid financing (United Nations, 2003). Donors realized that simply providing more money was not enough—the money also had to be spent in a more efficient manner. The OECD took the lead and organized a series of international meetings on the subject. The result was the 2005 Paris Declaration, which laid out the five fundamental requirements for effective aid. This was followed by the Accra Agenda for speeding up their implementation (OECD, 2008a). These principles have subsequently been endorsed by over 100 countries. If high-level politicians take the time to attend meetings on aid effectiveness, even the strongest aid enthusiast would accept that it's a sign there are significant problems with aid as it is currently practised.

There is nothing new about the recommendations of the Paris Declaration. The only factor that has really changed is a broad realization that such changes are now necessary. All the recently rediscovered elements of a successful aid project were established at the Alma Ata meeting in 1978. The following brief summary lists the proposed areas of change under the five headings of the Paris Declaration:

Ownership

Developing countries must be the leaders of their own development projects. This means all levels of society should be involved, not just government elites. This, in turn, implies that donors will often have to invest in building the capacity needed to provide local people with a voice. The Declaration's target was that three-quarters of developing countries should have their own national development strategy by 2010.

Alignment

Basically, aid should be used for the benefit and convenience of the recipient, not the donor. Aid policies should be aligned with the needs of the recipient, promised flows should be disbursed on time with less fluctuation, and aid should not be tied to goods and services within the donor country. In addition, donors should, where possible, use local systems for managing and monitoring aid. Again, this implies that donors must pay attention to strengthening such structures.

Harmonization

The current proliferation of aid agencies means that some countries are overwhelmed with the conflicting requirements of each donor. Apart from being inefficient, it is also costly. Donors must coordinate their visits and reporting needs so that the burden of aid projects is reduced. In addition, donors should avoid overlap by joining forces to fund particular broad segments, identified by the recipient, such as supporting a national education plan.

Results-Based Management

The move toward measuring results is a major advance in the general management of aid (Ravallion, 2009). Accurate monitoring data is vital to help allocate funds where they are best used, to detect problems in a project early on, and also to improve the design of future projects. This is an absolutely vital component for improved aid effectiveness.

Mutual Accountability

Accountability is essential, not just between donor and recipient, but also between recipient government and its citizens. Again, donors must be prepared to invest in local structures for monitoring results.

SUMMARY

In 2015, net official development assistance (ODA) flows from member countries of the Development Assistance Committee (DAC) were US$131.6 billion, representing 0.3% of gross national income (GNI). Although aid from most DAC countries falls well below the original target of 0.7 percent GNI, it still represents a great deal of money. Donor countries spend aid money through bilateral or multilateral channels. Aid can be placed into five very broad groups: economic aid, health aid, civil society aid, disaster relief, and climate aid. The presence of large non-OECD donors like China and India is introducing external competition into what used to be a DAC monopoly. For example, estimated development co-operation flows by 29 providers beyond the DAC reached US$33 billion in 2014. In addition, increases in alternative funds, such as remittance income, foreign direct investment, and private philanthropy, all allow developing countries more choice and fewer conditions when looking for sources of external funding. In 2015, worldwide remittance flows are estimated to have exceeded US$601 billion. Of that amount, developing countries were estimated to receive about US$441 billion, nearly three times the amount of official development assistance. The United States is by far the largest remittance-sending country, with an estimated US$56.3 billion in recorded outflows in 2014. Saudi Arabia ranks as the second largest.

Once aid money leaves an external donor's hand, it follows a complicated path before it reaches the intended recipient. In the last decade substantive efforts have been made to improve the quantity and quality of aid. Firstly, aid should be used for the benefit and convenience of the recipient, not the donor. Secondly, aid policies should be aligned with the needs of the recipient, and donors should, where possible, use local systems for managing and monitoring aid. Again, this implies that donors must pay attention to strengthening such structures. Thirdly, there must be harmonization where donors coordinate their visits and reporting needs so that the burden of aid projects is reduced. Fourthly, there must be a move toward measuring results. Finally, there must be mutual accountability. The target under SDG 17 to "revitalize the global partnership for sustainable development" emphasizes the importance of increasing financial resources for developing countries from multiple sources, assisting developing countries in attaining long-term debt sustainability, working in partnership, ensuring policy coherence, and respecting country ownership.

DISCUSSION QUESTIONS

1. What is DAC? How much influence does DAC play in international aid?
2. Imagine you are asked to chair DAC. What recommendations would you put in place to make aid more effective?
3. What was the Paris Declaration? What are its five overarching principles?
4. Why is remittance income very high? Which countries receive the highest remittance income?
5. What is the difference between bilateral and multilateral aid? Which do you think is more effective?
6. What does it mean for aid to be accountable? Does aid encourage corruption and dependency? Why or why not?
7. Which countries give the highest amount of aid in terms of percentage of GNI? How does that change if you were just evaluating the actual amount? Why does the difference matter?

8. In your opinion, are OECD countries giving enough aid to developing countries?
9. What is tied aid, and why is it important to untie aid?
10. What does it mean for aid to be transparent?

RECOMMENDED READING

Collier, P. 2007. *The bottom billion*. Pub: Oxford University Press.

Easterly, W. (Ed.). 2008. *Reinventing foreign aid*. Pub: MIT Press.

Moyo, D. 2009. *Dead aid: Why aid is not working and how there is a better way for Africa*. Pub: Farrar, Strauss, and Giroux.

Sachs, J. 2005. *The end of poverty*. Pub: Penguin Books.

REFERENCES

Acharya, et al. 2004. Aid proliferation: How responsible are the donors? Institute of Development Studies, working paper 214.

AGCCF. 2011. UN Advisory Group on Climate Change Financing. Retrieved from: www.climatefund.info/climate_fund_info.

AusAID. 2003. The contribution of Australian aid to Papua New Guinea's development 1975–2000. AusAID Evaluation and Review Series no. 34. Retrieved from: www.ausaid.gov.au/publications/pdf/qas34_contribution.pdf.

Barrientos, A., et al. 2006. Reducing child poverty with cash transfers: A sure thing? *Development Policy Review*, 24: 537–552. Retrieved from: www.eldis.org/vfile/upload/1/document/0708/DOC23659.pdf.

Bill and Melinda Gates Foundation. 2011. Retrieved from: www.gatesfoundation.org.

BRAC. 2012. Bangladesh Rural Advancement Committee. Retrieved from: www.brac.net.

Burall, S., et al. 2006. Reforming the international aid architecture: Options and ways forward. Overseas Development Institute, working paper 278.

Burnside, C., et al. 2004. Aid, policies, and growth: Revisiting the evidence. World Bank working paper no. 3251. Retrieved from: http://ideas.repec.org/p/wbk/wbrwps/3251.html.

Cabral, L. 2010. Sector-based approaches in agriculture. ODI briefing paper. Retrieved from: www.odi.org.uk/resources/download/4636.pdf.

Chanana, D. 2009. India as an emerging donor. *Economic and Political Weekly*, 44: 11–14.

Chinese Aid. 2011. Information Office of the State Council's White Paper on Chinese Foreign Aid. Retrieved from: http://news.xinhuanet.com/english2010/china/2011-04/21/c_13839683.htm.

CIDA. 2012. Retrieved from: www.acdi-cida.gc.ca.

Clemens, M., et al. 2004. Counting chickens when they hatch: The short-term effect of aid on growth. Centre for Global Development working paper no. 4. Retrieved from: www.cgdev.org/content/publications/detail/2744/.

Climate Funds. 2011. Retrieved from: www.climatefund.info/climate_fund_info.

Collier, P., et al. 2001. Can the world cut poverty in half? How policy reform and effective aid can meet international development goals. *World Development*, 29: 1787–1802.

Collier, P., et al. 2004. Aid, policy, and growth in post-conflict societies. *European Economic Review*, 48, 1125–1145.

DAC. 2010. Report on multilateral aid. Retrieved from: www.oecd.org/dataoecd/23/17/45828572.pdf.

Dalgaard, C.-J., et al. 2003. On the empirics of foreign aid and growth. Economic Policy Research Unit, University of Copenhagen. Retrieved from: www.econ.ku.dk/epru/files/wp/wp-03-13.pdf.

DCD-DAC. 2011. Development Co-operation Directorate. Retrieved from: www.oecd.org/dac.

Debt2Health. 2007. Innovative financing of the Global Fund. Retrieved from: www.theglobalfund.org/documents/publications/other/D2H/Debt2Health.pdf.

DFID. 2011. Department for International Development Multilateral Aid Review. Retrieved from: www.dfid.gov.uk/Documents/publications1/mar/multilateral_aid_review.pdf.

DFID. 2012. Retrieved from: www.dfid.gov.uk.

Easterly, W. 2002. *The elusive quest for growth: Economists' adventures and misadventures in the tropics*. Pub: MIT Press.

EITI. 2011. Extractive Industries Transparency Initiative. Retrieved from: http://eiti.org.

ESA. 2011. European Space Agency. Retrieved from: www.esa.int/esaSC/SEM75BS1VED_index_0.html.

EURODAD. 2008. Global vertical programmes. The reality of aid. Retrieved from: www.eurodad.org/uploadedFiles/Whats_New/Reports/realitycheck_jul2008_final.pdf.

GAVI. 2010. Alliance progress report 2010. Retrieved from: www.gavialliance.org.

George C. Marshall Foundation. 2009. Retrieved from: www.marshallfoundation.org.

Global Fund to Fight Aids, Tuberculosis, and Malaria. 2012. Retrieved from: www.theglobalfund.org.

Greenhill, R. 2006. Real aid 2: Making technical assistance work, 2006. Actionaid International. Retrieved from: www.actionaid.org.uk/doc_lib/real_aid2.pdf.

Hansen, H., et al. 2001. Aid and growth regressions. *Journal of Development Economics*, 64: 547–570.

Hewitt, A., et al. 2004. The international aid system 2005–2010: Forces for and against change. Overseas Development Institute, working paper 235.

Holmes, R., et al. 2008. Cash transfers in Sierra Leone: Are they appropriate, affordable, or feasible? ODI Project briefing paper no. 8. Retrieved from: www.odi.org.uk/resources/download/443.pdf.

Hudson Institute. 2011. The 2011 Index of Global Philanthropy and Remittances. Retrieved from: http://gpr.hudson.org.

IBRD. 2005. Global development finance: Mobilizing finance and managing vulnerability. Retrieved from: http://siteresources.worldbank.org/GDFINT/Resources/334952-1257197866375/gdf05complete.pdf.

IFFim. 2011. The value of innovative financing in saving children's lives. Retrieved from: www.iffim.org.

Lavergne, R. 2003. Program-based approaches: Questions and answers on a new way of doing business in CIDA. Retrieved from: http://g2lg.gop.pk/Portal/index2.php?option=com_docman&task=doc_view&gid=205&Itemid=105.

MCC. 2011. Millennium Challenge Corporation. Retrieved from: www.mcc.gov/pages/about.

McCall, M., et al. 1999. Selection, training, and support of relief workers. *British Medical Journal*, 318: 113–116.

Mohapatra, S., et al. 2011. Outlook for remittance flows 2011–2013. World Bank migration and development brief 16. Retrieved from: http://siteresources.worldbank.org/EXTDECPROSPECTS/Resources/476882-1157133580628MigrationandDevelopmentBrief16.pdf.

Murphy, R. et al. 2006. Government policy and the effectiveness of foreign aid. UBS Investment bank. Retrieved from: http://fmwww.bc.edu/ec-p/wp647.pdf.

Nzenza-Shand, S. 1997. *Songs to an African sunset.* Pub: Lonely Planet.

OECD. 2002. Foreign direct investment for development: Maximizing benefits, minimizing costs. Committee on International and Multinational Enterprises. Retrieved from: www.oecd.org/dataoecd/47/51/1959815.pdf.

OECD. 2006. Survey on harmonization and alignment of donor practices: Measuring aid harmonization and alignment in 14 partner countries. *OECD-DAC Journal*, 6 (Suppl. 1).

OECD. 2008a. The Paris Declaration on Aid Effectiveness and the Accra Agenda for Action. Retrieved from: www.oecd.org/dataoecd/11/41/34428351.pdf.

OECD. 2008b. Is it ODA? OECD Factsheet. Retrieved from: www.oecd.org/dataoecd/21/21/34086975.pdf.

OECD. 2010. Statistical annex for development cooperation. Retrieved from: www.oecd.org/dac/stats/dcrannex.

OECD. 2011. Paris Declaration and Accra Agenda for Action. Retrieved from: www.oecd.org/document/18/0,3343,en_2649_3236398_35401554_1_1_1_1,00.html.

OECD. 2012. Retrieved from: www.oecd.org.

OECD. 2015. Multilateral aid 2015: Better partnerships for a post-2015 world. Pub: OECD Publishing, Paris. Retrieved from: http://dx.doi.org/10.1787/9789264235212-en.

OECD. 2016a. Organisation for Economic Co-operation and Development, International Development Statistics (database). Retrieved from: https://data.oecd.org/.

OECD. 2016b. Development co-operation report 2016: The Sustainable Development Goals as business opportunities. Pub: OECD Publishing, Paris. Retrieved from: http://dx.doi.org/10.1787/dcr-2016-14-en.

Radelet, S. 2006. A primer on foreign aid. Centre for Global Development working paper no.

92. Retrieved from: www.cgdev.org/content/publications/detail/8846.

Rajan, R., et al. 2005. Aid and growth: What does the cross-country data really show? IMF working paper 05/127. Retrieved from: www.imf.org/external/pubs/ft/wp/2005/wp05127.pdf.

Ravallion, M. 2009. Evaluation in the practice of development. *World Bank Research Observer*, 24: 29–53.

Reddy, S., et al. 2006. Achieving the Millennium Development Goals: What's wrong with the existing analytical models? DESA working paper no. 30. Retrieved from: www.un.org/esa/desa/papers/2006/wp30_2006.pdf.

Rodrick, D., et al. 2004. From Hindu growth to productivity surge: The mystery of the Indian growth transition. IMF working paper 04/77. Retrieved from: www.imf.org/external/pubs/ft/wp/2004/wp0477.pdf.

Roodman, D. 2007. The anarchy of numbers: Aid, development, and cross-country empirics. Centre for Global Development working paper no. 32. Retrieved from: www.cgdev.org/content/publications/detail/2745/.

Rusheng, D. 2006. The course of China's rural reform. International Food Policy Research Institute. Retrieved from: www.ifpri.org/sites/default/files/publications/oc52.pdf.

Sandor, E., et al. 2009. Innovative financing to fund development: Progress and prospects. OECD Development Co-operation Directorate Issues Brief. Retrieved from: www.oecd.org/dataoecd/56/47/44087344.pdf.

Sharma, K. 2009. The impact of remittances on economic insecurity, 2009. Retrieved from: www.un.org/esa/desa/papers/2009/wp78_2009.pdf.

SIDA. 2003. Mapping of sector-wide approaches in health. Retrieved from: www.hlsp.org/LinkClick.aspx?fileticket=b1WL9AUfC-Y%3D&tabid=1809&mid=3507.

TEC. 2007. Joint evaluation of the international response to the Indian Ocean tsunami. Retrieved from: www.alnap.org/pool/files/Syn_Report_Sum.pdf.

UNCTAD. 2008. Budget support: A reformed approach or old wine in new skins? Retrieved from: www.unctad.org/en/docs/osgdp20085_en.pdf.

UNCTAD. 2011. The statistical division of the UN Conference on Trade and Development. Retrieved from: http://unctadstat.unctad.org.

UNITAID. 2009. Annual report 2009. Retrieved from: www.unitaid.eu.

United Nations. 2003. Monterrey Concensus on financing for development. Retrieved from: www.un.org/esa/ffd/monterrey/MonterreyConsensus.pdf.

USAID. 1998. Real progress: Fifty years of USAID in Costa Rica. USAID Program and Operations Assessment Report no. 23. Retrieved from: www.uvm.edu/rsenr/rm230/costarica/Fifty%20years%20of%20USAID%20in%20Costa%20Rica.pdf.

USAID. 2012. Retrieved from: www.usaid.gov.

Warrener, D. 2004. Current thinking in the UK on general budget support. Synthesis Paper 4.

Retrieved from: www.odi.org.uk/resources/download/2838.pdf.

WCD. 2000. World Commission on Dams: Kariba dam, Zambia, and Zimbabwe. Retrieved from: www.adb.org/water/topics/dams/pdf/cszzmain.pdf.

Winters, M. 2012. The obstacles to foreign aid harmonization: Lessons from decentralization support in Indonesia. *Studies in Comparative International Development*, 3: 316–341.

World Bank. 2011. Migration and remittances site. Retrieved from: www.worldbank.org/migration.

World Bank. 2016a. Migration and remittances factbook 2016 (3rd ed.). Retrieved from: https://openknowledge.worldbank.org/handle/10986/23743.

World Bank. 2016b. Migration and remittances, recent developments and outlook. Migration and Development Brief 26.

CHAPTER 12

Primary Health Care Strategies: The Essential Foundation

Some argue that primary health care was an experiment that failed; others contend that it was never truly tested.

—Lesley Magnussen, 2004

OBJECTIVES

Anyone studying global health will soon get used to a steady stream of abbreviations; PHC (primary health care) will be one of the most common. In practice, PHC is used to describe everything from an overall philosophy of national health care down to the distribution of a couple of packets of oral rehydration solution. For newcomers to the aid industry, it is very important to have a good idea about what does and does not constitute PHC. The subject has passed in and out of fashion over the last three decades. It is currently being rediscovered despite its slightly "old-fashioned" reputation. While opinions might change, the value of PHC does not. For all of those 30 years, it has acted as a fundamental guiding principle behind much of the health planning for developing countries. From the MDGs to the integrated management of childhood illnesses, PHC is a central feature of health initiatives. Consequently, this chapter will look carefully at the early development of the principles of PHC and their subsequent implementation around the world. After completing this chapter, you should be able to:

- understand the central importance of preventive medicine and health promotion strategies in the maintenance of population health
- appreciate the practical problems associated with implementing primary health care initiatives
- understand the evolution of primary health care strategies and their contribution to current maternal and child care initiatives
- understand the organization and funding of developing world health services

INTRODUCTION

An ounce of prevention is worth a pound of cure.

—Benjamin Franklin, 1736

Primary health care is a bit like love; nobody can describe it accurately, but a lot of people are certain that they have it. Health Canada defines PHC as all the services beyond conventional medicine that contribute to health (Health Canada, 2006). That's fine, but since they include income, housing, education, and the environment, it becomes a bit too inclusive to be of much value. Basically, PHC includes just about everything. The WHO/UNICEF's bureaucratic definition, clearly developed by a large committee, is not much better. In its narrowest definition, PHC is the provision of competent medical treatment for the common diseases in a community and represents the first point of contact between the population and health care services. In this form it is also called "primary medical care" (PHCRIS, 2011).

The broader concept of comprehensive PHC, developed at the 1978 meeting at Alma Ata, is based on a deeper understanding of the socio-economic roots underlying ill health. It defines PHC as

> essential health care based on practical, scientifically sound and socially acceptable methods and technology made universally accessible to individuals and families in the community through their full participation and at a cost that the community and country can afford to maintain at every stage of their development in the spirit of self-reliance and self-determination. It forms an integral part both of the country's health system, of which it is the central function and main focus, and of the overall social and economic development of the community. It is the first level of contact of individuals, the family and community with the national health system bringing health care as close as possible to where people live and work, and constitutes the first element of a continuing health care process. (WHO, 1978)

Rather than concentrating simply on medical treatments, PHC is extended to include the promotion of health based on the philosophy of equity, appropriate technology, and community involvement. These are not just trendy phrases to be taken lightly—PHC is a definable and highly valuable philosophy of treatment that deserves to be studied carefully. The fundamental difference from curative medicine is its emphasis on prevention rather than treatment, and the inclusion of local people in their own treatment plans. Emphasis is also placed on making sure that any therapies are universally acceptable, affordable, and technically appropriate. Of all the health care systems around the world, Cuba and, to a great extent, Canada remain closest to the philosophical ideals of the original Alma Ata Declaration.

Unfortunately, PHC is tarred with the same brush as public health—it has the reputation of being a bit boring, even a bit old-fashioned. When medical students get to the epidemiology part of their training, the lessons of preventive medicine are reinforced by trooping them round the local sewage-treatment plant and the waste dump. Predictably, interest levels are low compared to the thrills of the cardiac surgery rotation. However, once they qualify, it doesn't take them long to realize that smoking prevention is a lot better than coronary artery bypass surgery. Exactly the same lesson had to be learned by the aid industry. After spending 20 years trying to improve population health using Western medicine, it became clear that this approach wasn't working. During the 1970s, the World Health Assembly made a commitment to reverse this trend. The Assembly believed that development assistance and modern scientific advances should be able to provide a minimal standard of dignified living for every person in the world by the turn of the century. The slogan for this movement subsequently became "Health for all by the year 2000." The foundation for achieving this ambitious goal was to be primary health care.

A number of developing countries, particularly China, India, and some from Latin America, had already accumulated years of experience in tackling their own health problems with very limited financial resources. Their experience suggested

Box 12.1 History Notes

Miguel Sabido (1937–)

Miguel Sabido was working for a Mexican television company in the 1970s when he had the idea of using soap operas to spread health information. In essence, it was a technological update of the far older practice of using parables and myths to spread a social message. The first series introduced the topic of family planning. It was developed on the theory that humans base their behaviours on role models—in this case, the stars of telenovelas in Latin America. The method allowed previously taboo subjects to be discussed openly. Its success led to others, which addressed HIV/AIDS, family violence, and alcohol abuse. Education given through a medium that was accessible to much of the population rapidly caught on. The Sabido method is now termed "educational entertainment" (also "edutainment"), and is widely used as a public health tool around the world. In Tanzania, the radio soap opera "Twende no Wakati" ("Let's Be Modern") was credited with having a significant effect on contraceptive use. It became one of the most popular programs in the country. Follow the reference for more information: PMC (2011).

that preventive health initiatives were considerably more cost effective than those based solely on curative medicine. Each country differed, but a general consensus was reached about the most valuable elements of preventive care. These included an emphasis on breastfeeding, improved sanitation and clean water, access to basic medical care, immunizations, fertility-control information, and (most revolutionary of all) the inclusion of the poor in planning the solutions to their own health problems. By the 1970s, harsh practical experience had persuaded even the most technocratically minded developed countries that it was time to look for other solutions to the problem of ill health in the world's developing regions.

Under the energetic leadership of WHO's director-general Halfdan Mahler, the principles of what came to be called primary health care gained worldwide acceptance. The final result was an international meeting at Alma Ata in 1978, by the end of which there was universal support for the ambitious goal of "Health for all by 2000," based on worldwide implementation of the principles of primary health care (Baum, 2007). Inevitably, the dream of changing the world's medical system was easier in theory than in practice. However, despite problems of implementation and years of divisive argument between the comprehensive and selective PHC camps, a great deal of good was still achieved. More recent experience (particularly with the HIV/AIDS epidemic) has shown that effective initiatives must be aimed at multiple layers of a problem. Treatment and prevention are not antagonistic, but are simply part of a continuum, all parts of which need to be included in the final plan. It has taken over 30 years, but it is now clear that if a project is planned without using the elements clearly outlined in the philosophy of PHC, then that project's chances of success are slim—PHC rules!

THE DEVELOPMENT OF PRIMARY HEALTH CARE

> We recommend that, in laying out new towns and villages, and in extending those already laid out, ample provision be made for a supply, in purity and abundance, of light, air, and water; for drainage and sewerage, for paving, and for cleanliness.
>
> —Lemuel Shattuck, *Report of the Sanitary Commission of Massachussetts*, 1850

The Historical Development of Basic Hygiene and Health Care

While the benefits of basic medical care and sanitation were adopted at Alma Ata in 1978, these were certainly not new discoveries—a knowledge of basic hygiene had been around for a long time. Many centuries earlier, Roman military surgeons cleaned open wounds with vinegar, boiled surgical instruments, built ventilated hospitals with under-floor heating, and even isolated patients with fevers (Kennedy, 2004). From Augustus's time, military doctors were well paid and some probably lived in homes with sewage disposal and running water. It is a mystery why it took the rest of Europe so long to relearn these lessons after Rome fell in the 5th century. It was not until the mid-19th century that Virchow, Florence Nightingale, and Chadwick introduced the notion of public health to Europe, particularly the need for cleanliness, good housing, and nutrition (Schneider et al., 2008).

On the other side of the Atlantic, Lemuel Shattuck was making similar discoveries in America. Shattuck had already made significant contributions to the organization of public schooling before moving to Boston to work as a publisher. After persuading the Massachusetts legislature to introduce registration of births and deaths, he was subsequently appointed as head of a committee to study the sanitary conditions in the State of Massachusetts. The subsequent report (Shattuck et al., 1850) was an extraordinary document that was 100 years ahead of its time. One of the committee's recommendations is quoted at the start of this section. Others included the promotion of child health, improvements in housing, introduction of community health workers, and an emphasis on community participation through the establishment of sanitary associations. Some of the historical aspects of hygiene and public health are also discussed in Chapter 8.

The Early Days of the Aid Industry

As mentioned above, the broad topic of public health tends to have an image problem; it is just not very exciting. Anyone who has ever tried to teach the benefits of sewage treatment to medical students will understand this point. For a range of reasons, including the power of the medical establishment and the public perception of a need for medication, curative medicine always seems to overshadow preventive medicine (Seear, 2004). This was certainly the pattern when the modern era of aid started in the 1950s. Imposed health initiatives emphasized high technology and urban-based curative care in hospitals, famously described by Professor Morley as "disease palaces." Similarly, when newly independent countries started running their own health care systems in the 1950s and 1960s, they inherited the same type of health systems from their former colonial rulers. Either way, preventive strategies were not given a lot of emphasis at that time.

The public health programs of the day concentrated on vertical eradication programs, most noticeably against smallpox, yaws, and malaria. These programs were usually not integrated within the health services of the individual countries or even with each other; each usually had its own budget and staff. Although progress was made against a few individual diseases (most notably smallpox, but also yaws and tuberculosis), it was clear to many that this was an inefficient way to address the health needs of a population. These were some of the principal problems:

- Relatively high-technology, urban-based hospitals with sub-specialty services consumed disproportionate amounts of the national health budget.
- These large hospitals were usually concentrated in major cities and contributed little to the health of rural populations.
- The overall philosophy of imposed care rather than inclusive prevention strategies excluded the population from contributing to their own health.

By 1970, it was clear to many countries that curative medicine had significant limitations, particularly for their rural populations. Several countries responded by introducing various forms of village health centres, often staffed by nurse clinicians or medical orderlies. In 1975, a joint WHO/UNICEF report (Djukanovich et al., 1975) was produced which examined successful primary health care systems in a variety of countries, including Cuba, China, Tanzania, and Venezuela. Again, the conclusion was that Western medical systems were not adequate to meet the health of developing world populations. A somewhat romanticized version of the Chinese experience with "barefoot doctors" was particularly influential at the time (Sidel, 1972).

The literature of the day also reflected the growing realization that reorganization of developing world health services was long overdue. The highly influential 1974 report by Health Canada, known as the Lalonde Report (Lalonde, 1974), was the first acknowledgement by an industrialized country that medical care was only a small contributor to population health (far behind lifestyle effects and environmental influences). The report identified four variables that affected health (individual variation, environment, lifestyle, health care) and emphasized that governments should take a far broader approach toward improving population health. Ivan Illich's popular book, *Medical Nemesis* (Illich, 1975), went further in

Box 12.2 Moment of Insight

United States	Cuba	Dominican Republic
GDP per capita:	GDP per capita:	GDP per capita:
US$55,837	< US$7,000	< US$7,000
Infant mortality rate:	Infant mortality rate:	Infant mortality rate:
6.5	4.0	26

Source: World Bank. 2016. World Bank statistical database. Retrieved from: http://data.worldbank.org/indicator/SP.DYN.IMRT.IN.

asserting that medical care was not only almost irrelevant to health, but in areas where it consumed a large portion of the budget, it was even detrimental to population health. The level of interest in alternative approaches to health was so high that an international conference was called to discuss primary health care in 1978 (Cueto, 2004).

Alma Ata Declaration

> An acceptable level of health for all people of the world by the year 2000 can be obtained through a fuller and better use of the world's resources, a considerable part of which is now spent on armaments and military conflicts.
>
> —*Alma Ata Declaration, 1978*

The director-general of the WHO, Halfdan Mahler, was a leading proponent of PHC. During a speech in 1976, he first introduced the concept that the comprehensive introduction of preventive health methods could conceivably lead to widespread improvements in world health by the end of the century. This optimistic goal caught the popular imagination and was subsequently termed "Health for all by 2000." It was clearly time for a large meeting to decide exactly how this aim would be achieved (WHO, 1981). There was initially disagreement between the major communist powers about the site of the meeting. It was ultimately held in Alma Ata, the capital of Kazakhstan, after the Soviet Union agreed to cover the organizational expenses. Although the Chinese had been among the major proponents of PHC, they ultimately refused to attend. The meeting was the biggest single-issue international forum that had ever been held. It was attended by 134 governments and 67 international organizations (Cueto, 2004). After years of preceding preparatory discussions, delegates were well prepared for the topics. Not surprisingly, the resolutions were accepted unanimously. This consensus was subsequently confirmed at a meeting of the World Health Assembly the following year.

The eight elements constituting primary health care, plus the basic philosophical principles upon which those elements were based, are summarized in tables 12.2 and 12.1 respectively. Basically, Alma Ata was no less than an attempt to refashion the health systems of developing countries. It is not an exaggeration to say that there was a sense of euphoria following the meeting. The idea of health for all captured the spirit of the time; a brave new world seemed possible where poverty and avoidable ill health could be eradicated through widespread application of the principles of PHC. In many ways, it was similar to the current debate surrounding the "big push" approach advocated by Sachs (2005). Inevitably, pragmatic reality soon started to lower those initial idealistic expectations. It should be added that this methodology

Table 12.1: The basic principles of primary health care

Equity:	Equal access for all people regardless of income.
Community participation:	There must be meaningful involvement of the community in the planning, implementation, and maintenance of their own health services.
Health promotion:	This is the concept of providing people with the information to control and improve their own health.
Intersectoral coordination:	PHC extends beyond provision of health care and requires coordinated action by all sectors involved in that population's health, including agriculture, education, housing, and industry.
Appropriate technology:	In keeping with the principle of self-reliance, the technology associated with health care should be scientifically sound, adapted to local needs, robust, and easily maintained.

Table 12.2: The eight elements of primary health care

Education:	Health promotion and education given in local language
Nutrition:	Promotion of breastfeeding as the norm for all babies, plus nutrition supplements for high-risk children
Sanitation:	Universal access to clean drinking water and safe waste dis
Maternal and child health:	Maternal and child care to include antenatal care, under-fi clinics, and family planning
Immunization:	Universal access to WHO-recommended vaccination schedule
Disease control:	Prevention and control of endemic diseases backed by local epidemiological research
Medical care:	Appropriate treatment of common diseases and injuries
Essential drugs:	Reliable supplies of cheap and appropriate drugs tailored to local requirements

(particularly the emphasis on community involvement and the importance of prevention as well as cure) is equally applicable to developed countries. This became increasingly obvious once the HIV/AIDS epidemic started to spread.

After Alma Ata: Selective versus Comprehensive PHC

> There is nothing more difficult to take in hand, more perilous to conduct, or more uncertain in its success, than to take the lead in the introduction of a new order of things, because the innovator has for enemies all those who have done well under the old conditions and lukewarm defenders in those who may do well under the new.
>
> —*Niccolò Machiavelli, The Prince, 1513*

Even the greatest proponents of PHC would have to admit that the complete reorganization of the world's health services was a rather ambitious aim! Were the organizers of this revolution utopian hippy dreamers or serious social scientists? The stage was set for a long fight over practical implementation. Apart from the need for huge investments in money and work, real political will is needed to overcome opposition from vested interests, particularly the medical establishment, the pharmaceutical industry, and the status quo of the aid industry, represented particularly by the World Bank's opinion (Hall et al., 2003). Whether it was called an attack on established medicine or second-rate care for developing populations, PHC met strong opposition from the start.

Less than a year after Alma Ata, two researchers from the Rockefeller Foundation published a paper that analyzed the principal causes of death among the world's children (Walsh et al., 1979). They suggested that it would be more realistic if proven elements of PHC could be directed toward the principal lethal diseases. They were not critical of the all-inclusive PHC approach (now termed "comprehensive PHC"), but their pragmatic recommendation of selective therapies became influential in the implementation of Alma Ata's original plan (now called "selective PHC").

The Rockefeller Foundation subsequently held a meeting of major organizations at Bellagio, which included Robert McNamara, the head of the World Bank, and James Grant, the future director of UNICEF. The meeting adopted the notion of selective PHC, initially proposed by Walsh and Warren. The selective PHC pragmatists and the comprehensive PHC idealists subsequently feuded for the next decade while wasting a good deal of time and energy (Magnussen et al., 2004). With a few exceptions, most countries settled for some form of watered-down PHC, so it could be said that the selective pragmatists won. Whether the children of the developing world won or lost is still a matter of debate (Sanders, 2004). However, with progress toward the MDGs stalled in almost every sub-Saharan country, it is interesting to see how those original PHC ideals are suddenly being "rediscovered." The title of the 2008 World Health Report said it all: "Primary Health Care (Now More than Ever)" (WHO, 2008a).

Progress in Selective PHC

Under the leadership of Grant, UNICEF embraced selective PHC. For unrecorded reasons, they selected four of the elements of PHC: growth monitoring, oral rehydration, breastfeeding, and immunization (GOBI). The so-called "child survival revolution" was based on this GOBI strategy. Belated realization that women were important for the health of children led to the addition of three Fs to the strategy: Female education, Family spacing, and Food supplements for pregnant women. This focused approach to a cost-effective package of services was subsequently used in other areas, particularly in the Integrated Management of Childhood Illnesses.

In practice, even GOBI–FFF did not achieve widespread adoption (Kuhn, 1990). Limitations of money and political will meant that many countries simply concentrated on immunization and oral rehydration. Although these two therapies have probably saved millions of children's lives, their use is far from the original ideals of comprehensive PHC.

Despite the limited scope of selective PHC, enormous good was still achieved. Immunization and hygiene were the two most cost-effective therapies—both paid dividends in terms of child health. The introduction of clean water, sanitation, and the distribution of oral rehydration solution supplies coincided with a drop in annual diarrhea deaths from 4.5 million in 1980 to half a million in 2015 (UN, 2015). Similarly, the steady rise in immunization coverage happened at a time when cases of vaccine-preventable diseases fell sharply. Measles has nearly been eradicated from southern Africa and polio has almost been eradicated from the world. These are, of course, only two parts of a larger picture of selective PHC. Once others are included, such as family planning, antenatal care, vitamin A and zinc supplementation, breastfeeding, and female education, the final result has been an enormous benefit to the world's poorest women and children. The reduction in infant and child mortality since 1980 has been little short of dramatic. It is always important to be careful when linking two events in a cause-and-effect manner, but it seems safe to conclude that basic PHC has saved tens of millions of children's lives since it was first introduced.

Progress in Comprehensive PHC

A few countries, such as China, Cuba, Sri Lanka, and Kerala state in India, followed the principles of comprehensive PHC; all have much better population health indices than might be predicted from their per capita income. Cuba's socialized health care system provides free basic services for all citizens, and places emphasis on preventive medicine and public participation in health care. Cuba's child mortality rates and life expectancy are comparable to those of much richer countries and are very much better than other countries with similar per capita incomes (see "Moment of Insight"). These lessons were either ignored or forgotten, so, following the slow progress toward the MDGs in the poorest countries, it has been necessary to reinvent PHC for a new generation.

Some large NGOs adopted the philosophy of PHC with great success. Examples include the Comprehensive Rural Health Project in India, which is also known as Jamkhed (CRHP, 2011), and the Bangladesh Rehabilitation Assistance Committee (BRAC, 2011). Both organizations were started before the Alma Ata meeting, but subsequently adopted PHC methodology. BRAC has subsequently grown into one of the largest NGOs in the world and now exports aid projects to countries outside Bangladesh.

The Future for PHC

Unfortunately, the high ideals of the Alma Ata meeting were not met. While the health of women and children has improved greatly since the original meeting, we are still a long way from "health for all." As it turned out, the Millennium Summit (organized to discuss the poor state of world health) was held in the very year that Alma Ata had predicted there would be universal health for all. In retrospect, most countries exchanged a poorly funded imitation of Western medicine for a poorly funded imitation of PHC. The fact that neither system worked very well is not a criticism of either Western medicine or PHC; it simply represents the inevitable results of underfunding and poor health service organization.

With the general realization that progress toward the MDGs had stalled in many countries, particularly in sub-Saharan Africa, there was a renewed interest in the application of PHC methodologies. This rediscovery of PHC was reflected in the publication of two major reports in 2008 on the 30th anniversary of Alma Ata. Despite enormous social and economic changes during those three decades, both the World Health Report (WHO, 2008a) and the report of the Commission on Social Determinants of Health (WHO, 2008b) reaffirmed the continuing relevance of PHC for a modern world. Influential editorials (Lawn et al., 2008) and review articles (Koivusalo et al., 2008) around that time played the same theme. Some countries had already been through this process. Following early enthusiasm for PHC, both China (Yip et al., 2008) and India subsequently developed modern market-based health systems for their urban rich, but their rural poor had been left far behind. India's National Rural Health Mission, based on PHC principles, is an attempt to reduce the health gap between the rich and poor on a national scale.

In reviewing the SDGs, there is no direct reference to PHC, either because it was a serious oversight or, more optimistically, because primary health care is so integral and interwoven in the path toward the SDGs (Pettigrew et al., 2015). Regardless, PHCs need very strong measurement standards to continually improve them, standards that are lacking in many developing countries. We don't need to look beyond the recent Ebola outbreak in West Africa to notice the weakness of national health systems to effectively cope with such outbreaks. A new initiative, the Primary Health Care Performance Initiative (PHCPI) was launched by the Bill and Melinda Gates Foundation, World Bank Group, and World Health Organization on the sidelines of the UN General Assembly in September 2015 to catalyze improvements in primary health care in low- and middle-income countries. The initiative brings together health system managers, practitioners, advocates, and country policy-makers to help countries track key performance indicators for their PHC systems in order to enhance accountability and provide decision-makers with essential information to drive improvements (PHCPI, 2016).

CLINICAL ELEMENTS OF PRIMARY HEALTH CARE

> If I were to compose an epitaph on medicine throughout the 20th century, it would read, "Brilliant in its discoveries, superb in its technological breakthroughs, but woefully inept in its application to those most in need ..."
>
> *—Rex Fendall, 1972*

The basic components of PHC, outlined at Alma Ata, are widely used in overseas health initiatives. With time, terms change and PHC may be lost within new enthusiasms such as "big pushes" or "vertical programs," but the fundamental essence of the initiatives remains the same. Anyone working overseas will soon encounter programs designed around one or more of these basic elements, so it is important to have some detailed background information on each of them.

Immunization

> I should not fail to write to some of our doctors very particularly about it, if I knew any one of them that I thought had virtue enough to destroy such a considerable branch of their revenue, for the good of mankind.
>
> *—Lady Mary Montagu (1689–1762), describing the benefits of smallpox vaccination in Turkey*

Immunization has been one of the undeniable success stories of the aid industry. Earlier vaccine-based initiatives eradicated polio from the Western hemisphere. The more recent multi-agency Global Polio Eradication Initiative (GPEI, 2010) has managed to reduce the incidence to less than 2,000 new cases a year. Its aim of eradicating the disease entirely is optimistic because of the instability of the regions still affected, but it has made enormous progress. Measles-related deaths have followed a similar course. While the Joint Measles Initiative has likely saved over a million children's lives since it started in 1999, measles remains a major cause of death in young children (JMI, 2011). The work needed for a global campaign is extraordinary and usually not appreciated. For example, between 2000 and 2008, worldwide measles vaccine coverage rose to 83 percent. This required the administration of 686 million doses of vaccine during that period. This is only one of several vaccines given! As a result of similar campaigns, other infectious diseases of children, such as whooping cough, neonatal tetanus (from maternal vaccination), childhood tetanus, and diphtheria, are now all rare diseases in large parts of the developing world (WHO, 2010). Huge problems still exist in terms of sustainable funding and increasing coverage, but immunization remains the most cost-effective and equitable form of development aid.

The original Expanded Program on Immunization (EPI) grew out of the success of the smallpox eradication program. It started in 1974, so it predated Alma

Ata by many years. At the time, reliable vaccines were available for six diseases (diphtheria, pertussis, tetanus, measles, polio, and tuberculosis), but only a small fraction of the world's children had access to full coverage. Passive protection of newborns against tetanus was also achieved by including tetanus immunization for pregnant women as part of routine antenatal care. Immunization targets were not part of the formal MDGs or SDGs, but there is no shortage of goals and strategies developed in other areas. The current extensive WHO/UNICEF plan for the future of vaccinations is summarized in the Global Immunisation Vision and Strategy (GIVS, 2011). Further information is also available on WHO's Immunization, Vaccines, and Biologicals website (WHO, 2011).

It is estimated that vaccination saves roughly 2.5 million children's lives each year (Oxfam, 2011). This makes vaccination programs very attractive investments for a wide range of donors. Apart from the public-private partnerships targeting polio and measles that have already been mentioned, the original EPI attracted enough partners that it was able to relaunch itself in 1999 as the Global Alliance for Vaccines and Immunisation (GAVI, 2011). This influential group now includes UNICEF, the WHO, the Bill and Melinda Gates Foundation, the World Bank, plus others. Apart from providing funds to purchase vaccines and support the cost of immunization programs, GAVI also supports the introduction of new vaccines. It initially concentrated on Hemophilus influenza and hepatitis B, but has subsequently requested funding for rotavirus, pneumococcal conjugate, meningococcal conjugate, and, most recently, human papilloma virus (Oxfam, 2011).

Although immunization is cost effective, that does not mean it is cheap, particularly the new vaccines. Most of the routine vaccines for the poorest countries are either bought by UNICEF or by the poor countries themselves. Vaccine production is principally in the hands of five large companies, which limits competition. These firms follow a policy of tiered pricing, which means the poorest countries pay the lowest price—often only a tenth or less of the cost to rich markets. For example, the GAVI/UNICEF price for 7-valent pneumococcal vaccine is US$7, while the public sector price in the United States is US$275 (Oxfam, 2011). The role of GAVI has been to help pay for the introduction of new vaccines and also to act as a negotiator for the lowest prices, predominantly for low-income countries. While it has been successful, it is held back by funding shortfalls. In May 2012, the Global Vaccine Action Plan was launched, which is a framework approved by the World Health Assembly to achieve the Decade of Vaccines vision (2011–2020) by delivering universal access to immunization. The goal is to prevent millions of deaths by 2020 through more equitable access to existing vaccines for people in all communities.

Breastfeeding

> Breastfeeding is a natural safety net against the worst effects of poverty.
>
> —*James Grant, director, UNICEF*

For many reasons, exclusive breastfeeding is by far the best and safest nutritional source for babies in the developing world. Apart from the obvious advantages of bonding and nutrition, breastfeeding protects the infant from a range of infectious dangers, particularly gastroenteritis. It has clearly been shown that the mortality of bottle-fed children living in poverty is several times higher than that of exclusively breastfed infants. The topic of breastfeeding is covered in detail in Chapter 6.

Concerns about declining breastfeeding rates in the developing world led to the Innocenti Declaration on the promotion and support of breastfeeding (UNICEF, 2005) and the subsequent development of the Baby-Friendly Hospital Initiative in 1991 (WHO, 2009). Despite these initiatives and serious attempts to curb the unfair marketing practices of some baby formula companies, rates of exclusive breastfeeding in developing countries have remained low. In 2003, the WHO and UNICEF recognized this problem by initiating a renewed global strategy for infant and young-child feeding (WHO, 2007) that aims to revitalize efforts to promote adequate feeding of young children under developing world conditions.

Oral Rehydration Therapy

> The discovery that sodium transport and glucose transport are coupled in the small intestine so that glucose accelerates absorption of solute and water was potentially the most important medical advance this century.
>
> —*The Lancet, editorial, 1978*

The claim made by the editor of *The Lancet* (*The Lancet* editorial, 1978) may be an underestimate. In terms of the numbers of children saved, the discovery of oral rehydration solution (ORS) is one of the greatest medical advances of all time. Despite significant progress over the past decade, diarrheal diseases still kill 1.3 million children every year (WHO/UNICEF, 2009). Most of these deaths occur in children less than two years of age, almost all of whom lived in a developing country. Millions more survivors are chronically weakened by recurrent episodes of gastroenteritis that limit their growth, nutrition, and development potential. Fifty years ago, the main focus of diarrheal research was cholera. Huge epidemics still affected large areas of the world with high-fatality rates. At the time, medical opinion viewed oral rehydration as a treatment of last resort—much less useful than intravenous rehydration. In the 1950s, various concoctions of carrot soup

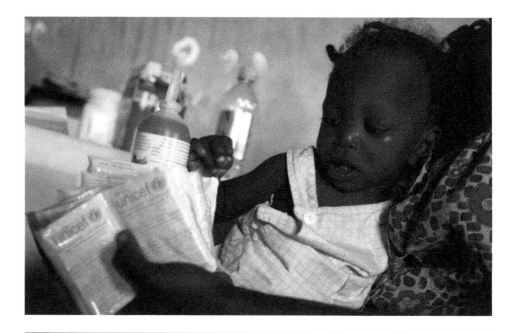

Photo 12.1: A Haitian child is treated with oral rehydration therapy during a cholera outbreak. The seemingly simple discovery that the addition of salt and sugar would increase the intestinal absorption of water has saved the lives of millions of children. In terms of lives saved, oral rehydration solution is one of the greatest medical discoveries ever made.

Source: UN Photo/Marco Dormino, with kind permission of the UN Photo Library (www.unmultimedia.org/photo).

(Selander, 1950) and dehydrated bananas were suggested, but conventional management involved administration of intravenous fluids. Apart from the fact that oral rehydration ultimately proved to be a better treatment, the equipment and personnel needed for intravenous therapy made it too expensive and cumbersome to be of value when treating hundreds of patients at a time.

Children were also invariably fasted for many days because of the belief that the intestinal lining was unable to absorb anything. Intravenous therapy was based on Darrow's early studies of water and electrolyte losses. By 1960, researchers had discovered that sugar and sodium are transported across the gut by a common mechanism, both in rats and later in humans (Philips, 1964). Young researchers from the National Institute of Health, working at the Cholera Research Laboratory in Dacca, built on this research and introduced the first formal studies of oral rehydration therapy in cholera by the mid-1960s (Hirschhorn et al., 1968). Similar work was achieved by researchers at the Johns Hopkins Center for Medical Research.

The Indo-Pakistan War of the period and the resulting social chaos was inevitably followed by a cholera epidemic. This terrible time provided ample opportunity to test the newly developed therapy against the full range of diarrheal diseases (Ruxin, 1994). Published results rapidly gained attention. By 1979, UNICEF was distributing small sachets of ORS crystals worldwide. Although there are many reasons for the fall in diarrheal deaths since then, treatment with ORS has certainly been an important factor in that progress. In 1980, 4.6 million children died of diarrhea. By 2009, this mortality had been reduced by 70 percent. UNICEF has continued to distribute ORS, but also encourages local production and home preparation.

With time, the use of ORS has changed slightly, with greater emphasis being placed on uninterrupted feeding. Prior to this, it had been recommended that food should be withheld, but it was found that this contributed to weight loss during the disease episode. There has also been considerable debate concerning the optimum levels of sugar and particularly sodium in the ORS mix. However, the fundamental basis of treatment is unchanged (Victoria et al., 2000). Unless the child is unconscious, the majority of children can be managed through the episode with careful nursing and oral therapy. It should always be remembered that provision of ORS is in no way a cure for the underlying social disruption that produced the diarrhea in the first place. The provision of ORS is a valuable therapeutic tool, but it can be defined as PHC only when it is part of a larger coordinated strategy aimed at all levels of the problem, including sanitation, clean water initiatives, education, and provision of ORS when necessary.

Hygiene

An ounce of prevention is a ton of work.

—Paul Frame, 1996

The word "hygiene" is derived from the name of Asclepius's daughter Hygieia. She was looked on as the goddess of personal health. In Victorian times, the word was used to mean public health. In PHC terms, it covers personal hygiene, acceptable housing standards, provision of clean water, and sanitation. The topic is covered in detail in Chapter 8. When selective forms of PHC were first being developed, the major cause of under-five death was diarrhea. Control programs were established that concentrated on the provision of clean water and oral rehydration solutions. While progress was certainly made, this remains a perfect example of the limitations of selective versus comprehensive initiatives. Selective provision of clean water has raised levels of access to clean water, but standards of sanitation lag far behind because sanitation wasn't "on the list." A comprehensive approach to child health requires much more than clean water. It must include slum clearance, modern sewage management, and education about washing and personal hygiene, starting in school.

Family Planning

> Population increases in a geometric ratio, while the means of subsistence increases in an arithmetic ratio.
>
> —*Thomas Malthus (1766–1834)*

Any attempt to control family size must inevitably clash with a wide range of ingrained taboos, social rules, laws, and cultural traditions. It is a complex and contentious topic that does not resolve itself into the simplistic provision of contraceptives. Even a cursory Internet search will turn up some very strange views. Some of these opinions will seem less paranoid if it is remembered that family-planning programs often consist of rich White people telling poor non-White people to have fewer children. Given the colonial past, this often well-intentioned policy can be viewed in a number of ways by those previously colonized. Conspiracy theories abound. Once political and religious views are added to the mix, the rhetoric can become heated. The situation can be defused, to some extent, by placing less emphasis on contraception as the only means of controlling population growth. It also helps to steer clear of the topic of abortion.

Over the last 50 years, population growth rates have slowed almost everywhere in the world. Developing countries now appear to be following a trend that began in Europe around the time of the Industrial Revolution. The model for the steady drop in fertility rate that appears to accompany improved prosperity was first devised by Thompson (1929). The four stages are shown graphically in Figure 12.1. Prior to the Industrial Revolution, the population in currently developed countries remained low and relatively stable because of high birth and death rates. As living standards began to improve, death rates fell steadily, probably due to improvements in food supply and public health. What is not so understandable is that fertility rates also started to drop sharply about a decade later. During this period, the population increased since death rates fell faster and earlier than birth rates. Once birth and death rates reached stable low levels, the population found a new equilibrium. In a few countries, such as Japan and Italy, there appears to be a fifth stage during which the birth rate falls so far that the population gradually decreases with time.

It is not likely that contraception had a major impact on this decline, since rapid decreases in fertility were observed in Italy and Ireland during periods when

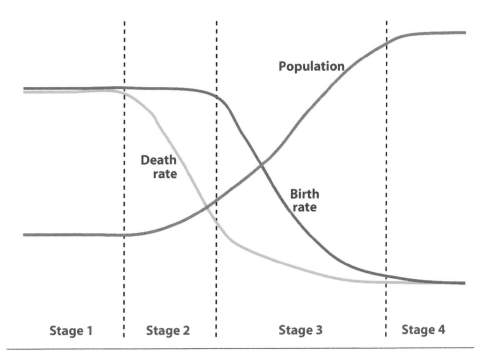

Figure 12.1: The demographic trend: As prosperity slowly rises, a country's death rate usually falls faster than its birth rate. Population rises until a new equilibrium is reached. In a few industrialized countries, a fifth stage has been reached where birth rates fall below death rates so that the population starts to fall.

Source: Thompson, W. 1929. Population. *American Journal of Sociology,* 34: 959–975.

contraception was illegal. Lifetime fertility starts to drop sharply once the under-five mortality rate falls below about 50 per 1,000 live births (less than 5 percent). Clearly, a full explanation of the drop in fertility rate is complicated. Improvements in female education change women's attitudes to the obligations of child-bearing. Once a society starts to value women, they become increasingly influential in making family-planning decisions. There is also a close association between increasing female literacy and reducing fertility. While contraception is part of the picture, it is probably no more important than the influence of television or films on changes in generally accepted values. The success of educational soap operas, developed by Miguel Sabido in Mexico, has shown that significant changes in personal beliefs can be affected by television programs (see History Notes text box).

Family-planning programs, such as the International Planned Parenthood Foundation and the United Nations Family Planning Association, have worked for decades to supply women in developing countries with contraceptives and family-planning advice. This task is not easy in conservative societies, particularly when the topic of induced abortion is raised. It is estimated that there are roughly 42 million induced abortions every year. Thirty-five million occur in developing countries with a rate of 29 per 1,000 births, compared to 7 million in developed countries with a rate of 26 per 1,000 births (Sedgh et al., 2007). Interestingly, illegality does not affect the abortion rate. The only significant result of legal sanction is to increase the number of women injured or killed by unsafe procedures. About 55 percent of abortions in developing countries are unsafe compared to 8 percent in developed countries. Worldwide each year, unsafe abortions result in 5 million women admitted to hospital with complications and 47,000 deaths (Singh, 2006).

Most developing countries now have national family-planning programs, but they are usually limited to contraception and sterilization. Sexuality and fertility involve the most complex of human relations; simplistic approaches, built solely on contraception, are unlikely to have lasting effects (Bangaarts et al., 2002). At a societal level, women must be able to make progress in terms of social status and education that allows them to manage their own health and sexual decisions. They must also be provided with family-planning services that cover the full range of reproductive health problems, including infertility management, treatment for sexually transmitted diseases, and domestic violence.

Equally complex problems include the provision of sex education for children in school. This is essential to prepare them for safe sexual relations as adults, particularly in a world altered by the HIV epidemic. As with any other aspect of female health, education is at the core. As women gain education, they are able to make informed decisions for themselves. As female literacy increases, lifetime fertility drops, age at first child increases, and teenage pregnancy rate decreases. Prevention of adolescent pregnancy and reduction of sexually transmitted diseases will require social acceptance of sex education and contraceptive services for teenagers. This is a huge challenge, both for conservative cultures and for conservative funding agencies.

SUMMARY

Primary health care is—or should be—a central feature of any initiative aimed at improving population health. Unfortunately, the features of PHC are often misunderstood and the topic is dismissed as old-fashioned public health—boring stuff that's of some value, but nowhere near as important as the marvels of modern medicine. Lack of progress toward MDGs in the poorest countries reopened the PHC debate. So, like it or not, PHC is on its way back. Anyone involved in global health should have a detailed understanding of the topic. The most important point to remember is that PHC is not just a shopping list of cost-effective therapies fashioned to meet local causes of mortality. The major treatment methods included within PHC are education and health promotion, nutrition, sanitation, maternal and child health, family planning, immunization, disease control, medical care, and essential drugs. The main principles behind PHC as outlined in Table 12.1 emphasize how it differs from conventional medical care. Those principles include a sense of equity (rich and poor should get the same treatment), health promotion (preventive measures are at least as important as treatment), and, above all else, community participation (poor people must be involved in planning solutions to their own problems). Much useful work can be done with selective therapies, but to get to the root of a problem, projects should be multi-level, with planning and implementation steps designed around the basic foundation of PHC.

Despite the importance of PHC, it is all too often the weakest link in the health system of many middle- and low-income countries, and there is insufficient capacity both to measure and to correct the inadequacies of PHCs in middle- and low-income countries. However, the recent creation of the Primary Health Care Performance Initiative (PHCPI), which was launched on the sidelines of the UN General Assembly in September 2015 by the Bill and Melinda Gates Foundation, World Bank Group, and World Health Organization, should help focus more attention on PHC in low- and middle-income countries. This initiative brings together country policy-makers, health system managers, practitioners, advocates, and other development partners to catalyze improvements in PHC through improved measurement metrics and knowledge-sharing.

DISCUSSION QUESTIONS

1. How would you define PHC? What are the basic principles of PHC?
2. Why is PHC a highly valuable philosophy of treatment that deserves to be studied carefully?
3. What are the practical problems associated with implementing PHC initiatives? How can these problems be overcome?
4. What is the fundamental difference between PHC and curative medicine?
5. Experience suggests that preventive health initiatives are considerably more cost effective than those based solely on curative medicine. Why?
6. What is the GOBI-FFF?
7. What is Selective PHC? What are its benefits?
8. Why do you think PHC is not mentioned in the SDGs?
9. What were some of the fundamental problems of aid?
10. What you would consider some of the early success stories of the aid industry?

RECOMMENDED READING

Hays, J. 2010. *The burden of disease: Epidemics and human response in Western history.* Pub: Rutgers University Press.

Johns Hopkins Primary Care Policy Centre. 2015. Primary care assessment tools. Available at: www.jhsph.edu/research/centers-and-institutes/johns-hopkins-primary-care-policy-center/pca_tools.html.

Rosen, G. 1993. *History of public health.* Pub: Johns Hopkins University Press.

Schneider, D., et al. (Eds.). 2008. *Public health: The development of a discipline.* Pub: Rutgers University Press.

Werner, D., et al. 1997. *Questioning the solution: The politics of primary health care.* Pub: Health Wrights.

Whiteford, L., et al. 2009. *Primary health care in Cuba: The other revolution.* Pub: Rowman and Littlefield.

WHO. 2008a. World health report 2008—primary health care (now more than ever). Retrieved from: www.who.int/whr/2008/en/.

Wilson, P., et al. 2005. *Combating AIDS in the developing world.* Pub: Earthscan Publications.

REFERENCES

Bangaarts, J., et al. 2002. Future trends in contraceptive prevalence and method mix in the developing world. *Studies in Family Planning,* 33: 24–36.

Baum, F. 2007. Health for all now! Reviving the spirit of Alma Ata in the 21st century. *Social Medicine,* 2: 34–41.

BRAC. 2011. Bangladesh Rehabilitation Assistance Committee. Retrieved from: www.brac.net/.

CRHP. 2011. Comprehensive Rural Health Project. Retrieved from: www.jamkhed.org/index.shtml.

Cueto, M. 2004. The origins of primary health care and selective primary health care. *American Journal of Public Health,* 94: 1864–1874.

Djukanovich, V., et al. (Eds.). 1975. *Alternative approaches to meeting basic health needs of populations in developing countries: A joint UNICEF/WHO study.* Pub: World Health Organization.

GAVI. 2011. Global Alliance for Vaccines and Immunizations. Retrieved from: www.vaccinealliance.org.

GIVS. 2011. WHO/UNICEF Global Immunization Vision and Strategy. Retrieved from: www.who.int/immunization/givs/en/index.html.

GPEI. 2010. Global Polio Eradication Initiative. Retrieved from: www.polioeradication.org.

Hall, J., et al. 2003. Health for all beyond 2000: The demise of the Alma Ata Declaration and primary health care in developing countries. *Medical Journal of Australia*, 178: 17–20.

Health Canada. 2006. About primary health care. Retrieved from: www.hc-sc.gc.ca/hcs-sss/prim/about-apropos-eng.php.

Hirschhorn, N., et al. 1968. Decrease in net stool output in cholera during intestinal perfusion with glucose-containing solutions. *New England Journal of Medicine*, 279: 176–181.

Illich, I. 1975. *Medical nemesis: The expropriation of health*. Pub: Pantheon Books.

JMI. 2011. Joint Measles Initiative. Retrieved from: www.measlesinitiative.org.

Kennedy, M. 2004. *A brief history of disease, science, and medicine*. Pub: Asklepiad Press.

Koivusalo, M., et al. 2008. Reclaiming primary health care—why does Alma Ata still matter? *Global Social Policy*, 8: 147–166.

Kuhn, L., et al. 1990. Village health workers and GOBI-FFF: An evaluation of a rural program. *South African Medical Journal*, 77: 471–475.

Lalonde, M. 1974. A new perspective on the health of Canadians: A working document. Pub: Government of Canada. Retrieved from: www.hc-sc.gc.ca/hcs-sss/pubs/system-regime/1974-lalonde/index-eng.php.

The Lancet editorial. 1978. Water with sugar and salt. *The Lancet*, 2: 300–301.

Lawn, J., et al. 2008. Alma-Ata 30 years on: Revolutionary, relevant, and time to revitalize. *The Lancet*, 372: 917–927.

Magnussen, L., et al. 2004. Comprehensive versus selective primary health care: Lessons for global health policy. *Health Affairs*, 23: 167–176.

NRHM. 2010. National Rural Health Mission. Government of India. Retrieved from: http://mohfw.nic.in/NRHM.htm.

O'Ryan, M., et al. 2005. A millennium update on pediatric diarrheal illness in the developing world. *Seminars in Pediatric Infectious Disease*, 16: 125–136.

Oxfam. 2011. Giving countries the best shot: An overview of vaccine access and R and D. Retrieved from: www.oxfam.org/sites/www.oxfam.org/files/giving-developing-countries-best-shot-vaccines-2010-05.pdf.

Pettigrew, L. M., et al. 2015. Primary health care and the Sustainable Development Goals. *The Lancet*, 386(10009): 2119–2121.

PHCPI. 2016. Primary Health Care Performance Initiative. Retrieved from: http://phcperformanceinitiative.org/about-us/about-phcpi.

PHCRIS. 2011. Primary Health Care Research and Information Service. Retrieved from: www.phcris.org.au.

Philips, R. 1964. Water and electrolyte losses in cholera. *Federation Proceedings*, 23: 705–712.

PMC. 2011. Sabido methodology. Retrieved from: www.populationmedia.org/what/sabido-method.

Population Media Center. 2011. Sabido methodology—background. Retrieved from: www.populationmedia.org/what/sabido-method/.

Ruxin, J. 1994. Magic bullet: The history of oral rehydration therapy. *Medical History*, 38: 363–397.

Sachs, J. 2005. *The end of poverty: Economic possibilities for our time*. Pub: Penguin Press.

Sanders, D. 2004. Twenty-five years of primary health care: Lessons learned and proposals for revitalization. Retrieved from: www.asksource.info/rtf/phc-sanders.RTF.

Schneider, D., et al. (Eds.). 2008. *Public health: The development of a discipline*. Pub: Rutgers University Press.

Sedgh, G., et al. 2007. Induced abortion: Rates and trends worldwide. *The Lancet*, 370: 1338–1345.

Seear, M. 2004. History's lessons. *Canadian Medical Association Journal*, 171: 1487–1488.

Selander, P. 1950. Carrot soup in the treatment of infantile diarrhea. *Journal of Pediatrics*, 36: 742–745.

Shattuck, L., et al. 1850. Report of a general plan for the promotion of public and personal health. Pub: Massachusetts State Printers. Retrieved from: www.deltaomega.org/shattuck.pdf.

Sidel, V. 1972. The barefoot doctors of the People's Republic of China. *New England Journal of Medicine*, 286: 1292–1300.

Singh, S. 2006. Hospital admissions resulting from unsafe abortions: Estimates from 13 developing countries. *The Lancet*, 368: 1887–1892.

Thompson, W. 1929. Population. *American Journal of Sociology*, 34: 959–975.

UN. 2012. Department of Economic and Social Affairs. Statistics and indicators on women and men. Retrieved from: http://unstats.un.org/unsd/demographic/products/indwm/default.htm.

UN. 2015. United Nations Levels & trends in child mortality report. Estimates developed by the UN Inter-agency Group for Child Mortality Estimation. Retrieved from: www.who.int/maternal_child_adolescent/documents/levels_trends_child_mortality_2015/en/.

UNICEF. 2005. Celebrating the Innocenti Declaration. Retrieved from: www.unicefirc.org/publications/pdf/1990-2005-gb.pdf.

UNICEF. 2012. Child health statistical tables. Retrieved from: www.childinfo.org/statistical_tables.html .

Victoria, C., et al. 2000. Reducing deaths from diarrhea through oral rehydration therapy. *Bulletin of the World Health Organization*, 78: 1246–1255.

Walsh, J., et al. 1979. Selective primary health care: An interim strategy for disease control in developing countries. *New England Journal of Medicine*, 301: 967–974.

WHO. 1978. Declaration of Alma-Ata International Conference on Primary Health Care, Alma-Ata, USSR, 6–12 September 1978. Retrieved from: http://apps.who.int/medicinedocs/documents/s21370en/s21370en.pdf.

WHO. 1981. Global strategy for the year 2000. Retrieved from: whqlibdoc.who.int/publications/9241800038.pdf.

WHO. 2007. Planning guide for national implementation of the global strategy for infant and young child feeding. Retrieved from: www.who.int/nutrition/publications/infantfeeding/9789241595193/en/index.html.

WHO. 2008a. World health report 2008—primary health care (now more than ever). Retrieved from: www.who.int/whr/2008/en/.

WHO. 2008b. Commission on Social Determinants of Health. Final report. Retrieved from: www.who.int/social_determinants/thecommission/finalreport/en/index.html.

WHO. 2009. The Baby-Friendly Hospital Initiative. Retrieved from: www.who.int/nutrition/topics/bfhi/en/index.html.

WHO. 2010. Vaccine-preventable diseases: Monitoring system. 2010 global report. Retrieved from: whqlibdoc.who.int/hq/2010/WHO_IVB_2010_eng.pdf.

WHO. 2011. World Health Organization: Immunization, vaccines, and biologicals. Retrieved from: www.who.int/immunization.

WHO/UNICEF. 2009. Diarrhea: Why children are still dying and what can be done. Retrieved from: www.childinfo.org/files/diarrhoea_hires.pdf.

WHO/UNICEF. 2011. Progress on sanitation and drinking water: 2010 update. Retrieved from: www.who.int/water_sanitation_health/publications/9789241563956/en/index.html.

Wolfson, L., et al. 2008. Estimating the costs of achieving the Global Immunization Vision and Strategy, 2006–2015. *Bulletin of the World Health Organization*, 86: 29–39.

World Bank. 2012. World Bank statistical database. Retrieved from: http://data.worldbank.org.

World Bank. 2016. World Bank statistical database. Retrieved from: http://data.worldbank.org/indicator/SP.DYN.IMRT.IN.

Yip, W., et al. 2008. The Chinese health system at a crossroads. *Health Affairs*, 27: 460–468.

CHAPTER 13

Curative Medical Care and Targeted Programs

The art of medicine consists of amusing the patient while nature cures the disease.

—*Voltaire*

OBJECTIVES

Although almost 6 million children die before their fifth birthday each year, and hundreds of thousands of women die or are injured during delivery, there are surprisingly few causes of this terrible burden of disease. Students working in the field of child health will see recurrent cases of children with pneumonia, acute diarrhea, malnutrition, and HIV infection. Those involved with the care of adults will encounter infectious diseases that reflect underlying poor social conditions. While recognizing that long-term solutions to these health problems lie in the field of public health, such changes occur slowly and are of no use when confronted with an acutely ill patient. This module is devoted to the topic of medical treatment—ranging from the most basic clinic care up to billion-dollar multi-agency eradication programs. It also looks at the framework needed for an effective health delivery system and the problem of finding safe and affordable medications. After completing this chapter, you should be able to:

- appreciate the part that traditional curative medicine has to play in controlling the major diseases of poverty
- understand the medical treatments available for the major infectious diseases of adults and children
- understand the use of essential health packages and the return of vertical disease control programs
- understand the minimum requirements for safe pregnancy-related health care
- appreciate the developing world's need for improved access to safe, affordable, and effective drugs
- understand the organization and funding of a national health service

INTRODUCTION

> The desire to take medicine is perhaps the greatest feature which distinguishes men from animals.
>
> *—William Osler, 1907*

Although access to good-quality medical care might be life-saving for individual patients, in terms of cost efficiency, far greater population health advantages are gained from investments in clean water, schooling, and sewage disposal. However, until the day arrives when everyone has access to the basic requirements for a healthy life, health professionals in underdeveloped countries will still have long queues of patients needing medical treatment. Such therapies are often simple and do not require extensive medical training to understand or administer. Prevention and cure are not antagonistic but are both necessary parts of an effective disease management program. When used in partnership with preventive strategies, curative care is an essential element in health initiatives. This chapter will examine the commonly used treatment protocols, plus the funding and supply of the necessary essential drugs. We will also review the organization and funding of health services in developing countries.

The methods used to control the three main infectious diseases provide good examples of the place of curative care. Management programs for HIV/AIDS require drug treatment, but to be effective, this must be only one part of a larger package that includes a concerted education campaign at a national level. Similarly, tuberculosis drug treatment must be augmented with contact tracing, testing of high-risk populations, and a similar emphasis on disease education. Finally, drug treatment of malaria must be accompanied by vector control through area spraying and regular use of treated bed nets. The only major disease on which social change has had little effect is maternal mortality. Pregnancy-related emergencies occur suddenly and unpredictably. The only way to improve maternal health statistics is to provide all pregnant women with easy access to good-quality obstetric care. Unfortunately, women's health has been given a shamefully low priority and it is only very recently that significant worldwide efforts have been made to improve pregnancy outcomes for women in developing countries, such as the Every Woman Every Child Movement, which mobilizes and strengthens international and national action by governments, the UN, multilaterals, the private sector, and civil society to address the major health challenges facing women, children, and adolescents (Every Woman Every Child, 2015).

Over the last five or six decades, the approach to the provision of health services in developing countries has followed differing trends. This history was

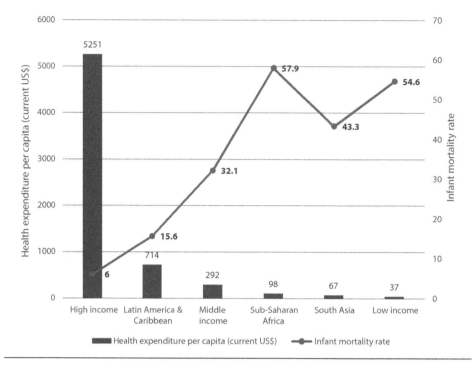

Figure 13.1: Health expenditure in US$ per capita (left axis) and infant mortality rate (right axis) for select regions of the world in 2014

Source: WHO GHE. 2016. World Health Organization Global Health Expenditure database. Retrieved from: http://apps.who.int/nha/database.

covered in detail in Chapter 2, but it is worth repeating the main points again. The initial response to widespread ill health was to export Western-style curative care models. In the 1960s and 1970s, newly independent countries simply continued that old colonial system, usually with less funding. The ultimate failure of urban hospitals to reduce disease in rural areas led to the 1978 Alma Ata meeting and a switch to more preventive strategies under the banner of PHC. The vagueness and failings around the "Health for all by 2000" goal led to another call for health care reform starting in the early 1990s (World Bank, 1993). While this movement has produced many alternative models (contracting out to NGOs, decentralized management structures, private health care, personal health insurance, etc.), no clear winner has emerged. In reality, many of the poorest countries simply have dilapidated remnants of an earlier district health system. Poor health services are one of the biggest single obstacles to meeting the SDG health targets.

Vast amounts of money are spent on health care, even by developing countries. Good health care costs a lot of money, but if a country doesn't invest

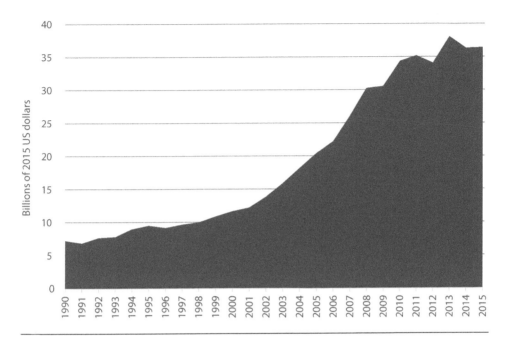

Figure 13.2: Trends in development assistance for health, for different world regions, over the last 25 years

Source: IHME. 2016. Institute for Health Metrics and Evaluation. Financing global health 2010. Retrieved from: www.healthdata.org/policy-report/financing-global-health-2015-development-assistance-steady-path-new-global-goals.

in health, the adverse results are easily measurable, particularly in conditions where conventional medical treatments are important. For example, there is a clear relationship between infant mortalities and a country's health care funding (Figure 13.1). Current world values for health care spending range from more than US$9,403 per capita in the United States to below US$50 per capita in many of the poorest countries (World Bank, 2016). As mentioned in Chapter 3, the principal determinants of population health are non-medical in nature. However, a certain level of funding is needed to maintain population health, and many of the poorest countries are far below that minimum level. Following meetings on health financing in Bamako in 1987 and Abuja in 1989, developing countries agreed to increase their health funding to 15 percent of GDP. This optimistic goal was not reached, but both internal health expenditure and external health aid have increased steadily in the subsequent period. In 2015, US$36.4 billion of development assistance for health (DAH) was disbursed, marking the fifth consecutive year of little change in the amount of resources provided by global health development partners (Dieleman et al., 2016). Between 2000 and 2009,

DAH increased at 11.3 percent per year (regarded as the golden age of global health financing), whereas between 2010 and 2015, annual growth was just 1.2 percent (Figure 13.2).

Finally, medical treatment requires effective medications, and this brings two new problems. Firstly, modern drugs are often prohibitively expensive for poor populations, particularly the newer antiretroviral medications. Once again, the rich drug manufacturing countries have been very slow to ensure that developing world populations have access to affordable drugs, although the situation is improving. Secondly, those drugs must be of high quality. Dispensed medications may be substandard for many reasons, including decomposition during storage, repackaging of time-expired drugs, adulteration with inactive or even toxic substances, and criminal drug counterfeiting. Sophisticated drug counterfeiting is likely to become a growing problem over the next few years, particularly where expensive drugs are concerned. Ensuring a supply of safe, effective, and affordable medications has become an increasingly important subject over the last decade.

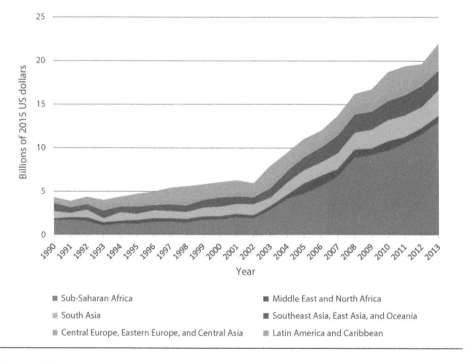

Figure 13.3: Trends in government health spending, for different world regions, over the last 20 years; the original data is based on estimates by the WHO

Source: IHME. 2016. Institute for Health Metrics and Evaluation. Financing global health 2010. Retrieved from: www.healthdata.org/policy-report/financing-global-health-2015-development-assistance-steady-path-new-global-goals.

THE ORGANIZATION AND FUNDING OF HEALTH SERVICES IN DEVELOPING COUNTRIES

> There will come a time when the Ministry of Health is the only Ministry we can afford to have and we still won't be able to afford the Ministry of Health.
>
> *—Dalton McGuinty, premier of Ontario, 2004*

Over the last 60 years, a number of theoretical and political trends have influenced the delivery of health services in developing countries. Until the Alma Ata meeting in 1978, the predominant system was based on a curative Western model. After Alma Ata, the emphasis shifted from cure to prevention under the PHC model. Although the PHC era has never been officially declared closed, it has been obvious over the last 15 years that serious attempts at reorganizing health care systems are long overdue. This more recent trend is usually dated to the 1993 World Development Report (World Bank, 1993), which raised the need for extensive changes, both in the services provided and in the administration and funding methods used to pay for those services. The WHO's subsequent World Health Report in 2000 continued the theme of health system improvement with a more practical approach that examined the various ways that health care delivery could be upgraded. The emphasis on cost efficiency and outcome measurement reflected the recent move, at that time, toward measuring health burdens and basing management plans on the results of clinically relevant research.

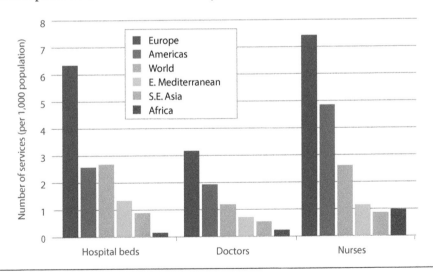

Figure 13.4: Supply of basic medical services in different world regions

Source: Peters, D., et al. Poverty and access to health care in developing countries. Annals of the New York Academy of Science, 1136(2008): 161–171.

The Western and PHC models have both slowly given way to a newer, more results-based approach (at least in theory). For want of a better term, the current trend is, perhaps, best called the "business model." Unfortunately, in the poorest countries, progress has been slow. Grand plans for improving global health sound good in planning meetings, but when clinics are badly maintained and have demoralized staff and poor supplies, implementing such plans is almost impossible. Sadly, such health services are most common in the very countries that have the greatest need for competent health care. There is huge inequity in the supply of medical services in different parts of the world (Figure 13.4). Since the early 1990s there has been general agreement that health systems need to be improved, but how is that process to be achieved? In order to design an "ideal" health system for a developing world population, it is necessary to examine three broad questions: (1) What services should be provided? (2) How will it all be paid for? (3) How should the system be organized? Obviously, answering each of these questions would fill several books, but useful summaries of the main points can be made within those headings.

The Traditional District Health Service

Before studying the different elements of a health service, it is worth starting by looking at the most common type of delivery system found in low-income countries. Given a small budget and a large rural population, there aren't many possibilities that will meet those restrictions. While there are obvious differences between countries, the usual framework is often a remnant of an older colonial model that the country inherited at independence. The basic element is a peripheral clinic that is able to meet most basic needs. More complex cases are then referred to an intermediate-level district hospital with, in some richer countries, final referral to a large national referral hospital. In colonial days, such an arrangement was called a district health system (DHS). Apart from meeting the demands of common sense, the DHS also received support from the WHO's earlier Harare Declaration on the health framework needed to meet the goal of "Health for all by 2000" (WHO, 1987). Since then, the goal has changed to the MDGs and more recently to the SDGs for 2030, but the conclusions of that report are still relevant today.

The fact that such a design has failed to meet current needs is a reflection of poor funding and mismanagement rather than a basic inadequacy in the concept. Given a tight budget, the health system designed for a poor country will inevitably be influenced by the management needs of the most common diseases. In its most basic form, such an approach may be limited to a fairly small package of cost-effective therapies. It is only much later that specialty services become possible, such as cardiac surgery, renal dialysis, and cancer treatment. Mental illnesses (particularly depression and substance abuse) are now so common that the provision of specific psychiatric services must be viewed as a necessity rather than an expensive luxury. The guide to the establishment of a district health service by the German group Gesellschaft fur Technische Zusammenarbeit (GTZ, 2004) is recommended reading. It gives a realistic idea of the cost and work needed to meet even the most basic health needs of a rural population.

General Organization of an Integrated District Health System

A district generally consists of around 250,000 people. There should be one clinic for every 10,000 people. An intermediate district hospital should provide one bed for every 1,000 people. Depending on the degree of decentralization allowed, the head of the district administrative committee should be elected from local people, while the regional director (over several districts) will be a government appointment. Involvement of local people in the district level committee is essential to ensure that services meet local needs. The main tasks of the regional and district administrative committees are given in Table 13.1. This "bare bones" list should make it obvious that even the most basic health system still requires a great deal of organization and money. Upgrading a dilapidated system sounds fine in theory, but in practice, it is a major undertaking in a poor country.

Table 13.1: The major responsibilities of regional and district administrations in an integrated district health system

Regional administration's responsibilities:	• implementation of national health policy
	• coordination and support of districts
	• budget administration and oversight
	• regional centre for nursing and health assistant training
	• major disease control coordination (HIV, TB, malaria)
	• capacity building to support decentralization
	• operational research
District administration's responsibilities:	• essential drug and vaccine procurement
	• decentralized budget management
	• coordination of targeted programs with local facilities
	• health centre staff management
	• building maintenance
	• collection of basic statistical data

The District Health Centre

The basic element of a DHS is the district health centre (Photo 13.1). It should be designed to meet the needs of about 10,000 people and should be less than 5 km from the majority of that population. Some countries have smaller services, such as village health posts, traditional birth attendants, and village health workers, but experience with minimally trained staff has not been positive. Unless there are particular local problems of remote access, the first contact with the health service should be through well-trained staff in formal health centres. The district administrator should be a doctor with public health training. The committee should also include representatives from local NGOs and organizers of vertical programs operating in the area. Targeted initiatives are now so common that they can overwhelm local capacity unless they are coordinated carefully. It is quite possible for a local health centre to have requests for drug programs against trachoma, schistosomiasis, filariasis,

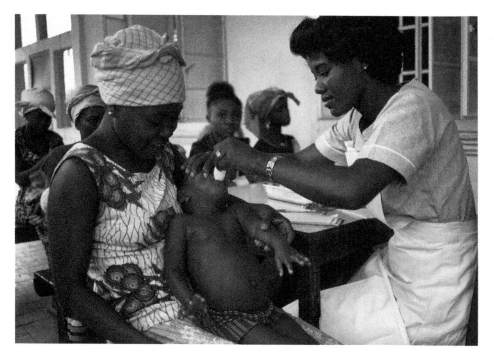

Photo 13.1: The basic element of a health care system—a well-run district health centre, staffed by trained nurses—is able to provide basic child care and uncomplicated deliveries. In this case, the clinic is in Freetown, Sierra Leone. Unfortunately, clinics are more often badly dilapidated, understaffed, and lacking even the most basic supplies. Poor rural services are a major obstacle to the implementation of health initiatives.

Source: UN Photo/B. Wolff, with kind permission of the UN Photo Library (www.unmultimedia. org/photo).

HIV, TB, and onchocerciasis, plus immunization days, bed net distribution, and house spraying. The major responsibilities of a health centre are listed below:

- curative care of common health problems (75 percent managed by nurses)
- obstetrics—antenatal care (tetanus, malaria treatment, nutrition supplements, monitoring, uncomplicated deliveries)
- child care—immunization, vitamin A, zinc, malaria treatment, newborn care, infant growth monitoring
- family-planning service
- education resource for community (hygiene, breastfeeding, safe sex, etc.)
- early referral of complicated cases
- simple laboratory service (glucometer, urine screen)
- basic dispensary following WHO's recommendations on essential drugs

The District Hospital

Experience suggests that less than 10 percent of all health centre patients will need referral. When they are referred, they should receive a good level of care, the most important feature of which should be access to safe anaesthesia and surgery. Without these services, the hospital is no more than a large health centre.

Table 13.2: The major services expected from a district hospital

Clinical responsibilities:	• basic surgery—obstetric, trauma, orthopedics, urology
	• safe general and local anaesthesia to support surgery and minor procedures
	• treatment of serious referred diseases—diabetes, HIV/AIDS, tuberculosis, heart failure
	• obstetrics—complicated pregnancies; includes housing for referred pregnant women waiting to deliver
	• dentistry
	• advanced eye care, including cataract surgery
	• mental health—increasingly important
Other essential services:	• diagnostic radiology—X-ray, ultrasound, plus technician training
	• laboratory services—basic chemical and microbiological tests, plus technician training
	• well-stocked and maintained pharmacy
	• hospital maintenance—workshop and technicians that also serve major maintenance needs of the health centres
	• training centre for the district—primary training and also upgrades for health centre staff
	• supervision of health centre standards
	• outpatient clinics

There must be a close working relationship between the hospital and district health centres. The hospital director may act as the head of the district administration committee. The hospital should have 150–200 beds with a nurse-to-bed ratio of 1:3. Wards should be divided into male, female, child, infectious diseases, and obstetrics. Many areas would consider a mental health unit an essential component. In addition to nurses, there should be at least three doctors, laboratory and radiology staff, plus administrators and general workers. Services should include radiology (X-ray and ultrasound), a clinical laboratory, equipment sterilization, laundry, maintenance, an outpatient clinic, a delivery room, an operating theatre, physiotherapy, a pharmacy, and administration offices. Investment in hospital sewage, water, waste disposal, and general cleanliness is absolutely central to safe operation. The main clinical and management responsibilities of a district hospital are given in Table 13.2.

What Services Should Be Provided?

Even a well-run district health system can provide only a certain level of treatment for the enormous range of human disease, so the difficult topic of rationing has to be faced. Some decisions are easy—diarrhea management is on the list of rationed treatments and modern cardiac surgery is not. But what about the thousands of conditions between these two extremes? Since health budgets in developing countries are limited, it is necessary to plan health interventions to achieve the greatest benefits for the least cost. Once risk factors have been identified, then it is possible to base cost-effective interventions on that information (WHO, 2008). As discussed in the last chapter on primary health care, the cost-effective package of therapies can be traced back to the arguments over selective health care and the work of Walsh et al. (1979) after Alma Ata. This led to the first large-scale essential package program, which was based on growth monitoring, oral rehydration, breastfeeding, and immunization (GOBI). While very narrow in its scope, the program did achieve success in the area of child mortality.

The influential 1993 World Development Report used this approach to identify a suggested basic package of treatments aimed at addressing the major risk factors found in the global study of disease. The report emphasized that limited budgets should be spent in the most cost-effective way and proposed two standard packages of health care aimed at getting the maximum benefit from a limited budget. These consisted of a public health package (expanded program on immunization, school health, micronutrient supplementation, and control programs for tobacco, alcohol, and HIV/AIDS) and a medical services package (tuberculosis treatment, reproductive health care, family planning, basic management for sick children, and treatment of sexually transmitted diseases). At the time, it was estimated that widespread implementation of these basic services would reduce mortality and morbidity in children by 20–30 percent and among adults by 10–20 percent.

The so-called US$12 basic package attracted criticism at the time. The average health spending by developing countries in 1993 was roughly US$4–$5 per capita; it was felt that more than doubling this budget was hopelessly unrealistic. Rather than being taken too literally, the package is better used as a reminder that cost-effectiveness analysis can lead to more equitable distribution of available health budgets.

Economic pressures mean that some form of rationing will always be necessary. In rich countries, such debates might involve the use of invasive care in a rapidly aging population, while administrators in poor countries must decide on the cost-effectiveness of expensive vaccines. Either way, some form of health care selection is here to stay. It is very important to realize that essential health packages are not viewed as a solution for weak management. No health delivery system will work well under those conditions. Packages are a pragmatic response to a tight budget—a guaranteed minimum. That minimum must be professional and competent, which, in turn, implies good standards of management, funding, and implementation up to that level. If a carefully constructed national plan is followed, the population's mortality and morbidity will decline, but there are no rapid fixes. Patients with complex problems that cannot be met will not be turned away, but they will not receive optimal therapy. As time passes, and health care expands within the country, fewer people will fall into that category.

Funding Developing World Health Services

> We have now just enshrined, as soon as I sign this bill, the core principle that everybody should have some basic security when it comes to their health care.
>
> —*Barack Obama, 2010*

There are almost as many health-funding mechanisms as there are countries around the world. Alternatives include tax-based funding (Canada, United Kingdom), mandatory health insurance (Germany, Japan, Costa Rica), voluntary private health insurance (United States, South Africa), community-based funding (Bamako Initiative, Thailand), direct out-of-pocket payments (much of the developing world), and overseas government or NGO funding (often against targeted initiatives). In rural areas of the developing world, income is so low that the tax base is not sufficient to support government health services or to pay for private care. Similarly, private insurance is still in its infancy in low-income developing countries. Even in the relatively prosperous Caribbean, it is estimated that only 12 percent of families are covered by health insurance and only 3 of 19 states offer some form of insurance (Barret et al., 2004). In practice, the poor must choose between underfunded, poorly supplied government clinics, or they must pay money to private practitioners and private pharmacists, or they must rely on the services of traditional healers (ranging from the Nganga of Zimbabwe to the Ayurvedic in India). In countries everywhere, uninsured families living in poverty run a constant risk of financial catastrophe caused by emergency medical expenses (Xu et al., 2003).

As a result of the financial crisis of the 1980s, many countries were obliged to impose user fees as part of the structural adjustment policies of the day. The WHO and UNICEF subsequently supported a meeting on health funding at Bamako in 1987. Although this meeting did lead to an agreement to use some form of cost recovery, it is often forgotten that greater emphasis was placed on improving health care standards and decentralizing management structures. Unfortunately, only the user fees were implemented. Raising money is not, of course, the only problem with funding. Once the money has been obtained, it has to be spent equitably and

Box 13.1 History Notes

Asclepius and Hippocrates (c. 4th century BC)

Hippocrates gets all the credit as the founder of modern medicine, but he referred to Asclepius as his superior. The two of them are credited with being the founders of modern Western medicine. Disentangling myth and reality is difficult, but it is generally accepted that both men were real people who lived in Greece around the 4th century BC—they might even have been contemporaries. Hippocrates was based on the island of Cos. He moved medicine away from superstition and started the long process of trying to sort out what was actually wrong with the patient. He based his therapies on the analysis of disease and the use of medications where necessary. It is not known how much of the large Hippocratic literature was actually written by him, but those works were influential for the next 2,000 years. The earlier habit of respecting ancient authority meant that physicians still believed in his doctrine of balancing humours well into the 19th century.

Asclepius's emphasis on exercise rather than medicine and his use of dream interpretation made him the founder of preventive medicine. Although his symbol of a snake wrapped around a wooden staff is still used today, he is less well known than Hippocrates. His daughter Hygieia is probably better known. Temples following his teaching are still standing, including a beautiful example on Cos, where Hippocrates may even have taught. His temples all have a running track, gymnasium, and spa. Patients had to spend the night in the temple, then report their dreams to the priests the next day. Perhaps he was a bit of a showman, but he probably did less harm than the conventional doctors of the day, who recommended purging and bleeding. Follow the reference for more details: Seear (2004).

efficiently. User fees, if used wisely, can occasionally be shown to have benefits, but they also have the inevitable result of reducing health care utilization by the poor, who cannot afford even the smallest fees (Uzochukwu et al., 2004). Increasing the costs associated with illness can force the poorest families to choose between food and medicine. In many cases, the money raised is so small that by the time it has been collected and passed through several administrative hands, the final result is not worth all the effort.

There is now an increasing appreciation that health and education services for poor people should be seen as national investments rather than profit-making endeavours. While there is considerable pressure to eliminate user fees, they must be replaced by other forms of funding, otherwise services will deteriorate even further (Gilson et al., 2005). It has been estimated that removal of user fees in sub-Saharan Africa could prevent over 200,000 child deaths annually by giving affordable medical access to the poorest in the region (Jamas et al., 2005). However, this assumes that policy-makers substitute sufficient alternative financing. With the stimulus of the MDGs, health funding improved sharply in the last decade and a half. Poor countries have not met their health spending goal of 15 percent GDP, but all regions have increased their domestic spending, even in the poorest regions (Figure 13.3). Development assistance for health has followed a similar trend and has nearly doubled since the 1990s (Figure 13.2). Some countries use external funding as an opportunity to redirect health spending to other areas (Lu et al., 2010), but most countries have risen to the challenge of improving health care for their poorest citizens.

Despite all the variety in funding methods, they all ultimately rely on only two sources—public and private:

- *Public funding sources:* These include general taxes, such as VAT and customs charges, or more progressive taxes, such as income tax where payments are reduced for those with low income. Other public sources include deficit financing (borrowing), lotteries and betting taxes, and, finally, external development aid, which may make up 20 percent of the health budget in the poorest countries.
- *Private funding sources:* These include community self-help groups, direct user fees, private insurance, collective employment schemes, charities, NGOs, and donations.

For the future, higher-income developing countries will probably move toward a mixed model of tax-based, government-funded services along with private care funded out of pocket and by health insurance. Low-income areas of the world will continue to rely on government-funded clinic systems and a variety of targeted health initiatives, often externally funded by donors. Such programs are increasingly being integrated into existing health services. In fact, the first step for many vertical programs is capacity building so that local health services can accommodate their planned initiative. User fees for the poorest people will, hopefully, be largely removed. It is also hoped that the resulting funding gap will be replaced by increased government spending.

Organization of Health Services in the Developing World

> Men are forever creating organizations for their own convenience and forever finding themselves the victims of their home-made monsters.
>
> —*Aldous Huxley*

Decentralization is the transfer of power from central authority out to the periphery. As usual, the process is far more complex in practice than in theory, which is probably one reason why progress toward this goal has been so slow. There has been rather more talk than action about improving health care standards through decentralization. It has been debated for more than 20 years, going back to the 1993 World Health Report. There is considerable support available for countries going through the process of health sector reform, but there is little to show for it in the poorest countries. The World Bank provides assistance through its Flagship Program on Health Sector Reform and Sustainable Financing (World Bank, 2011b). A joint Pan American Health Organization and USAID initiative supports a similar program called the Latin America and Caribbean Regional Health Sector Reform Initiative. Services offered include rational pharmaceutical choices, management and leadership training, and quality-assurance techniques.

There are many arguments in favour of decentralization, but the simplest one is that it is just not possible to sit in a central government office and gain any clear idea about the diverse needs of health districts spread across the country. Those peripheral centres know their own business and are the best ones to make management and budget decisions for their areas. The next best argument is that money given to the central ministry of health passes through many hands before the final small change reaches the peripheries, which is one of the reasons why central governments are opposed to the scheme. Cutting out the middle layers of bureaucracy is likely to improve the cash available for district operations. However, decentralization should not be viewed as an easy solution. Success requires managerial capacity, established systems of accountability, and transfer of sufficient funds to meet the local requirements.

Box 13.2 Moment of Insight

Overseas development aid given in 2010:	US pet-related expenses in 2010:
France: US$12.9 billion	Food: US$18.8 billion
Germany: US$12.7 billion	Supplies: US$11.0 billion
Japan: US$11.0 billion	Veterinary care: US$13.0 billion
Netherlands: US$6.2 billion	Grooming and boarding: US$3.6 billion
Spain: US$5.8 billion	Animal purchase: US$2.2 billion
Total US$48.6 billion	**Total US$48.6 billion**

Source: OECD. 2011. International development statistics. Retrieved from: www.oecd.org/dataoecd/50/17/5037721.htm.

Source: APPA. 2011. American Pet Products Association. Industry statistics and trends. Retrieved from: www.americanpetproducts.org/press_industrytrends.asp.

It is best to view decentralization as a continuum rather than an "all or nothing" process since it means different things to different countries, depending on the responsibilities that are involved. The most extreme form would be the complete devolution of political, financial, and administrative decision-making to locally elected management groups. The least effective version is simply the transfer of administrative authority from the central ministry of health to regional offices within the same ministry. Between these extremes lie many shades of grey concerning who has the authority over budget, administration, and broad decision-making. Not surprisingly, research findings will vary, depending on the type of decentralization involved. While decentralization of funding has been shown to be beneficial for maternal and child health in Bolivia (PHR, 2000) or immunization services in Zambia (Blas et al., 2001), it is, as usual, not altogether simple. A large World Bank study of the effects of decentralization on childhood immunization showed that decentralization improved immunization rates in low-income countries, but reduced coverage rates in middle-income countries (Khaleghian, 2004).

Decentralization requires competent management at the district level or the process will fail. For example, patients follow the available services, so decentralization produces a heavier patient load in peripheral clinics; this requires increased staff and training. Government funding must be sufficient to meet these peripheral needs for personnel and supply costs, and the associated bureaucracy must be streamlined so that payments are provided on time (PHR, 2000). Continuing government oversight is necessary to ensure that projects are not hijacked by local elites, and also that patients are not double-charged for services that have already been paid for by the government. Despite its potential problems, the trend for the future organization of government health care in developing countries will probably be increasing decentralization.

CONTROLLING INFECTIOUS DISEASES WITH TARGETED PROGRAMS

> You have erased from the calendar of human afflictions one of its greatest. Future nations will know by history only that the loathsome smallpox has existed.
>
> *—Thomas Jefferson to Edward Jenner, 1806*

Targeted Programs: The Dream of Eradication

One of the biggest innovations in aid over the last decade has been the emergence of targeted programs (also called vertical or global programs). While their origins can be traced back to the early disease-eradication programs of the 1960s, they have changed in everything but name compared to those first large-scale initiatives. The most obvious difference has been in funding sources. The emergence of private funds, advocacy groups, and non-traditional funding sources has introduced a sense of competition and innovation into the world of aid. These programs are so varied in terms of aims, management, implementation, and funding that simple generalizations are not applicable. If they have a common denominator, it is a belief that some problems are too large to be dealt with at a regional level and need a multi-agency grand "push" to solve. This is the current wisdom, but it doesn't mean that vertical approaches are without problems. Overlap with similar programs, questions of accountability and ownership, plus the difficult issue of integrating a vertical program with existing medical services, must all be addressed. In the poorest countries, this last problem is probably overemphasized. Local services are often so poor that integration is more of a theoretical rather than a practical problem.

While this section concentrates on health initiatives, it is important to understand that many multi-agency programs are also aimed at non-medical problems where management can be considered a global public good. Examples of well-known programs that target infectious diseases include: the Global Fund to Fight AIDS, TB, and Malaria (Global Fund, 2011), the Global Alliance for Vaccines and Immunization (GAVI, 2011), and the Stop Tuberculosis Partnership (StopTB, 2011). There are many lesser-known programs aimed at onchocerciasis, measles, trachoma, filariasis, and leprosy. Non-medical targeted programs include: the

Consultative Group on International Agricultural Research (CGIAR, 2011), the Global Environment Facility (GEF, 2011), and the Fund for the Implementation of the Montreal Protocol (MLF, 2011). As with medical projects, there are numerous smaller funds and groups aimed at topics such as international trade, conservation, and research in social sciences.

The dream of targeted medical projects is complete eradication of a human infectious disease. Unfortunately, this doesn't happen very often, so modern programs must learn from earlier international efforts against yaws, malaria, and yellow fever, and accept less ambitious goals. Following the eradication of smallpox in 1979, the Carter Center established a task force to examine which other major infectious agents might also be eradicated (ITFDE, 2011). They decided that seven diseases would fit into this category: measles, mumps, rubella, polio, filariasis, cysticercosis, and dracunculiasis. The process acted as a stimulus for the WHO that eventually led to the eradication and elimination programs that are established today. The task force's terminology for degrees of control is still used:

- *Eradication:* Reduction of the disease incidence to zero without the need for further control measures; so far, the only human disease to be eradicated is smallpox, but SARS may also fall into this category if it doesn't return within a few years. One other infectious disease, called Rinderpest, has been removed, but it got less attention because it was a disease of cattle. The WHO announced eradication of this virus in 2011 with surprisingly little fanfare (GREP, 2011).

- *Elimination:* Eradication of a disease from one part of the globe, e.g., polio and malaria in the Western hemisphere. The term is increasingly being used to mean the control of a disease to the level that it is no longer a public health menace. Examples include reducing new cases of leprosy below 1 per 10,000 population, or the significant reduction of onchocerciasis in West Africa.

- *Control:* Reduction of transmission to minimal levels, but with the need for continuing control measures, which implies there is a large non-human reservoir of infection that will always be present. Examples include tetanus and influenza A.

The enormous expense needed to get over the final hurdle between elimination and eradication has changed attitudes in recent years. Polio is a good example, where the predicted year of eradication has been steadily put back as intermittent wars and social chaos stubbornly prevent the last few hundred cases a year from being cleared up. Under these circumstances, many have argued that elimination

Table 13.3: The 10 infectious diseases currently targeted for elimination or eradication

DISEASE	TARGET
Polio	Global eradication
Dracunculiasis (Guinea worm)	Global eradication
Onchocerciasis (river blindness)	Elimination in the Americas
Lymphatic filariasis (elephantiasis)	Elimination as public health hazard
Chlamydia conjunctivitis (trachoma)	Elimination of blinding trachoma
Leprosy	Elimination as public health hazard
American trypanosomiasis (Chagas disease)	Elimination in the Americas
Visceral leishmaniasis (kala azar)	Elimination in Southeast Asia
Endemic treponematosis (yaws)	Elimination in Southeast Asia
African trypanosomiasis (sleeping sickness)	Elimination as public health hazard

Note: All, except polio, are on the WHO's list of neglected tropical diseases.

Source: National Academies. 2011. *The causes and impacts of neglected tropical and zoonotic diseases: Opportunities for integrated intervention strategies.* Pub: National Academies Press.

is as far as a program should go until slowly rising progress in the region finally allows complete eradication at some stage in the future (Thompson et al., 2007). The WHO is the only international body that can declare a disease either eradicated or eliminated, and it is also the only organization with the mandate to determine which infectious diseases are suitable targets for such programs.

Of the 10 diseases currently scheduled for elimination or eradication (Table 13.3), 9 of them are included within the WHO's list of neglected tropical diseases (WHO, 2010). This represents a significant shift in attention toward diseases of the world's poorest people. The only non-neglected disease on the list is polio. The three main infectious diseases (HIV, TB, malaria) are, of course, the subjects of intense control measures. All three are discussed in detail in Chapter 8. All three are difficult organisms to stop, so unless there is a breakthrough in developing an effective vaccine, it will be quite a while before it is possible to talk about control or elimination for any of them. Five of the largest control programs are described below. Two others (visceral leishmaniasis and African trypanosomiasis) are covered in Chapter 8.

Polio

> When I was about 9, I had polio, and people were very frightened for their children, so you tended to be isolated. I was paralyzed for a while, so I watched television.
>
> —*Francis Ford Coppola*

Polio is a highly contagious infection caused by the poliovirus (WHO, 2011b). It is an ancient disease—easily recognizable cases are seen in ancient Egyptian wall paintings. It is spread mainly by fecally contaminated water and food, but it can also be transmitted by respiratory secretions. An infected person can excrete virus in stool for weeks, so in endemic countries, almost all adults have been infected at some stage. It most commonly affects the old and young, hence its former name, infantile paralysis. From the mid-19th to the mid-20th century, epidemics swept through cities around the world, most commonly in summer and fall. After infection, the virus multiplies in the gut before spreading throughout the body following an incubation period of one to two weeks. Over 90 percent of infected hosts sense nothing more than a mild, flu-like illness. In about 1 percent of cases, the virus travels along nerves into the spinal cord and brain. It has a particular capacity to destroy cells called motor neurons, which leads to paralysis in the muscles served by that infected region. Roughly half of paralyzed patients recover fully. There is no cure, but some improvement was obtained through injection of serum containing antibodies from previously infected patients.

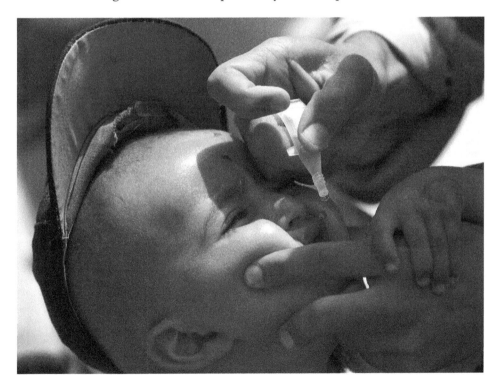

Photo 13.2: A young child receives oral polio vaccine in an Indian clinic; India was declared polio-free in 2014.

Source: With kind permission of the UN Photo Library (www.unmultimedia.org/photo).

It is easy to forget that polio was a dreaded disease within the recent past. Prior to vaccination in the 1950s, there were 20,000 cases each year in the US. It affected rich and poor alike—the best-known person affected by paralytic polio was US President Franklin Roosevelt. Its near eradication is one of the great success stories of international aid. The virus was isolated in 1908, but practical vaccines were not developed until the 1950s. Salk's first vaccine was based on inactivated virus given by injection. Sabin's later vaccine was a live attenuated virus that could be given orally. Following vaccination, the child excretes the virus, so other close contacts will be passively vaccinated by fecal-oral spread. Oral vaccine is the one more commonly used in large population programs. The very small risk that oral polio vaccine might reactivate and cause clinical disease has meant that many countries prefer to use the inactivated vaccine given by injection.

The international program against polio has been active for over 25 years. It is run by a coalition of groups that includes the WHO, UNICEF, the International Rotary, and the US CDC (GPEI, 2011). Within this time, an incredible amount of work has been done, including vaccinating 2.5 billion children (Photo 13.2). The annual number of cases worldwide has fallen from around 350,000 in the 1980s to 1,000–2,000 each year for the past 10 years. Unfortunately, those last cases are stubborn. Globally, the world is very close to reaching the goal of polio eradication. As of August 11, 2016, only 21 wild polio cases have been reported in 2016, compared to 34 cases at the same point last year. Four out of the six WHO Regions of the world have been certified polio-free. Pakistan and Afghanistan are the only two countries in the world that have never stopped transmission of polio (WHO, 2016).

Dracunculiasis (Guinea Worm)

It has never been a question of if we can rid the world of this ancient disease—but when.

—Stephen O'Brien, UK International Development minister, 2011

Dracunculiasis is a parasitic disease caused by a nematode called *Dracunculus medinensis*. It is another ancient disease of humans. The practice of slowly pulling the worm from the body by winding it around a stick is possibly the source of the traditional medical symbol of a serpent wrapped around a staff of wood. The larvae live inside small water crustaceans. When they are ingested with contaminated water, the crustaceans are killed, leaving the larvae to multiply. They pierce the wall of the gut and wander around until they reach the muscles of the leg, where the female can grow to 0.5–1 m long. The tail emerges from the skin when the host walks in water so eggs can be ejected and the cycle continued. There is no medical treatment for the worms. They can sometimes be slowly pulled from the leg over two days if the tail can be caught. They cause extreme pain and chronic ulcerating infections. The cycle can be broken by treating water sources with larvicide or, more simply, by filtering out the crustaceans before drinking contaminated water.

Along with polio, Guinea worm is the second disease selected for eradication. The international program is run by a joint agency consisting of the WHO, UNICEF, CDC, and the Carter Center. It is estimated that there were 3.5 million cases worldwide when the program started in 1986. By 2010, that had fallen to 1,800 cases in only four remaining countries (Sudan, Mali, Ethiopia, and Ghana). If current progress continues, the prospects for eradication look good. This has been achieved with no medication or vaccine. An important feature of the program is the use of trained local people as educators and also for case reporting.

Onchocerciasis (River Blindness) [1]

River blindness is caused by a parasitic infection by the nematode *Onchocerca volvulus*. It is the second-most common infectious cause of blindness after trachoma. The larval form is spread by the bite of the blackfly, which lives near fast-flowing rivers. The larvae develop into adults, over months, within nodules under the skin. Adults then live for years, producing thousands of micro-filariae every day. The body's reaction to these tiny organisms produces intense skin itching and cumulative eye irritation, which eventually leads to blindness. There are no drugs that kill the adults, but ivermectin, introduced in 1988, kills the micro-filariae and prevents the female from producing more. A single dose provides protection for a year. The parasite has a symbiotic relationship with bacteria called *Wolbachia*, which likely induce most of the inflammatory reaction. Daily use of tetracycline for six weeks is effective, but is not of value for mass treatment programs. It is estimated that 37 million people are infected in Africa within a band of 20 countries in West Africa. There is a smaller focus in Yemen. In South America, about half a million people are at risk in six countries.

Until ivermectin was available, control relied on vector reduction by spraying and the use of a less effective drug called DEC. The River Blindness Foundation in the Americas subsequently joined the Carter Center, together with the World Bank, the WHO, and others, to form a broad Onchocerciasis Control Program (Carter Center, 2011b) covering Africa and the Americas. The continued use of spraying and twice-yearly ivermectin (generously donated by Merck) has greatly reduced the transmission of onchocerciasis. At current rates of progress, the Carter Center has predicted that onchocerciasis transmission could be halted in the Americas before 2015, but could only be controlled in most regions of West Africa.

Lymphatic Filariasis (Elephantiasis)

> Many people in Malabar have very large legs, swollen to a great size.... They have no pain, nor do they take notice of this infirmity.
>
> —*Tome Pires, 1515*

Lymphatic filariasis is caused by infection with one of three nematodes within the same broad filarial group as Guinea worm. *Wucheraria bancrofti* is by far the most common cause. The larvae are spread by mosquito bites. They develop into adults within the lymphatic system of the body and, together with the body's inflammatory response, produce chronic lymph obstruction. The affected limb slowly swells to enormous size, hence the term "elephantiasis." The WHO estimates that over a billion people are at risk of infection in 80 countries spread throughout the tropics. Over 120 million are infected, with about 40 million suffering from disabling limb swelling. Two-thirds of cases are in Southeast Asia, and most of the remainder are in Africa, particularly Nigeria. The control program was started by the WHO in 2000 (WHO, 2011c). It is based on mass drug treatment with albendazole to kill the adult worms and ivermectin to kill the micro-filariae and reduce their production (which also reduces transmission). GlaxoSmithKline and Merck have donated the necessary drugs. In some areas, DEC is substituted, either as a once-yearly treatment or as DEC-fortified table salt. Progress has been good in many areas. China and the Republic of Korea have both eliminated the disease as a public health hazard.

Chlamydia Conjunctivitis (Trachoma)

Trachoma is caused by a bacterial infection of the cornea by *Chlamydia trachomatis*. It is found throughout the developed world and is the most common infectious cause of lost vision. It is another disease that has parasitized humans since ancient times. It used to be very common in Europe and wasn't completely eradicated until the 1950s. The bacteria are spread by flies, close contact with other infected children, and poor sanitary standards. Recurrent infections eventually damage the cornea and eyelid until sight is impaired. It is estimated that over 40 million people are infected, up to a million of whom have lost their sight (National Academies, 2011). The WHO's elimination program is based on the SAFE strategy (Surgery, Antibiotics, Face washing, Environmental improvement). The necessary antibiotic, zithromax, is donated by Pfizer. The aim is to reduce scarring trachoma below 1 in 1,000 and to eliminate blinding trachoma completely by 2020. The Alliance for Global Elimination of Trachoma was started in 1997 and consists of the WHO, plus the Edna McConnell Clark Foundation, the Carter Center, and Pfizer (WHO, 2011d).

THE MANAGEMENT OF PEDIATRIC DISEASES

The world is turned by the breath of schoolchildren.

—Babylonian Talmud, 119b

Children are important—a society's future progress and prosperity are largely dependent on the investment placed in child health care and education. The quote from the Talmud, above, is only one of many on the subject. It was written down centuries ago and had been passed on through oral tradition for centuries before that. It is difficult to understand why such an important idea, first brought up around a campfire thousands of years ago, has taken so long to become an international priority. Measured in terms of the care given to children in the poorest countries, the development assistance industry scores an A for research, epidemiology, and treatment, but close to an F for implementation. Workers in these various areas have found out what kills so many children each year and they have also devised highly effective treatment protocols. Unfortunately, the practical application of that knowledge has been inhibited by dilapidated health delivery systems in very poor regions.

With the introduction of programs aimed at vaccine-preventable diseases, diarrhea, and pneumonia, millions of child deaths have been averted over the last 20 years (annual deaths over 12 million in 1980s to below 6 million at last count). By now we have been through the same cycle three times—the Child Survival Revolution of the 1980s, the Integrated Management of Childhood Illness in the 1990s, and now the Partnership for Maternal, Newborn, and Child Health in the 2000s. On each occasion, the rediscovery that mortality is caused by only a few diseases prompts the design of an essential care package, which then runs into the same problem of implementation because of poor health systems. In order to understand the past accelerated effort to meet the health aims of the MDGs in 2015, it is necessary to look at the challenges faced by earlier initiatives.

1980s: The Child Survival Revolution

As discussed in Chapter 12, the debate over the implementation of primary health care eventually led to the adoption of selective PHC. These packages of cost-effective measures were limited in scope, but represented a big improvement over the existing standards of the day. In 1982, UNICEF, under the leadership of James Grant, announced a Child Survival Revolution based on the package known as GOBI (growth monitoring, oral rehydration, breastfeeding, and immunization). The idea caught on and UNICEF was soon joined by the WHO, the UNDP, and the World Bank to form the Taskforce for Child Survival and Development.

With time, the basic package was slowly expanded to include programs targeting diarrheal diseases, acute respiratory diseases, an expanded immunization program, vitamin A supplementation, treated bed nets, and others (Bryce et al., 2003). Taken together, a great deal was achieved. Stepping up immunization to reach 80 percent of the world's children was the biggest peacetime mobilization ever seen. However, by the early 1990s, there was a sense that progress had stalled.

1990s: The Integrated Management of Childhood Illness

Although vertical programs saved a lot of lives, they were never meant to be a substitute for comprehensive clinic systems, also known as horizontal care (Oluwole et al., 1999). The WHO recognized the need for an integrated system where care for the major childhood diseases could be given by well-trained staff in well-managed clinics. The ambitious plan that grew out of this development was launched in the mid-1990s as the Integrated Management of Childhood Illness (IMCI). This joint WHO/UNICEF initiative was intended to be a major advance in the care of children in developed countries (El Arifeen et al., 2004). The IMCI clinical guidelines are tailored to the major diseases of young children (pneumonia, diarrheal diseases, measles, malaria, and malnutrition). Based on the initial assessment by the health care worker, a child is classified under three colour codes: pink (urgent referral after initial treatment), yellow (treatment in the clinic), or green (treatment at home). The guidelines do not attempt to address the full range of childhood illnesses. For example, they do not describe management of acute emergencies, such as burns and poisonings.

Even the most inclusive treatment package is still only a superficial approach to medical problems that have their roots in poor living conditions, poverty, and lack of education. The IMCI recognizes this by also placing emphasis on education for parents and advocacy for improved standards of local health services. Emphasis is on health care workers counselling parents. Topics include home management of specific illnesses (how to take antibiotics or ORS), nutrition practices, fluids, and when to return to the clinic. If health care workers are given training to improve their communication and education skills, there are measurable improvements in parents' child care at home (Pelto et al., 2004). The IMCI program also takes a broader approach to the improvement of local health care services. These vary in different countries, but they range from organizing referral transportation to home care visits and counselling. An excellent example of an ancillary service is the large Lady Health Worker Program, which reaches 30 million people in rural Pakistan (Douthwaite et al., 2005).

The IMCI program was a model for a carefully introduced initiative. It was initially started in a small group of countries, and the early stages were closely monitored by a dedicated evaluation group (MCE, 2006). Unfortunately, results have fallen far short of expectations. In Tanzania, where it was introduced as part of a general program to strengthen health services and staff training was supported, it was shown to reduce child mortality (Schellenberg et al., 2004). However, this was the exception, not the rule. While IMCI has nominally been adopted by many countries, it has not been supported either financially or organizationally so that national coverage levels remain very low. IMCI's clinical training program has been praised and its plan of management can work if supported and widely implemented. In the reality of a very poor country, no management plan can overcome inadequate health delivery systems. This remains the principal barrier to improved child health.

2000s: Partnership for Maternal, Newborn, and Child Health

Toward the end of the 20th century, it was clear that advances in child health were slowing. By the year 2000, despite the discovery and implementation of highly effective therapies, there were still over 10 million deaths annually in children under five years. They died from the same six diseases in the same 40–50 countries of Africa and Southeast Asia. Within those countries, children from the poorest families were most likely to die (Figure 13.5). Any realistic long-term solution obviously needed to be more broadly based than was possible with single-issue vertical programs. The MDGs set the scene for the current coordinated plan against child mortality. Apart from the specific child health goal (target 4), there were also relevant associated goals for poverty reduction (target 1), maternal health (target 5), and sanitation and housing (target 7) (UN, 2011). All of these separate issues must be improved to achieve the best levels of child health, which are now fully reflected in the new SDGs.

The next step occurred when *The Lancet* published an influential series of papers on child health in 2003 (*The Lancet* Series, 2003). A similar series of articles was published the following year concerning early infant mortality (*The Lancet* Series, 2004). They were based on the findings of an expert panel known as the Bellagio Group (Bellagio Group, 2003). They had more data to analyze than the earlier researchers at Alma Ata (Walsh et al., 1979), but their findings were the same—there are well-described therapies that are known to reduce early and late child mortality. If these were widely implemented, it was calculated that two-thirds of the current mortality could be eliminated (Bhutta et al., 2010). That simple fact needs to be emphasized—23 interventions could collectively save 6

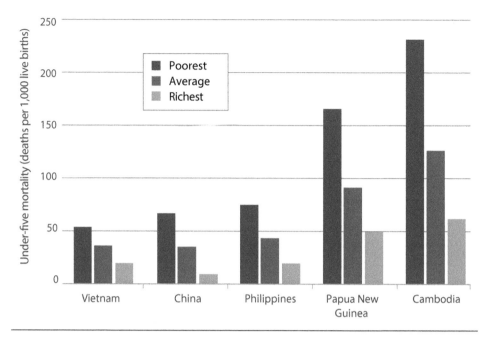

Figure 13.5: Under-five mortality rates from the richest to the poorest in five Asian countries

Source: ESCAP. 2011. Economic and Social Commission for Asia and Pacific. Statistical yearbook. Retrieved from: www.unescap.org/stat/data/syb2011/.

million children a year! Others have subsequently calculated that this could be achieved for not much more that US$5 billion per year or about US$900 per life saved (Bryce, 2003).

Since then there has been continued progress. The Child Health Epidemiology Reference Group, established in 2001, continues to provide a firm basis of high-class scientific data to support outcome evaluation (CHERG, 2011). A large group of organizations, including the WHO and UNICEF, formed the Partnership for Maternal, Newborn, and Child Health (PMNCH, 2011). This group has the ability to influence countries to increase their finance and resources for health care systems. The group also generates regular progress reports (PMNCH, 2011). Health spending by developing countries is rising (Figure 13.3) and so is health-directed aid from donor countries (Figure 13.2). Finally, the most recent estimates suggest that annual under-five mortality is approaching 6 million. This is still a shameful death total, but there are now real hopes that the fight against child mortality has been re-energized so that even the poorest countries will be able to meet the SDG targets on under-five mortality as 25 per 1,000 live births.

PREGNANCY-RELATED MEDICAL CARE

$13 to $20 billion a year could be saved in health care costs by demedicalizing childbirth, developing midwifery, and encouraging breastfeeding.

—Frank Oski

Complications of pregnancy and childbirth are the leading causes of death among women of reproductive age in most parts of the developing world. Although there have been recent improvements in maternal health statistics (see Chapter 10), 1,000 women still die of pregnancy-related causes every single day. A woman's lifetime risk of dying while pregnant ranges from 1 in 10,000 in some Scandinavian countries to 1 in 20 or worse in Afghanistan and parts of sub-Saharan Africa. The political will to do anything significant about this problem has been slow to develop (Hogberg, 2005). It was less than 20 years ago that the UN held a conference in Cairo, where plans for measurable reductions in maternal deaths were discussed (UN, 1994). The result was an ambitious 20-year plan focusing on improving infant, child, and maternal mortality through improved reproductive health services. Prior to the Cairo conference, a partnership of donor governments, NGOs, and a range of women's health groups launched the global initiative for safe motherhood at a meeting in Nairobi (Safe Motherhood, 2010). The initiative promotes diverse interventions aimed at improving the health of women and their children. The group is also a vigorous advocate for governments and donor agencies to make safe motherhood a major priority in their development plans.

Reducing these numbers does not require exotic technology. Basic measures needed include access to trained midwives, drugs like magnesium sulphate for eclampsia and oxytocin for post-delivery bleeding, and communications to ask for assistance and transportation to an established emergency obstetric centre (Adam, 2005). The Cairo conference intended to fund one-third of the necessary expenses from donors and the remainder from developing countries. Unfortunately, both sides have fallen below expectation so that no region in the developing world has met the goals of the Cairo conference's program of action. The increasing AIDS epidemic has also tended to divert money away from specific child and maternal health projects. The following elements are a central part of safe pregnancy-related care.

Antenatal Care

Routine antenatal visits were introduced in Britain during the 1930s with the hope that maternal mortality could be reduced by early identification of high-risk women. Subsequent research showed that many of the traditional elements of antenatal care (height and weight monitoring, blood pressure measurements) were surprisingly poor at predicting severe problems at time of delivery. The emphasis of antenatal care then shifted away from prediction and more toward improving maternal health, with obvious benefits to the mother, but also for the survival and health of the subsequent children. The early detection and treatment of anemia, malaria, poor nutrition, and sexually transmitted diseases, plus education for the mother, are the most important features of effective antenatal care (USAID, 2007). The main features should include:

- *Routine care:* The WHO recommends four visits, with the first one starting in the first trimester. If problems are detected, the number of visits should increase. Regular visits are an opportunity to offer education to groups of mothers on subjects such as personal care, nutrition, rest, child spacing, family planning, exclusive breastfeeding, and basic care of the infant to reduce the risk of neonatal tetanus. The mother should be counselled regarding where she plans to deliver and the need for a skilled attendant.
- *Focused care:* All pregnant women should be immunized with tetanus toxoid to reduce the risk of neonatal tetanus, and they should all be checked for anemia. This is the most common avoidable problem of pregnancy and should be treated with dietary counselling and iron-plus-folate supplementation.
- *Other investigations:* Depending on local disease patterns, other focused interventions should include: protection against malaria by intermittent treatment and provision of a treated bed net; presumptive treatment for hookworm; vitamin A and iodine supplementation in high-risk areas; screening for STDs, including HIV, plus prophylaxis and treatment where necessary.

Obstetric emergencies are often unpredictable and can be managed only by providing trained attendants, backed up by referral emergency services. The shift in focus toward improved delivery care involves much higher investments in staff, training, and equipment compared to the relatively low cost of routine antenatal care. Consequently, in many developing countries, the coverage for delivery care lags well behind the provision of antenatal care.

Delivery Care

The importance of a trained birth attendant in reducing maternal mortality is frequently emphasized (WHO, 2003). While a midwife is essential, it is important to remember that simply providing an attendant is only one part of the full picture. Every labour and delivery should certainly be supervised by a health worker with the skills needed to handle normal deliveries and the training to recognize when a woman has to be transferred. However, when problems are identified, there must be a system in place to provide the next level of care (WHO, 2005). Clearly, this requires a regional centre with the capacity for handling Caesarean sections and blood transfusion. A well-maintained ambulance, plus driver and communications, are also important to speed the process. In many parts of the developing world, delivery services are improving in the cities, but rural areas are still badly under-serviced. Where government services are inadequate, private delivery services, of variable quality, are meeting the demand (USAID, 2010).

Post-Delivery Care

The newborn baby should be dried, wrapped, and kept with the mother. Early baths are not necessary for the child. Early breastfeeding should be encouraged; colostrum should not be discarded. Hospital and clinic policies toward breast-feeding should be guided by the recommendations of the Baby-Friendly Initiative (UNICEF, 2006). Minimum resuscitation equipment for a newborn should in-clude clean umbilical cord care, tube and mask resuscitation (using air, not oxygen), and antibiotics for infants showing signs of sepsis.

Antenatal treatment and delivery care are not, of course, the end of preg-nancy-related health care. A comprehensive maternal health service should also provide treatment for sexually transmitted diseases and a wide range of health education opportunities. This must all be backed up by a general societal approach that values women and understands the need to invest in maternal health. It is particularly important that young mothers have access to family-planning services. Overall, roughly two-thirds of women in stable relationships use regular contra-ception throughout the developing world, but this ranges from 84 percent in East Asia to 23 percent in sub-Saharan Africa. Women's ability to plan and space their children contributes greatly to their health and well-being.

ACCESS TO ESSENTIAL DRUGS

I firmly believe that if the whole material medica could be sent to the bottom of the sea, it would be all the better for mankind and all the worse for the fishes.

—*Oliver Wendell Holmes, 1860*

The quote above contains a fair bit of truth. Of all the tens of thousands of prescrip-tion and non-prescription drugs listed in the pharmacies of developed countries, only a surprisingly small number are of any real value. When the World Health

Organization first brought out its suggested essential drug list in 1977, it was possible to run a regional hospital with not much more than 100 drugs, which included intravenous fluids and vaccines. Obviously, a few new drugs will be added to the list each year—treatments for malaria, TB, HIV/AIDS, and common bacterial and parasitic diseases are all good examples—but even the most recent list contains not much more than 300 drugs (WHO, 2011a).

Easy access to effective drugs is an important part of health care in the developing world, but it has received attention only fairly recently (DFID, 2004). There are two main problems affecting the supply of effective drugs: affordability and availability. Even a short course of cheap antibiotics can be prohibitively expensive for a poor rural family. This has always been a problem, but has been a particular issue over the last decade because of the cost of antiretroviral therapy. The second problem is that research and development into developing effective world drugs are not likely to produce large profits for drug companies. The drug eflornithine was an effective, much less toxic alternative for the treatment of West African trypanosomiasis, yet its only manufacturer stopped its production for sleeping sickness, but continued making it as a facial hair remover. This decision was reversed in response to political pressure, and Sanofi-Aventis now donates the drug for sleeping sickness treatment (Wickware, 2002).

Drug Affordability

The World Health Organization and Médecins sans Frontières (MSF, 2011a) have been leading advocates for access to affordable medicines. Since 1999, MSF has led a campaign to lower drug costs through increased use of generic alternatives, voluntary discounts by drug manufacturers, and local production in some countries. They also emphasize the need for increased research into "unprofitable" tropical diseases, such as tuberculosis, malaria, sleeping sickness, and leishmaniasis. The subject came to a head in 2001 when South Africa decided to import generic antiviral drugs for use in its fight against its HIV epidemic. At the time, triple therapy cost US$10,000 per patient per year. An Indian generic company offered the same regime for US$300 per person per year. South Africa intended to use the generic drugs only for its own patients, but 39 of the world's largest pharmaceutical companies took the South African government to court to stop the country from using cheap alternatives (Sidley, 2001). There was widespread criticism of the drug companies' action, including a resolution from the European Union Parliament calling for them to drop their case. After it became obvious that they would have to publish their profits and justify their pricing, they abandoned the case.

Unfortunately, the subject is complicated because patent restrictions on essential medicines are only one small part of ongoing debates surrounding world trade. Most developing countries signed on for a set of trade rules that included pharmaceutical patents in 1995. However, there is some flexibility in the Trade-Related Aspects of Intellectual Property Rights (TRIPS) agreements. The World Trade Organization's 2001 Doha Declaration specifically states that "the TRIPS Agreement does not and should not prevent members from taking measures to protect public health." This Doha loophole applies only to countries with domestic pharmaceutical manufacturing capacity. There is no general agreement on how poor countries without manufacturing capacity can obtain licences to import HIV drugs from countries such as Brazil and India. Small countries lacking money and political influence are currently relying on first-generation antiretrovirals. As time passes and viral resistance increases, the issue will be raised again as the price of newer drugs becomes an issue. More recently, increased drug financing through the Global Fund and the President's Emergency Fund, combined with advocacy from the Clinton Foundation, has certainly improved access to HIV drugs, but the problem of patent rights and graded pricing for different countries is by no means solved (MSF, 2011b).

Drug Quality and Availability

Public health services in many developing countries are often in poor condition, particularly in rural areas. An overall lack of basic services and supplies can exacerbate local people's inability to receive adequate drug treatment for their illnesses. Numerous studies have shown that drugs in developing world markets are often repackaged expired drugs or, in some cases, have no pharmacological activity at all (Dondorp et al., 2004). In poorer districts where power is in short supply, drugs that require refrigeration (such as vaccines) may degrade rapidly in warm temperatures.

While local laws may stipulate that only hospital clinics and pharmacists can dispense medication, there is often little control over drug distribution. Informal dispensers usually lack sufficient knowledge about correct drug use and dosage; they may also be involved in straightforward deception in order to peddle worthless medications. Poor consumers who cannot pay for a visit to a doctor or clinic end up relying on anecdotal evidence supplied by dispensers. As a result, scarce money is spent on useless medicine. Due to the influx of Western pharmaceuticals and lack of government control, people are often able to purchase Western medicines without having to queue in crowded clinics. Instead, medications are bought and administered without a prescription, often on the advice of a shopkeeper or friend.

The cumulative effect of poor manufacturing standards, poor storage, repackaging of expired drugs, and criminal counterfeiting is significant. The WHO estimates that counterfeit drugs alone make up 10 percent of worldwide supplies, with much of the fake drugs ending up in developing countries. There has been considerable interest in counterfeiting—the WHO held the first conference on the subject in Rome in 2006 (Attaran et al., 2011). The literature is surprisingly poor considering all the excitement on the subject. At present, the available studies certainly support the existence of counterfeiting in some markets, but relabelling of expired drugs and simple degradation during storage are likely far more common causes of poor drug quality in most areas (Seear et al., 2011). There is a need for a great deal more focused research in this important area of clinical medicine.

SUMMARY

In 2015, US$36.4 billion in development assistance for health (DAH) was disbursed, an increase of 0.3 percent over 2014 levels. Over the last five or six decades, the approach to the provision of health services in developing countries has followed differing trends. The initial response to widespread ill health was to export Western-style curative care models. The ultimate failure of urban hospitals to reduce disease in rural areas led to the 1978 Alma Ata meeting and a switch to more preventive strategies under the banner of primary health care. The vagueness and failings around the "Health for all by 2000" goal led to another call for health care reform starting in the early 1990s. While this movement has produced many alternative models (contracting out to NGOs, decentralized management structures, private health care, personal health insurance, etc.), no clear winner has emerged. In reality, many of the poorest countries simply have dilapidated remnants of an earlier district health system.

One of the biggest innovations in aid over the last decade has been the emergence of targeted programs (also called vertical or global programs). While their origins can be traced back to the early disease-eradication programs of the 1960s, they have changed in everything but name compared to those first large-scale initiatives. Examples of well-known programs that target infectious diseases include: the Global Fund to Fight AIDS, TB, and Malaria, the Global Alliance for Vaccines and Immunization, and the Stop Tuberculosis Partnership. There are many lesser-known programs aimed at leprosy, onchocerciasis, measles, trachoma, and filariasis. The dream of targeted medical projects is complete eradication of a human infectious disease. Unfortunately, this does not happen very often, so modern programs must learn from earlier international efforts against yaws, malaria, and yellow fever, and accept less ambitious goals. Following the eradication of smallpox in 1979, the Carter Center established a task force to examine which other major infectious agents might also be eradicated. They decided that seven diseases would fit into this category: measles, mumps, rubella, polio, filariasis, cysticercosis, and dracunculiasis. The process acted as a stimulus for the WHO that eventually led to the eradication and elimination programs that are established today. The enormous expense needed to get over the final hurdle between elimination and eradication has changed attitudes in recent years. Polio is a good example, where the predicted year of eradication has been steadily put back as intermittent wars and social chaos stubbornly prevent the last few hundred cases a year from being cleared up. Under these circumstances, many have argued that elimination is as far as a program should go until slowly rising progress in the region finally allows complete eradication at some stage in the future. The WHO is the only international body that can declare a disease either eradicated or eliminated, and it is also the only organization with the mandate to determine which infectious diseases are suitable targets for such programs.

DISCUSSION QUESTIONS

1. Until the Alma Ata meeting in 1978, the predominant system to initial response to widespread ill health was based on a curative Western model. What changed after the Alma Ata meeting?

2. What are some questions to keep in mind when designing an "ideal" health system for a developing world population? Why are such questions important?

3. What are the essential elements for the successful organization of an integrated district health system?

4. What are the major clinical responsibilities of a District Health Centre? What is the Integrated Management of Childhood Illnesses (IMCI)?

5. Name a few of the health-funding mechanisms that exist. What are the pros and cons of each?

6. What are targeted or vertical programs? Why are they important in global health?

7. What is the difference between eradication and elimination?

8. Why does polio remain endemic in a few countries, such as Afghanistan and Pakistan?

9. What is river blindness? What is the most common infectious cause of blindness?

10. What are the main features of effective antenatal care? What are the leading causes of death among women of reproductive age in most parts of the developing world?

RECOMMENDED READING

Crisp, N. 2010. *Turning the world upside down: The search for global health in the 21st century*. Pub: Hodder Arnold.

Gandy, M., & Zumla, A. (Eds.). 2003. *The return of the white plague: Global poverty and the new tuberculosis*. Pub: Verso.

Ghosh, J., et al. (Eds.). 2003. *HIV and AIDS in Africa: Beyond epidemiology*. Pub: Blackwell.

Leach, B., Palluzi, J., & Munderi, P. 2005. *Prescription for healthy development: Increasing access to medicines*. Pub: Earthscan.

Levine, R. 2007. *Case studies in global health: Millions saved*. Pub: Jones and Bartlett.

Seear, M. 2000. *Manual of tropical pediatrics*. Pub: Cambridge University Press.

Teklehaumanot, A., et al. 2005. *Coming to grips with malaria in the new millennium*. Pub: Earthscan.

REFERENCES

Adam, T., et al. 2005. Cost effectiveness analysis of strategies for maternal and neonatal health in developing countries. *Brit Med Journal*, 331: 1107–1112.

APPA. 2011. American Pet Products Association: Industry statistics and trends. Retrieved from: www.americanpetproducts.org/press_industrytrends.asp.

Attaran, A., et al. 2011. Why and how to make an international crime of medicine counterfeiting. *Journal of International Criminal Justice*, 9: 953–957.

Barret, R., et al. 2004. Health financing innovations in the Caribbean: EHPO and the National Health Fund of Jamaica. Inter-American Development Bank. Retrieved from: idbdocs. iadb.org/wsdocs/getdocument.aspx?docnum=823515.

Bellagio Group. 2003. The Bellagio Study Group on child survival. *The Lancet*, 362: 323–327.

Bhutta, Z., et al. 2010. Countdown to 2015 decade report (2000–2010): Taking stock of maternal, newborn, and child survival. *The Lancet*, 375: 2032–2044.

Blas, E., et al. 2001. User payment, decentralization, and health service utilization in Zambia. *Health Policy and Planning*, 16: 19–28.

Bryce, J., et al. 2003. Reducing child mortality: Can public health deliver? *The Lancet*, 362: 159–164.

Carter Center. 2011a. Guinea worm disease eradication. Retrieved from: www.cartercenter. org/health/guinea_worm/mini_site/index.html.

Carter Center. 2011b. River blindness program. Retrieved from: www.cartercenter.org/health/ river_blindness/index.html.

Carter Center. 2011c. Lymphatic filariasis program. Retrieved from: www.cartercenter.org/health/lf/index.html.

CDC. 2010. CDC's Centre for Global Health: Dracunculiasis. Retrieved from: http://dpd.cdc.gov/dpdx/html/Dracunculiasis.htm.

CGIAR. 2011. The Consultative Group on International Agricultural Research. Retrieved from: www.cgiar.org/.

CHERG. 2011. Child Health Epidemiology Reference Group. Retrieved from: http://cherg.org/main.html.

DFID. 2004. Access to medicines in under-served markets. Retrieved from: www.dfid.gov.uk/pubs/files/dfidsynthesispaper.pdf.

Dieleman, J. L., et al. 2016. Development assistance for health: Past trends, associations, and the future of international financial flows for health. *The Lancet,* 387(10037): 2536–2544. doi:10.1016/S0140-6736(16)30168-4.

Dondorp, A., et al. 2004. Fake antimalarials in Southeast Asia are a major impediment to malaria control: Multinational cross-sectional survey on the prevalence of fake antimalarials. *Tropical Medicine and International Health,* 9: 1241–1246.

Douthwaite, M., et al. 2005. Increasing contraceptive use in rural Pakistan: An evaluation of the Lady Health Worker Program. *Health Policy and Planning,* 2: 20–25.

El Arifeen, S., et al. 2004. Integrated Management of Childhood Illness (IMCI) in Bangladesh: Early findings from a cluster-randomized study. *The Lancet,* 364: 1595–1602.

ESCAP. 2011. Economic and Social Commission for Asia and Pacific. Statistical yearbook. Retrieved from: www.unescap.org/stat/data/syb2011/.

Every Woman Every Child. 2015. Saving lives, protecting futures: Progress report on the global strategy for women's and children's health. Retrieved from: http://everywomaneverychild.org/images/EWEC_Progress_Report_FINAL_3.pdf.

Frenk, J., et al. 2006. Comprehensive reform to improve health system performance in Mexico. *The Lancet,* 368: 1524–1534.

GAVI. 2011. The Global Alliance for Vaccines and Immunization. Retrieved from: www.gavialliance.org/.

GEF. 2011. The Global Environment Facility. Retrieved from: www.thegef.org/gef/.

Gilson, L., et al. 2005. Removing user fees for primary care in Africa: The need for careful action. *British Medical Journal,* 331: 762–765.

Global Fund. 2011. The Global Fund to fight AIDS, TB, and Malaria. Retrieved from: www.theglobalfund.org/en/.

GPEI. 2011. Global Polio Eradication Initiative. Retrieved from: www.polioeradication.org/.

GREP. 2011. Global Rinderpest Eradication Programme. Retrieved from: www.fao.org/ag/againfo/resources/documents/AH/GREP_flyer.pdf.

GTZ. 2004. The district health system: Experiences and prospects in Africa. Retrieved from: www.afronets.org/files/district-health-en.pdf.

Hansen, P., et al. 2008. Measuring and managing progress in the establishment of basic health services: The Afghanistan health sector balanced scorecard. *International Journal of Health Planning and Management*, 23: 107–117.

Hogberg, U. 2005. The World Health Report 2005: "Make every mother and child count"—including Africans. *Scandinavian Journal of Public Health*, 33: 409–411.

IHME. 2016. Institute for Health Metrics and Evaluation. Financing global health 2010. Retrieved from: www.healthdata.org/policy-report/financing-global-health-2015-development-assistance-steady-path-new-global-goals.

IMB. 2011. Independent Monitoring Board for the Global Polio Eradication Initiative. Retrieved from: www.polioeradication.org/Portals/0/Document/Aboutus/Governance/IMB/4IMBMeeting/IMBReportOctober2011.pdf.

ITFDE. 2011. The International Taskforce for Disease Eradication. Retrieved from: www.cartercenter.org/health/itfde/index.html.

Jamas, C., et al. 2005. Impact on child mortality of removing user fees: Simulation model. *British Medical Journal*, 331: 747–749.

Khaleghian, P. 2004. Decentralization and public services: The case of immunization. *Social Science and Medicine*, 59: 163–183.

The Lancet Series. 2003. *The Lancet*, 361: 2226–2234; *The Lancet*, 362: 65–71; 159–164; 233–241; 323–327.

The Lancet Series. 2004. *The Lancet*, 365: 891–900; 977–988; 1087–1098; 1189–1197.

Lele, U., et al. 2007. The changing aid architecture: Can global initiatives eradicate poverty? Retrieved from: www.oecd.org/dataoecd/60/54/37034781.pdf.

Lu, C., et al. 2010. Public funding of health in developing countries: A cross-national systematic analysis. *The Lancet*, 375: 1375–1387.

MCE. 2006. Multi-Country Evaluation of IMCI. Retrieved from: www.who.int/imci-mce/.

MLF. 2011. The Multilateral Fund for the Implementation of the Montreal Protocol. Retrieved from: www.multilateralfund.org/default.aspx.

MSF. 2011a. Campaign for access to essential medicines. Retrieved from: www.accessmed-msf.org.

MSF. 2011b. Untangling the web of antiretroviral price reductions. Retrieved from: http://utw.msfaccess.org/.

National Academies. 2011. *The causes and impacts of neglected tropical and zoonotic diseases: Opportunities for integrated intervention strategies*. Pub: National Academies Press.

OECD. 2011. International development statistics. Retrieved from: www.oecd.org/dataoecd/50/17/5037721.htm.

Oluwole, D., et al. 1999. Management of childhood illness in Africa. *British Medical Journal*, 320: 594–595.

Pelto, G., et al. 2004. Nutrition counseling training changes physician behaviour and improves caregiver knowledge acquisition. *Journal of Nutrition*, 134: 357–362.

Peters, D., et al. 2008. Poverty and access to health care in developing countries. *Annals of the New York Academy of Science*, 1136: 161–171.

PHR. 2000. Reducing maternal and child mortality in Bolivia. Retrieved from: www.healthsystems2020.org/content/resource/detail/811/.

PMNCH. 2010. Decade report (2000–2010): Taking stock of maternal, newborn, and child survival. Retrieved from: www.countdown2015mnch.org/.

PMNCH. 2011. The Partnership for Maternal, Newborn, and Child Health. Retrieved from: www.who.int/pmnch/about/en/.

Safe Motherhood. 2010. Safe Motherhood inter-agency group. Retrieved from: www.safemotherhood.org.

Schellenberg, A., et al. 2004. Effectiveness and costs of facility-based integrated management of childhood illness (IMCI) in Tanzania. *The Lancet*, 364: 1583–1594.

Seear, M. 2004. History's lessons. *Canadian Medical Association Journal*, 171: 1487.

Seear, M., et al. 2011. The need for better data about counterfeit drugs in developing countries. *Journal of Clinical Pharmacology and Therapeutics*, 36: 488–495.

Sidley, P. 2001. Drug companies sue South African government over generics. *British Medical Journal*, 322: 447–450.

StopTB. 2011. The Stop TB partnership. Retrieved from: www.stoptb.org/.

Thompson, K., et al. 2007. Eradication versus control for poliomyelitis: An economic review. *The Lancet*, 369: 1363–1371.

UN. 1994. United Nations International Conference on Population and Development. Retrieved from: www.iisd.ca/cairo.html.

UN. 2011. The Millennium Development Goals. Retrieved from: www.un.org/millenniumgoals/environ.shtml.

UNICEF. 2006. Baby-Friendly Hospital Initiative. Retrieved from: www.unicef.org/programme/breastfeeding/baby.htm.

USAID. 2007. Focused antenatal care: Providing integrated, individualized care during pregnancy. Retrieved from: www.accesstohealth.org/toolres/pdfs/ACCESStechbrief_FANC.pdf.

USAID. 2010. Private delivery care in developing countries: Trends and determinants. Retrieved from: www.measuredhs.com/pubs/pdf/WP76/WP76.pdf.

Uzochukwu, B., et al. 2004. Socio-economic differences and health seeking behaviour: A case study of four local government areas operating the Bamako initiative program in southeast Nigeria. *International Journal of Equity in Health*, 3: 6–12.

Walsh, J., et al. 1979. Selective primary health care: An interim strategy for disease control in developing countries. *New England Journal of Medicine*, 301: 967–974.

WHO. 1987. The 1987 Harare Declaration: Declaration on strengthening district health systems based on primary health care. Retrieved from: whqlibdoc.who.int/hq/1987/WHO_SHS_DHS.pdf.

WHO. 2000. World health report. Health systems: Improving performance. Retrieved from: www.who.int/whr/2000/en/.

WHO. 2003. Managing complications in pregnancy and childbirth. Retrieved from: www.who.int/making_pregnancy_safer/documents/9241545879/en/.

WHO. 2005. World health report 2005—make every mother and child count. Retrieved from: www.who.int/whr/2005/en/.

WHO. 2008. Essential health packages. Draft Technical brief no. 2. Retrieved from: www.who.int/healthsystems/topics/delivery/technical_brief_ehp.pdf.

WHO. 2010. Working to overcome the global impact of neglected tropical diseases. Retrieved from: whqlibdoc.who.int/publications/2010/9789241564090_eng.pdf.

WHO. 2011a. The WHO model list of essential medicines. Retrieved from: whqlibdoc.who.int/hq/2011/a95053_eng.pdf.

WHO. 2011b. Poliomyelitis. Fact sheet no. 114. Retrieved from: www.who.int/mediacentre/factsheets/fs114/en/.

WHO. 2011c. The global program to eliminate lymphatic filariasis. Retrieved from: www.who.int/lymphatic_filariasis/disease/en/.

WHO. 2011d. The alliance for the global elimination of trachoma by 2020. Retrieved from: www.who.int/blindness/causes/trachoma/en/index.html.

WHO. 2011e. Integrated management of childhood illness. Retrieved from: www.who.int/child_adolescent_health/topics/prevention_care/child/imci/en.

WHO. 2016. Government of Nigeria reports 2 wild polio cases, first since July 2014. New cases come on the two-year anniversary since the last confirmed case of polio was reported in Africa. Retrieved from: www.who.int/mediacentre/news/releases/2016/nigeria-polio/en/.

WHO GHE. 2016. World Health Organization Global Health Expenditure database. Retrieved from: http://apps.who.int/nha/database.

Wickware, P. 2002. Resurrecting the resurrection drug. *Nature Medicine,* 8: 908–909.

World Bank. 1993. World development report: Investing in health. Retrieved from: http://go.worldbank.org/66EFVCNW90.

World Bank. 2016. World Development Indicators. Retrieved from: http://data.worldbank.org/indicator/SH.XPD.PCAP.

Xu, K., et al. 2003. Household catastrophic health expenditure: A multi-country analysis. *The Lancet,* 362: 111–117.

CHAPTER 14

Poverty Reduction, Debt Relief, and Economic Growth

The ladder of development hovers overhead, and the poorest of the poor are stuck beneath it. They lack the minimum amount of capital necessary to get a foothold, and therefore need a boost up to the first rung.

—*Jeffrey D. Sachs, The End of Poverty, 2005*

OBJECTIVES

Lack of money and a huge debt burden are major contributors to the misery and ill health that afflict populations throughout the developing world. A good knowledge of both is central to an understanding of global health. Although the statistics concerning the extent of absolute poverty and the size of the developing world debt, discussed in Chapter 5, are quite overwhelming, solutions are available. However, they must be based on careful research specific to that country and the subsequent plans need to be supported over years. Above all, the poor themselves must be given a voice in the solutions to their own problems. This might seem obvious, but it is only within the last 10–15 years that the poor have been given a central place in the debate. After completing this chapter, you should be able to:

- appreciate the central part that poverty relief plays in achieving the broader Sustainable Development Goals (SDGs)
- understand the major methods used to combat poverty
- understand the origins of the current debt relief mechanisms
- understand the controversies surrounding various economic theories of economic growth

INTRODUCTION

Some people think that poor people are lazy. Actually, it takes a lot of work to survive when you are dirt-poor.

—Muhammad Yunus, 2006 Nobel Peace Prize

The first goal of the SDGs is to "end poverty in all its forms everywhere" with the following targets:

- By 2030, eradicate extreme poverty for all people everywhere, currently measured as people living on less than US$1.25 a day
- By 2030, reduce at least by half the proportion of men, women, and children of all ages living in poverty in all its dimensions according to national definitions
- Implement nationally appropriate social protection systems and measures for all, including floors, and by 2030 achieve substantial coverage of the poor and the vulnerable
- By 2030, ensure that all men and women, in particular the poor and the vulnerable, have equal rights to economic resources, as well as access to basic services, ownership and control over land and other forms of property, inheritance, natural resources, appropriate new technology, and financial services, including microfinance
- By 2030, build the resilience of the poor and those in vulnerable situations and reduce their exposure and vulnerability to climate-related extreme events and other economic, social, and environmental shocks and disasters
- Ensure significant mobilization of resources from a variety of sources, including through enhanced development co-operation, in order to provide adequate and predictable means for developing countries, in particular least developed countries, to implement programs and policies to end poverty in all its dimensions
- Create sound policy frameworks at the national, regional, and international levels, based on pro-poor and gender-sensitive development strategies, to support accelerated investment in poverty eradication actions

The first person to study the factors contributing to economic growth was the Scottish philosopher Adam Smith. His book, published in 1776, *An Inquiry into the Nature and Causes of the Wealth of Nations*, tries to answer the obvious question: Why are some countries rich and others poor? His observations on the importance of healthy workers and the role of government are still relevant today. Once some of the features of rich countries are defined, the next step is to transfer those discoveries to poor countries so they can catch up—sounds easy. For the last five or six decades, with varying degrees of success, that is what the aid industry has been trying to do. Unfortunately, while much has been written on the subject, there is still no universal agreement about the place of aid in stimulating economic growth (Doucouliagos et al., 2010). In fact, there are plenty of respected economists who believe that aid actually makes economic growth worse (Moyo, 2009). Despite the vocal group who feel aid (as currently structured) has a negative effect on growth, the increase in development assistance over the last few years presumably indicates that most donor countries feel it is worthwhile.

In practice, most aid is spent on projects that are not likely to show short-term economic returns (immunization programs, food aid, disaster relief, etc.), so economic growth is a poor proxy for aid effectiveness. Aid spent on maternal health should be monitored by measures of maternal health, not GDP per capita. The fact that immunization programs have no short-term economic benefits does not mean they have no value. Aid is not even the main source of money for projects expected to produce economic growth. Alternatives include remittance income, direct foreign investment, export earnings, and bank loans. Aid may be more useful when targeted for technical assistance, specific infrastructure construction, and to help governments develop policies and legislation to support economic growth. Apart from keeping economists occupied, the aid-growth debate has reached its expiry date.

If we bypass the aid effectiveness debate and accept that development assistance, with all its problems, is a necessary part of poverty reduction, there is still further disagreement about the type of pro-growth policies that should be supported. There is, of course, no single formula that will fit the wide variations between different countries, but a broad framework would be a helpful starting point. The "one size fits all" economic reforms, introduced during the era of structural adjustment, were widely viewed as unsuccessful for the simple reason that they were not adjusted for each debtor country's unique circumstances (Birdsall et al., 2011). Clearly, it is better to tailor a set of policies to fit a country's particular needs, but what should those policies be? The list of possibilities is a long one—getting women into the workforce, agricultural extension, higher education, trade reforms, health initiatives, manufacturing zones, new roads and ports, communication technology, etc. Do you concentrate on specific areas that have been shown to work by careful prospective research (Banerjee, 2007) or try to speed things up by using a "big push" shotgun approach and hope that you included the right ones?

Smith was writing at the dawn of the Industrial Revolution, just when economic growth was taking off in England. With the exception of a few discoveries, such as gunpowder and telescopes, the technological achievements of early 18th-century

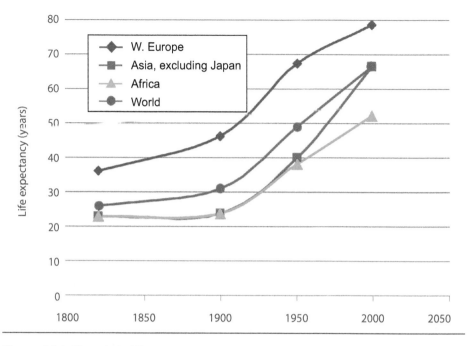

Figure 14.1: Trends in life expectancy for different world regions over the last two centuries

Source: Maddison, A. 2001. The world economy: A millennial perspective. OECD Development Centre. Retrieved from: www.nkeconwatch.com/nk-uploads/theworldeconomy.pdf.

England were little better than those of ancient Rome. The discovery of steam power led to a revolution in transport and manufacturing that allowed unprecedented growth in population and income. Advances in agriculture sustained that growing population. In 200 years, the spread of this new technology allowed life expectancy in the richest countries to increase by 50 years (Figure 14.1) and average world income to increase tenfold (Figure 14.2). Prior to this period, life was much the same everywhere—fairly short and miserable. After the Industrial Revolution, the income of increasingly industrialized nations outstripped those without access to the new technology. Within the last 50 years, an enormous and increasingly prosperous global middle class has narrowed that gap, but the poorest performing countries of sub-Saharan Africa and Asia—Collier's "bottom billion" (Collier, 2007)—have continued to lag far behind.

Despite the advances of the last 50 years, 18–20 percent of the world's population still live in extreme poverty. For many reasons, this situation should be viewed as a global emergency. Apart from the humanitarian impulse to help people living lives of hunger and ill health, there are also pragmatic, selfish reasons to act. Poor countries are at high risk of internal conflict and state failure.

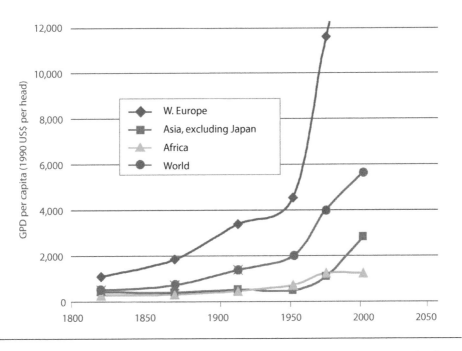

Figure 14.2: Trends in GDP per capita for different world regions over the last two centuries

Source: Maddison, A. 2001. The world economy: A millennial perspective. OECD Development Centre. Retrieved from: www.nkeconwatch.com/nk-uploads/theworldeconomy.pdf.

They are a danger to themselves and surrounding countries and also act as a source of drug and human smuggling, health threats, and environmental disasters—poverty is bad news for everyone. The fundamental solution is economic growth (Dollar et al., 2001). This seemingly simple statement raises a great deal of controversy because of concerns about how that increased wealth gets down to the poorest. Does prosperity trickle down due to invisible market forces that have nothing to do with government policies, or is legislation necessary to make sure the money doesn't end up with elites? Basically, does a rising tide lift all boats or just the yachts? Dollar et al.'s original study showed a tight correlation between growth and poverty reduction, but others found a far looser relationship, implying that the redistribution of wealth is very unequal in some growing countries. China and India are good examples—both have grown rapidly and lifted millions out of poverty. China's initial level of inequality was much lower than India's and its policies appear to have ensured better pro-poor growth, although inequality has worsened in recent years (Ravallion, 2009). The best indicator of unfair economic growth is a country's level of inequality prior to economic growth (Ravallion, 2001).

History will likely be unkind in its assessment of the aid industry's approaches to poverty and debt management between the time of Mexico's payment default in 1982 and the Gleneagles meeting in 2005. Ideologically driven economic interventions were enforced long after it was clear they were a failure. During much of this period, the poor were largely ignored as economic belt-tightening was recommended by short-term consultants. The adverse effects of budget cuts for health, education, or reduced food subsidies fell hardest upon the poor and their children. How many suffered directly or indirectly as a result of these policies over 20 years? No one knows, but it must be measured in many millions. Over the past decade, particularly with the establishment of the MDGs and the Enhanced Heavily Indebted Poor Countries initiative, there has been a growing understanding that improving the lives of the poor must be the primary aim of any long-term economic plan. The poor are important—aid must be targeted toward them and the planning of that aid must include their input at every level. It must be hoped that we are at a new beginning in our approach to the poorest people on this shared planet.

In Chapter 5, we looked at the origins, magnitude, and adverse health effects of general poverty and also the development of the vast debt accumulated by many developing countries. In this chapter, we'll examine the practical side of these issues. What can be done to help? Poverty alleviation and, to a lesser extent, debt relief have attracted decades of research, analysis, and commentary, but it is only surprisingly recently that significant and measurable progress has been made with either. Making significant gains against endemic poverty is a slow process and, like any economic topic, there is no shortage of arguments about the best method to use. However, a few things are certain—poverty relief must be based on clear plans sustained over many years and should be combined, when possible, with improvements in human rights. Significant attempts to reduce the developing world's debt have also been slow to develop and have been influenced more by ideology than serious outcome analysis. The extraordinary level of worldwide popular support for the topic of debt relief helped to influence rich G8 countries to make significant debt concessions at the 2005 Gleneagles G8 meeting, but there is still a long way to go!

POVERTY ALLEVIATION

> To give aid to every poor man is far beyond the reach and power of every man. Care of the poor is incumbent on society as a whole.
>
> *—Baruch de Spinoza, 1677*

Although poverty is an inevitable common denominator contributing to the ill health of developing world populations, this is not by any means the full story.

As mentioned before, the origins of that poverty usually lie within some form of social injustice. The causes vary depending on the country, but whenever there is widespread poverty, there is also usually obvious oppression or discrimination (Feachem, 2000). Clearly, long-term sustainable solutions are very difficult unless there are accompanying improvements in any underlying social inequity. Unfortunately, large-scale shifts in society occur slowly. However, while the social wheels are turning, there are approaches that can be used to make the burden of poverty more bearable. This section will examine some of the major means of reducing poverty. Whatever initiative is used, planners must always remember that benefits are measured in years; quick fixes do not exist. Effective programs must be based on careful research relevant to the specific country and backed by long-term commitments of money and skilled assistance (Sachs, 2005).

Figure 14.1 shows how health benefits (assessed by life expectancy) slowly accumulate in different world regions after prolonged and consistent pro-poor economic growth. It is important to note that the operative word is "slowly," which is significant. Improvements are measured in decades. After implementing sustainable projects aimed at access to health and education for the poor, plus an emphasis on economic growth, it later becomes difficult to tell which developments are "cause" and which are "effect." Better-educated and healthier parents have better-educated and healthier children. The process grinds on, slowly gathering speed until, many years later, there is a generation of healthy children who can barely believe the deprivations that their grandparents and great-grandparents suffered through. The results of development work take a long time to bear fruit, which is one of many reasons why short-term projects are of value only to the participants.

It should always be remembered that all the current wealthy countries have been through a period when their standards of health and living conditions were no different from those of any of today's developing countries. That is all the more reason why they should be keen to help poor countries climb out of poverty—not through the obligation of charity, but out of a sense of shared past experience. The following initiatives all include increased prosperity as a major end point.

Pro-Poor Growth

> In a state that is desirous of being saved from the greatest of all plague, there should exist among the citizens neither extreme poverty nor again excessive wealth.
>
> —*Plato, Laws, 5th century bc*

Buckle up before driving through this topic; the literature is extensive, technical, and very contentious (Eastwood et al., 2000). This section addresses the simple question:

Is economic growth automatically good for the poorest section of that country's society, or does increased prosperity simply increase inequality, i.e., the rich get richer, but the poor stay the same (Fuentes, 2005)? This debate is a common one, particularly among those who study the broader effects of global markets. It is generally accepted that all developing countries that have achieved sustained economic growth over the last two or three decades have also reduced their absolute poverty levels (PGRP, 2005). Measures of economic disparity within a country, such as the Gini index, remain relatively stable over long periods, showing that economic growth is distributed throughout all segments of a population—not always equally—but at least some of that prosperity eventually trickles down to the poorest (Dollar et al., 2001).

The arguments begin once the types of economic growth are analyzed. For many years, the emphasis of the major international financial institutes was upon pure economic growth. This wasn't growth at the expense of the poor, it was growth that didn't even acknowledge that the poor existed. The topic of structural adjustment policies is central to the development of pro-poor policies because it was largely their failure that prompted current policies aimed at poverty reduction. Starting around 1980, the increasing inability of poor countries to meet their international debt repayments gave the IMF and World Bank an unusual degree of influence over the internal economic policies of many developing countries. Both institutions increasingly tied their loans to a range of interventions that came to

Box 14.1 History Notes

Norman Borlaug (1914–2009)

Norman Borlaug was one of the major scientists of the 20th century, but his name is not well known. He was awarded the Nobel Peace Prize in 1970 for his central role in the agricultural advances that, collectively, are called the Green Revolution. He was born in a small Norwegian-American town and was educated in a small one-room school. He saw the reality of widespread hunger during the Depression in the US and this shaped his future research interests. After training as a plant pathologist and geneticist, he helped establish a wheat research program in Mexico with Rockefeller Foundation support. After making thousands of plant crossings, the research laboratory developed higher-yield, disease-resistant strains. In 20 years, these new cultivars allowed Mexico to go from an importer to an exporter of grain. The improved yields and resistance of crops developed in the centre (later including maize and rice) have spread better nutrition and prosperity across large parts of the developing world, particularly India and other Asian countries. Borlaug's discoveries have been credited with saving a billion lives! Due to these advances, from 1950 onwards, Malthaus was proved wrong—annual increase in food production exceeded population growth without increasing the area planted. Follow the reference for more information, including recent criticism of the Green Revolution: Norman Borlaug Heritage Foundation (2011).

be called structural adjustment policies (SAPs) (Ismi, 2004). Unfortunately, SAPs often included belt-tightening policies, such as reduced food subsidies and cuts in education and health budgets. Unfortunately, it wasn't the expensive external consultants whose belts were being tightened. The biggest criticism of the "adjustment" years is that there is little or no evidence to suggest that these interventions were beneficial and plenty to suggest they were measurably harmful (Easterly, 2001).

Beginning with an influential early critique by UNICEF (1987), criticism of structural adjustments slowly grew. Two of the most vocal opponents were actually senior staff of the World Bank. The Bank's chief economist, Josef Stiglitz (subsequent Nobel Prize winner), criticized imposed economic restructuring and said that the policy had failed (Stiglitz, 2002). He resigned over the issue in 1999. Another of the World Bank's senior economists, William Easterly, has written a series of well-known books critical of aid policies; he also parted company with the World Bank over his opinions (Easterly, 2002). As we shall see later in this chapter, the IMF and the World Bank slowly softened their approach. The current Poverty Reduction Strategy was a response to this criticism, so it is important to understand the history. The poor are now included in a country's long-term economic restructuring plan. Is the World Bank turning into a soft and cuddly organization staffed by aging hippies? Perhaps not, but a recent chief economist, Francois Bourguignon, published extensively on the need for reducing inequality by redistributing profits (Bourguignon, 2003).

It is important to remember that the effects of economic policy changes are complex and, of course, unexpected adverse effects will inevitably fall upon the poorest of a country's population. Relationships between trade legislation, tax reform, privatization of public utilities, cost-recovery strategies, and their ultimate effects upon poverty are endlessly complex. Writing at a time when Europe is on the edge of a recession, it is clear that we don't know how to stop our own developed countries from swinging in and out of recession, so our attempts to meddle with other countries should be tempered by some degree of humility and care. An investigation by an independent organization has been cautiously optimistic about the process of poverty restructuring strategies in developing countries (Driscoll et al., 2005).

It has taken a long time for the topic of income inequality to enter the aid-growth debate (Beck et al., 2004). Directly targeting the poor involves redistributing wealth. This concept has proved rather too socialist for some tastes. The subject was certainly not openly discussed during the years of the Cold War—perhaps that is why the euphemism "pro-poor growth" is applied to the concept rather than "economic redistribution." As usual, the term needs defining since it means different things to different people. For some, pro-poor growth means that the poor should, at the very least, have the same growth as the rest of the country. Others accept the term only if the poor are growing faster than the national average. There is no

framework for pro-poor growth that works in all cases, but the Canadian government's priorities include: a focus on private business, agricultural development,
education at all levels, improved health of working people, improved living conditions and sanitation, and access to affordable transport and energy (CIDA, 2011).

Microfinancing

> When combined with information and communication technologies, micro-credit can
> unleash new opportunities for the world's poorest entrepreneurs and thereby revitalize
> the village economies they serve.
>
> *—Madeleine Albright, 2004*

When it comes to financial services, such as access to credit, savings accounts,
money transfers, and insurance, the needs of the poor are no different from those
of the rich—they just have less money to pay for those services. Without these
services, small savings have to be converted into livestock or jewellery. Houses and
possessions cannot be insured, and remittances from overseas are reduced by high
service charges. Since remittance income now greatly exceeds foreign aid volumes,
this is a particularly important issue. In the absence of credit facilities, the poor can
obtain money only through moneylenders, who usually charge high rates, or from

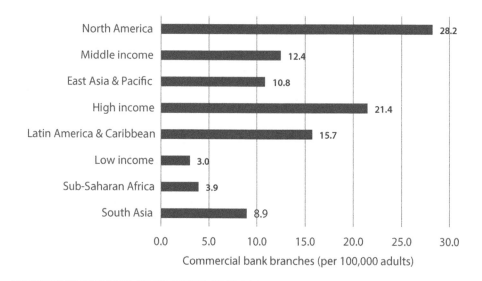

Figure 14.3: Access to banking, measured by commercial bank branches (per
100,000 adults) for different regions of the world; contrasting high- vs. low-
income countries

Source: World Bank. 2016. World Development Indicators. Retrieved from: http://databank.worldbank.
org/data/reports.aspx?source=2&series=FB.CBK.BRCH.P5&country.

pawnshops. In fact, the oldest financial institution in North or South America is a pawnshop on Mexico City Central Square, established in 1775 by the Spanish Crown. Access to credit is important for economic growth at all levels of society. For example, there is a close relationship between access to bank accounts and a country's income level (Figure 14.3). While micro-credit schemes attract most attention, it is important to remember that the poor need access to the full range of conventional banking services.

After small starts in the early 1970s, so-called microfinance or micro-credit schemes have gained in popularity to the point that they are now considered a major means of helping the poorest to escape their poverty. The first on the scene was probably Opportunity International, a non-profit NGO, which began lending small amounts in 1971 to the poor of Colombia. ACCION International made its first loans in Brazil, followed by the Grameen Bank in 1976 in Bangladesh (Grameen Bank, 2011). Its founder, Muhammad Yunus, was a professor of economics at Chittagong University. He started lending money to the poor in local

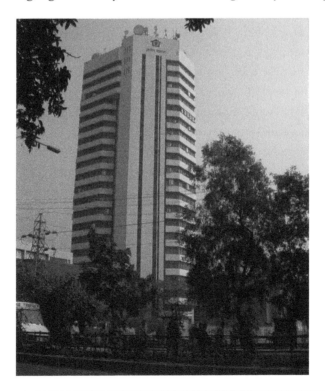

Photo 14.1: The Grameen Bank is now one of the biggest buildings in Dhaka, Bangladesh. The organization has come a very long way from Professor Yunus's first small loans made to local people around Chittagong in the early 1970s.

Source: Photo courtesy of Wikimedia Commons.

villages in an attempt to protect them from loan sharks. The idea caught on! The bank now employs over 20,000 people and has branches throughout Bangladesh (Photo 14.1). To date, it has loaned billions of dollars to poor people. His autobiography is essential reading (Yunus, 2003). He has been awarded numerous international prizes, including the 2006 Nobel Peace Prize. He was recently edged out of the bank through what looked like political jealousy, but he still has plenty to do. The broader Grameen group has helped introduce microfinance around the world, including a pilot project in the US. Grameen is also involved in businesses for the poor, ranging from fisheries to cellphones.

The early micro-credit model was often based on forming the lenders into groups, which had to meet at regular intervals. Hard collateral was replaced by the social pressures from within a group. Clearly, this was not a flexible model for individuals. As time passed, services such as savings, financial transfers, and insurance have grown. Banking services more recently resemble a conventional commercial bank except that they exist for the poor. Banco Sol in Bolivia is one example in Latin America. Using small loans, families can begin projects like drying fish or selling kerosene. Large loans up to US$200 can be used to start a small store, buy fertilizers and seed, or buy a bull for breeding. Once a small lender establishes a loan repayment history, then larger loans become available.

Although micro-credit has an established place in aid projects, there is surprisingly little hard epidemiological and research data on their operations and outcomes. Types of lending institutions are so broad that there are no accurate statistics for their numbers. They are certainly measured in the tens of thousands; obviously some are good and, equally, some are bad. One sign of the increased importance of banking for the poor is the emergence of rating agencies that provide relatively objective measures of different banks (M-CRIL, 2011). Microfinancing is now profitable enough that it has even attracted large commercial banks over the last few years (USAID, 2005).

High-Quality Education for All

> Education is not the filling of a pail but the lighting of a fire.
>
> —*Unknown*

Lack of education is not the only factor that keeps poor people poor and unhealthy, but it is certainly a major contributor. From numerous perspectives, educating children (and removing gender disparity in education) has endless measurable advantages. Education raises economic productivity, lowers infant mortality, improves the nutritional status and health of adults and children, reduces poverty, and helps control the spread of HIV/AIDS and other diseases. Lack of education is particularly harmful for girls. Along with immunization, education initiatives produce the best "bang" for a development "buck." Not surprisingly, the SDGs include a new global education goal (SDG 4) to ensure inclusive and equitable quality education and promote lifelong learning opportunities for all. The goal has seven targets and three means of implementation:

- By 2030, ensure that all girls and boys complete free, equitable, and quality primary and secondary education leading to relevant and effective learning outcomes
- By 2030, ensure that all girls and boys have access to quality early childhood development, care, and pre-primary education so that they are ready for primary education
- By 2030, ensure equal access for all women and men to affordable and quality technical, vocational, and tertiary education, including university
- By 2030, substantially increase the number of youth and adults who have relevant skills, including technical and vocational skills, for employment, decent jobs, and entrepreneurship
- By 2030, eliminate gender disparities in education and ensure equal access to all levels of education and vocational training for the vulnerable, including persons with disabilities, indigenous peoples, and children in vulnerable situations
- By 2030, ensure that all youth and a substantial proportion of adults, both men and women, achieve literacy and numeracy
- By 2030, ensure that all learners acquire the knowledge and skills needed to promote sustainable development, including, among others, through education for sustainable development and sustainable lifestyles, human rights, gender equality, promotion of a culture of peace and non-violence, global citizenship, and appreciation of cultural diversity and of culture's contribution to sustainable development
- Build and upgrade education facilities that are child, disability, and gender sensitive and provide safe, non-violent, inclusive, and effective learning environments for all
- By 2020, substantially expand globally the number of scholarships available to developing countries, in particular least developed countries, small island developing States, and African countries, for enrolment in higher education, including vocational training and information and communications technology, technical, engineering, and scientific programs, in developed countries and other developing countries

- By 2030, substantially increase the supply of qualified teachers, including through international co-operation for teacher training in developing countries, especially least developed countries and small island developing States

Significant progress has been made, particularly in primary school enrolment and gender disparity in the last 15 years (Figure 14.4). The number of children missing from school is below 100 million for the first time since records were kept. In developing countries, participation in education rose to 82 percent in 2013 as opposed to 62 percent in 2000. There are numerous explanations for the incomplete progress, but they should not disguise the fact that well-intentioned countries can make huge improvements in the face of very difficult circumstances. Uganda and Afghanistan have both greatly increased their enrolment and reduced gender disparity despite considerable obstacles.

Good-quality education is expensive and the benefits take years to appear, but it is worth the wait. India's first Nobel laureate, Rabindranath Tagore, came from a rich family, but he was an enlightened man. He wrote extensively on the subjects of poverty and education. In 1901, he established a school (Santiniketan). Many years later, a young child called Amartya Sen received his first basic schooling there. He went on to make significant contributions to the field of poverty research, for which he was also awarded a Nobel Prize.

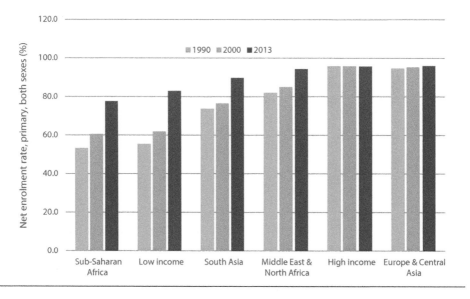

Figure 14.4: Trends in primary school enrolment between 1990 and 2013 in different world regions

Source: World Bank. 2016b. World Development Indicators. Retrieved from: http://databank.worldbank.org/data/reports.aspx?source=2&series=SE.PRM.NENR&country.

In the Philippines, a mobile teaching program for poor families in the remote northern areas is designed to address the same problems. Only 50 years ago in Canada, remote rural communities received some of their education from mobile schools transported there by rail. In Brazil, voucher systems have been introduced, aimed at allowing poor children to attend schools that have extra capacity (Denes, 2003). In some areas, this has been part of a larger scheme to reduce the number of children who have to work to support their families (called Bolsa Escola). The family is paid as long as the child stays in school. Although there are many ways to expose poor children to education, they all share the same basic premise—equitable education is the fundamental foundation upon which all other poverty alleviation interventions must be built.

The problems of providing education to poor people are identical to those found in providing adequate health care. The only approach that appears to work is to decentralize education, and place management and administration of the bulk of funding in the hands of local people. Several models exist around the world. In Bangladesh, the Bangladesh Rural Advancement Committee (BRAC, 2011) runs a non-formal primary education program that has now grown to be the largest education group in the world. Its founder, Sir Fazle Abed, appears to have much in common with another Bangladeshi, Professor Yunus. From very small beginnings, his organization has grown into an international aid agency that provides assistance to many developing countries. Administration of their schools is provided by village management committees and parent-teachers' associations. Most teachers are women and at least half of the pupils are girls. Accommodation is usually modest, with earth floors and basic teaching materials.

Agricultural Improvement

> I know of no pursuit in which more real and important services can be rendered to any country than by improving its agriculture.
>
> —*George Washington, 1794*

Until recently, agricultural improvement has received less emphasis than it deserves. In prosperous countries, fewer than 20 percent of the population live in rural areas. This fraction rises steadily in poorer countries until in the very poorest countries agriculture provides employment for most of the population (Figure 14.5). In Africa, agriculture provides employment for 60–70 percent of the population. It produces half of the exports and an equally significant proportion of the gross national income. Clearly, any improvement in agricultural output is the ideal form of pro-poor growth. It benefits the country, but also disproportionately improves life for the rural

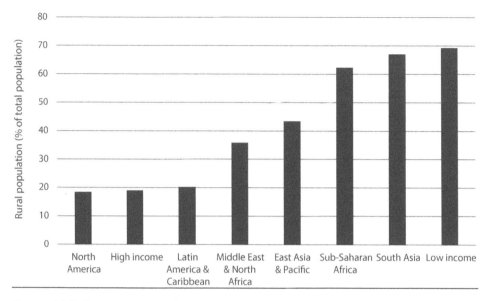

Figure 14.5: Percentage of the population living in rural areas, by region

Source: World Bank. 2016c. World Development Indicators. Retrieved from: http://data.worldbank.org/indicator/SP.RUR.TOTL.ZS.

poor. It has been shown that a 1 percent increase in agricultural yield can reduce severe poverty by between 0.6 and 1.2 percent (Irz et al., 2001). During the 1960s and 1970s, the introduction of high-yield seeds pioneered by Dr. Norman Borlaug, combined with modern farming methods, produced a revolution in food production throughout India and South Asia, now widely called the Green Revolution. Since that time, annual food production has continued to outpace population growth even though the total area under cultivation has declined (Davies, 2003). For many reasons, particularly the shortage of irrigation, these advances could not be adopted in sub-Saharan Africa. Newer discoveries in agricultural techniques, particularly in dry land farming and the development of new seeds, now mean that those advances can be applied to areas of the world with less reliable water supplies, such as sub-Saharan Africa and Central Asia (Djurfeldt et al., 2005).

Repeating the Green Revolution in Africa and Central Asia would pay huge dividends in economic growth, but it is a complex and difficult task (Dawson et al., 2016). Some of the many obstacles include access for the poor to land and water, investment for rural road upgrades, storage and distribution facilities, irrigation, and farm machinery. The problems are further complicated by adverse national agricultural policies, international trade barriers, and low commodity prices. Taken together, agricultural improvement can hardly be viewed as an instant solution. However, it is a vital step and these problems are individually manageable.

International aid agencies such as the British Department of International Development are already showing a renewed interest in investment in agriculture (DFID, 2003). There is also a growing international emphasis on the need to liberalize agricultural trade, particularly in the European Union and North America.

The principal requirements are:

- *Land reform:* Ownership or, at very least, secure lease of good, productive land
- *Financial services:* Micro-credit to cover seasonal costs, and insurance services to reduce risks caused by crop failures
- *Agricultural services:* Access to affordable seeds, fertilizer, plus irrigation and machinery, all backed up by expert education

None of these tasks is easy, but if sustained investment can be assured, then it is possible that the Green Revolution, with all of its extended benefits, could be reproduced in some of the poorest parts of the world. The World Bank's 2008 report on agriculture's place in development is essential reading (World Bank, 2008).

Trade Liberalization and Aid for Trade

> The problem is that the human development potential inherent in trade is diminished by a combination of unfair rules and structural inequalities within and between countries.
>
> —*UNDP, Human Development Report, 2005*

Over three-quarters of the world's poor obtain their small income from agriculture. Most of the remainder work in labour-intensive sweatshops in one form or another. Output from these industries must confront an indescribably complex set of national and international tariffs and trade barriers that affect every single exported item. A much-quoted example of the complexities of trade is the effect of enforced trade liberalization upon rice farmers. During the structural adjustment policy era, the IMF and the World Bank often attached conditions to developing countries asking for loans. In 1995, for example, the IMF induced Haiti to cut its import rice tariff from 35 percent to 3 percent, with the result that rice imports increased greatly over the next decade. Although urban Haitian consumers obtained a small benefit from the drop in imported rice cost, the indigenous Haitian rice growers suffered greatly through loss of a market. The only clear winners were the major rice exporters in the United States (Oxfam, 2005).

What is the best course in such a complex situation? Local consumers need affordable food, but local producers also need to survive. In a strong market economy,

---

Box 14.2 Moment of Insight

Bellagio Study Group's estimate of the cost to save 6 million children's lives every year by implementing known effective therapies:	Canadian population 34.5 million
	Per capita daily cost for Canada to meet Bellagio Study Group's recommendations:
US$5.1 billion	**40 cents**

Source: Bryce, J., et al. Can the world afford to save the lives of 6 million children each year? *The Lancet*, 365(2005): 2193–2200.

---

the attitude would be that rice farmers should become competitive. While they modernize in response to external pressures, the country can rely on a host of other manufacturing areas for income. In a poor country reliant on only a few agricultural products, overnight changes to tariffs can be a disaster. There aren't other producers able to carry the country while agriculture modernizes. Under those circumstances, important local producers are preferentially supported and the poor get high food prices. Among the lessons learned from the economic success of China and India is that trade liberalization must be a stepwise process. It took developed economies many decades to open their markets and developing countries are no different. There are no overnight changes that will produce economic success.

Although large countries like China, Brazil, and India can make economic gains from selling to their enormous internal markets, it is generally believed that for long-term economic growth, a country needs to manufacture goods and then trade those products internationally (ODI, 2010). A country's manufacturing base must first be ensured before slowly liberalizing trade barriers. This was the approach used by China and India. It certainly worked for them, so the aid industry has hopped on the bandwagon and designed its current approach to economic growth around this general model. The result is called aid for trade (AfT) and it has become a major part of the aid framework over the last decade. It was first raised as a specific issue at the 2002 Monterrey conference on financing for development (WFTO, 2009). Prior to this time, efforts had largely been aimed at optimizing trade policy and regulations, referred to as trade-related technical assistance. This narrow form of AfT, based largely on legislative reform, was tied to success in the world trade talks.

Although the worst examples of unfair trade have improved over the last few years, the international trade playing field can hardly be described as level. For example, the Common Agricultural Policy (CAP) is a system of subsidies for Europe's farmers. Agricultural subsidies are currently above US$350 billion per year in Europe alone. The result is an artificial reduction in the true cost of producing foods such as sugar, milk, soya beans, maize, poultry, and cattle. Unrealistically cheap surpluses can then be dumped on any country that does not have tariff restrictions to protect its own farmers. It should be added that cumulative advances in trade have made this debate less relevant than it might have been 10 years ago. Trade barriers are of importance only once there are goods to trade—manufacturing is now the emphasis. As with any economic debate, opinions differ.

Trying to obtain an agreement that covers all the trade barriers on all the imported and exported goods in all of the countries of the world seems a rather optimistic task. In 2001, the World Trade Organization (WTO) weighed into this mess with the optimistic hope of sorting out everything, including subsidies on agriculture; non-agricultural market access (NAMA, which includes everything from gem production to industrial goods); access to services like electric power, health care, and education; and trade-related intellectual poverty rights (TRIPS). The first round of talks was held in Doha, Qatar in 2001. The subsequent negotiations are called the Doha Development Agenda (DDA). The first talks in Doha, unfortunately, reached no agreement and produced considerable friction. After two years, another attempt was made with a meeting in Cancun. The outcome in Cancun was even worse—talks collapsed after a few days. Europe (particularly led by France), Japan, and the United States pressed for trade liberalization, while increasingly influential developing countries insisted upon protection for their young industries.

The WTO looked for a while as if it would collapse into smaller interest groups, such as the so-called G20 (large developing countries led by China, India, Brazil, and South Africa), the G90 (a group of the least-developed countries), the Africa-Caribbean and Pacific Group (ACP), and the African group. Up to this point, almost nothing had been achieved except for one small agreement under the TRIPS heading that allowed developing countries to import cheap generic versions of anti-HIV drugs. Some agreements on agricultural subsidies were reached in Hong Kong in 2005, but the most important development was that the WTO endorsed the development of more comprehensive AfT initiatives. The Doha process came to a halt in Geneva in 2008 over unresolved issues between Brazil, India, and the US. The topic, once again, was agricultural subsidies. The talks have not subsequently been restarted.

The expanded form of AfT recommended by the WTO task force goes beyond trade policy and regulations and includes investment in trade-related infrastructure, building production capacity, and technical assistance to help countries plan a suitable trade policy. A good example of the application of sequenced growth is provided by Mauritius. Since independence, it has gone from a poor nation dependent on agriculture (principally sugar) to a middle-income country with a current growth rate of 4.0 percent, life expectancy of 75 years, and GDP per capita of US$14,000. The country started with a preferential sugar export agreement with Europe. The income was invested in textile manufacturing (they do not have an army). The profits from the textile export processing zone were then invested into a diversified economy. This was backed by a stable government and suitable support for health and sanitation improvements. It is now an increasingly prosperous middle-income country with many lessons for other countries with similar starting points.

Human Rights Legislation

> Where, after all, do universal human rights begin? In small places close to home. Such as the places where every man, woman and child seeks equal justice, equal opportunity, equal dignity, without discrimination.
>
> —*Eleanor Roosevelt, 1948*

Over the last two decades, research has increasingly shown that poor people are not just short of money, they are short of everything that even remotely resembles the basic needs for a restful life. Quite apart from hunger and ill health, poverty carries with it feelings of helplessness and constant fear. At first glance, human rights legislation might not seem to be closely related to poverty alleviation, but it is, in fact, an absolutely necessary foundation. No agricultural interventions are possible until the poor have guaranteed access to land and water rights. Similarly, fair employment initiatives require protective labour laws. A community cannot take full part in any large-scale initiative until everyone feels free in terms of religious observance and has access to fair legal process, effective property laws, and protection from corrupt state officials. Women and children are particularly at risk of abuse and require specific human rights legislation tailored to their unique needs (Foresti et al., 2010).

This is an area where legislation acts as a catalyst to speed up changes and improve the general sense of safety that the poor experience. Numerous historical examples exist demonstrating the value of human rights legislation in the gradual improvement in health for populations of currently developed countries. In the United Kingdom, infant mortality in 1900 was as bad as it is in any developing country today. Infant mortality has fallen steadily in the subsequent century for many reasons, but at least part of the solution was the consistent series of legislation aimed at improving access to health for the poor (Figure 14.6), such as the Midwives Act in 1902, the National Insurance Act in 1911, the Poor Law in 1927, the Family Allowance Act in 1945, and the National Health Service Act in 1946.

The vital importance of legislated human rights is exemplified by the United Nations. Human rights were emphasized in that organization's founding charter shortly after World War II, and its first major international success was the

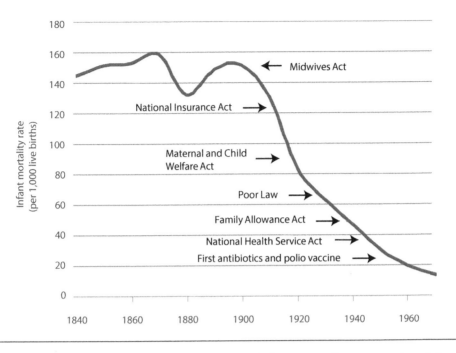

Figure 14.6: Historical relationship between infant mortality rate and social legislation in the United Kingdom

Source: McKeown, T. 1980. *The role of medicine: Dream, mirage, or nemesis?* Pub: Princeton University Press.

adoption of the Universal Declaration on Human Rights in 1948 (Photo 14.2). This was later followed by two further covenants on human rights, adopted in 1966. Together, these now comprise the International Bill of Rights, which has had a profound effect upon the constitutions and laws of many countries around the world. Other major human rights achievements have been the agreement on the basic rights of all children in 1990 and the formal establishment of an international criminal court in 2002. Even the Human Rights Commission itself became a victim of the move toward decent behaviour. It lost all credibility by allowing membership to countries with terrible records of human rights violations. It was replaced by the smaller Human Rights Council.

Of course, lip service to legislation is of no use without the will to enforce that legislation. For example, the new South African constitution is an enlightened document that enshrines the rights of women, yet on a daily basis women are exposed to abuse, violence, and rape throughout that country's informal settlements. Legislated protection for the poor and the weakest members of society is an essential foundation on which prosperity can be built. The topic is important; the whole of Chapter 15 is devoted to the subject of establishing civil and peaceful society.

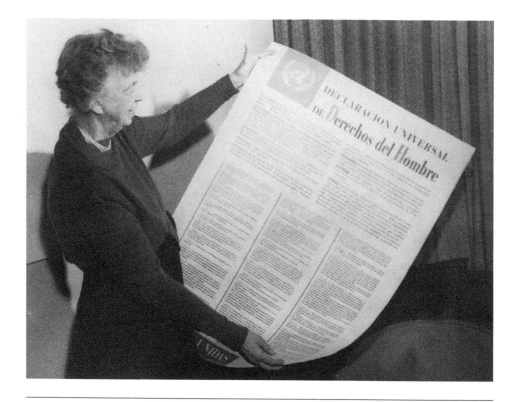

Photo 14.2: This famous image from 1949 shows the former first lady, Eleanor Roosevelt, holding a Spanish version of the United Nations' Universal Declaration of Human Rights.

Source: Photo courtesy of Wikimedia Commons.

Other Elements of Pro-Poor Growth

Access to Energy

One of the reasons that the Industrial Revolution started in Britain was the abundant supply of coal to power the new technology of steam engines. No meaningful growth can occur without an affordable power supply. Energy is needed for household cooking, lighting, and heating; to power small industries and enterprises; to run health centres; to light schools; to power communication technologies; and to fuel transport systems. Renewable energy can play an important role in meeting these development challenges, especially in rural areas where access to grid electricity is a distant prospect. The poorest people who need power the most are the very ones that don't have it—probably well over a billion people have only limited access to any form of power other than firewood. As renewable energy technology becomes more affordable, emerging markets are developing local capacity. For example, China, India, and

Brazil all have homegrown markets for biofuels and wind power. In volcanic areas of Africa, pilot plants for geothermal energy production exist in Kenya and Ethiopia.

Extensions to an electricity grid are expensive—roughly US$15,000–$20,000 per kilometre. High cost and low demand mean that it will take a long time before rural areas can rely on grid electricity. Local alternatives exist to serve small users or a local village user grid. These include solar home systems, small hydro-power generators linked to a village grid, biofuel generators, and wind pumps. These all have the advantage that they use available energy sources (wind, water, sun, and biomass). The recent moves by the private sector to provide services to the poor have meant that private-sector power generation is becoming more common. India currently stands fifth in the world as a generator of wind-powered electricity—almost all is generated by private companies (OECD, 2008).

Affordable Transport

Safe and affordable transport is an essential requirement for economic growth. Efficient transport greatly reduces agricultural marketing costs—agricultural improvements will not occur unless farmers can get their crops to distant markets without spoiling. Transport also allows them to bring in seeds and fertilizer more cheaply, and it helps the family access health care and their children to get to school. The benefits of improved transport are enormous and can be measured in terms of agricultural output, child education, and reduced maternal mortality. Investments in roads pay large dividends. Development agencies have adopted rural accessibility as a reliable indicator of economic growth and poverty reduction. For example, the World Bank uses the proportion of rural people living within 2 km of an all-season road as a measure of transport's contribution to achieving the MDGs. It is also important to remember that by 2020, half the world's population will live in cities, so the efficiency of urban transport is also vital. In a large city, huge numbers of products and passengers must be moved every day. Clearly, from village to large city, efficient transport is an essential requirement for a country's future.

With the spread of global markets, it is necessary to plan transport on a regional basis. For efficient movement of goods, people, and ideas, intercity travel must be facilitated. Large urban areas must also be connected to their food source in the rural regions in order to keep food prices down and limit the need for imports. On that topic, neighbours must also co-operate in common transport plans to improve access to local markets and seaports to improve both regional and international trade. Planning at this level requires a lot more than roads and must include harmonized customs operations in order to reduce delays and transport costs. Transportation systems are complex. They not only facilitate the movement of people and goods, but also have wide-ranging impacts on land use, economic growth, and quality of life (SSATP, 2009).

The Private Sector

The term "bottom of the pyramid," or BoP, is used in economics to describe the poorest socio-economic group. In global terms, the poorest people have very little, but they form a very large group of consumers. The more than 2 billion people who live on less than US$2.50 per day are now viewed as a business opportunity by the private sector. The book *The Fortune at the Bottom of the Pyramid* by C. Prahalad popularized the notion that there are profits to be made serving the needs of the poor. If such businesses are built around local people, then local benefits of economic growth can be found. The idea is catching on and tends to be described by the term "market-based solutions" (Monitor, 2011). Employing the poor to work in businesses aimed at the poor is the most direct form of pro-poor growth.

Starting a business in a very poor area with tiny profit margins is not an easy undertaking. As experience is gained, it seems likely that a completely new business model will need to be developed in order to turn a profit. There will be a good deal of trial and error, but there are already success stories to study:

- *Voltic Cool Pac:* Ghana's leading drinking water producer developed 500 mL sachets for low-income consumers: they sell for 3 cents. With such a small profit margin, the company had to develop a decentralized production process. They use local street hawkers to sell the sachets. They currently employ nearly 10,000 hawkers and sell 480,000 sachets every day (Supply Chain, 2011).
- *Jeppe College of Commerce and Computer Studies:* The Jeppe schools in South Africa offer narrow courses aimed at unemployed high school graduates looking for jobs in service industries. They cover expected payment defaults by accepting both poor and middle-income students. They also offer job placement assistance. They currently serve about 700,000 students (JCCCS, 2010).
- *Afro-Ki:* This company provides storage, processing, and transport for agricultural produce in Uganda. They serve 7,000 small farmers and are able to guarantee a forward price and timely payment. They provide seeds at a subsidized rate, allowing a significant increase in farm profits (Masakure et al., 2005).
- *Kilimo Salama:* This Kenyan company sells agricultural insurance to poor farmers who have little money to spare for extra protection. The insurance is sold by local fertilizer suppliers that the farmers trust and is usually bundled with the fertilizer costs. They currently serve 11,000 farmers (Kilimo Salama, 2011).

Healthy Workers: The Pro-Poor Health Approach

Is poverty caused by widespread ill health or is ill health the result of poverty? Obviously the correct answer is *yes*. Either way, healthy workers are a necessary component of economic growth. That does not imply that the only reason for health initiatives is to get people to work more efficiently. Health is a basic human right, so health projects are an end in themselves. However, if one of the intangible results of improved health happens to be prosperity, then that's a fair side effect to accept. The importance of health as a driver of prosperity was first emphasized in a report by the WHO's Commission on Macroeconomics and Health, chaired by Professor Sachs (WHO, 2002). The commission pointed out numerous links between health and economic development:

- *Increased productivity:* Healthy workers are more productive, miss less work, and, consequently, tend to earn more money.
- *Higher investment:* Higher productivity attracts more investment in local industry. A country considered safe from malaria and other diseases is more attractive to external companies and their employees.
- *Cycle of health:* Healthy children go to school regularly. Educated children ultimately earn more money and as adults, they have healthier children themselves.
- *Family savings:* Healthy adults earn more, save more, and set aside cash for capital projects such as housing improvements.
- *Behavioural changes:* Numerous unpredictable benefits result from improved education. The results are often difficult to explain, but they are real. For example, educated girls have lower teen pregnancy rates, lower fertility rates, and healthier, heavier children.

THE DEVELOPMENT OF THE MODERN DEBT RELIEF MECHANISM

Like some physicians, we were too busy—and too sure of ourselves—to listen to patients with their own ideas. Too busy, sometimes, even to look at the individual countries and their circumstances. The economists and development experts of the Third World, many of them brilliant and highly educated, were sometimes treated like children. Our bedside manner was dreadful; and, as one patient after another couldn't help noticing, the medicine we dispensed abroad was, in important aspects, not really the same stuff we drank at home.

—*J. Stiglitz, Globalization and its Discontents, 2004*

The history of the developing world debt is covered in detail in Chapter 5. This section looks at the international response to the debt crisis after it finally came to a head in 1982 with Mexico's default on its debt service payments. This was the first global financial disaster since 1929, so there was a great deal of debate about the best way to respond. Not surprisingly, there was a good deal of trial and error before

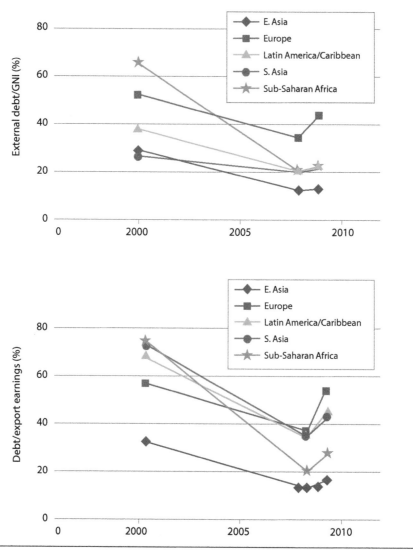

Figure 14.7: Recent trends in debt ratios for various regions of the world. Top: external debt/gross national income. Bottom: external debt/export earnings. The financial crisis of 2008 produced a measurable deterioration in all regions.

Source: World Bank. 2011b. Debt sustainability framework for low-income countries (DSF). Retrieved from: http://go.worldbank.org/A5VFXZCCW0.

a workable plan finally emerged. Each successive step—from structural adjustment policies to the Heavily Indebted Poor Countries Initiatives to Gleneagles and the Multilateral Debt Relief Initiative—built on its predecessors, so it is important to understand the history of this process. Current debt relief initiatives have produced measurable improvements in the debt ratios of the poorest countries. The indices for sub-Saharan African countries are now far better than those of developed European countries (Figure 14.7). The debt service costs/export earnings in many African countries are now below 5 percent, so while there is room for progress, the debt relief mechanism has produced benefits. Before looking at the history of debt relief, it is important to get some of the terms sorted out as they can become confusing. Most importantly, debt is held by three groups:

- *Multilateral debt:* This is lending by international financial institutions (IFIs). These are large banks supported by various numbers of international governments. The best known are the International Monetary Fund and the World Bank. There are many others, including the Islamic Development Bank, the Nordic Development Bank, and the Africa Development Fund. These institutions are backed by government guarantees so are considered preferred creditors; that is, they are paid out first before other creditors.
- *Bilateral aid:* This is money given by governments to governments. It includes bank debt that is insured by governmental institutions such as the export credit guarantees given by Britain, France, Sweden, and others.
- *Private loans:* These are private sector banks that loan money without government guarantees.

1982: Start of the Debt Crisis

> During the long macroeconomic crisis that started at the end of the 1970s, poverty considerations were set aside. The neoliberal stream that dominated the 1980s downplayed distribution and poverty and insisted on re-establishing market mechanisms to promote growth.
>
> —*James Wolfenson, then president of the World Bank, 2004*

In the mid-1970s, it was clear to a few commentators that the economies of several developing countries were in serious danger of collapse. Trouble began with a steadily rising oil price. In succession, the Yom Kippur War, the Arab oil embargo, the Iranian revolution, and the Iran-Iraq war all contrived to drive the price steadily higher. These profits (called "petrodollars") were recklessly invested in developing countries with little or no bank regulation and controls (Perkins, 2005).

The rising oil price also triggered a recession in the West, leading to a drop in the commodity prices that supported many developing economies. At a time when developing countries were saddled with increasing petrodollar loans, their ability to pay the interest was reduced by a drop in commodity prices and a rise in interest rates. The market did not listen to these warnings and, as was the case in 1929, the final collapse of this financial house of cards seemed to come as a great surprise (Eichengreen et al., 1992). Greater detail about the history behind the developing world debt is given in Chapter 5.

The crisis is often dated to August 1982, when Mexico's minister of finance announced Mexico would be unable to meet its debt repayment. This was only the tip of the iceberg. By October 1983, 26 more countries, owing a total of US$239 billion, were in a similar position. As a result, several of the world's largest banks faced the real prospect of major defaults and subsequent bank failures. During the first phase of response, from 1982 to 1985, rich countries reacted to the possibility of default by simply providing new loans. Private lenders wanted to reduce their exposure since the commercial banks were already in enough trouble. However, the largest creditors, represented by the Paris Club, the IMF, and other multilateral development banks, stepped in with more loans. They initially viewed the crisis as being due to an acute shortage of cash that would be solved by pouring in more money. It was claimed that this would allow poor countries to "grow" out of their debt.

By 1985, it was obvious that developing countries were not "growing" out of their debt, but were sinking below the weight of new short-term loans. It also slowly became obvious that the problem was not liquidity but simply a case of excessive debt; clearly, a new approach was necessary. Without some form of debt relief, many countries would never be able to emerge from their crisis. Tony Blair and George Bush did not come up with the idea of debt forgiveness in 2005 at Gleneagles; the concept had been around for more than 20 years (Daseking et al., 1999). Debt relief, in various forms, slowly became part of a variety of concessions and interventions during this period. It was subsequently a bumpy road between Mexico's default in 1982 and Gleneagles in 2005. The major twists and turns are outlined below.

1985: Baker and Brady Plans, Paris Club Terms, and SAPs

The mid-1980s was a confusing period as the various creditors tried new ways to help countries deal with their debts and repayments. The American government came up with the Baker and then the Brady plans. The IMF went further and further with its structural adjustment policies (SAPs), while the Paris Club countries tried a variety of rescheduling terms that changed with each annual meeting. It should be stressed that no matter what approach was used, the aim of those various initiatives was always to help the country become a better debt payer. The emphasis was always on repayment of debt; the poor came in a distant second. The concepts of forgiving debt and actually planning initiatives that would help improve the health of the poorest of those countries were slow to develop.

- *Baker and Brady plans (Vasquez, 1996):* The first of these plans was suggested in 1985 by then US Treasury secretary James Baker. Besides increased lending, the topic of conditionality was introduced. Interventions such as tax reduction, privatization of state-owned enterprises, and reduction of trade barriers were attempted. By 1988, it was apparent that this plan was not working, so the next secretary, James Brady, brought in a revised plan. This was one of the earliest attempts to provide real debt relief. New loans could be obtained below market interest rates and some commercial debts were written off. Various loan options were available to enable countries to extend their payback period. By 1994, 18 countries had agreed to Brady deals for a total debt forgiveness estimated at US$60 billion, spread over countries that were predominantly from Latin America.
- *Paris Club approach (Powell, 2000):* In 1987, the United Kingdom argued that Paris Club commercial loans to poor countries should be rescheduled at below market interest rates. Over the following years, at a variety of meetings, the rescheduling terms and amount of debt relief were slowly increased (Toronto terms, London terms, Naples terms, and, most recently, Lyon terms).
- *The IMF approach:* As early as 1980, the IMF had tested various structural adjustment programs in the Philippines, Turkey, and Costa Rica. Over the next two decades, structural adjustment programs were extended to most of the developing world, which gave the IMF extraordinary (almost colonial) power to influence and remodel the economies of sovereign states.

The general theory behind structural adjustment policies was straightforward: earn more and spend less. Interventions used in different countries were surprisingly similar—in fact, this "cookie-cutter" approach was one of the major criticisms of the SAP process. In general, interventions included currency devaluation, cutbacks in government expenditure, elimination of subsidies and price controls, a drop in wages, the opening up of markets for foreign competition, an emphasis on export-oriented industry, and privatization of government industries (Stiglitz, 2002). Poor countries had little option when confronted with these changes to their economies. Without the approval of the IMF, they would not be able to obtain credit from any other source. Although the IMF is made up of 184 countries, its voting structure is skewed toward the richest nations. Voting percentage is proportional to the money a country pledges to the IMF. Consequently, the poorest countries have little influence over IMF policy.

The universality of the debt crisis meant that the IMF gained extraordinary power to control the economic organization of many of the world's poorest countries. The whole program was criticized as a form of recolonization—basically restructuring the world's economy on an IMF model. This might have been justified if SAPs were shown to work, but, unfortunately, evidence of any benefit is hard to find. The final result was a worsening of life for the world's poor. SAPs have been criticized on many grounds, but the principal one is the inability to find any country in which the economic adjustments have clearly led to improved economic performance. The SAP Review International Network (SAPRIN) has published a detailed review of the problems associated with this period of IMF and World Bank policies (SAPRI, 2004).

Criticisms of SAPs grew steadily, but it was not until 1998 that the IMF commissioned external and internal reviews of its programs. Both were critical and revealed that the debt burden of countries implementing SAPs actually doubled between 1985 and 1995. Targets were not reached on reducing budget deficits or on raising government revenue. Although it was clear that many developing countries urgently needed economic reform, those changes should be tailored to fit each country rather than forcing everyone into a "one size fits all" model. The SAPs were deeply flawed and from the poor's perspective, they were a disaster. The poor played absolutely no part in the economic plan—even their governments had little say in what have been called "off the shelf austerity measures flown in directly from Washington." The perceived inflexibility of the IMF ultimately led to calls for reductions in its power. The chastened IMF that finally emerged is probably little consolation to the millions upon millions of people whose lives had been adversely affected by its policies (Wolfenson & Bourguignon, 2004).

1996: Heavily Indebted Poor Countries (HIPC) Initiative

> The Bank's philosophy has changed, moving toward country specific and flexible analysis and away from the twin dogmas of pervasive state control (1960s–1970s) and unregulated markets (1980s–early 1990s ...). Even the understanding of poverty has broadened from a narrow focus on income and consumption to a multidimensional notion of education, health, social and political participation, personal security and freedom, environmental quality and so forth.
>
> —*James Wolfenson, then president of the World Bank, 2004*

In response to the growing level of criticism of SAPs, the World Bank and IMF established the first Heavily Indebted Poor Countries Initiative (HIPC-1) in October

1996. It was designed to provide a "robust exit from the burden of unsustainable debt." Although it was introduced as a major new response to the poorest countries, this was not entirely accurate. The main aim of the program was still to reduce debt only to the level where a country would become able to continue paying back interest. The reputation of the World Bank and the IMF had been badly damaged by the widely accepted failure of the structural adjustment era. Not surprisingly, there was plenty of cynicism about this new and improved approach to debt management.

With time (and a lot more criticism), the HIPC program changed significantly. However, the basic qualifying criteria and monitoring processes have stayed the same, so they are covered here. Countries must first qualify for HIPC consideration by meeting a variety of criteria designed to ensure that they have unsustainable debts and are likely to comply with the necessary planning and implementation steps. Not every poor country meets these criteria. Sudan, Somalia, and Eritrea are now admitted to the first stage of the procedure, but Zimbabwe is still excluded. Eligibility criteria include the following:

- The country should have extreme poverty, and poor social development and health indicators; its exports would be dependent on a few primary commodities; and it would rely heavily on financial aid.
- The country must have a track record of implementing IMF and World Bank economic reforms. Countries are still required to follow these interventions in order to qualify for debt relief.
- The country should have an unsustainable debt burden (usually defined as total debt to export ratio above 150 percent) and should also have been given maximum relief by other routes, particularly the Paris Club group of creditors.

Using these criteria, 40 countries have to date been declared eligible for HIPC assistance (IMF, 2011a). The eligible country now enters a two-stage process. In the first three-year period, it has to establish a record of economic reform (under HIPC-1, this was simply SAPs by another name). If this was achieved to the satisfaction of the IMF and the World Bank, then a 67 percent relief of eligible debt was granted by Paris Club creditors. All other creditors (non-OECD bilateral creditors and commercial banks) are supposed to give comparable reductions. This is called the decision point. If this does not produce a sustainable debt, the country moves into a second three-year period, during which time support is given from international financial institutions for further reforms and debt reduction. At the end of this period (the completion point), the country becomes eligible for an 80 percent reduction in Paris Club debt.

Criticism of HIPC-1 was widespread. The most significant objection was that HIPC reforms were exactly the same as the ones that had failed when they had been called SAPs (OED, 2003). In the first three years of the program, developing world debt climbed from US$2.2 trillion up to US$2.6 trillion, while economic output fell slightly. The World Bank bowed to pressure and commissioned internal and external reviews, both of which were critical. The subsequent response was the Enhanced HIPC Program announced in 1999 (also called HIPC-2).

1999: Enhanced HIPC and PRSPs

The biggest change under HIPC-2 has been the introduction of Poverty Reduction Strategy Papers (PRSP) (IMF, 2011b). During the first three-year period leading to the decision point, a broad range of groups (including the poor) are gathered together to plan the country's future economic course. This is, of course, intended to include the provision of pro-poor choices in the grand plan. Rather than having to accept imposed external reforms, the PRSP is generated by the eligible country. It is intended to act as the blueprint for progress through the second third-year period. Completion of a PRSP is one of the provisions that must be met by the decision point. There is some optimism in the literature in support of the PRSP process, particularly when countries have had time to get experience with the new rules (Booth, 2005).

After meeting reforms agreed upon at the decision point, the country must adopt and implement its national PRSP for a full year. At that time, the country has reached completion and is eligible for more debt relief. Of the 40 HIPC countries, 32 are receiving full debt relief from the IMF and other creditors after reaching their completion points. Four others have passed their first decision point, so they have also received some debt relief, while another four are in the early stages of the process. The estimated program costs of US$75 billion are met roughly equally by the IMF (through its multilateral donors) and bilateral creditors. Prior to the HIPC Initiative, the average poor country was spending more on debt servicing than on health and education combined. After reaching completion points, average health and education spending is roughly five times higher than debt servicing. As stated above, average debt ratios for sub-Saharan African countries are considerably better than those for European countries (Figure 14.7).

The eight countries still in the early stages of the HIPC process all face major common problems of severe poverty, poor governance, and internal conflict. External support from the international donor community is important to help these countries progress. The IMF, the World Bank, and other large creditors have met their debt relief obligations under the HIPC-2 agreement. Unfortunately, many smaller institutions have lagged far behind with granting debt relief. As of 2016, debt reduction packages under the HIPC Initiative had been approved for 36 countries, which has provided US$76 billion in debt service relief. Thirty of these countries are in Africa (IMF 2016).

2000: Pressure for Debt Cancellation

Although the HIPC Initiative does provide debt relief, it still does not provide complete forgiveness of debt. Open public discussion about the full cancellation of all debts has been a very late development. Oddly enough, President George W. Bush was one of the first people to ask for large-scale debt cancellation. In his case, it was to obtain billions of dollars in debt relief for postwar Iraq. Much of the credit for this increase in popular support has to be given to various pressure groups, particularly Jubilee 2000 (Jubilee, 2011), Make Poverty History, and the widely watched Live 8 concerts.

About 20 years ago, G8 meetings hardly made the news, but by 2000, these annual meetings attracted huge levels of protest and popular debate, much of it aimed at debt relief. It is difficult to know whether debt relief became a major G8 topic because of altruism among world leaders or whether these elected officials were simply responding to the popular opinion of the voting public. It is also possible that the devastation caused by the Boxing Day 2004 tsunami had a significant effect on the debate. Discussion of debt cancellation for affected countries increased general interest in the topic. No matter what the reasons were, substantive discussion of debt relief is finally a reality. Relieving the developing world's debt burden was at the top of the agenda at the 2005 G8 summit meeting in Britain.

2005: Gleneagles Meeting, MDRI, and the Future

The 2005 Gleneagles G8 meeting resulted in the first serious attempt to write off debts of the poorest countries. A total of US$40 billion of debt was written off for 18 of the poorest countries in the world that had already completed HIPC programs. In total, it is estimated they will save US$1.5 billion a year in debt repayments. Nine more HIPC countries qualified within the next few months, which took the total of debt relief to US$55 billion. In addition, the meeting also agreed upon a doubling of aid to Africa from US$25 billion to $50 billion. The success of the initial G8 debt relief proposal led to the development of the Multilateral Debt Relief Initiative (MDRI). Under this agreement, countries that successfully reach the HIPC completion point are given full debt relief from three organizations—the World Bank, the IMF, and the African Development Fund (IMF, 2011c).

Unlike the HIPC agreement, MDRI does not include debt relief from other bi-lateral or bank creditors. The initial three founding agencies were later joined by the Inter-American Development Bank.

The HIPC/MDRI process is closely monitored to ensure that govern-ment finances freed up by debt relief are spent on social programs (IDA/IMF, 2010). Another significant step was the establishment in early 2005 of the Debt Sustainability Framework for low-income countries. This joint WB-IMF initiative is intended to monitor a country's debt and assess its ability to service further loans so that future unsustainable debt can hopefully be avoided. The program also offers guidance to lending institutions to ensure not only that loans are consistent with a country's development priorities, but that the repayments are sustainable given realistic economic projections (World Bank, 2011b).

SUMMARY

Although about 1 billion people rose out of extreme poverty between 2000 and 2015, about 702 million people still live in extreme poverty, representing about 10 percent of the world's population. One in five persons in developing regions live on less than US$1.25 per day. The overwhelming majority of people living on less than US$1.25 a day live in one of two regions: South Asia or sub-Saharan Africa. For many reasons, this situation should be viewed as a global emergency. Lack of money and a huge debt burden are major contributors to the misery and ill health that afflict populations throughout the developing world. The poor themselves must be given a voice in the solutions to their own problems, but it is only within the last 10–15 years that they have had a central place in the conversation. Apart from the humanitarian impulse to help people living with hunger and ill health, there are also pragmatic, selfish reasons to act. Poor coun-tries are at high risk of internal conflict and state failure. They are a danger to themselves and surrounding countries, and also are a source of drug and human smuggling, environmental disasters, and health threats, as we saw with the recent Ebola crisis in West Africa. The fundamental solution is economic growth. This seemingly simple statement raises a great deal of controversy because of concerns about how that increased wealth gets down to the poorest in order to sustainably end extreme poverty. Poverty relief policy efforts need to focus more directly on the poorest among the poor. Current debt relief initiatives have produced mea-surable improvements in the debt ratios of the poorest countries. These include the structural adjustment policies, Heavily Indebted Poor Countries Initiatives, Gleneagles, and the Multilateral Debt Relief Initiative.

DISCUSSION QUESTIONS

1. How does poverty relief play a central role in achieving the broader Sustainable Development Goals?
2. Why is poverty an inevitable common denominator contributing to the ill health of developing world populations?
3. How is lack of education a factor that keeps poor people poor and unhealthy?
4. How is microfinancing important in poverty alleviation? What has been the impact of the Grameen Bank in poverty alleviation?
5. What is the Green Revolution? What was its impact on poverty alleviation?
6. How does education raise economic productivity, lower infant mortality, and improve the nutritional status and health of adults and children?
7. Is there a connection between access to energy and poverty? Explain.
8. What are the major methods used to combat poverty? Which do you think would be most critical to achieving the SDG goal on poverty by 2030?
9. What were the origins of the current debt relief mechanisms?
10. The World Bank and IMF established the first Heavily Indebted Poor Countries Initiative (HIPC-1) in October 1996. Why?

RECOMMENDED READING

Armendariz, B., et al. 2010. *The economics of microfinance* (2nd ed.). Pub: MIT Press.

Collier, P. 2007. *The bottom billion: Why the poorest countries are failing and what can be done about it.* Pub: Oxford University Press.

Federico, G. 2005. *Feeding the world: An economic history of world agriculture, 1800–2000.* Pub: Princeton University Press.

Fogel, R. 2004. *The escape from hunger and premature death, 1700–2100: Europe, America, and the Third World.* Pub: Cambridge University Press.

Yunus, M. 2003. *Banker to the poor: Micro-lending and the battle against world poverty.* Pub: Public Affairs.

REFERENCES

Banerjee, A. 2007. *Making aid work.* Pub: MIT Press.

Beck, T., et al. 2004. Finance, inequality, and poverty: Cross-country evidence. World Bank Research Paper no. 3338. Retrieved from: www.aeaweb.org/assa/2005/0108_0800_0302.pdf.

Birdsall, N., et al. 2011. The post-Washington concensus. *Foreign Affairs*, 90: 45–53.

Booth D. 2005. Missing links in the politics of development: Learning from the PRSP experiment. Overseas Development Institute working paper no. 256. Retrieved from: www.odi.org.uk/resources/docs/2003.pdf.

Bourguignon, F. 2003. The poverty-growth-inequality triangle. Retrieved from: http://go.worldbank.org/WYJBJ44NN0.

BRAC. 2011. Bangladesh Rural Advancement Committee. Retrieved from: www.brac.net.

Bryce, J., et al. 2005. Can the world afford to save the lives of 6 million children each year? *The Lancet*, 365: 2193–2200.

CIDA. 2011. Stimulating sustainable economic growth. Retrieved from: acdi-cida.gc.ca/acdi-cida/ACDI-CIDA.nsf/eng/FRA-101515146-QKD.

Daseking, C., et al. 1999. From Toronto terms to the HIPC Initiative: A brief history of debt relief for low-income countries. IMF working paper no. 142. Retrieved from: www.imf.org/external/pubs/ft/wp/1999/wp99142.pdf.

Davies, W. 2003. An historical perspective from the Green Revolution to the gene revolution. *Nutrition Reviews*, 61: 124–134.

Dawson, N. et al. 2016. Green Revolution in Sub-Saharan Africa: Implications of imposed innovation for the wellbeing of rural smallholders. *World Development*, 78: 204–218.

Denes, C. 2003. Bolsa Escola: Redefining poverty and development in Brazil. *International Education Journal*, 4: 137–146.

DFID. 2003. Agriculture and poverty reduction: Unlocking the potential. Retrieved from: www.dfid.gov.uk/pubs/files/agri-poverty-reduction.pdf.

Djurfeldt, G., et al. 2005. *The African food crisis: Lessons from the Asian green revolution*. Pub: CABI Publishing.

Dollar, D., et al. 2001. Growth is good for the poor. World Bank Policy Research paper no. 2587. Retrieved from: http://go.worldbank.org/NQD3WT7RG0.

Doucouliagos, H., et al. 2010. Conditional aid effectiveness: A meta study. *Journal of International Development*, 22: 391–410.

Driscoll, R., et al. 2005. Second-generation poverty reduction strategies: New opportunities and emerging issues. *Development Policy Review*, 23: 5–25.

Easterly, W. 2001. The effect of IMF and World Bank programmes on poverty. UN University, discussion paper no. 102. Retrieved from: www.wider.unu.edu/stc/repec/pdfs/dp2001/dp2001-102.pdf.

Easterly, W. 2002. *The elusive quest for growth*. Pub: MIT Press.

Eastwood, R., et al. 2000. Pro-poor growth and pro-growth poverty reduction: Meaning, evidence, and policy implications. *Asian Development Review*, 18(2). Retrieved from: www.adb.org/Poverty/Forum/pdf/Lipton.pdf.

Eichengreen, B., et al. (Eds.). 1992. *The international debt crisis in historical perspective*. Pub: MIT Press.

Feachem, R. 2000. Poverty and inequity: A proper focus for the new century. *Bull World Health Organ*, 78: 1–2.

Foresti, M., et al. 2010. Human rights and pro-poor growth. Retrieved from: www.odi.org.uk/resources/download/4613.pdf.

Fuentes, R. 2005. Poverty, pro-poor growth, and simulated inequality reduction. HDR preparatory report. Retrieved from: http://ideas.repec.org/p/hdr/hdocpa/hdocpa-2005-11.html.

Grameen Bank. 2011. Bank for the poor. Retrieved from: www.grameen-info.org/.

Hufbauer, G., et al. 2006. The Doha round after Hong Kong. Retrieved from: www.iie.com/publications/pb/pb06-2.pdf.

IBRD. 2009. Banking the poor. Retrieved from: www.cgap.org/gm/document-1.9.7730/Banking%20the%20Poor.pdf.

IDA/IMF. 2010. HIPC Initiative and MDRI—status of implementation. Retrieved from: www.imf.org/external/np/pp/eng/2008/091208.pdf.

IMF. 2011a. Debt relief under the HIPC Initiative. Retrieved from: www.imf.org/external/np/exr/facts/hipc.htm.

IMF. 2011b. Poverty reduction strategy papers. Retrieved from: www.imf.org/external/np/prsp/prsp.aspx.

IMF. 2011c. The Multilateral Debt Relief Initiative. Retrieved from: www.imf.org/external/np/exr/facts/mdri.htm.

IMF. 2016. Debt relief under the Heavily Indebted Poor Countries (HIPC) Initiative. Retrieved from: www.imf.org/en/About/Factsheets/Sheets/2016/08/01/16/11/Debt-Relief-Under-the-Heavily-Indebted-Poor-Countries-Initiative.

Irz, X., et al. 2001. Agricultural productivity growth and poverty alleviation. *Development Policy Review*, 19: 449–466.

Ismi, A. 2004. Impoverishing a continent: The World Bank and the IMF in Africa. Halifax: Canadian Centre for Policy Alternatives. Retrieved from: www.policyalternatives.ca.

JCCCS. 2010. Jeppe College of Commerce and Computer Studies. Retrieved from: www.jeppecollege.co.za/.

Jubilee. 2011. Jubilee Debt Campaign. Retrieved from: www.jubileedebtcampaign.org.uk/.

Kilimo Salama. 2011. Micro-insurance for farmers. Retrieved from: http://kilimosalama.wordpress.com/about/.

Maddison, A. 2001. The world economy: A millennial perspective. OECD Development Centre. Retrieved from: www.nkeconwatch.com/nk-uploads/theworldeconomy.pdf.

Masakure, O., et al. 2005. Why do small-scale producers choose to produce under contract? *World Development*, 33: 1721–1733.

McKeown, T. 1980. *The role of medicine: Dream, mirage, or nemesis?* Pub: Princeton University Press.

M-CRIL. 2011. Micro-Credit Ratings International Ltd. Retrieved from: www.m-cril.com/.

Monitor. 2011. Promise and progress: Market-based solutions to poverty in Africa. Retrieved from: www.businessinsociety.eu/market-based-solutions-to-poverty-in-africa.

Moyo, D. 2009. *Dead aid: Why aid is not working and how there is a better way for Africa*. Pub: Farrar, Straus, and Giroux.

Norman Borlaug Heritage Foundation. 2011. Retrieved from: www.normanborlaug.org.

ODI. 2010. Trade and pro-poor growth. Retrieved from: www.oecd.org/dataoecd/37/8/47466544.pdf.

OECD. 2008. Natural resources and pro-poor growth. DAC guidelines. Retrieved from: www.oecd.org/dataoecd/61/43/42440224.pdf.

OED. 2003. Debt relief for the poorest: An OED review of the HIPC Initiative. WB Operations Evaluation Department. Retrieved from: http://lnweb90.worldbank.org/oed/oeddoclib.nsf/DocUNIDViewForJavaSearch/86DD1E3DCA61E0B985256CD700665B1C.

Oxfam. 2005. Kicking down the door: How upcoming WTO talks threaten farmers in poor countries. Oxfam briefing paper no. 72. Retrieved from: www.fao.org/monitoringprogress/docs/WTO_2005.pdf.

Perkins, J. 2005. *Confessions of an economic hit man*. Pub: Berrett-Koehler.

PGRP. 2005. Pro-poor growth in the 1990s: Lessons and insights from 14 countries. Pro-poor Growth Research Programme. Retrieved from: http://go.worldbank.org/W7RLTE9D80.

Powell, R. 2000. Debt relief for poor countries. *Finance and Development*, 37: 5-9.

Ravallion, M. 2001. Can high-inequality developing countries escape absolute poverty? World Bank Policy Research working paper no. 1775. Retrieved from: http://ideas.repec.org/p/wbk/wbrwps/1775.html.

Ravallion, M. 2009. A comparative perspective on poverty reduction in Brazil, China, and India. World Bank Development Research Group, paper no. 5080. Retrieved from: http://go.worldbank.org/X6YNKVZ8F0.

Sachs, J. 2005. *The end of poverty: Economic possibilities for our time*. Pub: Penguin Press.

SAPRI. 2004. *The SAP Review International Network Report: The policy roots of economic crisis, poverty, and inequality*. Pub: Zed Books.

SSATP. 2009. Sub-Saharan Africa Transport Policy. A framework for a pro-growth, pro-poor transport strategy. Retrieved from: http://go.worldbank.org/5GT0JCEDK0.

Stiglitz, J. 2002. *Globalization and its discontents*. Pub: Norton and Co.

Supply Chain. 2011. Voltic success story—decentralized bottling in Ghana. Retrieved from: www.thesupplychainlab.com/blog/africa/voltic-success-story-decentralized-bottling-in-ghana/.

UN. 2010. The Millennium Development Goals report. Retrieved from: www.un.org/millenniumgoals/pdf/MDG%20Report%202010%20En%20r15%20-low%20res%2020100615%20-.pdf.

UNICEF. 1987. *Adjustment with a human face*. Pub: Clarendon Press.

USAID. 2005. Banking at the base of the pyramid: A microfinance primer for commercial banks. Retrieved from: http://pdf.usaid.gov/pdf_docs/PNADD677.pdf.

Vasquez, I. 1996. The Brady plan and market-based solutions to debt crises. *The Cato Journal*, 16: 233–243. Retrieved from: www.cato.org/pubs/journal/cj16n2/cj16n2-4.pdf.

Weisbrot, M., et al. 2002. The relative impact of trade liberalization on developing countries. Retrieved from: www.cepr.net/documents/publications/trade_2002_06_12.pdf.

WFTO. 2009. World Fair Trade Organisation: Aid for Trade. Retrieved from: www.wfto.com/index.php?option=com_content&task=view&id=1030&Itemid=293.

WHO. 2002. Report of the Commission on Macroeconomics and Health. Investing in health for economic development. Retrieved from: http://whqlibdoc.who.int/publications/2001/924154550x.pdf.

Wolfenson, J., & Bourguignon, F. 2004. Development and poverty reduction: Looking back, looking ahead. Retrieved from: siteresources.worldbank.org/PRESIDENTSITE/Resources/jdw_bourguignon_english.pd.

World Bank. 2008. World development report: Agriculture for development. Retrieved from: http://siteresources.worldbank.org/INTWDR2008/Resources/WDR_00_book.pdf.

World Bank. 2011a. Global development finance: External debt of developing countries. Retrieved from: http://data.worldbank.org/data-catalog/global-development-finance.

World Bank. 2011b. Debt sustainability framework for low-income countries (DSF). Retrieved from: http://go.worldbank.org/A5VFXZCCW0.

World Bank. 2011c. World Development Indicators database. Retrieved from: http://data.worldbank.org/indicator.

Yunus, M. 2003. *Banker to the poor: Micro-lending and the battle against world poverty.* Pub: Public Affairs.

CHAPTER 15

Building Peace, Good Governance, and Social Capital

Peace and justice are two sides of the same coin.

—Dwight D. Eisenhower, 1957

OBJECTIVES

In the same way that health is not just an absence of disease, true peace consists of a great deal more than the absence of war (although that's a good starting point). A peaceful civil society requires representative government, fair rule of law, citizen participation, and broad human rights. All of these essential supports must be backed by an educated, healthy population whose values, attitudes, and behaviours all reflect a culture of peace. Developing such a society is a slow process—systems for democracy and justice don't appear overnight. However, even in the worst dictatorships, the international community can use its influence to promote peace and improve government actions toward its unfortunate citizens. About a quarter of the world's population live under conditions that are almost unimaginable for someone brought up in a developed country. The methods used to build peace and social capital within such regions vary widely and are largely dictated by the degree of social chaos. Responses may vary from military intervention in the worst cases, through post-conflict reconstruction, to government capacity building and support of civil society organizations in more stable countries. After completing this chapter, you should be able to:

- appreciate the importance of peace as a foundation for the development of a healthy and prosperous society
- understand the history of military intervention and its likely future importance in the response to dangerously unstable countries
- understand the development of the International Criminal Court and its importance in influencing the behaviour of tyrants
- understand the current approach to rebuilding countries emerging from conflict
- understand the theory and practice of improving social capital in developing countries

INTRODUCTION

There will be no more mindless democracy in this country.

—Alyaksandr Lukashenka, president of Belarus, commenting about riots after rigged elections in 2011

Despite steady improvements in health and prosperity over the last few decades, a large fraction of the world's population still live under conditions that would not be tolerated for one minute by people living in a democracy. Of all the injustices that poor people have to endure, the most significant is the lack of freedom to choose their own government. Presidents for life, military dictatorships, one-party states, or a theocracy backed by secret police—the concept of losing power because of an election has no meaning for any of them. By turns, their rule is corrupt, incompetent, or simply indifferent. In fact, some governments act toward their citizens as if they were an enemy. The inevitable results are poverty, ill health, and high rates of internal violence. While solutions exist for each of these individual problems, no lasting and profound changes will occur until the underlying injustice and instability that caused them are improved. The move toward full democracy is a slow one, so the first priorities are peace, "good enough" governance (Grindle, 2007) that at least isn't harmful to its people, and the development of a civil society where private citizens' groups are allowed some influence in the governing process.

The desire to be free is deeply rooted in human nature—people will eventually rise against even the most oppressive regimes. From the murder of Caligula by his own guards in ancient Rome to recent pictures of Gaddafi's body in a meat locker, history is full of the squalid deaths of tyrants who thought they would rule forever. The citizens' groups risking their lives in protests across the Arab world have managed to remove the governments of Egypt, Tunisia, and Libya, and Syria's is probably not far behind. In essence, they are no different from the protests and violence in Europe during the 1980s and 1990s that brought new regimes to Poland, East Germany, and Czechoslovakia. The establishment of the International Criminal Court will hopefully mean that this process can be achieved with less bloodshed in the future. The day may come when many more dictators, like the currently indicted al-Bashir of Sudan, will meet less dramatic but equally terminal ends to their careers in jail.

During the Cold War, both sides of the ideological struggle turned a blind eye to despotism. Leaders who would now be indicted by the International Criminal Court were actually given financial and military support. The attitudes of the time are summed up by the quote about Somoza, attributed to President Truman: "He's a bastard, but he's our bastard." The collapse of the Soviet Union

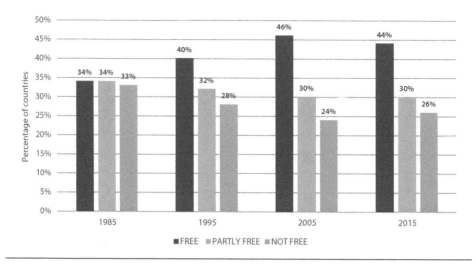

Figure 15.1: Trends in percentages of countries classified as free, partly free, or not free, 1985, 1995, 2005, and 2015

Source: Freedom House. 2016. Freedom in the world 2016. Anxious dictators, wavering democracies: Global freedom under pressure. Retrieved from: https://freedomhouse.org/report/freedom-world-2016/overview-essay-anxious-dictators-wavering-democracies.

in the early 1990s meant that support for brutal regimes was withdrawn. In terms of governance, this was a period of revolutionary change. Once money and arms dried up, tyrants toppled and long-festering wars ended in Central America. For the first time, standards of governance could be openly discussed and even enforced. When Freedom House started classifying countries in the early 1970s, only a quarter of them were considered to be free. In the last four decades this has improved significantly (Figure 15.1). In their most recent annual report, half of the world's 195 countries are now considered to be free (Freedom House, 2016). While military interventions and civil uprisings have rid the world of the insane rules of Amin, Pol Pot, and Nguema, roughly a quarter of all countries are still governed by regimes whose attitudes to democracy are summed up by the quote at the beginning of this section.

A common phrase used to describe the unfortunate people caught in the world's worst-governed countries is derived from Paul Collier's influential book, *The Bottom Billion* (Collier, 2007). The only problem is that the number is too small by at least half a billion people. Of the 195 countries studied by Freedom House in 2015, 86 are said to be free, 59 are partly free, and 50 are not free. Those 50 countries represent at least a quarter of the world's countries and stand at 2.6 billion people, or 36 percent of the global population, though it is important to note that more than half of this number live in China (Freedom House, 2016). Since measures of poor

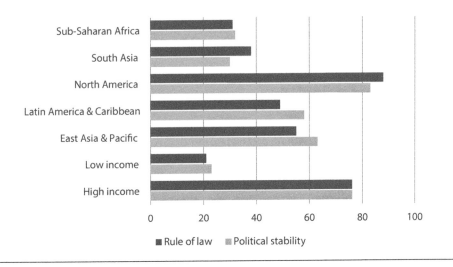

Figure 15.2: Rule of law and political stability by regions of the world, including low-income and high-income countries

Source: World Bank. 2016. Worldwide governance indicators. Retrieved from: http://info.worldbank.org/governance/wgi/index.aspx#reports.

governance are closely associated with poverty (Figure 15.2), the World Bank's classification of 215 countries and territories, based on GNI per capita, is also a fair indicator of government standards (World Bank, 2016):

- *Low income:* US$1,025 per capita or less; 31 countries, including Bangladesh, Haiti, Malawi, Sudan, and Tajikistan
- *Lower-middle income:* US$1,026 to $4,035; 52 countries, including Egypt, Iraq, Philippines, Vietnam, and Zambia
- *Upper-middle income:* US$4,036 to $12,475; 56 countries, including Argentina, Brazil, China, Namibia, and Russia
- *High income:* US$12,476 or more; 79 countries, including Australia, Canada, the UK, Germany, Italy, and France

Whether the GNI per capita categories are superimposed on plots of health, longevity, or nutrition, the same 50 countries, with roughly 1.5 billion people, appear at the bottom of every list. Bad governance is not confined only to the poorest countries, but low scores are an invariable finding within the low-income category. Some landlocked countries with poor natural resources, like Nepal or Malawi, will be poor no matter who is in charge. Others find ways to thrive despite the grasping corruption of their rulers. However, an unjust government is a large part of the problem in the world's lowest quartile. Bad governments are harmful not only to their populace, but now that aid is increasingly allocated on the basis of good governance, the possibility exists that the international community will increasingly bypass high-risk countries and invest in more stable places where aid stands a fair chance of producing measurable benefits.

This chapter examines the options available to improve peace and governance. They range from military intervention in response to severe crises, to restoring stability after a peace settlement, to developing a civil society in more stable low-income countries. Without significant improvements in peace and the quality of governance, the poorest countries risk being left far behind as the rest of the world becomes increasingly prosperous.

ESTABLISHING PEACE (PEACEMAKING)

Peace is always beautiful.

—*Walt Whitman, Leaves of Grass, 1855*

During the last few decades, more people have been lifted out of poverty than at any time in past history. India and China head the list because of their enormous populations, but this has been a worldwide phenomenon. Obviously, the causes are complex and incompletely understood, but it's fair to say that the spread of peace during this period has been an important enabling factor. A large part of that outbreak of peace is explained by the end of the Cold War. Although Russia and America never fought each other directly (they were probably fairly close over Cuba), the broad ideological struggle between East and West spawned dozens of wars among their proxies. Examples range from the Korean and Vietnam Wars down to chronic conflicts between right and left in Central America, marked by horrifying abuses of human rights (Gaddis, 2005). By the time Gorbachev introduced the Perestroika and Glasnost reforms in Russia during the late 1980s, these wars had collectively killed millions of people. Considering the damage done by the Cold War (from the McCarthy era to nuclear proliferation), its ending was an anticlimax; everyone just seemed to lose interest in the whole pointless exercise around the same time. The exact causes have received surprisingly little study, probably out of embarrassment. The final end of the Cold War is usually dated to 1990 with the fall of the Berlin Wall.

The passage of time has meant that people have largely forgotten about the results of the thawed relationship between East and West, but it was a truly revolutionary period in history. Apart from allowing advances in nuclear disarmament, the end of the Cold War was beneficial in terms of peace in countries plagued by chronic internal violence. While there is a close temporal relationship between the

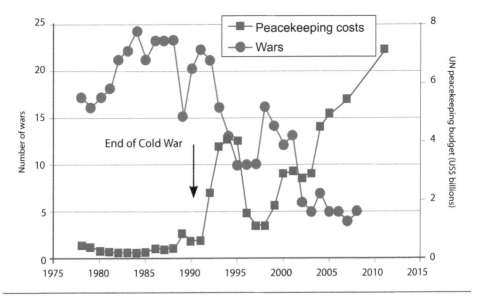

Figure 15.3: Trends in the number of wars (defined as conflicts causing more than 1,000 deaths per year) and the cost of United Nations peacekeeping operations (US$ billions) over the last 40 years

Sources: Human Security Report. 2010. Retrieved from: www.hsrgroup.org/human-security-reports/20092010/overview.aspx; Renner, M. 2006., Peacekeeping expenditures in current vs. real terms: 1947–2005, Worldwatch Institute. Retrieved from: http://www.globalpolicy.org/images/pdfs/Z/pk_tables/currentreal.pdf.

decline in global conflict and the end of the Cold War (Figure 15.3), it is overly simplistic to attribute this only to the withdrawal of financial and military support from either Russia or America. At best, this support was usually only a minor factor. The principal change was a new air of co-operation at the level of the Security Council in the UN. Once it was possible to pass resolutions without veto, the UN was free to try a range of peacemaking initiatives that included increasingly complex peacekeeping operations, multi-party mediation, and the application of multilateral sanctions (Figure 15.4). This was also a time of increasing democratization and rising prosperity, both of which also contribute to the spread of peace because weak states with high poverty rates are at far higher risk of violence.

Peacemaking (to be distinguished from peacekeeping) is a cost-effective strategy in terms of money and lives saved per dollar invested. A widely reported study by Collier et al. (2004) estimated that the average cost of civil war, in terms of military expenses and lost economic growth, was US$54 billion. Anything that can reduce that terrible waste of lives and money is a good way to invest aid resources. It has been estimated that every US$1 spent on conflict prevention ultimately generates over US$4 in savings to the international community

(Chalmers, 2004). As a result of these benefits, peacekeeping has grown into a very big business. For example, the UN now maintains the second-largest number of deployed soldiers after America. The 2010–2011 UN budget for peacekeeping alone was over US$7 billion (Figure 15.3). Clearly, it is in everyone's best interests to persuade and sometimes even to force warring parties to settle for peace. The following peacemaking initiatives are used.

Mediation

> Discourage litigation. Persuade your neighbors to compromise whenever you can.
>
> *—Abraham Lincoln, 1850*

The most common method used to end conflicts is mediation by governments and other interested third parties (Sisk, 2009). Despite its internal problems, the broad membership of the United Nations makes it the most obvious first choice. The UN department responsible for mediation and peacekeeping is the Department of Political Affairs (DPA, 2016). It maintains several offices in high-risk countries in Africa and the Middle East. Many other organizations with local influence may also be involved. Examples include ex-colonial rulers, religious organizations, private organizations such as the Carter Center, and groups collectively known as the Friends of UN. The first Friends group consisted of the UN ambassadors from Spain, Mexico, Venezuela, and Colombia. They were instrumental in obtaining a peace settlement in El Salvador (Whitfield, 2007). Similar influential groups have become increasingly common in the last 20 years (Figure 15.4).

There are so many factors that might affect the potential success of mediation that it is difficult to make broad comments applicable to all situations. Some of the major variables include UN or regional organization involvement, major power support for either side, the willingness of parties to co-operate, the duration of the war, ethnic or religious differences between combatants, relative military strengths, the threat of external military intervention, the number of deaths, the broader strategic importance of the war, etc. Establishing a system that might predict the wars most likely to respond to mediation is clearly unrealistic. If there is no guidance for the best use of mediation, it is at least worth looking at the success rate. If success includes everything from full settlement to at least a ceasefire, the limited data suggest that diplomatic interventions are often successful. In Regan et al.'s (2009) study of over 400 mediations, about 40 percent ended in a settlement and the majority of the remainder at least achieved a ceasefire. In a smaller study of mediation in 35 wars since 1990, Beber (2010) found that diplomacy achieved some form of peaceful settlement in about half the cases.

Multilateral Sanctions

> It is not enough merely to make sanctions "smarter," the challenge is to achieve consensus about the precise and specific aims of the sanctions, adjust the instruments accordingly and then provide the necessary means.
>
> *—Kofi Annan, 2000*

In keeping with mediation efforts, the application of international sanctions also took off rapidly after the end of the Cold War (Figure 15.4). While sanctions are commonly employed to induce behavioural change, there is a widespread perception that they are often ineffective, are poorly enforced, only harm the poor, and encourage corruption. A good example was the early use of sanctions against the Rhodesian government in 1966. Enforcement was poor because the South African regime at the time helped to break the blockade. Sanctions forced the Smith regime to expand industrial capacity, which actually strengthened the country, while the embargo on medications simply harmed the poor. The subsequent response was to design sanctions that affected only the country's rulers—termed "smart sanctions" (Drezner, 2003). Unfortunately, these have also had problems. Apart from the current failure of targeted sanctions to change Iran's nuclear policy, the most obvious failure was the "oil for food" program in

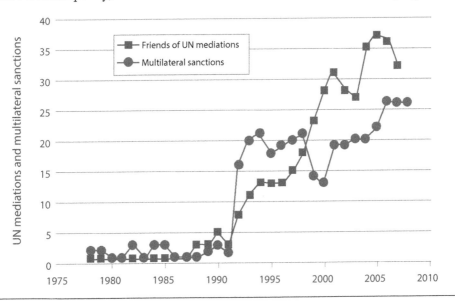

Figure 15.4: Trends in the use of mediation and multilateral sanctions over the last 40 years

Sources: Human Security Report. 2010. Retrieved from: www.hsrgroup.org/human-security-reports/20092010/overview.aspx; Whitfield, T. 2007. *Friends indeed: The United Nations, groups of friends, and the resolution of conflict.* Pub: US Institute of Peace.

Iraq. In order to mitigate the harmful effects of sanctions against Iraq's poor, the country was allowed to sell oil in exchange for a steady supply of food for the Iraqi people. Subsequent enquiries by the US Senate and the Independent Inquiry Committee under Volcker (IIC, 2005) found the program was riddled with corruption—billions of dollars were unaccounted for.

Over time, various forms of sanctions have been used, including a general embargo (Iraq), targeted economic sanctions (Iran), trade restrictions of various forms (Cuba), arms embargo (Congo), termination of foreign aid (North Korea), and financial restrictions against political leaders (Sudan). Sanctions are also imposed for different reasons—to induce regime change, to stop human rights abuses, to stop nuclear proliferation, and also to persuade combatants to start peace negotiations. Obviously, the final picture is complicated. As with studies of mediation, conclusions about effectiveness depend on the definitions used by researchers. However, a long-term study of sanctions going back to 1915 concluded that economic sanctions were of some help in only about a third of cases (Hufbauer et al., 2007). This result is not so much a criticism of sanctions as a policy, but more an indication that monitoring and enforcement have frequently been inadequate. A more recent study, which hopefully reflects better management, has shown that sanctions significantly shorten the length of civil wars. The study also showed that multilateral sanctions were more effective than unilateral embargos (Escriba-Folch, 2008). Since the next step in conflict resolution involves the complexity and expense of military intervention, sanctions are likely to remain a feature of international diplomacy despite their current reputation. It is hoped that more effort will be placed in their enforcement in future.

Military Intervention

> From time to time, the tree of liberty must be watered with the blood of tyrants.
>
> —*Thomas Jefferson, 1787*

The failure of the League of Nations to prevent World War II led to the end of that organization, but, more importantly, it prompted the newly formed United Nations to include some military "teeth" in its constitution. The UN body responsible for international peace and security is the five-member permanent Security Council. Under Chapter VII of the UN Charter, the UN (acting through the permanent Security Council) is allowed to take various actions, including military intervention, to restore international peace and security. Each member has the power of veto over the others and it was the frequent use of this veto by the US and Russia that paralyzed the UN during the Cold War. Attention was focused on Chapter VII powers after the failure of the international community to intervene in the

Rwandan massacre. In response to a request by Kofi Annan for a review of the UN's responsibilities, the Canadian government responded by starting the International Commission on Intervention and State Sovereignty. Its report, *Responsibility to Protect* (ICISS, 2001), has been highly influential. The report stressed that it is a state's right and responsibility to maintain peace and security within its own borders. However, if it fails in this responsibility, the international community should act in a timely manner to protect the safety of the population.

The idea of the responsibility to protect (often shortened to RtoP) was subsequently discussed widely by UN states. At the 2005 World Summit meeting, the concept of the obligation to prevent mass atrocities was universally accepted by all states. It is still not part of international law, but it is now widely accepted as a norm of international behaviour. The practical application of RtoP was further expanded by the secretary-general's report on its implementation in 2009 (UN, 2009). The question of sovereignty has been largely solved—if a government commits atrocities against its citizens, it is now generally accepted that the larger community can intervene. However, the problem of selectivity remains. Why use air power in Libya, but not in Syria? Why use external force to liberate Kuwait, but view Chechnya as a sovereign responsibility of Russia? These questions are still under active debate, but it is reasonable to suggest that a common attitude would be that just because the UN doesn't intervene in every civil war does not mean it shouldn't intervene in any of them.

Box 15.1 History Notes

Lester Pearson (1897–1972)

Pearson was born in a small Ontario town. He graduated early from school and entered the University of Toronto, but his studies were interrupted by World War I. He initially served in the Medical Corps, but later transferred to the Flying Corps. After the war he studied history at Oxford before returning to Canada. After teaching for a few years, he entered the Canadian Foreign Service. He advanced rapidly so that by 1945, he was Canadian ambassador to Washington and in 1946 was minister for external affairs in the St. Laurent government. He went on to become prime minister of Canada for a five-year term, but is probably better remembered for his international work. He played an important role in the establishment of NATO and the UN. During the Suez Crisis of 1956, his diplomacy is credited with averting larger spread of the war. His idea for an international police force for the area made him the founder of the UN Emergency Force and also the originator of international peacekeeping efforts. For this work he was awarded the Nobel Peace Prize in 1957. After his retirement, he was made chairman of the Commission on International Development (also known as the Pearson Commission), an effort at the time to increase development financing. Based on mathematical models of the day, the committee recommended the well-known 0.7 percent GDP as the national goal for aid funding. This was adopted by the UN in 1970. For more information, follow the link: Foreign Affairs (2008).

The well-publicized failures of earlier military missions in Rwanda and Somalia and the chaos of the Iraq war were followed by a period of disillusionment with armed interventions. The UN responded to their obvious operational deficiencies by commissioning an external enquiry (UN, 2001), which has resulted in real organizational change. In addition to this sense of change at the UN and the move toward the concept of RtoP, there were also some successful interventions to hold up as examples. The NATO-led bombing campaign in Kosovo was controversial, but it did, at very least, force the withdrawal of Serbian forces and allow peacekeepers to enter the region. Around the same time, a small British intervention in Sierra Leone managed to halt the brutal activity of the Revolutionary United Front and return the country to peace in a short, well-organized campaign. The recent UN multinational force that provided air and naval support for Libya's revolution, and the armed intervention that ended the violence in Ivory Coast, were both considered to be successes. Despite the complexity, expense, and risk of military interventions, recent experience would suggest that they may be more frequently used in the future.

POST-CONFLICT RECONSTRUCTION (PEACEBUILDING)

Peacebuilding involves a range of measures targeted to reduce the risk of relapsing into conflict, in countries emerging from war, by strengthening national capacities at all levels, addressing key causes of conflict and laying the foundations for sustainable peace and development.

—*UN Peacebuilding Commission, 2009*

As discussed in Chapter 4, colonial wars, interstate wars, and large-scale conflicts killing more than 1,000 people a year have become steadily less common over the last two decades. The principal form of violent conflict is now almost exclusively civil war within states marked by poor (or even absent) government; widespread poverty; the presence of ethnic, tribal, or religious intolerance; and a history of earlier conflict. The end of the Cold War allowed a more complex debate about the results of internal violence. The effects of war on women, children, and the landless poor now dominated the debate, rather than geopolitical advantage. The triumph of human rights over ideological allegiance can be dated to the 1994 Human Development Report (UNDP, 1994) in which the authors stated that the best way to achieve lasting security was to focus on "freedom from want" and "freedom from fear."

This "new" approach, which viewed violence, malnutrition, poverty, and ill health as part of an interrelated whole, represented a quiet revolution at the UN. Peace can be built only on a foundation of good governance, prosperity, and good

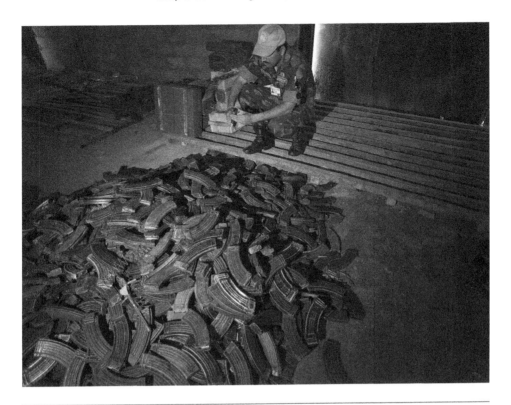

Photo 15.1: A UN peacekeeper, from an Indian battalion, examines AK-47 magazines collected during the demobilization process in North Kivu, the Democratic Republic of Congo.

Source: UN Photo/Martine Perret, with kind permission of the UN Photo Library (www. unmultimedia.org/photo).

health—you don't get one without the others. Such ideas were at the basis of the UN's Charter of Human Rights when it formed after World War II, but that early and open optimism was lost under the paralyzing effects of the Cold War. It took nearly 50 years before those ideas surfaced again. The results can be seen in the MDGs, the Responsibility to Protect debate, serious reform of the Human Rights Council, and the establishment of the Peacebuilding Commission in 2005 (UN, 2011a). Hopefully, the time when it was possible for Libya, under Gadhafi, to hold the chair of the Commission on Human Rights, will never be seen again.

Whether measured by its effects on society, the economy, or on fragile neighbours, civil wars have terrible consequences. The economic results alone are startling. The economist Paul Collier estimated that the cost of new civil wars each year was greater than annual foreign aid (Collier, 2007). Clearly, it is in everyone's interests to control intra-state violence. Since the majority of "new" wars are simply old wars that had just stopped for a while, it is obvious that a peace settlement is only the first step in a complex multidisciplinary process that aims to reduce the future risk of violence (sometimes called a peace operation). The importance of conflict prevention is reflected in the money spent by multilateral agencies—as noted earlier, the UN's peacekeeping budget alone was US$7 billion for 2010–2011. The World Bank's allocation to post-conflict states—including grants, loans, the Post-Conflict Fund, and the Low Income under Stress Fund—has now grown to 25 percent of its total budget. The UN Development Programme (UNDP) spends approximately 15 percent of its budget on peacekeeping (Nakaya, 2009). Many large donors, such as the UK and the US, also have their own bilateral peacekeeping funds. So what is all this money spent on?

The Initial Reconstruction Response

> Peace is not the product of a victory or a command. It has no finishing line, no final deadline, no fixed definition of achievement. Peace is a never-ending process, the work of many decisions.
>
> —*Oscar Arias, 1987*

Since the international community has placed greater emphasis on establishing and then maintaining peace, there is no shortage of examples to study. Afghanistan, Iraq, Sierra Leone, Bosnia, Haiti, Lebanon, and many others are all at various stages of the difficult journey from internal violence to peace, representative government, and increasing prosperity (Photo 15.1). Each country has its own unique set of causes behind the violence and varying degrees of government capacity, so it is not possible to make a simple framework to follow. NYU's Center of International Cooperation's review of the challenges of reconstruction is a good starting point (NYU, 2008). One thing is certain—a management model that imagines a smooth continuum from humanitarian assistance to security to reconstruction of facilities, finally followed by governance and economic development, will not work. These are complex situations that may change daily, but some very broad comments can be made:

- This is not a place for bureaucracy. The response organization must be flexible enough to take advantage of sudden opportunities. This is an argument in favour of establishing a professional, well-trained organization that does nothing else other than reconstruction work—the UNDP or the World Bank would be the most likely sponsoring organizations.
- The need for long-term security and the time taken to establish local governance capacity are such that any reconstruction response must plan for years of significant involvement. Ten years is the minimum expected engagement time.

- In a complex environment where there is limited faith on all sides, it is vital that all agreements and undertakings are fulfilled by the response team. Variability in engagement due to slow or volatile financial support is harmful to partnerships. It is vital that reliable and long-term financing is available.
- The assistance must not favour any side in the conflict and must also be free from any political or military objectives.

The first problem may simply be gaining access to the country. For example, after Cyclone Nargis, it took three weeks of diplomacy before the Burmese government would even allow humanitarian teams to enter the country. Once established, the first priority in many cases will be the provision of food. This needs to be planned carefully in order to avoid depressing local agricultural markets. Whenever possible, it is cheaper to access food from the neighbouring region rather than laboriously shipping it in from North America. If local food production can meet demand, one alternative is either to give local people direct cash payments or to establish food-for-work programs. One of the biggest examples of such an arrangement is Ethiopia's Productive Safety Net Program (Gilligan et al., 2008). The longer-term distribution of money and food carry considerable organizational problems and can be arranged only with full agreement and support from local authorities.

Obtaining funding is obviously a major issue. There is a multitude of sources to choose from. Their use depends on the size of grant required and

Box 15.2 Moment of Insight

School deworming programs give a child effective protection from hookworm, round-worm, whipworm, and schistosomiasis for 12 months. Drug costs:	Cost to park for two-and-a-half minutes in downtown Vancouver:
One tablet of praziquantel: 20 cents One tablet of albendazole: 5 cents	
Annual cost to protect a child from debilitating effects of worms:	
25 cents	**25 cents**
Source: WHO. 2003. School deworming. Retrieved from www.who.int/wormcontrol/documents/en/at_a_glance.pdf.	*Source:* I. Glynn & J. Glynn, The life and death of smallpox (Pub: Cambridge University Press, 2004).

the organizational capacity of the country. The Emergency Response Fund, run by the UN's Office for the Coordination of Humanitarian Affairs, and the Peacebuilding Fund, controlled by the UN's Peacebuilding Commission, are both commonly used in the early stages of peacebuilding. Long-term financing is now increasingly provided from a common basket of funds that accept money from multiple donors. Examples include Common Humanitarian Funds used in Central African Republic and the Multi-Donor Trust Funds established in Sudan (DFID, 2010).

When it comes to the longer-term issues of maintaining security, fostering economic development, resuscitating public services (health and education), improving food security and agriculture, and improving government capacity, it is worth studying the common problems outlined in the NYU study commissioned by the UK's development agency (NYU, 2008). A study of past reconstruction projects revealed the following common weaknesses:

- There is commonly a lack of support for local capacity, whether it is governmental or private. Whatever initiatives are introduced, there must be an emphasis on local ownership and management, with training provided if necessary. Whenever possible, local people must be given the leadership.
- Peace agreements need to be enforced, monitored, and generally looked after carefully. This important step is often forgotten, which leads to separation of the parties and a drift back to violence.
- In the early chaos following peace, there is a tendency to concentrate on the problems at hand rather than taking the time to form a rough strategy that includes broad aspects such as governance, peace, development, and humanitarian concerns.
- Slow and volatile funding sources endanger the smooth implementation of long-term projects. Stable funding is essential.
- The people involved in the various elements of the response are not always uniformly professional. Peacekeeping troops must be well trained and adequately equipped to meet likely responses. Expert advisers and teachers are necessary for government and economic capacity building. Their training and experience must be adequate to meet the complex demands of state rebuilding.
- Economic recovery is better based on new ideas than on older structures whose inequities may have been one of the sources of conflict in the past (UNDP, 2008).

Disarmament, Demobilization, and Reintegration (DDR)

> Ultimately, DDR is the first step in construction of the new order, rather than the last step of something that has ceased to be.
>
> *—Virginia Gamba, 2006*

Peacekeeping has become considerably more sophisticated over the last 20 years. It has grown from a few soldiers armed with little more than the UN's reputation to a complex, multi-agency process that ranges from peacekeeping to economic development. An important part of modern reconstruction is the disarmament and reintegration of former combatants, often known as DDR. DDR operations have become more common over the last 10 years. There are examples in all the world's regions, but most are in sub-Saharan Africa. The main elements include the following (Carames et al., 2009):

- *Disarmament:* The process of collecting and documenting arms, ammunition, and explosives. They may then be stored, destroyed, or given to the new national security force.
- *Demobilization:* This step involves the decommissioning of combatants. They may first have to gather in camps or barracks while they are registered and then discharged in a controlled manner.
- *Reintegration:* This is a complex process that is not just confined to vocational training. There are also difficult issues of social reconciliation to confront.

There are numerous difficulties confronting a disarmament program, so its success is far from a guarantee. If one side has been beaten militarily, then disarmament is largely enforced, but in the event of a ceasefire where both sides still have military capability, unequal disarmament will leave one side vulnerable. This requires a good deal of trust in a situation where trust is in short supply. Another problem is the practical difficulty of keeping hardened fighters interested in the business of earning a living in a poor country. For example, the people fighting in West Africa's shifting wars often started out as children who were kidnapped and forced to participate in civil wars within Liberia, Sierra Leone, Guinea, and Burkina Faso. They then drifted into a life of fighting for money wherever another war broke out in the region. War simply offered the best economic opportunity. Breaking this cycle with vocational training and resettlement into civilian life is not easy (Dufka, 2005). The most common cause of unsuccessful programs is the failure to provide combatants with a well-planned, well-funded way out of poverty that does not involve fighting. The largest and most detailed guide to achieving this aim is published by the UN's Department of Political Affairs (DPA, 2006).

Entry into a DDR program may be dependent on having a weapon to hand in. If the entry criteria are set too low, then the program will be flooded with people claiming to be ex-fighters in order to benefit from the shelter, food, and training offered to demobilized combatants. In fact, it is this favourable treatment for people who carried out the fighting that remains a very contentious ethical problem facing any peacebuilding process. However, the pragmatic issue remains—if they are not reintegrated, the risk of slipping back into war will be increased. As with many other aspects of foreign aid, DDR seems like a good idea in theory, but there is surprisingly little evidence confirming its effectiveness. Given the problems facing such programs, it should not be surprising to find that a study in Sierra Leone found little effect of DDR (Humphreys et al., 2007), while another in Liberia, using similar methodology, found a positive effect (Pugel, 2007). Both studies emphasized the need for good planning and management, reliable funding, and national ownership of the program.

Peacekeeping

Today, we have more than 110,000 men and women deployed in conflict zones around the world. They come from nearly 120 countries—an all-time high, reflecting confidence in United Nations peacekeeping.

—*Ban Ki-moon, 8th Secretary-General of the United Nations, 2008*

Peacekeeping has already been discussed in Chapter 4, but it is an important subject that can stand some repetition. The UN's peacekeeping force (under the guidance of the Department of Peacekeeping Operations) has grown steadily over the last few decades (DPKO, 2016). It has gone from a small, lightly armed force to the second-largest deployment of armed soldiers after the US. After 1990 when the UN's Security Council was freed from constant veto, the number of operations increased sharply. The UN currently has 16 operations around the world, with a similar number run by non-UN forces. UN and non-UN interventions are not mutually exclusive, but often form part of a continuum. Initial peace-enforcement forces (e.g., the US in Haiti or Australia in East Timor) may gradually hand over control to UN forces as the situation settles. The UN currently fields over 120,000 soldiers, police, and various volunteers. The biggest providers of troops are Bangladesh, Pakistan, India, and Nigeria.

The cost of peacekeeping has obviously risen steadily over this period, and it is now about US$7 billion per year (Figure 15.3). The biggest financial contributors are the US, Japan, the UK, and Germany. It is generally felt that the UN provides military services at lower cost than those provided by NATO forces. It has been shown that peacekeeping operations can significantly reduce the risk of return to war (Collier et al., 2004). They are also a highly cost-effective use of foreign aid resources (Collier et al., 2006). Despite past successes, UN peacekeeping has not been free from controversy—in particular, the spectacular failures to prevent loss of lives in Rwanda and Bosnia. To its credit, the organization reduced operations in the late 1990s while waiting for the results of the external Brahimi review. The recommendations were predictable—soldiers in high-risk areas should be better trained and equipped, and standards of preparation and planning should be improved. The UN has responded with changes to its peacekeeping policies, restructuring of the peacekeeping department, and the introduction of strict new rules governing the conduct of soldiers in the field (UN, 2011b).

Prosecuting Human Rights Abusers

> The principal goal of the International Criminal Court is to deter other people from committing crimes.
>
> —*Fatou Bensouda, deputy prosecutor, International Criminal Court, 2008*

In the years since the end of World War II, there has been an explosion of human rights treaties. From the early Declaration of Human Rights in 1948 to subsequent conventions against slavery and torture, the international community has been strong on legislation, but weak on enforcement. However, in the last 20 years, this has changed quite rapidly. Lutz et al. (2008) were able to document 43 prosecutions of heads of state between 1990 and 2008. Rather than holding states accountable, courts are now beginning to hold individuals criminally responsible for atrocities against civilians. This so-called revolution in accountability (Sriram, 2003) is used against the worst forms of human rights violations, such as torture, genocide, and the use of rape and mutilation as a means of war. The aim is not just revenge, there is also a desire to avoid such horrors in the future. Prosecution is only one form of deterrence; others include truth commissions (South Africa), genocide museums (Cambodia), and reparations (Canadian residential schools). Prosecution is the only one that carries a punishment.

Even if tyrants manage to avoid prosecution through age (such as Pinochet) or death (Milosevich), the process is still harmful to them in terms of legal costs, lost earnings in detention, and loss of prestige and international legitimacy. Prosecution is harmful to the accused, but, of equal importance, does prosecution of leaders deter others from similar acts? Until recently, there was no research to answer this question, but a study by Kim et al. (2010) has added valuable insights into the effects of human rights prosecutions. Prior to 1970, they showed there was almost no chance of bringing charges against a head of state for crimes against humanity.

Using a large database of human rights prosecutions, they showed that the increasing risk of prosecution has had a measurable effect on the degree of repression. In addition, countries with human rights prosecutions are subsequently less repressive than those who have not been through the process. Countries are also less repressive if their regional neighbours have had prosecutions. Holding leaders to account for terrible crimes against humanity has numerous tangible and intangible benefits and results. This development has been one of the major advances in international health since the end of World War II.

In the past, if those accused of crimes against humanity could not be prosecuted in their own national court systems, there was no independent international court to take over the task. The establishment of the International Criminal Court in 2002 now provides a permanent international court to try crimes against humanity (ICC, 2011). The first calls for an international court date back to the Nuremberg and Tokyo war crimes trials following World War II. The outrages in the former Yugoslavia and also in Rwanda in the 1990s were so shocking that international tribunals were organized to try those guilty of the worst crimes. International support for the process subsequently resulted in the 1998 Rome Statute, which provides the legal framework for the ICC. It was ratified by 120 countries and came into force in 2002. Recent prominent people indicted by the court include Sudan's President al-Bashir (who has not surrendered), Libya's Gaddafi (subsequently killed), his son Saif al-Islam (arrested for trial in Libya), and Ivory Coast's Gbagbo (now under trial by the ICC). The claim that the ICC is biased against African countries is weakened by the fact that three African signatories to the Rome treaty have referred cases to the court (Uganda, the Democratic Republic of Congo, and Central African Republic).

STATE-BUILDING

> A feature of internal conflicts is the collapse of state institutions, especially the police and judiciary, with resulting paralysis of governance, a breakdown of law and order, and general banditry and chaos. Not only are the functions of government suspended, but its assets are destroyed and looted.
>
> —*Boutros Boutros-Ghali, former UN secretary-general, 1994*

By this stage, the mechanisms described in the preceding sections have allowed the international community to cajole or even force warring parties to stop fighting. Peace then allows the large aid agencies to help the country build a foundation of normality with delivery of basic services such as water, food, and security. The next step is the daunting task of building a stable state on a foundation that can provide its population with protection, growing prosperity, and, above all else, a way out of recurrent relapses into further violence. It is worth remembering that most of the current developed countries had to face identical struggles during their slow progress toward prosperity—it is also worth remembering that the journey from tzars, kings, and emperors to stable, prosperous democracies took two or three centuries of violent history. Clearly, state-building is a slow process that requires individualized planning and long-term investment. The benefits of stability and peace are so great that state-building should be viewed as one of the most important aspects of foreign aid. The consequences of failure are typified by Sudan, which has suffered decades of recurrent violence, refugees, starvation, and, ultimately, the destabilization of an entire region.

The end of the Cold War dramatically changed international attitudes toward oppressive governments. Apart from allowing the end of support for a range of tyrants from Suharto to the Greek colonels, it also marked a new era of openness in discussing the approach to "fragile" or "failed" states. This dialogue has now grown to become a major focus of modern aid. Unfortunately, repairing a failed state takes a long time, so prospective research takes many years to generate useful guidelines. While there is no shortage of reviews (DFID, 2005), recommendations (Englebert, 2008), classifications, and scoring systems (Rice et al., 2008), there is still far from a clear consensus on the correct way to repair a broken country. Simply trying to rebuild post-conflict countries using a strictly Western model of democracy and market-based economy is unlikely to survive pragmatic reality. Some form of hybrid system that includes past practices is inevitable. For example, a democratic government structure may not be accepted without the establishment of an unelected council of elders (e.g., Somaliland and Afghanistan), and economic reforms may have to tolerate some remnant of state ownership (e.g., Mozambique and Guyana).

Establishing a simple definition that encompasses all post-conflict fragile states is not possible because of the broad range of variables unique to each country. The Brookings Institution has published a multi-component scoring system that provides some comparison of different countries, but measurement error and subjective bias will always limit the practical value of component scores (Rice et al., 2008). In terms of planning interventions, nothing can replace the need for expert analysis based on detailed local knowledge. When it comes to ease of partnership, Britain's Department of International Development divides fragile states into four categories based on their governance capacity and willingness to co-operate (DFID, 2005):

- good partners with a functional government structure and enthusiasm to co-operate with the international community; examples include postwar Croatia, Bosnia-Herzegovina, and South Africa

- weak but willing states that have emerged from destructive wars with badly damaged capacity, but an effective peace agreement and a willingness to rebuild; examples include Mozambique, Libya, and El Salvador
- repressive states with some governance capacity, but little apparent interest in partnerships that benefit their people; examples include Central African Republic, Burma, and North Korea
- failed states where decades of war have left the country with no functioning administration outside the major cities and limited ability to form international partnerships; examples include Somalia and the Democratic Republic of Congo

The challenge of helping the fragile states within these various groups is the greatest dilemma facing the aid community. The majority of the world is moving ahead rapidly while these states, which have around 20 percent of the world's population, are increasingly left far behind. This does not mean that poor people are found only in fragile states—severe poverty still exists side by side with extraordinary wealth in many countries, including China, India, and Brazil. The marks of a fragile state are not just the presence of poverty, but the lack of progress or any real hope that things will be significantly better in the future. By any measure, their populations are disadvantaged when compared to middle-income countries. This means fewer children in school, widespread lack of access to hygiene and clean water, and high rates of poverty and maternal and child mortality. While there is no magic formula for rebuilding failed states, the establishment of peace, using the methods discussed earlier, followed by strengthening government capacity, is the broad route to take. How best to improve governance is a matter of debate; the following methods are used.

Developing Civil Society

At its most general level, civil society refers to all people, activities, relationships, and formal and informal groups that are not part of the process of government.

—R. Riddell, 2007

Of all the interventions designed to improve governance standards, "establishing civil society" is the term that will be heard most commonly. As with many fashionable terms, its definition is difficult because it means different things to different people. Broadly speaking, civil society is the "place" between government and the general population where private citizens join together to promote and protect a huge number of special interests. Such groups range from parent-teacher associations to Amnesty International. In free countries, someone somewhere is raising a petition to protect something you've likely never heard of. The endless variety of civil society represents the most basic right of a citizen and it is an essential part of a strong society. In developing countries, groups focus on more immediate issues, such as human rights, crime, violence, and access to information. NGOs specializing in civil society work are usually referred to as CSOs (civil society organizations). In countries with weak governments emerging from civil war, donors face a dilemma when it comes to administering aid. Using NGOs and local CSOs may be the only way to deliver aid with any reliability during the initial recovery phase, but this risks alienating the existing remnants of government. Of course, NGOs are not free from internal squabbles or local tribal and religious biases, so the rebuilding period is a minefield of potential problems.

The current enthusiasm for improving governance through the support of civil society organizations started with its rapid growth in the 1990s. The theoretical value of such a policy was articulated by the World Bank's influential paper in 1999, which laid out the broad principles governing the World Bank's engagement with developing countries in the new millennium (World Bank, 2010). This Comprehensive Development Framework subsequently influenced the design of the Poverty Reduction Strategy process introduced the following year. Its influence can also be seen in the design of the MDGs around the same time. Among other recommendations, it emphasized the need for partnerships between government and civil society and also for the active involvement of citizens in the planning and implementation of aid projects. The subsequent "meteoric career" for civil society (Brouwers, 2011) can be dated from that time.

Unfortunately, prodding governments into action is not an easy task, even under the best of circumstances. While there are examples of successful policy changes resulting from civil society pressure (UN, 2007), studies have shown that funding for CSO advocacy groups often has only a limited impact on government behaviour (Robinson et al., 2005). While no one argues against the need for the active involvement of citizens in the broad governmental process, implementing this in practice is a different matter. The widespread citizens' demonstrations across the Arab world have produced extraordinary changes in previously repressive governments, and they show what can be achieved when desperate people take to the streets. However, less extreme citizen responses, such as advertising campaigns, negotiations with various levels of government, sit-ins, and marches, will inevitably have less effect on entrenched powers (IDS, 2008). It has been suggested that policy change should not be the only measured end point. While funding citizens' groups to have open discussion about their main concerns may not have much effect on government policy, the process itself may be beneficial. It is possible that the main advantage of civil society involvement may simply be better levels of civility. The following section gives a few examples of successful changes in government policy that resulted from civil society lobbying actions.

Civil Society in Action

A representative and responsive government is composed of so many different elements that it is difficult to know where to start when taking on the job of building a strong system. The following sections gives examples where citizens' groups of various sorts have managed to make significant changes in governance in the areas of democratic representation, delivery of public services, the rule of law, and the fight against corruption. All have their problems, but it is the accumulation of these imperfect small advances that finally add up to a stable, peaceful society.

Democratic Representation
- *South Africa:* Although the South African constitution mandates civil society participation in local government, surveys in the 1990s revealed engagement was poor, with little knowledge of the process among local governments or CSOs. The government's response was to pass the Municipal Systems Act in 2000, which required municipalities to include the public in local development planning (IDASA, 2011). Experience showed that progress did occur, but forming truly productive links between government and the community was a slow process that required commitment from both sides. Representation for traditionally less advantaged groups, such as women, children, and the disabled, was also slow to develop.
- *Palestine:* During the early days of the Palestine Authority in the mid-1990s, women had little say or active involvement in the political process. In response, Palestinian women formed the Women's Affairs Technical Committee (WATC) in order to lobby for gender-related legislation and the protection of women's rights (UN, 2010). Their pressure through media campaigns and lobbying the legislative council led to the creation of a Ministry for Women's Affairs and also a guaranteed quota for women on local councils. While there are now women in public life, their full participation is sometimes resisted and a large gender gap persists.

Delivery of Public Services
- *Romania:* In Romania, the minority Roma make up over 10 percent of the population. They suffer significantly worse health than the majority

because of discrimination, poverty, and lack of access to education and health care. In response, the Roma Centre for Social Intervention and Studies (CRISS) started the Roma Health Mediator program in 1997. They trained local Roma to act as mediators between their communities and the health system (ENAR, 2007). While the health mediator system has been successful across the country in helping communities access medical care and health insurance, the program has not been backed by national legislation that guarantees greater inclusion of Roma in society.

- *Uganda:* The Karamojong are a semi-nomadic people living in northern Uganda. In the 1990s, their literacy rates were very low because of poor school enrolment. The Alternative Basic Education for Karamoja program (ABEK) was established to provide schooling compatible with their way of life. Before schooling was started, it was necessary to address deep-seated distrust of government. In addition to basic reading, writing, and numeracy, the children are also taught about livestock, crops, and home management. ABEK has been a successful project. Enrolment has increased greatly and girls outnumber boys in school. Many children are now going on to join the formal school system. Problems include poor security in the region and the need for sustainable funding.

Rule of Law

- *Malawi:* As a result of underfunding and poorly trained staff, Malawi's prisons were overcrowded with remand prisoners who were being held without charge. Most prisoners were unaware of their rights and had little chance of obtaining legal representation. In 2000, an NGO-sponsored pilot scheme, based on 12 trained paralegal staff, was started to improve the capacity of the justice system. Paralegals worked with the police to process cases faster, and they also worked in the prisons to educate prisoners about their rights. Priority is given to vulnerable groups, such as women, juveniles, and the mentally ill. The Paralegal Advisory Service (PAS) was successful and later expanded in partnership with the prison service (Kerrigan, 2002). In five years, PAS helped obtain the release of 2,000 prisoners who had been illegally detained, and halved the number of remand prisoners in the prison population.
- *Chile:* During the Chilean military dictatorship of the 1970s and 1980s, government repression affected hundreds of thousands of people. Many of them were left with severe long-term mental and physical health problems. In response to lobbying by victims' groups, the Ministry of Health

established the Program of Reparation and Comprehensive Care (PRAIS) for survivors of torture. It provides victims and their families with free medical care and also offers free mental health care from specially trained teams (Bacic, 2002). Apart from providing health care, PRAIS has given the victims a national voice. The main problems are growing numbers of eligible people and lack of funding.

Combating Corruption

- *Botswana:* Although Botswana has a history of stable democratic government, it was hit by a series of corruption scandals in the early 1990s. Failure of the government to take any serious action resulted in pressure from public groups, particularly the country's free media. After considerable national debate, the government responded by establishing the Directorate of Corruption and Economic Crime (TI, 2001). The Directorate has a broad mandate that includes investigation of corruption, public education, and prevention. While it has successfully prosecuted many cases and has raised public awareness of anti-corruption mechanisms, the Directorate is not fully independent since it has to report to the president and must rely on the attorney general's office to agree to a prosecution.
- *India:* Embezzlement of public funds at the local government level is common in India. In the 1990s, detecting and preventing corruption was particularly difficult because Indian states did not reveal budget documents. A workers' and farmers' organization, called MKSS, pressured authorities in Rajasthan to allow the public the right to information about local government finances. After a long battle, the Rajasthan Right to Information Act came into force in 2001. Open auditing of public expenditures was successful in improving the flow of money to public projects. It spread to other states and became national law in 2005. Access to information is still far from a full inclusion of the poor in local governance, but it is a good first step.

SUMMARY

Of the 195 countries studied by Freedom House, a total of 50 countries are deemed Not Free, representing 26 percent of the world's countries and 2.6 billion people. A peaceful civil society requires representative government, fair rule of law, citizen participation, and broad human rights. All of these essential supports must be backed by an educated, healthy population whose values, attitudes, and behaviours all reflect a culture of peace. Peace can be built only on a foundation of good governance, prosperity, and good health. Such ideas were at the basis of the UN's Charter of Human Rights. Some regions of the world enjoy sustained levels of peace and security, while others fall into seemingly never-ending cycles of conflict and violence. The benefits of stability and peace are so great that state-building should be viewed as one of the most important aspects of foreign aid. The consequences of failure are typified by the country of Sudan, which has suffered decades of recurrent violence, refugees, starvation, and, ultimately, the destabilization of an entire region. Furthermore, peace allows large aid agencies to help build a foundation of normality with the delivery of basic services such as water, food, and security. After a time of conflict, the next step is the daunting task of building a stable state on a foundation that can provide its population with protection, growing prosperity, and above all else, a way out of recurrent relapses into further violence. Good governance is critical for peace and social capital can be done by "establishing a civil society" where private citizens join together to promote and protect a huge number of special interests. The 16th SDG highlights the critical nature of peaceful societies: "Promote peaceful and inclusive societies for sustainable development, provide access to justice for all and build effective, accountable and inclusive institutions at all levels." This SDG aims to significantly reduce all forms of violence, and to work with governments and communities to find lasting solutions to conflict and insecurity, as indicated in one of the targets, to "promote the rule of law at the national and international levels and ensure equal access to justice for all." Strengthening the rule of law, promoting human rights, and strengthening the participation of developing countries in the institutions of global governance are key to the process of establishing peaceful and healthy societies.

DISCUSSION QUESTIONS

1. Why is peace important as a foundation for the development of a healthy and prosperous society?

2. Why do a large fraction of the world's population still live under conditions that would not be tolerated for one minute by people living in a democracy?

3. How would you evaluate the history of military intervention in the response to dangerously unstable countries?

4. What are the current approaches to rebuilding countries emerging from conflict? Which approaches do you consider most effective?

5. What are some of the significant issues that arise in trying to build peace and good governance in developing countries? Why do these issues exist?

6.   What are the factors that might affect the potential success of mediation?

7.   What UN body is responsible for international peace and security?

8.   What has been the importance of the International Criminal Court in influencing the behaviour of tyrants?

9.   What is RtoP? DDR?

10.   How important is SDG 16 in relation to peace, justice, and effective, accountable, and inclusive institutions? What are its key targets, and do you think they will be achieved by 2030?

11.   Provide examples where citizens' groups have managed to make significant changes in governance in the areas of democratic representation, delivery of public services, the rule of law, and the fight against corruption.

RECOMMENDED READING

Crocker, C., et al. (Eds.). 2007. *Leashing the dogs of war: Conflict management in a divided world*. Pub: US Institute of Peace.

Fortna, V. 2008. *Does peacekeeping work? Shaping belligerents' choices after civil war*. Pub: Princeton University Press.

Hufbauer, G., et al. 2007. *Economic sanctions reconsidered* (3rd ed.). Pub: Institute for International Economics.

Lutz, E., et al. 2008. *Prosecuting heads of state*. Pub: Cambridge University Press.

Mdulo, N., et al. (Eds.). 2010. *Failed and failing states: The challenges for African reconstruction*. Pub: Cambridge Scholars Publishing.

Muggah, R. (Ed.). 2009. *Security and post-conflict reconstruction: Dealing with fighters in the aftermath of war*. Pub: Routledge.

Sisk, T. 2009. *International mediation in civil wars: Bargaining with bullets*. Pub: Routledge.

REFERENCES

Bacic, R. 2002. Dealing with the past: Chile—human rights and human wrongs. *Race and Class*, 44: 17–31.

Beber, B. 2010. The (non) efficacy of multi-party mediation in wars since 1990. New York University. Retrieved from: https://files.nyu.edu/bb89/public/files/Beber_MultipartyMediation.pdf.

Brookings Institution. 2004. Poverty and the right to know: Using information to demand equity and justice. Retrieved from: www.brookings.edu/comm/events/20041028.pdf.

Brouwers, R. 2011. When civics go "governance": On the role and relevance of civic organizations in the policy arena. Retrieved from: www.hivos.nl/eng/Hivos-Knowledge-Programme/Themes/Civil-Society-Building/Publications/Synthesis-studies/When-Civics-go-Governance.

Carames, A., et al. 2009. Analysis of the world's disarmament, demobilization, and reintegration programs in 2008. Bellaterra School for a Culture of Peace. Retrieved from: http://escolapau.uab.cat/img/programas/desarme/ddr/ddr2009i.pdf.

Chalmers, M. 2004. Spending to save? An analysis of the cost effectiveness of conflict prevention. Retrieved from: www.csae.ox.ac.uk/conferences/2004-BB/papers/Chalmers-CSAE-BB2004.pdf.

Collier, P., et al. 2004. The challenge of reducing the global incidence of civil war. Centre for the Study of African Economies. Retrieved from: www.copenhagenconsensus.com/Files/Filer/CC/Papers/Conflicts_230404.pdf.

Collier, P., et al. 2006. Post-conflict risks. Centre for the Study of African Economies. Retrieved from: www.csae.ox.ac.uk/workingpapers/pdfs/2006-12text.pdf.

Collier, P. 2007. *The bottom billion.* Pub: Oxford University Press.

CSIS. 2002. Centre for Strategic and International Studies: Post-conflict reconstruction. Retrieved from: http://csis.org/images/stories/pcr/framework.pdf.

DFID. 2005. Why we need to work more effectively in fragile states. Retrieved from: www.jica.go.jp/cdstudy/library/pdf/20071101_11.pdf.

DFID. 2010. Working effectively in conflict-affected and fragile situations. Retrieved from: www.dfid.gov.uk/Documents/publications1/governance/building-peaceful-states-G.pdf.

DPA. 2006. Operational guidance note: Disarmament, demobilisation, and reintegration. UN Department of Political Affairs. Retrieved from: http://reliefweb.int/node/23698.

DPA. 2016. UN Department of Political Affairs. Retrieved from: http://www.un.org/undpa/en.

DPKO. 2016. Department of Peacekeeping Operations. Retrieved from: www.un.org/en/peacekeeping/about/dpko/.

Drezner, D. 2003. How smart are smart sanctions? *International Studies Review,* 5: 107–110.

Dufka, C. 2005. Youth, poverty, and blood: The lethal legacy of West Africa's regional warriors. Human Rights Watch. Retrieved from: http://allafrica.com/peaceafrica/resources/view/00010617.pdf.

ENAR. 2007. The situation of Roma in Europe. European Network against Racism. Retrieved from: www.romadecade.org/files/downloads/General%20Resources/The%20situation%20of%20Roma%20in%20Europe%202007.pdf.

Englebert, P., et al. 2008. Postconflict resolution in Africa: Flawed ideas about failed states. *International Security,* 32: 106–139.

Escriba-Folch, A. 2008. Economic sanctions and the duration of civil conflicts. *Journal of Peace Research*, 47: 129–141.

Foreign Affairs. 2008. Lester B. Pearson. Retrieved from: www.international.gc.ca/about-a_propos/pearson_nobel.aspx?view=d.

Freedom House. 2011a. Freedom in the world: Comparative and historical data. Retrieved from: www.freedomhouse.org/template.cfm?page=439.

Freedom House. 2011b. Freedom in the world 2011. Retrieved from: www.freedomhouse.org/images/File/fiw/FIW_2011_Booklet.pdf.

Freedom House. 2016. Freedom in the world 2016. Anxious dictators, wavering democracies: Global freedom under pressure. Retrieved from: https://freedomhouse.org/report/freedom-world-2016/overview-essay-anxious-dictators-wavering-democracies.

Gaddis, J. 2005. *The Cold War*. Pub: Penguin Press.

Gilligan, D., et al. 2008. An analysis of Ethiopia's Productive Safety Net Program and its linkages. International Food Policy Research Institute. Retrieved from: www.csae.ox.ac.uk/conferences/2008-EDiA/papers/391-Taffesse.pdf.

Grindle, M. 2007. Good enough governance revisited. *Development Policy Review*, 25: 553–574.

Heldt, B., et al. 2005. Peacekeeping operations: Global patterns of intervention and success, 1948–2004. Folke Bernadotte Academy Research Report. Stockholm.

Hufbauer, G., et al. 2007. Economic sanctions reconsidered (3rd ed.). Pub: Institute for International Economics.

Human Security Report. 2010. Retrieved from: www.hsrgroup.org/human-security-reports/20092010/overview.aspx.

Humphreys, M., et al. 2007. Demobilization and reintegration. *Journal of Conflict Resolution*, 51: 531–567.

ICC. 2011. The International Criminal Court. Retrieved from: www.icc-cpi.int/Menus/ICC.

ICISS. 2001. International Commission on Intervention and State Sovereignty. The responsibility to protect. Retrieved from: http://responsibilitytoprotect.org/ICISS%20Report.pdf.

IDASA. 2011. Participatory governance at local level. Institute for Democracy in South Africa. Retrieved from: www.idasa.org/our_products/resources/output/participatory_governance_at/?pid=municipal_governance_in_sa.

IDS. 2008. Building responsive states: Citizen action and national policy change. Institute of Development Studies policy briefing. Retrieved from: www.ids.ac.uk/files/InFocus5.pdf.

IIC. 2005. Independent Inquiry Committee into manipulation of the Oil for Food Programme. Retrieved from: www.iic-offp.org/story27oct05.htm.

Kerrigan, F. 2002. Energizing the criminal justice system in Malawi: The Paralegal Advisory Service. Retrieved from: www.penalreform.org/publications/energising-criminal-justice-system-malawi-0.

Kim, H., et al. 2010. Explaining the deterrence effect of human rights prosecutions for transitional countries. *International Studies Quarterly*, 54: 939–963.

Lutz, E., et al. 2008. *Prosecuting heads of state*. Pub: Cambridge University Press.

Muggah, R. (Ed.). 2009. *Security and post-conflict reconstruction: Dealing with fighters in the aftermath of war*. Pub: Routledge.

Nakaya, S. 2009. Aid in post-conflict (non) state building: A synthesis. Bunche Institute for International Studies. Retrieved from: http://statesandsecurity.org/_pdfs/Nakaya.pdf.

NorAd. 2006. A review of the Alternative Basic Education program in Karamoja. Norwegian Aid agency. Retrieved from: www.norad.no/en/tools-and-publications/publications/publication?key=138659.

NYU. 2008. NYU Centre on International Cooperation. Recovering from war: Gaps in early action. Retrieved from: www.cic.nyu.edu/peacebuilding/docs/earlyrecoveryfinal.pdf.

Pugel, J. 2007. What the fighters say: A survey of ex-combatants in Liberia. UNDP Joint Implementation Unit. Retrieved from: www.lr.undp.org/UNDPwhatFightersSayLiberia-2006.pdf.

Regan, P., et al. 2009. Diplomatic interventions and civil war: A new dataset. *Journal of Peace Research*, 46: 135–146.

Renner, M. 2006. Peacekeeping expenditures in current vs. real terms: 1947–2005. Worldwatch Institute. Retrieved from: www.globalpolicy.org/images/pdfs/Z/pk_tables/currentreal.pdf.

Rice, S., et al. 2008. Index of state weakness in the developing world. Brookings Institution. Retrieved from: www.brookings.edu/~/media/Files/rc/reports/2008/02_weak_states_index/02_weak_states_index.pdf.

Robinson, M., et al. 2005. Civil society, democratization, and foreign aid in Africa. Institute of Development Studies. Retrieved from: www.ids.ac.uk/files/Dp383.pdf.

Sisk, T. 2009. *International mediation in civil wars: Bargaining with bullets*. Pub: Routledge.

Sriram, C. 2003. Revolutions in accountability: New approaches to past abuses. *American University International Law Review*, 19: 310–329.

TI. 2001. Transparency International. National integrity systems: Country study report, Botswana. Retrieved from: www.transparency.org/policy_research/nis/nis_reports_by_country.

UN. 2001. Report of the panel on UN peace operations. Retrieved from: www.un.org/peace/reports/peace_operations/.

UN. 2007. Good governance practices for the protection of human rights. Retrieved from: www.ohchr.org/Documents/Publications/GoodGovernance.pdf.

UN. 2009. Report of the secretary-general. Implementing the responsibility to protect. Retrieved from: http://globalr2p.org/pdf/SGR2PEng.pdf.

UN. 2010. Situation of and assistance to Palestinian women. Report of the secretary-general. Retrieved from: www.peacewomen.org/assets/file/PWandUN/CSW/55/csw55_sgreportonsituationofandassistancetopalestinianwomen_12.10.2010.pdf.

UN. 2011a. United Nations Peacebuilding Commission. Retrieved from: www.un.org/en/peacebuilding/index.asp.

UN. 2011b. Reform of peacekeeping. Retrieved from: www.un.org/en/peacekeeping/operations/reform.shtml.

UNDP. 1994. Human development report: New dimensions in human security. Retrieved from: http://hdr.undp.org/en/reports/global/hdr1994/chapters/.

UNDP. 2008. Post-conflict economic recovery: Enabling local ingenuity. Retrieved from: http://europeandcis.undp.org/home/show/3E355E78-F203-1EE9-B7C2F002B8A5F9B4.

Whitfield, T. 2007. *Friends indeed: The United Nations, groups of friends, and the resolution of conflict*. Pub: US Institute of Peace.

WHO. 2003. School deworming. Retrieved from: www.who.int/wormcontrol/documents/en/at_a_glance.pdf.

World Bank. 2010. Comprehensive development framework. Retrieved from: http://go.worldbank.org/N2NDBE5QL0.

World Bank. 2011a. World Development Indicators database. Retrieved from: http://data.worldbank.org/indicator.

World Bank. 2011b. Worldwide Governance Indicators. Retrieved from: http://info.worldbank.org/governance/wgi/index.asp.

World Bank. 2011c. How we classify countries. Retrieved from: http://data.worldbank.org/about/country-classifications.

World Bank. 2016. World Bank country and lending groups. Retrieved from: https://datahelpdesk.worldbank.org/knowledgebase/articles/906519.

PART V

OTHER ASPECTS OF GLOBAL HEALTH

CHAPTER 16

Natural and Humanitarian Disasters and Displaced Populations

When disaster strikes, it tears the curtain away from the festering problems that lie beneath.

—*Barack Obama, 2005*

OBJECTIVES

Taken together, humanitarian and natural disasters are surprisingly common. The last few years have witnessed some of the most lethal and certainly some of the most expensive disasters in history. Apart from the immediate death and injury caused by a disaster, the subsequent economic and social chaos (plus the effects of displaced populations) can be enormous. Poor building standards, lack of civil defence organizations, concentrations of population in high-risk areas, and lack of money are some of the reasons why developing countries can be so badly affected by disasters. After completing this chapter, you should be able to:

- appreciate the human and financial costs associated with wars and natural disasters
- understand the differences between refugees, migrants, and other types of displaced populations
- understand the harsh realities of life as a refugee and develop a list of priorities aimed at keeping a refugee population as healthy as possible
- understand the general organizational framework needed to manage a complex human emergency

INTRODUCTION

"God's work," he would say
When the rain pelted down
And the floods rushed in the rivers
And storms lashed the tree-tops
"God's work!"
God should play more.

—Ian McDonald, "God's Work," Essequito, 1992

Wars and natural disasters, and the forced migrant populations they produce, are constants in human history. On a global scale, the most common disaster facing a large number of developing countries is the need to care for displaced refugees fleeing an internal war. Major natural disasters are less common than humanitarian catastrophes, but their costs in terms of lives and economic collapse are usually much higher. When the recent earthquakes in Japan, Haiti, and Pakistan are combined with the humanitarian disasters currently affecting Sudan and Somalia, it is clear that these events are not rare. The human and financial costs of disasters are such that they can slow a developing country's progress for decades after the event. Their effects are felt worldwide, so disasters should be part of any study of global health. Since their burden falls disproportionately upon countries with limited resources, anyone working in a developing country should have a good idea of the health problems confronting a displaced population. This module looks at the causes behind large-scale population migrations (particularly natural and humanitarian disasters) and also reviews the international structures that have been developed to deal with these enormously complex problems.

This chapter will also examine the essential requirements needed to reduce mortality among a refugee population. While there is a very understandable human desire to help the survivors of a disaster, it is important to ensure that the response is organized and professional. Hard lessons learned from the Asian tsunami showed that the sudden influx of hundreds of uncoordinated groups is not the most efficient way to respond to a chaotic situation. The initial emergency aid for survivors, followed by the reconstruction of their shattered society, is an overwhelming job. Apart from money and materials, there is a need for well-trained experts in subjects ranging from nutrition and sanitation to construction and public planning. While the international disaster response agencies have achieved valuable work under very difficult conditions, it is widely accepted that there is room for improvement in the areas of coordination, professionalism, and standardization.

Until recently, the response to disasters has principally concentrated on the initial emergency management, but this emphasis is changing. Although earthquakes, storms, and volcanic eruptions cannot be avoided, their adverse effects can, to some extent, be predicted, and effective plans made to reduce those effects. Disaster mitigation is still a relatively new subject. It is based on specific risk analysis, local response strategies, and, most recently, on disaster insurance. It is hoped that improvements in the international disaster response, plus more widespread mitigation planning, will greatly reduce the burden of these terrible events.

NATURAL DISASTERS

> We had scarce sat down, when darkness overspread us, not like a moonless or cloudy night, but of a room when it is shut up and the lamp put out. You could hear the shrieks of women, the crying of children, and the shouts of men.
>
> —*Pliny, eyewitness account of the destruction of Pompeii, AD 79*

The Center for Research on Epidemiology of Disasters (CRED, 2011) was established in 1973 in Belgium. The organization collects data on all emergencies that have a significant human impact. In the absence of an internationally agreed-upon definition, they define a disaster as an event where at least one of the following criteria is met: there are over 10 deaths; more than 100 people are affected; a state of emergency is declared; or international assistance is requested. They split disasters into three categories:

- *Natural:* Earthquake, volcanic eruption, temperature extremes, floods, meteorological events, tsunami
- *Technological:* Principally accidents involving industry or mass transport
- *Humanitarian:* Complete social and economic collapse, usually following a civil war

Apart from having a reliable and easily accessible database, the centre also collects and publishes valuable health and nutrition data on conflict zones.

There is nothing new about disasters. The Minoan civilization was destroyed by the vast eruption and probable tsunami following the eruption of Santorini in 1600 BC. The early walls of Troy were toppled by earthquakes, and the first eyewitness account of a disaster was written by Pliny the Younger, who described the eruption of Vesuvius in AD 79 that buried Pompeii. His uncle died in the disaster while trying to save a family friend. Some disasters attract considerable attention, while others, in a world of short headlines, soon vanish from the news. It is very easy to forget even the most terrible examples of these catastrophes. Most are familiar with the recent Japanese earthquake, Hurricane Katrina, and the Asian tsunami,

Table 16.1: Major natural disasters in recent years

HURRICANES		
Cyclone Nargis, Burma	2008	138,000 dead; cost to region US$10 billion
Hurricane Katrina, US	2005	1,400 dead; huge social and economic consequences, including over US$200 billion in damages
Hurricane Mitch, Central America	1998	19,000 dead; enormous economic consequences for Central America: US$6 billion in damages
Cyclone Bhola, Bangladesh	1970	500,000 dead; largest ever natural disaster
EARTHQUAKES/TSUNAMIS		
Tōhoku earthquake, Japan	2011	20,000 dead or missing; over US$200 billion in damages
Haiti earthquake	2010	Total deaths disputed, but likely above 100,000; enormous social disruption
Sichuan earthquake, China	2008	85,000 dead and missing; over US$75 billion in damages
Kashmir earthquake, Pakistan	2005	80,000 dead; enormous damage to the region's infrastructure
Asian tsunami, Indonesia, Sri Lanka	2004	200,000 dead; immeasurable economic and social effects

Table 16.2: Major biological and industrial disasters of recent years

BIOLOGICAL DISASTERS		
Ebola outbreak in West Africa	2013–2016	Mainly in three West African countries (Liberia, Sierra Leone, and Guinea); about 28,700 cases and 11,300 deaths
West Africa meningitis (Meningococcus)	2009	Four African countries affected; 25,000 cases, 1,000 deaths
Avian influenza (H5N1 strain)	2003–present	Annual worldwide outbreaks since 2003; 300 human deaths, huge agricultural impact
SARS (Coronavirus)	2002	Rapid worldwide spread from China; 8,400 cases, 900 deaths
Hong Kong influenza (H3N2 strain)	1968	Rapid spread from South Asian focus; estimated 1 million deaths
INDUSTRIAL DISASTERS		
Lac-Mégantic rail disaster	2013	Derailment of an oil shipment train; 47 killed and 30 buildings destroyed
Fukushima nuclear disaster	2011	Level 7 reactor meltdown following Tohoku earthquake; no deaths
Gulf oil rig explosion and oil spill	2010	Huge economic and environmental effects; 11 killed in explosion
Chernobyl nuclear disaster	1986.	Reactor explosion; 31 killed and unknown future risk of radiation-related deaths
Bhopal disaster	1984	Methyl isocyanate release; 4,000 dead initially; many thousands more die over the following years

but how many remember Cyclone Nargis in 2008, which killed 138,000 people in Burma, or the Sichuan earthquake that happened only a few days afterwards, killing 85,000 people in China? Tables 16.1 and 16.2 list some of the worst disasters in various categories within recent years.

Major disasters are surprisingly common. As the global population grows, more people live in areas at high risk of recurring events such as floods, hurricanes, and earthquakes. Consequently, the total number of disasters affecting humans seems to be rising slowly each decade (Figure 16.1). For each person who dies, many times that number are injured or economically affected. Despite the chaos surrounding the Hurricane Katrina response, developed countries generally have the resources to minimize the adverse effects of natural disasters, but this comes with an impressive bill. The last 20 years have witnessed the most expensive disasters in history (Figure 16.2). Hurricane Andrew cost US$35 billion in 1992 and the 1995 Kobe earthquake caused US$100 billion in property damage, plus US$50 billion in reduced economic output. Hurricane Katrina caused US$100 billion damage in New Orleans alone; the final bill is still not in, but seems likely to approach US$200 billion (Schiermeier, 2006). According to the World Bank's estimated cost, the bill for the Japanese earthquake could be as high as US$235 billion, making it the costliest natural disaster in world history. (Zhang, 2011).

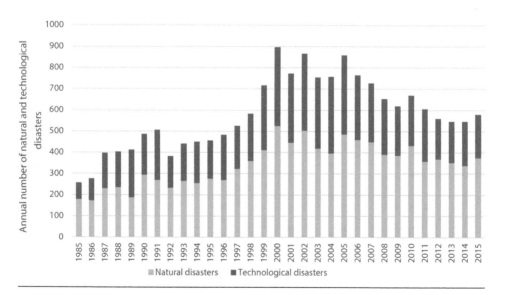

Figure 16.1: Trends in the annual number of technological and natural disasters combined over the last 30 years

Source: EM-DAT. 2016. Emergency Events Database, Centre for Research on the Epidemiology of Disasters. Retrieved from: www.emdat.be/advanced_search/index.html.

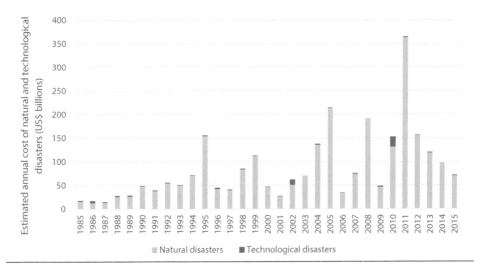

Figure 16.2: Trends in total annual damage estimates from natural and technological disasters over the last 30 years; costs caused by technological disasters were only a significant fraction of the total in 2002 due to a large oil spill from a Spanish tanker.

Source: EM-DAT. 2016. Emergency Events Database, Centre for Research on the Epidemiology of Disasters. Retrieved from: www.emdat.be/advanced_search/index.html.

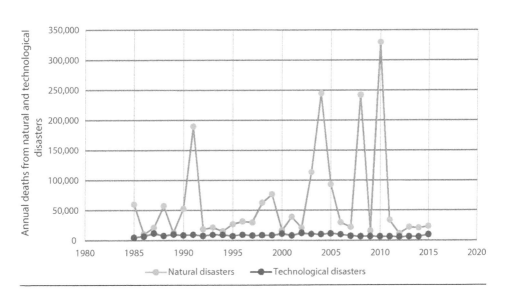

Figure 16.3: Trends in combined annual deaths from natural and technological disasters

Source: EM-DAT. 2016. Emergency Events Database, Centre for Research on the Epidemiology of Disasters. Retrieved from: www.emdat.be/advanced_search/index.html.

Disasters kill significant numbers of people each year (Figure 16.3) and the social repercussions of such events should not be underestimated. Again, recent years have seen some of the most lethal disasters in history. Taken together, the Asian tsunami, earthquakes in Haiti, Pakistan, and Japan, plus Cyclone Nargis, claimed hundreds of thousands of lives. When expressed as a rate, the chance of being killed in a disaster is small, but the death rate is not the best indicator of the final human and economic costs of disasters. In some instances, those costs are large enough to cause major political upheavals. Examples within recent history include Cyclone Bhola in 1970, which triggered the Bangladesh war of independence; the 1976 Tangshan earthquake, which is credited with bringing about the end of the Cultural Revolution; and the 2004 Asian tsunami, which hastened the end of the Sri Lankan civil war by weakening Tamil resistance.

A good summary of the effects of disasters is given in a report by Guha-Sapir et al. (2004). In the decade following 1994, the review estimates that more than 255 million people (range 68 million to 618 million) were affected by natural disasters every year, and the average annual mortality was 58,000 people (range 10,000 to 133,000). In the same time period, the damage caused by disasters cost US$67 billion per year (range US$28 billion to $230 billion). This cost has increased fourteen-fold since the 1950s. When the figures are averaged out, disasters cause roughly US$1 billion of damage, kill 1,000 people, and in some way adversely affect 5 million people every single week. During 2003, 1 in 25 people worldwide were affected by a natural disaster. The total number of people affected by the social and economic results of disasters is large and appears to be growing steadily. Anyone working overseas in a developing country should have a good practical knowledge of disaster response and the care necessary for displaced populations.

International Disaster Management

Eritrea received seven truckloads of expired Aspirin tablets that took six months to burn; a container full of unsolicited cardiovascular drugs with two months to expiry; and 30,000 bottles of expired amino acid infusion that could not be disposed of anywhere near the settlement because of the smell.

—*Hans Hogerzeil, 1998*

Apart from immediate injury and loss of life, the property damage associated with a disaster can destroy the complex infrastructure that supports public health. Without prompt action, outbreaks of common communicable diseases, such as gastroenteritis and measles, are a significant risk. The international community has responded to this challenge. International humanitarian assistance increased for the third consecutive year, reaching a record high of US$28.0 billion in 2015 (GHA, 2016).

People's desire to help others under these circumstances is quite understandable, but the enthusiasm of some responders greatly exceeds their competence. Health care is a serious undertaking at the best of times. Under suboptimal conditions of war and disaster, where teams may face very real physical danger, high levels of training, coordination, and continuous assessment are vital. The need for international standards governing the coordination and management of disaster response teams is an urgent priority. Within the last decade, there has also been an increasing focus on disaster mitigation. Prior to this, money and research had been predominantly devoted to the emergency response effort. However, the concept of mitigating disasters through risk assessment and management is now gaining increased attention and funding (HFA, 2005).

The United Nations agency responsible for coordinating emergency relief is the Office for the Coordination of Humanitarian Affairs (OCHA, 2011). It was formed in 1998 from the earlier UN Disaster Relief Coordinator. A separate department of OCHA called the Integrated Regional Information Network (IRIN, 2011) acts as a specialized news agency that provides an excellent source of news and analysis about current disasters. Emergencies are unpredictable, so the emergency relief coordinator in charge of OCHA has to have access to immediate funds for humanitarian disasters. This obvious requirement was met with the establishment of the Central Emergency Response Fund in 2006 (CERF, 2011). OCHA aims to have US$500 million available for rapid use. Despite hard economic times, donors have responded well, which allows OCHA to be a major initial responder to disasters around the world.

In general, once a disaster reaches the world's headlines, people are surprisingly generous; there is a feeling that something must be done and done quickly. This can lead to considerable inappropriate effort, such as airlifts of shoes, discarded clothing, and competing high-technology field hospitals, which may simply add to the chaos. Disaster management attracts a lot of research attention and is emerging as a specific medical subspecialty with at least two medical journals devoted to the topic. There are also several field handbooks guiding management priorities during a disaster. The handbooks, published by Médecins sans Frontières (MSF, 1997) and UNICEF (2005), both provide reliable guidelines for management priorities. The Sphere Project, formed in 1997, grew out of the extensive investigation of the humanitarian response to the Rwandan crisis. The organization has developed a useful handbook on the management of large disasters, but has also broken new ground by establishing standards of good practice and accountability (Sphere Project, 2011).

Common Problems with Disaster Responses

Emergency medical aid is not for amateurs.

—The Lancet editorial, 1997

Apart from cases of acute trauma during the initial emergency, there is nothing medically unique about disasters except the numbers involved. The sudden compression of large numbers of people into small areas, with poor sanitation and shelter, will inevitably lead to the usual diseases of poverty and overcrowding. As long as security can be assured, these problems are manageable using the basic principles of primary health care. This relief work should be done by agencies that are coordinated and, above all, staffed by people who know what they are doing (Photo 16.1). The basic essentials of management will be covered later in the chapter, but some general comments about the problems associated with emergency responses are necessary at this stage.

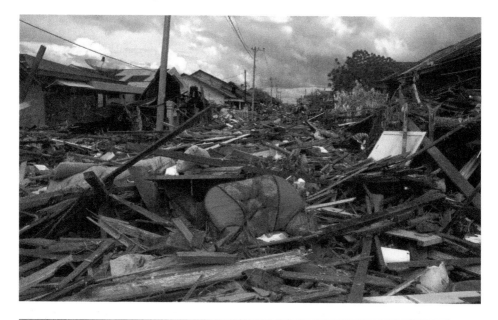

Photo 16.1: This is a scene of absolute devastation in Aceh province after the December 2004 Asian tsunami. Responding to a disaster of this magnitude and complexity requires well-trained, stable individuals from a variety of professional backgrounds, all backed by sustainable funding and logistic support.

Source: Jeffri Aries/Integrated Regional Information Network photo library (www.irinnews.org/photo).

Disasters are chaotic situations and large-scale emergency response efforts are still a relatively new development. Under these circumstances, it should be no surprise to learn that those efforts are frequently poorly coordinated and ineffective. This is not to say that the correct approach is a mystery. There is plenty of literature concerning best practice in humanitarian disasters. The first large-scale review of a disaster response was the comprehensive five-volume report produced by the Joint Evaluation of the Emergency Assistance to Rwanda (Dabelstein, 1996). Two organizations that grew out of those recommendations were the Sphere Project (2011) and the Active Learning Network for Accountability and Performance in Humanitarian Action (ALNAP, 2011). Both are dedicated to improving the standards of assistance provided to populations affected by disasters. Their work has helped establish clear standards for staff selection and training, team coordination, initial needs and outcome assessment, and project management. OCHA has produced similar recommendations (Adinolfi et al., 2005). Practical problems in the field are due to poor implementation of management standards that have been known for years. They are not due to lack of basic knowledge.

Although the extraordinary worldwide humanitarian response to the Indian Ocean tsunami mounted in early 2005 did have some positive end results, the process was far from perfect. It was so far from perfect, in fact, that the WHO organized a conference on the lessons to be learned from the international response as early as May 2005. The UN held a similar review process in August. The final reports from these two meetings contain many suggestions for improvements (McGarry et al., 2005). The most significant points are described below.

Coordination

During the initial disaster response period, there is clearly a need for coordination and order among the various agencies in the area. It is not widely appreciated how numerous and variable the responders can be. For example, during the Asian tsunami, over 300 agencies were registered with district health authorities in eastern Sri Lanka. Complicating matters further were numerous other groups fired with religious or political certainties that felt no need (and were under no obligation) to listen to anyone. This led to the absurd situation of different groups actually fighting over patients. While some coordinating organizations exist—examples include the UN's Inter-agency Standing Committee (IASC, 2011) and the UK's Disaster Emergency Committee (DEC, 2011)—there is still no umbrella group with the international mandate to control, manage, and, in some cases, limit the responding agencies.

Competence

The Lancet editorial quoted above should be noted. If someone isn't qualified to practise emergency medical care in his or her own country, there is no good reason why that person should be given permission to diagnose and manage critically ill people in a developing country. Emergencies are not places for untrained amateurs, and enthusiasm is no substitute for competence (*The Lancet*, 1996). The UN recommends not only that there should be far fewer disaster response agencies, but also that their quality (in terms of personnel training and internal management) should be much higher. India solved the problem by refusing to accept any foreign aid after the tsunami. The Sphere Project (2011) has made a good start by establishing minimum standards of training required by emergency responders, but recommendations are of no use without monitoring and implementation.

Needs Assessment

Many agencies start by performing an initial needs assessment. Unfortunately, these assessments are usually neither standardized nor shared. Multiple assessments not only waste time, but also subject stressed populations to repeated questioning by different groups. There is clearly a need for a unified disaster assessment system that identifies initial needs, but also includes long-term surveillance and outcome measurements. There are signs of improvement. The UN Disaster Assessment and Coordination team (UNDAC, 2011) consists of disaster management experts who can be rapidly deployed, within hours, to carry out an initial assessment of priority needs. The Field Assessment and Coordination Team (FACT, 2011) performs the same function for the International Federation of Red Cross and Red Crescent societies. Their assessment and coordination systems are compatible with those used by UNDAC.

Forensics

Most developing countries do not have the capacity to handle large numbers of casualties. The great majority of deaths in the Asian tsunami went unrecorded. In the rush to bury or cremate victims, adequate forensic information was not collected. There was also no standardization in forensic identification, which varied from Polaroid photos to DNA testing. The UN recommended that a pool of forensic pathologists should work to establish international standards for disaster victim identification and also for the safe storage of mass victims (Tun et al., 2005).

Women

Gender imbalances, present worldwide, are exacerbated by acute disasters. Families headed by female survivors are particularly vulnerable to poverty and ill health during the disaster recovery phase. The reproductive health and safety issues unique to women should be given particular priority following a disaster (IASC, 2006). These issues include feeding supplementation for pregnant women and an emphasis on security for women.

Psychological Trauma

There also needs to be a wider understanding of the psychological trauma and chronic mental illness associated with the survivors of major disasters. Whole communities can be devastated by the psychological effects of a disaster (IASC, 2007). Support and counselling can be established within the community, particularly within schools, but expert assistance is required to plan the necessary programs. "Counselling" is a term that has suffered from common use. Helping traumatized children to recover from psychological trauma requires long-term commitment and the assistance of professionally qualified staff. Properly planned, long-term initiatives (given in the local language by trained local staff) are an important part of the recovery process. However, sessions given by well-meaning but untrained short-term visitors may well do more harm than good. Once schools restarted in Sri Lanka following the tsunami, self-appointed counsellors became so disruptive that the education authority had to ban all foreigners from the schools. This complicated matters for legitimate professional teams.

Disaster Mitigation

> If people are constantly falling off a cliff, you could place ambulances under the cliff or build a fence on the top of the cliff. We are placing all too many ambulances under the cliff.
>
> —*Denis Burkitt*

By now it should be clear that the cumulative socio-economic effects of disasters are large enough that they should be viewed as a global concern. During the last several years, the world has witnessed some of the worst disasters in history, including the Asian tsunami; drought and famine in Somalia; hurricanes in the Gulf Coast and Central America; and earthquakes in Pakistan, Haiti, and Japan. Their direct and indirect effects are so great that, in some manner, their effects touch everyone. An exhaustive 2005 World Bank report on natural disaster hot spots revealed that over half of the world's population is exposed to one or more major natural hazards. It points out that between 1980 and 2003, the World Bank provided US\$14.4 billion in emergency lending to 20 developing world countries suffering from disasters (Dilley et al., 2005). The adverse economic effects of a large disaster add huge debts to a country, which slow its subsequent recovery and future development. Disasters

---

Box 16.1 Moment of Insight

Global Polio Eradication Program started in 1988.	Newest polio bivalent vaccine, introduced in 2010.
Number of children paralyzed every day, during introductory year:	Total number of cases reported that year in the entire world:
1,000	**1,000**

Source: Global Polio Eradication. 2011. Retrieved from: www.polioeradication.org/.

---

should not be viewed as rare occurrences that affect only a few thousand people. In many parts of the world, they are relatively common and they can affect the lives of millions of people, even whole countries. The planning and management needed to reduce disaster damage should now be an integral part of development aid programs (UNDP, 2004).

Attempts to reduce the damage caused by disasters are not new. The website of the UN's International Strategy for Disaster Reduction gives a useful historic timeline of the major events (ISDR, 2011). Interest picked up about 20 years ago with the declaration of the International Decade for Natural Disaster Reduction in 1990. The first strategy for disaster mitigation was developed in 1994, following a meeting in Yokohama (UN, 1994). These recommendations were updated at a 2005 meeting in Hyogo and are now widely referred to as the Hyogo Framework for Action (HFA, 2005). Interest in disaster mitigation is widespread, so there is plenty of information on the subject, including the annual World Disasters Report, published by the International Federation of Red Cross and Red Crescent (IFRC, 2010), and the ISDR's regular Global Assessment Reports on Disaster Risk Reduction (GAR, 2011).

It should be remembered that reducing disaster risk requires significant financial and administrative resources—plans are cheap, but implementation is not. Risk-reduction measures are more likely to be adopted if they can be shown to have socio-economic advantages other than a reduced disaster risk at some stage in the future. Examples would be a borehole program to reduce drought risk or community cyclone shelters used as schools. Unfortunately, the countries most in need of risk reduction are those that can least afford it. Consequently, risk-reduction projects are a growing factor in aid projects (UNDP, 2004). Disaster risk reduction is an enormous subject; it can be covered only briefly in this space, but there are several excellent sources for further research (Concern, 2005). In summary, disaster mitigation consists of three broad elements:

- *Risk analysis:* Risk management must be based on the identification of risk based on the best available science (Dilley et al., 2005). The principal hazards facing a country depend on the vulnerability of populations in high-risk areas, the availability of disaster response teams, building standards, and the country's previous history of meteorological and geological disasters. Based on this complex analysis, it is possible to arrive at estimates of degree of risk and the expected impact of the most likely natural disasters.
- *Disaster mitigation:* A comprehensive mitigation program requires coordinated initiatives established at many levels of society (Kreimer et al., 2000). Depending on the risk a country faces, mitigation might include land use regulations, such as limiting building within 100 m of the seashore, as was discussed in Sri Lanka; changes in building codes so that at least hospitals and schools meet earthquake requirements; and population warning systems such as sirens, radio broadcasts, and the currently discussed Pacific tsunami early warning system. Clearly, these must be backed up by enforcement and widespread population education. For example, education about earthquake response is a routine part of schooling in Japan and California. Every country should have a formal national disaster strategy based on their own estimate of risk and, of course, their available resources. The need for coordinated civil defence responses (and the use of army detachments) emphasizes the fact that efficient disaster preparedness can be achieved only with a sustained national effort. The development and testing of emergency evacuation plans should be a continuing and routine process.
- *Disaster risk insurance:* In order to stop countries from entering a spiral of economic depression, which may take decades to reverse, there are early moves to shift some of the financial burden onto disaster risk insurers (CCD, 2008). Regional insurance markets have been proposed that make the market size more attractive to the insurance industry and also lower the cost to individual countries. Another option, still in its infancy, is the issuing of disaster bonds. Following the establishment of the World Bank's MultiCat Program in 2009, Mexico was the first country to issue bonds as a form of disaster insurance (World Bank, 2009).

HUMANITARIAN DISASTERS

This is the excellent foppery of the world, that, when we are sick in fortune, often the surfeits of our own behaviour, we make guilty of our disasters, the sun, the moon, and the stars.

—*Shakespeare, King Lear*

The expression "complex humanitarian disaster" (also "complex disaster" or "complex emergency") was first used in the early 1990s by the United Nations to describe the increasing number of humanitarian crises typified by the chronic war and social disruption in Somalia and Sudan (Munslow et al., 1999). A complex humanitarian emergency may be defined as a situation in which:

- political authority and public services deteriorate or collapse completely as a result of internal ethnic, tribal, or religious conflicts
- widespread violence against civilians and mass starvation due to lack of food supply result in enormous population displacements
- inadequate public health services result in epidemics of communicable disease
- the chaos leads to macroeconomic collapse with general unemployment and destruction of the currency

It is commonly claimed that complex emergencies are largely the result of the political changes caused by the end of the Cold War. While it is true that the abrupt loss of external influence caused enormous changes in many countries, the results were not always negative. Some countries (such as Germany, Poland, South Africa, and Czechoslovakia) navigated these new political waters without disaster, while others (such as the former Yugoslavia, Afghanistan, and the former Zaire) did not. Complex disasters did not begin with the fall of the Berlin Wall in 1989; they have been around for centuries. The name might have changed, but there is nothing new about revolution and human brutality.

The chaos of the Russian Revolution, the years of war following the French Revolution, and the more recent Chinese Cultural Revolution are all examples of lethal combinations of continuous unrest, economic collapse, widespread starvation, and disintegrating political authority that are currently called complex emergencies. The loss of superpower support for various tyrants and puppet governments acted as a catalyst, in some countries, for long-simmering tensions to erupt into war, but this was not the only cause. When complicated by economic collapse, drought, and crop failure, some situations degenerated into intractable chronic emergencies; African states have been particularly badly affected. Examples include Burundi, Sierra Leone, Rwanda, the former Zaire, Liberia, and Guinea-Bissau (Lautze et al., 2004). Somalia's war has been so destructive that the state has actually failed. In the absence of an effective national government, the country has been divided up among warlords.

As discussed in Chapter 4, wars have changed in the last few decades. Conflicts fought between countries, such as the Iraq-Iran war of 30 years ago, are now uncommon. Civilians were certainly killed in "old-fashioned" wars, but they were usually not directly targeted. The mass indiscriminate bombings of cities in World War II started to change that attitude. Most modern conflicts now occur within countries and are often associated with deliberate targeting of civilians (including humanitarian workers). The very darkest side of human nature is reflected in brutal abuses of human rights, including mass murder, mutilations, sexual violence, and forced displacement of huge numbers of people (Fennell, 1998). Destruction of the usual economic and social structures necessary for a functioning society contributes to a permanent state of insecurity, where a small, powerful elite rules the subjugated majority.

The origins of the current famine in Somalia provide a good example of a complex disaster. Since the Barre government collapsed following civil war in 1991, there has been no unified national government. Unrecognized but functioning administrations exist in the north, but the south of the country is ruled by various armed factions. In the absence of any administrative or economic resources, the south cannot absorb the stress of drought. The complex mixture of poverty, civil war, lack of political organization, and agricultural collapse has resulted in famine, refugees, and the destabilization of neighbouring countries.

Humanitarian support for those affected is vital, but it is not a solution to the underlying problems. In the colonial past, revolutions have been justified in the name of freedom from oppression, but there are no heroes or noble sentiments behind these current wars (Collier et al., 2004). Modern conflicts are motivated by greed rather than grievance—greed for natural resources such as oil (Angola, Sudan) and diamonds (Sierra Leone, the Democratic Republic of Congo), or for power and control over historical opponents (Rwanda, Somalia).

The adverse health effects of chronic societal collapse are enormous. In southern Somalia, it is estimated that half of the population is malnourished. Family disruption, forced displacement, economic and agricultural failure, plus a range of other factors (including unplotted land mines and environmental destruction), all contribute to lives of absolute misery and ill health for the powerless majority. Long-term solutions can be achieved only through political and, more recently, military alternatives. Humanitarian interventions, based on models developed for natural disasters, can only scratch the surface of these problems by providing some support for starving displaced populations. There has been considerable criticism that humanitarian interventions might even make complex disasters worse (Macrae et al., 2001). The legal status afforded to refugee populations inadvertently protects combatants who are illegally mixed among those refugees. The value of food and donated goods acts as a further source of trouble.

Complex emergencies pose enormous ethical dilemmas for humanitarian agencies—the Rwandan genocide of 1994 was a good example. Once the Rwandan Patriotic Front, under Paul Kagame, started to regain control of the country, those responsible for the genocide fled with their families into neighbouring countries (particularly what was then eastern Zaire). It is estimated that there were 2 million refugees, a proportion of whom had been guilty of appalling crimes. A huge humanitarian effort was mounted to support these refugees under very difficult circumstances. Over the next two years, camps became militarized and were used as bases to launch attacks against the new Rwandan government (Terry, 2002). The international community failed to disarm the camps and simply reacted by withdrawing their support, leaving the United Nations High Commissioner for Refugees to do the best it could (Chaulia, 2002). The situation steadily worsened until, in 1996, combined attacks on the camps by Zairean rebels and Rwandan military killed unknown thousands of people (Banatrala et al., 1998). The entire area was destabilized and descended into chronic war that still drags on today.

The Great Lakes refugee crisis was a watershed for many large agencies; there was a definite loss of innocence where complex emergencies were concerned (Rieff, 2002). Did the humanitarian response actually contribute to the Congo wars, or was it simply a small part of an endlessly complex situation? The accusation that UNHCR was knowingly feeding murderers was answered by Sadako Ogata (the UN High Commissioner for Refugees at the time), who said, "There were also innocent refugees in the camps; more than half were women and children. Should we have said, 'You are related to murderers, so you are guilty too?'" Apart from the moral dilemmas, 26 UNHCR field personnel were also killed or missing.

The Evolution of Responses to Complex Emergencies

The beginning of the modern response to complex emergencies is probably dated to the intervention in the Biafran war at the end of the 1960s (Lautze et al., 2004). The inadequacy of the international response prompted a group of French doctors working in Biafra to start a new group, Médecins sans Frontières (MSF), which would concentrate on the victims rather than worrying about political implications. Their apolitical approach to disaster management was tested severely during the subsequent response to the Cambodian genocide in the late 1970s. Many NGOs, including MSF, had to start dealing with the ethical dilemmas caused by balancing impartiality against a desire to report the horrors they were witnessing. One of the founders of MSF, Bernard Kouchner, split with the leadership of MSF over this very subject and started a separate group, Médecins du Monde.

During the 1970s and 1980s, humanitarian agencies operated under the assumption that warring parties would follow the usual standards of international humanitarian law and would leave them alone to do their job. For a while, it looked as if this approach might even work. The signing of Operation Lifeline Sudan

Box 16.2 History Notes

Bernard Kouchner (1939–)

Kouchner was born in France and trained as a doctor and gastroenterologist. While working with the Red Cross during the Biafran war, he and a few colleagues became so disillusioned with the poor humanitarian responses of the day that they formed a new organization called Médecins sans Frontières (MSF) in 1971. This has grown to become a highly successful NGO that provides emergency support for refugees in many countries. MSF has subsequently broadened its scope and is also an influential advocate for affordable drug access. The organization was awarded the Nobel Peace Prize in 1999. Kouchner fell out with the leadership of MSF over the subject of whether aid agencies should comment on humanitarian abuses. In 1979 he organized a highly publicized "floating ambulance" for the aid of Vietnamese refugees (L'Île de Lumière). His understanding of the importance of public opinion is shown by his inclusion, on the boat, of journalists and photographers, along with doctors and nurses. He built on the success of that initiative by forming a separate group called Médecins du Monde (Doctors of the World). Apart from his humanitarian work, he has also been a successful politician. He has served as a member of the European Parliament, as well as the minister of health and the minister of foreign affairs in different French governments.

in 1989 allowed international agencies to provide basic medical care and food to remote populations affected by the fighting (Taylor-Robinson, 2002). Similar negotiations with other belligerent or obstructive governments were also successful, at least for short periods, in other areas of conflict, such as Angola and Sri Lanka. These "days of tranquility" sometimes lasted long enough to organize a mass immunization program or deliver a new crop to market.

Unfortunately, in the 1990s it became quite obvious in the chaos of Somalia and Rwanda that it would take more than the Geneva Convention to provide protection for civilians and humanitarian workers in war zones. In 1993, the first attempt to support humanitarian action with military backing was tried in Somalia. The operation, termed "Restore Hope," was initially successful in helping agencies to deal with the country's famine victims (Clarke et al., 1997). Unfortunately, after 24 Pakistani peacekeepers were killed by Somali militia, some months later, the force's impartiality was lost during the subsequent hunt for their leader. After the battle of Mogadishu, international forces were later withdrawn and the country settled back into anarchy and poverty, which have continued until today. Deaths among the multinational force had a significant effect on subsequent intervention decision-making.

As mentioned earlier in this chapter, lessons were learned from the humanitarian response in Rwanda. One change was an increasing emphasis on greater professionalism among agency staff. The establishment of various standards of conduct, particularly those developed by the Sphere Project (Walker, 2005), helped this process. The UN formed the Department of Humanitarian Affairs in 1992 with the aim of imposing some form of coordination on agencies responding to emergencies; in 1998, this became the Office for the Coordination of Humanitarian Affairs (OCHA). The ethical and practical dilemmas posed by governments that purposely wage war on their own populations have not been solved. A strong international court to settle international disputes, backed by an effective and permanent UN army, is a real possibility for the future, but a military presence is still no guarantee of success (Shawcross, 2001). There were UN troops in Rwanda during the genocide, but they were forbidden to get involved, and the declaration of a UN "safe haven" did not stop the massacre at Srebrenica.

There is also a subjective element in the definition of an emergency that depends, to some extent, on media access and public interest. For example, why send troops to Somalia in 1993 rather than Sudan, or to Sierra Leone in 1999 rather than a much earlier intervention in East Timor? There is an obvious reluctance to invade a sovereign state, but at some stage, intervention becomes a humanitarian necessity. Earlier intervention, with a credible force, would probably have saved tens of thousands of lives in Rwanda or East Timor. Unfortunately, such interventions carry a risk of casualties. For example, the deaths of Canadian troops in Afghanistan raise inevitable questions. Who wants their children to fight and die for a humanitarian ideal in a distant country, and, more pragmatically, who pays for it? The success of the International Criminal Court offers hope that some tyrants will pause before committing atrocities that might one day put them in a dock shared by Milosevic, Charles Taylor, and, very likely, some of the current perpetrators of violence against civilians in Syria and Libya.

DISPLACED POPULATIONS

Once a refugee, always a refugee.

—*Elie Weisel, 1986*

The last 25 years have seen some of the biggest migrations of refugee populations in history (Photo 16.2). An estimated 1 million Kurds left Iraq in 1991 and, in the space of a few weeks during the Rwandan genocide, neighbouring countries were flooded with an estimated 2 million refugees. In the late 1990s, hundreds of thousands more refugees were displaced by wars in Sudan, Sierra Leone, Liberia, and Indonesia. We are currently witnessing large and growing refugee populations in southern Somalia. Due to the conflict in Syria, there have been increased numbers of refugees in Turkey, Jordan, Lebanon, and Europe (World Bank, 2016). Unfortunately, refugees remain

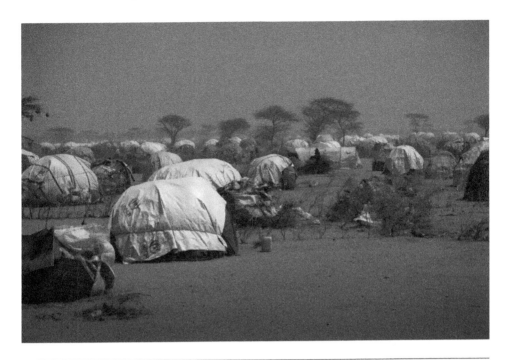

Photo 16.2: Temporary shelters in the Dagehaley camp in northeastern Kenya; this is one of three camps in the area around Dadaab. Collectively they make up the largest refugee camp in the world and currently contain close to half a million people. The camps give shelter for people fleeing wars and drought in East Africa, particularly Somalia.

Source: Kate Holt/Integrated Regional Information Network photo library (www.irinnews.org/photo).

as common as the civil wars that displace them. Refugees are defined as people who have left their country of origin because of well-founded fears of persecution due to race, religion, nationality, or political opinion. Table 16.3 gives definitions for the various types of displaced populations. People fleeing a natural disaster are called forced migrants. They are not defined as refugees under the Geneva Convention. By far the most common cause of population displacement is civil war.

Keeping track of refugee statistics is not easy. Those people who cross an international boundary may try to avoid attention, but reasonable estimates of numbers are available for these groups. However, probably at least equal numbers are displaced, but remain within their country of origin. These people are termed "internally displaced people" (IDP) and are much harder to count. They are also much harder to help because they still live within the borders of their original country. External assistance is affected by sovereignty issues, so they may remain at increased risk of continuing abuse. Other types of displaced people are identified,

Table 16.3: Definitions used to describe different types of displaced people

Refugee	A person forced out of his or her country due to persecution as defined in the Geneva Convention
Asylum seeker	Someone claiming refugee status, but whose claim has not been proved
Internally displaced person	A person who is forced to move due to persecution, but remains within his or her own country
Migrant	Voluntary movement to another country
Internal migrant	Voluntary movement within own country
Forced migrant	Involuntary movement caused by disaster, not persecution

including economic migrants, who cross to another country simply in search of a more prosperous life. Examples include Hispanic migrants (both legal and illegal) entering the United States and a large illegal immigrant population in Europe. Finally, the UN also uses the term "persons of concern" to describe populations at high risk of flight, usually due to a worsening security situation.

The UN agency responsible for refugees is the Office of the UN High Commissioner for Refugees (UNHCR, 2011a). The UNHCR was established in 1950 and the first convention relating to the status of refugees was passed in 1951. Its initial focus was on European refugees escaping the fighting of World War II, but its scope was expanded to a global mandate by a 1967 protocol. The UNHCR has given assistance to many tens of millions of people during its six decades of existence. The organization has been awarded the Nobel Peace Prize twice, most recently in 1981. The UNHCR is a large agency—apart from its important emergency response role, it also provides care and support for other categories of displaced people:

- *Returnees:* Assistance with repatriation to their own homes, as with the recent return of those displaced by the Swat Valley fighting in Pakistan; in intractable situations, UNHCR attempts to get the refugees included and integrated within the host country
- *Asylum seekers:* Assisting host countries to establish fair and fast evaluation procedures to determine which claimants are valid refugees
- *Displaced people:* Assistance with shelter and clean water during the initial emergency, but the UNHCR is also a valuable advocate for the refugees with their host country
- *Stateless people:* People without a passport or birth certificate are not always refugees, but live in a country without a citizen's usual rights, such as pension and health care; UNHCR works to reduce stateless numbers by encouraging countries to implement the long-standing UN convention on statelessness

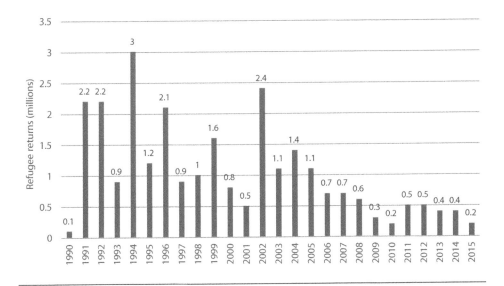

Figure 16.4: Trends in refugee returns over the last 25 years. In 2015, 201, 400 refugees returned to their countries of origin, with 57% receiving UNHCR assistance.

Source: UNHCR. 2016a. Global trends: Forced displacements in 2015. Retrieved from: www.unhcr.org/statistics/unhcrstats/576408cd7/unhcr-global-trends-2015.html.

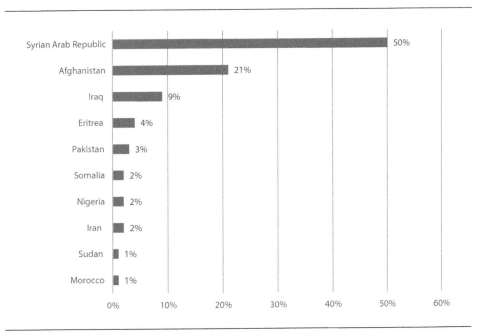

Figure 16.5: Top 10 nationalities of Mediterranean arrival in 2015

Source: UNHCR. 2016a. Global trends: Forced displacements in 2015. Retrieved from: www.unhcr.org/statistics/unhcrstats/576408cd7/unhcr-global-trends-2015.html.

The best source for epidemiological data on displaced people is the UNHCR's statistical division (UNHCR, 2016b). The total number of refugees and internally displaced persons protected or assisted by UNHCR was 52.6 million in 2015, compared to 46.7 million at the end of 2014 (UNHCR, 2016a). It is important to realize that these are the people UNHCR could reach—the true number is much higher. The greatest sources of refugees are the Syrian Arab Republic, Afghanistan, and Somalia, which produce well over half the total. For example, almost 75 percent of the refugees arriving at the Mediterranean in 2015 were Syrian Arab Republic and Afghanistan nationalities (Figure 16.5). While considerable attention is given to the numbers of refugees hosted by developed countries, this is only a small part of the total. Over 80 percent of refugees live in developing countries and their care represents a major economic burden. A good example is the strain placed on Kenya by large numbers of refugees from Somalia. The global number of refugees under UNHCR's mandate was estimated to be 16.1 million at the end of 2015, with the majority based in Africa and Europe (Figure 16.6). During the course of 2015, more than 12.4 million individuals were forced to leave their homes and seek protection elsewhere.

The Care and Management of Displaced Populations

Médecins sans Frontières has been an example of thoughtful management in the area of complex humanitarian emergencies since its earliest days in the 1970s. The organization responded to the challenges of caring for refugee populations by backing its field policies with relevant research, which to this day remains a revolutionary concept for some agencies. As early as 1987, MSF established an operational research centre to determine the best way to manage complex humanitarian emergencies (Epicentre, 2011). Its subsequent publications have allowed others working in the field to base their management on targeted research rather than dogma (Brown et al., 2008).

The first days and weeks of a disaster are chaotic times, which is all the more reason that aid agencies and their staff should be professional and well trained. It is convenient to divide the emergency into two broad groups—early and late—based on the crude mortality rate (CMR) (Burkholder et al., 1995). The CMR can be expressed as deaths per 1,000 per month (usually 1–2 in an average developing country) or as deaths per 10,000 population per day (usually less than 0.5). Depending on the baseline health of the affected population, the degree of violence they have faced, and the distance they have travelled, the early stage is marked by crude mortality rates as high as 20–40 times greater than normal. During this phase, management should be based on the well-established principles of primary health care, such as shelter, water, and food. The main priorities in the management of a large displaced population include:

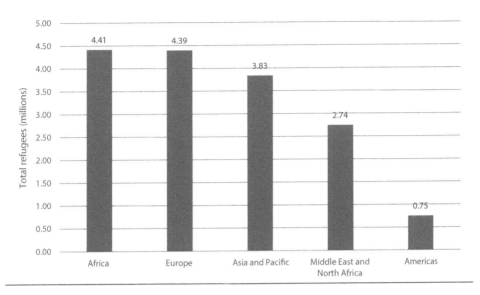

Figure 16.6: Refugee populations by UHNCR regions in 2015

Source: UNHCR. 2016a. Global trends: Forced displacements in 2015. Retrieved from: www.unhcr.org/ statistics/unhcrstats/576408cd7/unhcr-global-trends-2015.html.

- rapidly assess demographic and health status of the refugee population
- vaccinate all children against measles
- establish clean water supply
- establish sanitation system
- meet daily nutrition requirements
- establish nutrition rehabilitation program for the most seriously malnourished
- plan the site and establish the size and type of shelters
- source essential non-food supplies
- establish protocol-driven curative care for the common conditions
- establish a daily health surveillance system
- plan for a response to common epidemics
- survey the population for suitable qualified camp staff
- establish a security plan, particularly for women and children
- coordinate with partner agencies (Brown et al., 2008)

Once mortality rates fall to the usual background level, refugee camps slowly turn into organized towns. Table 16.4 gives some of the UNHCR minimum recommendations for camp construction. Acute infectious diseases remain important, but other problems now need attention, particularly tuberculosis, HIV, sexually

Table 16.4: UNHCR standards for refugee camps

Land	30–45 m²/person
Shelter	3.5 m²/person
Water	15–20 L/person/day
Food	2,100 kcal/person/day
Latrine	1 per family (5–10 people)
Water tap	1 per community (80–100 people)
Health centre	1 per camp (20,000 people)
Hospital	1 per 200,000 people
School	1 per 5,000 people

Source: UNHCR. 2006. Standards and indicators in UNHCR operations. Retrieved from: www. unhcr.org/40eaa9804.html.

transmitted diseases, mental illness, and violence against women and children. It is important to provide basic public health programs (such as family planning and basic maternal and child health care) and to establish means of employment (such as providing seeds and fertilizer for small holdings).

As mentioned above, there is nothing medically unique about the care of displaced populations. Although each situation will have its unique complexities, the basics of shelter, security, water, food, and essential health care remain as constants (Brown et al., 2008). The main management priorities are as follows.

Rapid Epidemiological Assessment

At least nine of the major relief organizations produce a disaster response manual (MSF, 1997; Sphere Project, 2011; UNICEF, 2005), each of which has its own version of an initial assessment protocol. There have been repeated calls for greater uniformity, but the collection and distribution of standardized information during the early stage of a disaster have not yet been achieved (Bradt et al., 2002). Careful information gathering (within the limitations imposed by the situation) is an essential first step in planning and managing a displaced population. Although there is little standardization, there is no shortage of literature. The WHO alone has produced a steady stream of reports, ranging from rapid evaluation techniques developed during the smallpox program to a more recent handbook (WHO, 1999). The following information should be collected:

- *Social/political situation:* Information needed includes the reasons behind the population displacement; the security situation in the original country and the host country; traditional relations between the host country and the original country; and whether the refugees are accepted, tolerated, or actively disliked by the host government.

- *The refugee population:* Basic demographic information should include an estimate of the total population and rough distribution by age and gender, particularly the numbers of vulnerable groups, such as unaccompanied children, the elderly, and pregnant women. Is the refugee population homogeneous or does it include warring parties within the camp? Are there remnants of previous health workers, police, or administrative personnel?
- *The camp:* Information needed includes the total area available, the climate of the region, a map of the site and local countryside, and the state of the roads. Information on the camp facilities should include the type of shelters, latrines, local water sources, and available power.
- *Population health:* Using information from health care workers and measurements of samples of children, the following health information should be available: crude mortality rate, frequency of the most common and expected diseases (such as measles, diarrheal diseases, pneumonia, and malaria), degree of malnutrition, and information about the population's past health (common diseases, degree of vaccination coverage).
- *Resources available:* Is health and social support available in the region, and what is the degree of willingness of the host population to support the refugees? What is the number of trained medical and support staff within the refugee population? What material is available to the refugees (pots, pans, food, clothing, water containers, wood or paraffin stoves)?

The initial assessment should be completed rapidly within a few days to allow agencies to make the first decision about whether they can, or even should, intervene. Once the aid effort is underway, some degree of continuous monitoring is essential and should be the sole task of one particular group to allow adjustments to be made in the recovery program.

Water, Sanitation, and Household Waste

WATER
The provision of water is a major problem facing refugee camps (Roberts et al., 2001). If tankers are required, then the monthly cost is significant. The bare minimum needed for some degree of hygiene and hydration is 5 L of water per person per day. A minimal supply of clean water will reduce the risk of diarrheal diseases, but will do nothing to limit hygiene-related diseases such as trachoma and scabies. In order to clean clothes, dishes, and maintain personal hygiene, it is necessary to provide 15–20 L per person per day (UNHCR, 2008). Water sources include wells, boreholes, and surface water. Failing this, water will have

to be transported using trucks and stored in large bladders. Turbid water can be treated by settlement with flocculation additives and subsequent chlorination. This procedure requires specially trained staff.

HUMAN SANITATION

Until the camp is organized, limited control of contamination can be obtained using a defecation field (UNHCR, 2009). With tape and stakes, a large field can be divided into strips. Starting with the strip furthest from the camp, a different area can be used for defecation every day. Unless some means of covering the field with soil can be found, this is only a very temporary approach. Until it is possible to provide each family with their own latrine, the best interim approach is to dig communal latrines, which are relatively quick and cheap to construct. One trench latrine should be available for 50 people.

The trench should be about 2 m deep and spanned by pairs of wooden boards. Each day, the contents should be covered by a layer of soil to reduce smell and flies. When the trench is full, a new trench is dug at another site. Although a trench is a simple structure, it requires daily cleaning and supervision or the population will not use it. Safe sanitation can be achieved only with the full co-operation of the community. It is important that the community is involved in the management of the waste disposal and the water storage systems. The routine care of the water and sanitation should be handed over to camp occupants as soon as suitable people can be trained.

HOUSEHOLD WASTE

This should be collected regularly and is best handled by a landfill system. Again, this is a task that should be handed over to the refugee population as soon as possible. Contaminated waste from health posts and clinics should be burned or buried deeply (Oxfam, 2008). A cemetery area should be available. Soap should be provided as part of the routine public health education for the camp. The basic need is one bar per person per month. If attention is not paid to waste disposal, then problems of flies, rats, and other vectors can become uncontrollable.

Nutrition

In the past, malnutrition has been a major problem in refugee camps due to underestimation of the basic requirements of the population and also lack of funds to buy sufficient food (WFP, 2002). Bare survival is obtained with 1,500–1,800 kilocalories per person per day, but the target should be 2,100 kilocalories per person per day. Once intake reaches 2,400 kilocalories, the need for supplementary feeding is much reduced. Although there have been great improvements in the feeding of displaced populations, current reports of the presence of scurvy and pellagra show that micronutrient deficiencies are still present (Young et al., 2004).

The UNHCR and the World Food Program's practice is to include fortified blended cereal in the food rations of all food aid–dependent populations. However, the best approach is to include a more diversified diet with provision of fresh vegetables and fruit. In situations where the population has access to local markets, they have been encouraged to sell or bargain a portion of their ration for fresh produce. With time, the development of family garden plots improves the food sufficiency of camp households. Selective feeding programs for high-risk groups, such as undernourished children and pregnant women, will also be necessary.

Young children are the most vulnerable section of the camp in terms of malnutrition, so nutritional surveys of the under-five-year-olds will provide a reasonable indication of the nutrition of the camp as a whole. Research by MSF has shown that the best single indicator of acute malnutrition is weight for height expressed as a z-score (Brown et al., 2008). If more than 5 percent of sampled children have a weight for height score below –2 z, this should act as a warning that the camp's nutrition is inadequate. A rising crude mortality rate may also be another indicator that nutrition is poor.

Shelter

For reasons of culture and social acceptance, it has been shown that refugees do best if they can build their own housing, as long as the necessary materials and organization are provided. In the short term, plastic sheeting stretched across rough wooden supports is the usual shelter that each family is able to construct. In cold climates, the wide daily variations in temperature and the lack of adequate shelter and clothing will soon have a major adverse affect on health. In addition to basic shelter, there should be provision of blankets and clothing. Once again, it is important that refugees should help to build their own housing. This reduces costs and ensures that it better meets their needs.

Tents may be necessary in the short term if local materials are not available (UNHCR, 2011b). The lifespan of a well-constructed tent is one to two years; adequate supplies of repair materials should be available. Ideally, the tent should provide enough height to allow occupants to stand upright and should have an outer flysheet to protect the tent underneath. Tents are difficult and expensive to heat and the risk of fire is significant. They are not ideal as cold-climate shelters, but there may be no options, as experience with the Pakistan earthquake showed. Shelters for Sri Lankan tsunami refugees were predominantly made of

UV-resistant, heavy-duty plastic sheeting. The large blue UNHCR tarpaulins were a common sight throughout the camps. Wooden support frames can be easily constructed using locally produced framing material.

Guiding the growth of the camp as it turns into a small town is obviously a complex undertaking. A good source of information is the guide produced by the University of Cambridge's Shelter Project (Corsellis et al., 2005). Although there are many design issues to consider, safety is a particularly important one. When planning the camp, there is a need to ensure that protection principles are taken into account from the start. Water sources, latrines, and communal areas should be well lit to reduce the risk of violence against women and children.

Environmental Issues

The question of the impact of refugee camps on the local environment is increasingly being examined. The use of firewood for cooking by a large number of refugees may have a significant effect on the ability of the local population to access firewood themselves for cooking (Lyytinen, 2009). Under these circumstances, women and children who leave the camp to scavenge firewood are placed at increased risk from attack. Environmental degradation is one of the major sources of potential conflict between refugees and the local population and, if such conflict occurs, it can have a major effect on the ability of aid agencies to conduct their work.

Basic Health Care

Apart from the effects of violence, the majority of mortality in the refugee camps is caused by a limited number of diseases. The most common disease is usually malnutrition, followed by diarrheal diseases, pneumonia, measles, and malaria (Wisner et al., 2003). The most serious of the potential epidemic illnesses are meningococcal meningitis and cholera. As with any developing world population, malnutrition can be a primary problem, but it may also greatly increase the mortality from other diseases. It is important to establish a basic daily mortality and morbidity disease surveillance system for the camp (Martin et al., 1994).

The most basic health services will consist of two components: peripheral health posts and community outreach services delivered by community health workers (Hafeez et al., 2004). With time, traditional birth attendants and others with training as health workers will probably be found within the population of the camp. With further training and supervision, they can play a valuable role by providing basic health education, identifying those who need treatment, and collecting health-monitoring data such as the number of deaths and their causes. Once trained, suitable ratios are 1 health care worker per 1,000 population and 1 traditional birth attendant per 3,000.

The basic health post needs to be a simple, clean building with the ability to treat common diseases. It should, at the very least, have supplies of effective malaria medication, oral rehydration solution, oral antibiotics, and storage facilities for measles vaccine. In populations with poor vaccination coverage, measles epidemics are a major health risk for children. During the early stages of the camp, measles vaccine and vitamin A should be given to all children below the age of 15 even if measles is not yet evident. Ideally, there should be 1 health post per 5,000 people.

As services become available, there should be a larger health centre for up to 20,000 people. The centre should be able to treat most cases except those requiring general anaesthetic and major obstetric emergencies. These can hopefully be managed through referral to existing local hospital services after suitable negotiations. Ideally, the health facility should be open 24 hours a day, with 8-hour shifts. There will also need to be 24-hour security arrangements. The facility should be able to care for uncomplicated deliveries, minor surgeries, short-term pediatric hospitalization, and basic wound dressing. A well-run unit will also act as a centre for epidemiological surveillance and health education initiatives.

SUMMARY

Humanitarian and natural disasters are surprisingly common. The last decade has witnessed some of the most lethal and certainly some of the most expensive disasters in history, such as the 2011 Tōhoku earthquake and tsunami, one of the costliest natural disasters in world history. Apart from the immediate death and injury caused by a disaster, the subsequent economic and social chaos can be enormous. People living in poverty are hardest hit by disasters due to poor building standards, lack of civil defence organizations, high concentrations of the population living in high-risk areas, and lack of money, making them more vulnerable to future disasters and deeper poverty. International humanitarian assistance is a vital resource for many people affected by crises. Large-scale emergencies increased the amount of international humanitarian assistance provided in 2015, which reached a record high of US$28.0 billion and represented the third consecutive annual increase. While there is a very understandable human desire to help the survivors of a disaster, it is important to ensure that the response is organized and professional. Hard lessons learned from the Asian tsunami showed that the sudden influx of hundreds of uncoordinated groups is not the most efficient way to respond to a chaotic situation. Disasters and chaotic situations also arise from conflicts such as those continuing in Syria, Iraq, and South Sudan, which have increased the number of those living in forced displacement. The United Nations agency responsible for coordinating emergency relief for major disasters is the Office for the Coordination of Humanitarian Affairs. The global number of refugees under UNHCR's mandate was estimated to be 16.1 million at the end of 2015, which is a 55 percent rise from 10.4 million in 2011. This increase was driven mainly by the conflict in Syria, which accounted for more than half of new refugees in 2015. The ability to cater to the needs of refugees is a key element of global health, and although each situation will have its unique complexities, the basics of shelter, security, water, food, sanitation, and essential health care remain as constants.

DISCUSSION QUESTIONS

1. What is a complex humanitarian emergency? What key elements of an effective organizational framework are needed to manage a complex humanitarian emergency?

2. Which United Nations agency is responsible for coordinating emergency relief? Imagine you are called to lead such an agency. What steps would you take to effectively coordinate emergency relief during an earthquake like the 2010 Haiti earthquake?

3. What are the human and financial costs associated with wars and natural disasters?

4. What is the difference between refugees, migrants, and other types of displaced populations? Why are these populations considered an important aspect and focus of global health?

5. Why are natural and technological disasters an important aspect of global health? What has been the trend in annual deaths from natural and technological disasters over the last decade?

6. Important lessons gleaned from the Asian tsunami showed that the sudden influx of hundreds of uncoordinated groups is not the most efficient way to respond to a chaotic situation. What is the most efficient way?

7. How does the beginning of the modern response to complex emergencies date back to the Biafran war at the end of the 1960s?

8. Imagine you are called to support a refugee population. What are the essential requirements needed to reduce mortality among such a population? What would be the major priorities to consider when catering to their needs?

9. Why is emergency medical aid not for amateurs?

10. Do you agree or disagree with the statement that if someone is not qualified to practise emergency medical care in his or her own country, there is no good reason why that person should be given permission to diagnose and manage critically ill people in a developing country?

RECOMMENDED READING

Briggs, S., et al. (Eds.). 2003. *Advanced disaster medical response manual for providers*. Pub: Harvard Medical International Trauma & Disaster Institute.

De Waal, A. 2002. *Famine crimes: Politics and the disaster relief industry in Africa*. Pub: Indiana University Press.

Elena Fiddian-Qasmiyeh, E., et al. (Eds.). 2014. *The Oxford Handbook of Refugee and Forced Migration Studies*. Pub: Oxford University Press.

Macrae, J. 2001. *Aiding recovery: The crisis of aid in chronic political emergencies*. Pub: Zed Books.

Médecins sans Frontières. 1996. *World in crisis: The politics of survival at the end of the 20th century*. Pub: Routledge.

Médecins sans Frontières. 1997. *Refugee health: An approach to emergency situations*. Pub: MacMillan.

Terry, F. 2002. *Condemned to repeat? The paradox of humanitarian action*. Pub: Cornell University Press.

REFERENCES

Adinolfi, C., et al. 2005. Humanitarian response review. Office for the Coordination of Humanitarian Affairs. Retrieved from: www.ennonline.net/resources/713.

ALNAP. 2011. Active Learning Network for Accountability and Performance in Humanitarian Action. Retrieved from: www.odi.org.uk/alnap.

Banatrala, N., et al. 1998. Mortality and morbidity among Rwandan refugees repatriated from Zaire, November 1996. *Prehospital Disaster Medicine*, 13: 17–21.

Bradt, D., et al. 2002. Rapid epidemiological assessment of health status in displaced populations: An evolution towards standardized minimum, essential data sets. *Prehospital Disaster Medicine*, 17: 178–185.

Brown, V., et al. 2008. Research in complex humanitarian emergencies: The Médecins sans Frontières/Epicentre experience. *PLoS Medicine*, 5: e89. Retrieved from: www.plos-medicine.org/article/info%3Adoi%2F10.1371%2Fjournal.pmed.0050089.

Burkholder, B., et al. 1995. Evolution of complex disasters. *The Lancet*, 346: 1012–1015.

CCD. 2008. The role of risk transfer and insurance in disaster risk reduction. Retrieved from: www.ccdcommission.org/Filer/pdf/pb_risk_transfer.pdf.

CERF. 2010. CERF annual report. Retrieved from: http://ochanet.unocha.org/p/Documents/CERFAnnRep_2010_Web.pdf.

CERF. 2011. Central Emergency Relief Fund. Retrieved from: ochaonline.un.org/Default.aspx?alias=ochaonline.un.org/cerf.

Chaulia, S. 2002. UNHCR's relief, rehabilitation, and repatriation of Rwandan refugees in Zaire (1994–1997). *The Journal of Humanitarian Assistance.* Retrieved from: www.jha.ac/articles/a086.htm.

Clarke, W., et al. 1997. *Learning from Somalia: The lessons of armed humanitarian intervention.* Pub: Westview Press.

Collier, P., et al. 2004. Greed and grievance in civil war. *Oxford Economic Papers,* 56: 563–595. Retrieved from: www.econ.nyu.edu/user/debraj/Courses/Readings/CollierHoeffler.pdf.

Concern. 2005. Approaches to disaster risk reduction. Retrieved from: www.concernusa.org/media/pdf/2007/10/Concern_ApproachestoDRR%20paper%20-%20final.pdf.

Corsellis, T., et al. 2005. *Transitional settlement, displaced populations.* Pub: Oxfam. Retrieved from: postconflict.unep.ch/liberia/displacement/documents/Corsellis_Vitale_Transitional_Settlement_Displaced_Populatio.pdf.

CRED. 2011. Centre for Research on the Epidemiology of Disasters. International Disaster Database. Retrieved from: www.emdat.be/database.

Dabelstein, N., 1996. Evaluating the international humanitarian system: Rationale, process, and management of the joint evaluation of the international response to the Rwandan genocide. *Disasters,* 20: 286–294.

DEC. 2011. Disasters Emergency Committee. Retrieved from: www.dec.org.uk.

Dilley, M., et al. 2005. Natural disaster hotspots: A global risk analysis. World Bank. Retrieved from: http://sedac.ciesin.columbia.edu/hazards/hotspots/synthesisreport.pdf.

EM-DAT. 2016. Emergency Events Database, Centre for Research on the Epidemiology of Disasters. Retrieved from: www.emdat.be/advanced_search/index.html.

Epicentre. 2011. MSF operational research centre. Retrieved from: www.epicentre.msf.org/.

FACT. 2011. Field Assessment and Coordination Team. Retrieved from: www.ifrc.org/en/what-we-do/disaster-management/.

Fennell, J. 1998. Hope suspended: Morality, politics, and war in Central Africa. *Disasters,* 22, 96–108.

GAR. 2011. Global Assessment Report on disaster risk reduction. Retrieved from: www.preventionweb.net/english/hyogo/gar/2011/en/home/index.html.

GHA. 2010. Global Humanitarian Report. Retrieved from: www.globalhumanitarianassistance.org/wp-content/uploads/2010/07/GHA_Report8.pdf.

GHA. 2016. Global Humanitarian Report. Retrieved from: www.globalhumanitarianassistance.org/report/gha2016/.

Global Polio Eradication. 2011. Retrieved from: www.polioeradication.org/.

Guha-Sapir, D., et al. 2004. *Thirty years of natural disasters, 1974–2003: The numbers.* Pub: Presses Universitaires de Louvain. Retrieved from: www.em-dat.net/documents/Publication/publication_2004_emdat.pdf.

HAC. 2009. Health Action in Crises. 5 year action plan progress report. Retrieved from: www.who.int/hac/events/5years_progress_report_brochure.pdf.

Hafeez, A., et al. 2004. Integrating health care for mothers and children in refugee camps and at district level. *British Medical Journal*, 328: 834–836.

HFA. 2005. Hyogo Framework for Action 2005–2015. Building the resilience of nations and communities to disasters. Retrieved from: www.unisdr.org/we/inform/publications/1037.

Hogerzeil, H., et al. 1998. Guidelines for drug donations. *British Medical Journal*, 314: 737–738.

IASC. 2006. Gender handbook in humanitarian action. Retrieved from: www.humanitarianinfo.org/iasc/.

IASC. 2007. IASC guidelines on mental health and psychosocial support in emergency settings. Retrieved from: www.humanitarianinfo.org/iasc/.

IASC. 2011. Inter Agency Standing Committee. Retrieved from: www.humanitarianinfo.org/iasc/.

IFRC. 2010. World disasters report. Focus on urban risk. Retrieved from: www.ifrc.org/Global/Publications/disasters/WDR/WDR2010-full.pdf.

IRIN. 2011. Integrated Regional Information Networks. Retrieved from: www.irinnews.org/.

ISDR. 2011. Milestones in the history of disaster risk reduction. Retrieved from: www.unisdr.org/who-we-are/history.

Kreimer, A., et al. 2000. Managing disaster risk in emerging economies. World Bank. Retrieved from: http://go.worldbank.org/7RZO0AV7P0.

The Lancet. 1996. Emergency medical aid is not for amateurs. *The Lancet*, 348: 1393–1394.

Lautze, S., et al. 2004. Assistance, protection, and governance networks in complex emergencies. *The Lancet*, 364: 2134–2141.

Lyytinen, E. 2009. Household energy in refugee and IDP camps. UNHCR research paper no. 172. Retrieved from: www.unhcr.org/4a1d2f422.pdf.

Macrae, J., et al. 2001. Apples, pears, and porridge: The origins and impact of the search for "coherence" between humanitarian and political responses to chronic political emergencies. *Disasters*, 25: 290–307.

Martin, A., et al. 1994. Infectious disease surveillance during emergency relief to Bhutanese refugees in Nepal. *JAMA*, 272: 377–381.

McGarry, N., et al. 2005. Health aspects of the tsunami disaster in Asia. *Prehospital Disaster Medicine*, 20: 368–377.

MSF. 1997. *Refugee health: An approach to emergency situations*. Pub: Macmillan.

Munslow, B., et al. 1999. Complex emergencies: The institutional impasse. *Third World Quarterly*, 20: 207–221.

OCHA. 2011. Office for the Coordination of Humanitarian Affairs. Retrieved from: www.unocha.org/.

Oxfam. 2008. Refugee camp waste management, collection, and disposal. Retrieved from: sheltercentre.org/sites/default/files/Domestic%20and%20Refugee%20Camp%20Waste%20Management%20Collection%20and%20Disposal%20(Oxfam).pdf.

Rieff, D. 2002. *A bed for the night: Humanitarianism in crisis*. Pub: Simon and Schuster.

Roberts, L., et al. 2001. Keeping water clean in a Malawi refugee camp: A randomized intervention trial. *Bulletin of the World Health Organization*, 79: 280–287.

Schiermeier, Q. 2006. The costs of global warming. *Nature*, 439: 374–375.

Shawcross, W. 2001. *Deliver us from evil: Warlords and peacekeepers in a world of endless conflict.* Pub: Bloomsbury Publishing.

Sphere Project. 2011. Sphere handbook. Retrieved from: www.sphereproject.org.

Taylor-Robinson, S. 2002. Operation Lifeline Sudan. *Journal of Medical Ethics*, 28: 49–51.

Terry, F. 2002. *Condemned to repeat? The paradox of humanitarian action.* Pub: Cornell University Press.

Tun, K., et al. 2005. Forensic aspects of disaster fatality management. *Prehospital Disaster Management*, 20: 455–458.

UN. 1994. Yokohama strategy and plan of action for a safer world. Retrieved from: www.unisdr.org/files/8241_doc6841contenido1.pdf.

UNDAC. 2011. UN Disaster Assessment and Coordination Team. Retrieved from: www.unocha.org/what-we-do/coordination-tools/undac/overview.

UNDP. 2004. Reducing disaster risk: A challenge for development. Retrieved from: www.undp.org/cpr/whats_new/rdr_english.pdf.

UNHCR. 2006. Standards and indicators in UNHCR operations. Retrieved from: www.unhcr.org/40eaa9804.html.

UNHCR. 2008. UNHCR field guide on water and sanitation services. Retrieved from: www.unhcr.org/49d080df2.html.

UNHCR. 2009. Excreta disposal in emergencies: A field manual. Retrieved from: www.unhcr.org/4a3391c46.html.

UNHCR. 2010. Global trends. Retrieved from: www.unhcr.org/4dfa11499.html.

UNHCR. 2011a. UN refugee agency. Retrieved from: www.unhcr.org/cgi-bin/texis/vtx/home.

UNHCR. 2011b. Family tent design. Retrieved from: www.unhcr.org/4d1b120d9.pdf.

UNHCR, 2016a. Global trends: Forced displacements in 2015. Retrieved from: www.unhcr.org/statistics/unhcrstats/576408cd7/unhcr-global-trends-2015.html.

UNHCR, 2016b. The UNHCR population statistics database. Retrieved from: http://popstats.unhcr.org/en/overview.

UNICEF. 2005. Emergency field handbook: A guide for UNICEF staff. Retrieved from: www.unicef.org/publications/files/UNICEF_EFH_2005.pdf.

Walker, P. 2005. Cracking the code: The genesis, use, and future of the code of conduct. *Disasters*, 29: 323–336.

WFP. 2002. World Food Programme emergency field operations pocketbook. Retrieved from: www.unicef.org/emerg/files/WFP_manual.pdf.

WHO. 1999. Rapid health assessment protocols for emergencies. Retrieved from: http://helid.digicollection.org/en/d/Jh0212e/.

Wisner, B., et al. (Eds.). 2003. Environmental health in emergencies and disasters. Chapter 11: Control of communicable diseases. Retrieved from: www.who.int/ water_sanitation_health/hygiene/emergencies/emergencies2002/en/.

World Bank. 2009. MultiCat Program: Insuring against natural disaster risk. Retrieved from: http://treasury.worldbank.org/bdm/pdf/Handouts_Finance/Financial_Solution_ MultiCat.pdf.

World Bank. 2016. Migration and remittances. Recent developments and outlook. Migration and development brief 26. Retrieved from: http://pubdocs.worldbank.org/ en/661301460400427908/MigrationandDevelopmentBrief26.pdf.

Young, H., et al. 2004. Public nutrition in complex emergencies. *The Lancet*, 364: 1899–1909.

Zhang, Bo. 2011. Top 5 Most Expensive Natural Disasters in History. Archived April 12, 2011. Retrieved from: www.accuweather.com/en/weather-news/ top-5-most-expensive-natural-d/47459.

CHAPTER 17

The Health and Rights of Indigenous Populations

It is not too much to say, that the intercourse of Europeans in general, without any exception in favour of the subjects of Great Britain, has been a source of many calamities to uncivilized nations. Too often, their territory has been usurped; their property seized; their numbers diminished ... they have been familiarized with the use of our most potent instruments for the subtle or the violent destruction of human life, viz. brandy and gunpowder.

—*House of Commons Select Committee Report on Aborigines, 1837*

OBJECTIVES

Indigenous or Aboriginal peoples are usually defined as those who inhabited a country or region prior to the arrival of later foreign immigrants. Such groups inhabit every corner of the Earth, from the Arctic to the South Pacific. Accurate data is a constant problem, but common estimates of their numbers range from 300 million to 350 million (roughly 5 percent of the world's population). Examples include the large Mayan groups of Central America, the Native populations of North and South America, and the broad Polynesian groups of New Zealand and other Pacific islands. Many Indigenous peoples have managed to retain their unique cultural and linguistic traditions despite depressingly similar colonial histories of discrimination and oppression. Although the situation for Indigenous peoples has improved with time, the size of the world's Indigenous population, combined with its high rate of significant health problems, makes this topic an important part of global health. After completing this chapter, you should be able to:

- appreciate the extent and diversity of the world's Indigenous populations
- understand the historical factors that lie behind the current poor health of many Indigenous populations
- understand the common health problems found among many Indigenous populations
- appreciate the slow move toward a charter of human rights for Indigenous peoples
- understand the approaches needed to improve the health of Indigenous populations

INTRODUCTION

> Indigenous Peoples never did the Europeans any harm whatever; on the contrary, they believed them to have descended from the heavens, at least until they or their fellow citizens have tasted, at the hands of these oppressors, a diet of robbery, murder, violence, and all other manner of trials and tribulations.
>
> *—Bartolome de las Casas, Spanish missionary, early proponent of Native rights, and author of*
> *A Short Account of the Destruction of the Indies, 1552*

No matter how they are defined, there are probably well over 300 million people around the world whose past histories distinguish them as descendants of pre-colonial inhabitants. Traditional Indigenous populations are custodians of an extraordinary range of languages and cultures that form an irreplaceable part of what it means to be a human. They make their own countries, and the world in general, a more interesting place to live. In addition, the enormous scientific (particularly pharmaceutical) value of some of their botanical knowledge has only recently been appreciated. A common history of invasion, colonization, and subsequent oppression means that the international community bears some responsibility for the current poor state of health of many Indigenous groups around the world. It is hoped that they recognize this responsibility and help to redress old wrongs by placing more emphasis on the health of Indigenous peoples in the future.

Many of the SDGs are relevant for Indigenous peoples and have direct linkages to the human rights commitments outlined in the UN Declaration on the Rights of Indigenous Peoples. The SDGs make six direct references to Indigenous peoples, including in SDG 2 related to agricultural output of Indigenous small-scale farmers, and SDG 4 on equal access to education for Indigenous children:

- Target 2.3: By 2030, double the agricultural productivity and incomes of small-scale food producers, in particular women, indigenous peoples, family farmers, pastoralists and fishers, including through secure and equal access to land, other productive resources and inputs, knowledge, financial services, markets and opportunities for value addition and non-farm employment.
- Target 4.5: By 2030, eliminate gender disparities in education and ensure equal access to all levels of education and vocational training for the vulnerable, including persons with disabilities, indigenous peoples, and children in vulnerable situations.

In addition to the aforementioned SDG targets, the health-related targets in SDG 3 are relevant for Indigenous health with respect to universal health coverage, access to high-quality essential health services, medicines, and vaccines.

There is no unambiguous definition of Indigenous peoples that clearly distinguishes between ethnic minorities and original inhabitants, but the outline given by Alderete (1999) provides a good starting point for discussion. Indigenous groups have the following characteristics:

- They are descendants of people who were in the territory of the country long before other groups of different cultures or ethnic origin arrived.
- Because of isolation from the dominant segment of the country's population, they have preserved customs and ancestral traditions, religion, dress, livelihood, and lifestyles that characterize them as Indigenous.
- They often live within a state structure that incorporates social and cultural characteristics alien to their own traditions.

Estimates of their numbers vary widely (IWGIA, 2010; World Bank, 2007). The most commonly quoted figure is 300 million people, composed of 5,000–6,000 different groups spread over 70 countries. Collectively, their contributions to the world have been extensive and usually underappreciated. Apart from lessons to be learned from their attitudes to the stewardship of the environment, many groups

Box 17.1 History Notes

Rigoberta Menchu (1959–)

Rigoberta Menchu is a controversial character. Following her widely read autobiography, published in 1982, and her subsequent Nobel Peace Prize in 1992, she has become a symbol of the discrimination and violence suffered by Indigenous peoples. Later research casts doubts on the accuracy of her book and has led to a "battle of books" between opposing intellectual factions. Although some of her claims were exaggerated, her family certainly suffered severely from the murderous Guatemalan army during the country's 35-year-long civil war. The true story contains more than enough evil without the need for elaboration. Her brother was not burned alive, as claimed; he was "only" shot to death. She also lost her mother, father, brothers, and other relatives through murder and torture.

Menchu was born in Guatemala. She is a member of the Quiché branch of the much broader Mayan population. After basic schooling, she became increasingly involved in protest movements against the oppression of peasants in Guatemala. By the time her oral autobiography was widely published in 1983, she had been forced to flee her country and live in Mexico. After the end of the war in 1996, Menchu continued her activism on behalf of Native peoples. In 2004, Guatemala's president invited Menchu to join his government as a monitor of the country's adherence to the negotiated peace treaty. She has subsequently worked to bring perpetrators to court, both in Guatemala and in Spain. For more information on this complex story, see Arias (2001).

have accumulated a knowledge of the pharmaceutical properties of plants that is of great contemporary value—so valuable that efforts are being made to protect and pay for the use of that knowledge (Brush et al., 1996).

Indigenous populations show extraordinary variation in their lifestyles, traditions, and cultures (DESA, 2015). They range from small communities, measured in tens of thousands (such as the San Bushmen of southern Africa), to populations in the millions (such as the diverse descendants of the Maya in Mexico and Central America. Unfortunately, during the long colonial history of the European powers, the collision of cultures between the new immigrants and existing populations was rarely a happy one (Coates, 2004). Many Aboriginal peoples share a common history of conquest, land appropriation, and depopulation until they became minorities in their own land. At best, they subsequently suffered from discrimination, and at worst, some groups lived through periods of terrible deprivation (DESA, 2015). For example, in Latin America, access to public services such as piped water are consistently lower for Indigenous groups than their non-Indigenous counterparts (Figure 17.1).

Despite the growing influence of Indigenous movements over the last 25 years, Aboriginal peoples all over the world still face the loss of their lands and ways of

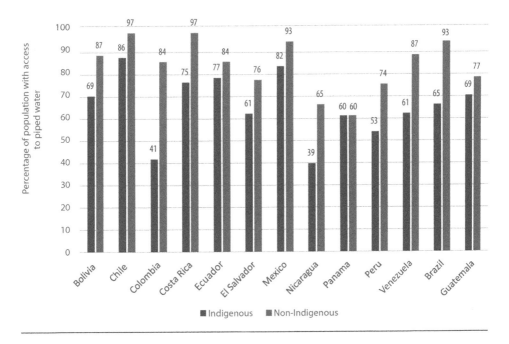

Figure 17.1: Access to public services by Indigenous status

Source: World Bank. 2015. Indigenous Latin America in the twenty-first century: The first decade. Retrieved from: https://openknowledge.worldbank.org/handle/10986/23751.

life. For example, the Ainu of Japan are struggling to preserve their culture in the midst of a modern technological society, and the Saami of northern Europe are seeking self-rule over traditional lands included within the borders of Sweden, Finland, Norway, and Russia. In the fairly recent past, Indigenous peoples in El Salvador and Guatemala have also been the targets of severe political violence that included widespread torture and murder.

In spite of the extraordinary cultural and ethnic diversity of Indigenous peoples around the world, there are often striking similarities between their social grievances and common health problems (Gracy et al., 2009). With time, Indigenous organizations have developed a voice for their people and the situation for many groups has improved. However, despite enlightened government policies and a great deal of financial investment, the health indices of Native populations in countries such as Canada, Australia, New Zealand, and the United States lag far behind national averages. It is still possible to find developing world conditions affecting

Table 17.1: Major milestones in establishing rights for Indigenous peoples

1840	New Zealand's Native Land Treaty is signed at Waitangi.
1920s	Native American and Mayan leaders both petition the early League of Nations on behalf of Indigenous peoples, but are denied access.
1975	New Zealand's government grants limited legal recognition of Waitangi treaty; extended recognition is granted in 1985.
1979	Denmark grants home rule to the largely Inuit Greenland.
1982	The first working group on Indigenous populations (WGIP) is formed as a subcommittee of the UN Economic and Social Council.
1985	The WGIP begin work on the draft of a Declaration of Rights of Indigenous Peoples. The draft is completed in 1993.
1989	International Labour Organization adopts Convention no. 169, emphasizing the rights of Indigenous groups to determine their own future.
1994	The UN General Assembly launches the International Decade of the World's Indigenous Peoples from 1995 to 2004.
1999	Canada forms the self-governing territory of Nunavut, with a largely Inuit population.
2000	The UN Permanent Forum on Indigenous Issues (UNPFII) is formally established.
2005	Second International Decade of the World's Indigenous People starts, with the theme "partnership for action and dignity."
2006	UNHCR passes the non-binding Declaration on Indigenous Rights, but without full consensus.
2007	The UN Declaration on the Rights of Indigenous Peoples is adopted by the UN General Assembly (www.un.org/esa/socdev/unpfii/en/declaration.html).
2009	Canada endorses the UN Declaration on Indigenous Rights.
2014	High-Level Plenary Meeting of the United Nations General Assembly, also known as the World Conference on Indigenous Peoples, is held.

Aboriginal communities in the reserves, settlements, and downtown cores of all these countries (King et al., 2009). A recent study examining the well-being of more than 154 million Indigenous and tribal peoples from 23 countries revealed evidence of poorer health and social outcomes for Indigenous peoples than for non-Indigenous populations using indicators such as life expectancy at birth, infant mortality, maternal mortality, child malnutrition, and a host of other health indicators (Anderson et al., 2016).

Current evidence suggests that the health status of many Indigenous groups is actually improving, but there is a long way to go before they have the same health measures as non-Indigenous people within their same country. Improvements in global communications will hopefully make it harder to exploit Indigenous groups without the rest of the world finding out. Communication advances also make it easier for small Indigenous groups to be heard (Kunitz, 2000). Maintaining those improvements in health will require coordinated interventions that must be supported over a long period (Durie, 2003). These include economic revival, specific Indigenous health research (including national plans to recognize and deal with the current deficiencies in Indigenous statistics), increased funding and resources for Indigenous peoples, and constitutional and legislative changes to improve their degree of self-determination (Freemantle et al., 2015).

With time, the voices of Indigenous populations are slowly being heard. Some of the highlights from the last 30 years are given in Table 17.1. Indigenous issues are now given attention by large international agencies, the most significant of which was the establishment of the Permanent Forum on Indigenous Issues at the United Nations (UNPFII, 2011). The UN Declaration on the Rights of Indigenous Peoples (UNPFII, 2007), which resulted from that forum, was signed by most countries in 2007. Universal consensus was delayed because of unresolved issues concerning autonomy, self-governance, and control of natural resources, but Canada, New Zealand, Australia, and the US now all support the document. When Denmark granted independent rule to Greenland in 1979, it marked a major step in self-determination for largely Indigenous communities. The establishment of a new territory in northern Canada (Nunavut, 2011a) has continued that trend. Other countries, including Norway and New Zealand, have also shown enlightened policies toward autonomy for their Indigenous populations.

MAJOR INDIGENOUS GROUPS

We are not myths of the past, ruins in a jungle or zoos. We are people and we want to be respected, not to be victims of intolerance and racism.

—*Rigoberta Menchu, 1992*

North American Native Peoples

There is a large (and growing) Indigenous population in North America. In Canada alone, the population of the three groups of Indigenous peoples—First Nations, Métis, and Inuit—is more than 1 million. The most recent US census review estimates there are 3.1 million American Indigenous people, ranging from Inuit and Aleut groups in Alaska to the wide diversity of Native groups that still exist across the American mainland (US Census Bureau, 2011). Based on a variety of archaeological sites (particularly Clovis, New Mexico), it was assumed, until fairly recently, that modern Native Americans crossed over from Siberia roughly 13,000–14,000 years ago. However, recent findings at Topper in South Carolina and other sites have raised contentious arguments that may end by moving that estimate back by thousands of years. The route of migration has also been challenged by theories that now include transatlantic and trans-Pacific alternatives.

The collision of cultures caused by the westward migration of largely European colonists produced a very sad history the effects of which are still apparent today. Collectively, these various raids, skirmishes, and battles are known as the Indian wars. They began with fights between English settlers and local Native tribes, starting from the earliest days of the Jamestown settlement around 1610. They ended with what is generally considered the final large engagement (more of a massacre than a battle) at Wounded Knee in 1890. In total, there were probably many thousands of separate incidents over this period; the best known is the destruction of Custer's forces at Little Big Horn. Although the death rate was low compared to the mortality from disease and forced relocation, many of the engagements were noted for their brutality. An extensive bibliography of the subject is available (Osborn, 2001).

In Canada, the history was much less violent, but was still far from ideal. Misguided policies of forced assimilation, through compulsory schooling, have left deep scars on Aboriginal society. It is estimated that between 1880 and the 1970s, more than 150,000 Indigenous children were removed from their homes and sent to residential schools, where their languages and cultures were suppressed (United Church, 2007). Excessive corporal punishment and even sexual predation resulted in an entire generation of Indigenous peoples who lost their identity. The resulting pattern of substance abuse, family violence, suicide, and social disruption is a common legacy of that policy; a legacy that may be found, for example, in First Nations communities across Canada (Adelson, 2005). The Truth and Reconciliation Commission of Canada (TRC) established in 2008 was a way to redress some of the wrongs done and respond to the abuse experienced by Indigenous peoples through the residential school system. The commission travelled throughout Canada to hear from Aboriginal people who had been taken from their families as children into these residential schools (TRC, 2015). The commission completed their work in December 2015 and provided a set of recommendations to advance the process of reconciliation between the federal/provincial/territorial governments and Indigenous peoples of Canada. These recommendations revolved around child welfare, education, language, culture, health, and justice (TRC, 2015).

Australia's Aboriginal Population

The Indigenous peoples of Australia are commonly called Aboriginals (Photo 17.1). They arrived in the country tens of thousands of years before the European settlers. They are a diverse group spread throughout Australia and some offshore regions, such as the Torres Strait Islands and Tasmania. Estimates of the pre-European population vary between 500,000 and 1 million, but this dropped sharply after the arrival of the Europeans. At one point, it was widely accepted that the

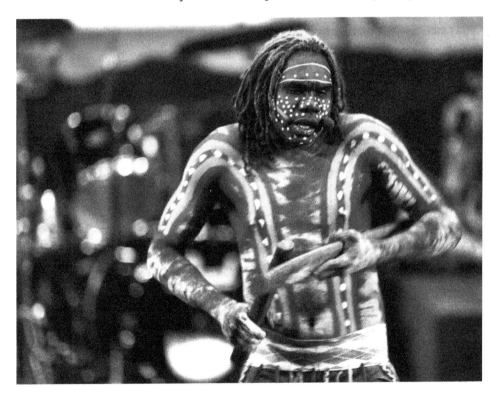

Photo 17.1: A member of Yothu Yindi, an Australian Aboriginal rock band, performs in 1993 during the opening ceremonies of the International Year of the World's Indigenous People.

Source: UN Photo/John Isaac, with kind permission of the UN Photo Library (www.unmultimedia. org/photo).

Aboriginal population would die out, but since the mid-1960s, their numbers have increased (ABS, 2011). The most recent estimate was roughly 517,000 for 2006. The Aboriginals are an ancient people who crossed a land bridge to Australia from Southeast Asia. Australian archaeological sites have provided the oldest human remains outside of Africa. A skeleton found at Mungo Lake is widely believed to be 40,000 years old, and the first people may have arrived 10,000 years before that.

Starting in the 17th century, the British transported convicted criminals to their colonies rather than housing them in jails. They initially used America, but switched to Australia following the American War of Independence. The first penal colony established in Australia was founded in 1788 in the area of Sydney. Inevitably, there were conflicts as the new settlers slowly took over the fertile parts of the country (Hughes, 1996). Aboriginals had no military tradition and no modern weapons, so these fights were little more than massacres. In Tasmania, the original population of several thousand people was reduced to a few hundred in a matter of years. The last surviving Tasmanian Aboriginal died in the late 19th century.

The combination of newly introduced diseases, loss of traditional land, and oppressive treatment caused a steep population decline well into the 20th century before it started to rebound. Australian Aboriginals were not allowed citizenship until 1967. Unfortunately, the government also followed a policy of forced assimilation similar to the Canadian practice. Until as late as 1972, large numbers of Aboriginal children were forcibly removed from their parents and either fostered into a European family or placed in residential care. The social results of this so-called "stolen generation" are exactly the same as those suffered by the North American Indigenous population—high rates of suicide, substance abuse, family violence, and ill health (Ring et al., 2002).

Maori and Polynesian Islanders

Despite the voyage of the *Kon-Tiki* and Thor Heyerdahl's early theory about the South American origin of Polynesian peoples, it is now widely accepted that the Polynesian settlers of Tonga, Samoa, Tahiti, Hawaii, the Marquesas, and New Zealand had their origins in Southeast Asia, probably around Taiwan. Slow eastward migration across the Pacific reached New Zealand (Aotearoa) by AD 800–1000. New Zealand's isolation meant that the first European colonists did not arrive until the early 19th century. Unfortunately, the introduction of firearms to the warlike Maori culture led to a series of murderous intertribal wars. In order to control the situation, the British government intervened in 1839; by 1840, Britain claimed the country as a colony at the Treaty of Waitangi. The agreement has subsequently been the source of a great deal of political controversy. More recently, the New Zealand government has been a pioneer in honouring early treaties by basing subsequent settlements on that early document (NZ History, 2011).

The peace imposed by the colonial treaty initially seemed beneficial for all, but it did not last. Inevitable conflicts over land erupted into war by 1845. The Maoris were no pushovers and soundly beat elite British troops on several occasions. Fighting lasted over 30 years before a final peace was reached. The Maori population in 1840 was estimated at 115,000, but the gradual loss of land and traditional practices led to a steady decline in that number. In keeping with the Australian experience, it was believed that Maori culture would cease to exist. Fortunately, Indigenous culture again proved more resilient than expected. Although health indicators such as obesity, diabetes, and family violence are higher than national averages (Bramley et al., 2006), the Maori people are largely well adapted in modern New Zealand society. Currently, over half a million people are classified as Maori; they make up roughly 15 percent of the population.

Circumpolar Indigenous Peoples

Indigenous groups previously referred to as "Eskimos" (now called Inuit in Canada, or Yupik in Russia and Alaska) are people who inhabit the High Arctic above the treeline. Related groups can be found in the Aleutians, northern Canada, Greenland, and northeastern Russia. Inuit arrived in North America long after Native American Indians and retained a distinctly different culture. Inuit are descended from the Thule people, who had populated Alaska by AD 500 and arrived in Canada by AD 1000, when they displaced the existing Dorset people (Glenbow, 2008).

Their adaptation to a harsh environment allowed them to avoid European contact until the 18th century, when whalers and, later, fur traders moved north. Inuit had little contact with the rest of Canada until the Canadian government began to establish a presence in the North during the 1940s. Communities have now abandoned their traditional seasonal camps and moved into permanent settlements, which are supported with medical care, social services, and a police presence. Some communities have had significant problems with substance abuse (particularly alcohol and glue sniffing), combined with a high rate of tuberculosis and other diseases associated with poverty (Bjerregaard et al., 2004). The current population of Inuit in Canada is 55,000; over half live in the new territory of Nunavut.

Inuit organizations have been very successful in lobbying for Indigenous rights. In 1977, the Inuit Circumpolar Conference (ICC) was created to represent the interests of Inuit groups in Canada, Greenland, Russia, and Alaska (ICC, 2011). The

Box 17.2 Moment of Insight

Cameroon	Kenya	Canada	Australia
Indigenous (Baka) life expectancy	Indigenous (Maasai) life expectancy	Indigenous (Inuit) life expectancy	Indigenous (Aboriginal or Torres Strait Islander) life expectancy
35.5 years	43.5	68.5 years	71.4
Non-indigenous life expectancy	Non-indigenous life expectancy	Non-indigenous life expectancy	Non-indigenous life expectancy
57 years	56.6 years	81 years	81.4 years
Gap **21.5 years**	**Gap** **13.1 years**	**Gap** **12.5 years**	**Gap** **10 years**

Source: Anderson, I., et al. 2016. Indigenous and tribal peoples' health (The Lancet–Lowitja Institute Global Collaboration): A population study. The Lancet, 388(10040), 131–157.

ICC promotes Inuit rights and interests at an international level. The Nunavut land claims agreement reached in 1993 ultimately led to the establishment of the territory of Nunavut in 1999, where Inuit form much of the population (Nunavut, 2011b).

Mayan and Central American Indigenous Groups

Central and Southern America have seen great Amerindian civilizations rise and fall. The current theory is that Indigenous groups migrated down through North America, but other theories (including a trans-Pacific route) have also been proposed. Some of those early peoples—such as the Olmec, Maya, and Aztec—developed civilizations with sophisticated knowledge of mathematics and astronomy. In some parts of Mexico, Belize, and Guatemala, Native American Indigenous groups form up to 50 percent of the population, although they certainly do not share 50 percent of the available wealth.

The arrival of three small ships, led by Columbus in 1492, forever altered the existing Indigenous culture. The subsequent story of murder, slavery, and introduced diseases is a dark chapter in human history (Stannard, 1992). Despite everything, the Mayan culture has proved resilient. Today, approximately 6 million Maya are spread principally through Mexico, Guatemala, Belize, and Honduras. Unfortunately, severe violence aimed at Maya is not just ancient history. The terrible events described by Rigoberta Menchu happened during the Guatemalan civil war, which ended only in 1996. As many as 200,000 Indigenous people lost their lives during that war (USDS, 2011). The Maya remain predominantly agricultural people and still suffer varying degrees of discrimination and the inevitable health problems that stem from marginalization within a richer society.

CANADA'S INDIGENOUS COMMUNITIES

It is often easier to become outraged by injustice half a world away than by oppression and discrimination half a block from home.

—*Carl T. Rowan (1925–2000), African American journalist*

The absence of significant public or political interest in Indigenous peoples, combined with the difficulty in finding even the most basic information about the reality of their lives, tends to make Aboriginal groups strangers in their own lands. It is not likely that the average person chatting over coffee in downtown Vancouver, Sydney, or Seattle spends much time worrying about Indigenous health even though there are probably inner-city Aboriginal people living lives of terrible deprivation just around the corner. With the exception of North America, New Zealand, Australia, and, to some extent, Latin America, the standards of published information concerning Indigenous populations are very poor (Bramley et al., 2004). For the enormous diversity of Indigenous groups in China, India, and Africa, accessible data is virtually non-existent. This section takes a careful look at the lives of Indigenous peoples in Canada simply because there is a good deal of epidemiological information available. Clearly they will differ from Aboriginal groups in other parts of the world, but the common threads of discrimination and ill health are so widespread that it will hopefully give useful insights into the lives of Aboriginal peoples in other countries.

It is not necessary to travel outside Canada to see the results of poverty and poor access to health care. Even though Canada has a free and fair society, jurisdictional disputes, cultural barriers, and geographic isolation still impede some Aboriginal peoples' access to adequate housing and health care. In general, the more remote communities, particularly those in the far North, fare the worst. The inevitable result is a lower level of health among Indigenous peoples in Canada (Figure 17.2). For example, cardiovascular disease is twice as common, Type 2 diabetes is five times as common, and tuberculosis is 10 times as common compared to non-Indigenous rates (HC-SC, 2010). Those Canadians interested in studying the health of developing world populations should start with a good understanding of the socio-economic and health standards of Indigenous peoples living within their own borders.

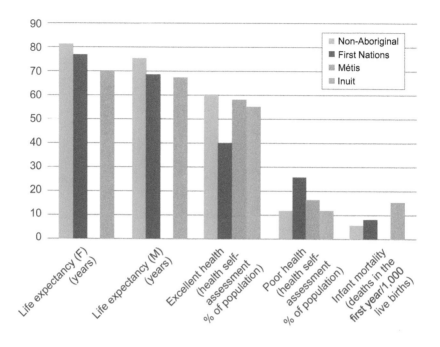

Figure 17.2: Basic health indicators for Indigenous populations in Canada

Source: HC-SC. 2011. Health Canada: First Nations, Inuit, and Aboriginal health. Retrieved from: www. hc-sc.gc.ca/fniah-spnia/index-eng.php.

Early legislation passed by the British Crown, such as the 1763 Proclamation on Aboriginal land title and the 1876 Indian Act, principally referred to First Nations, but it is important to appreciate that the Aboriginal population of Canada does not fit into one neat category. Based on the most recent five-yearly Aboriginal Peoples' Survey (StatCan, 2011a), there are roughly 1.2 million people of Aboriginal descent in Canada. They are represented throughout the country, ranging from 1 percent of the population in Ontario up to 85 percent of the population in Nunavut. The population is also young and growing. The 2008 census showed that half of the Aboriginal population was under the age of 25 (compared to less than a third in the non-Aboriginal population), and the birth rate was up to twice the national average. Average age of first pregnancy is also significantly lower than the Canadian average.

There are three main groups of Indigenous peoples in Canada: First Nations (65 percent), Métis (30 percent), and Inuit (5 percent). Aboriginal peoples registered as "Indian" under the Indian Act are more commonly referred to as First Nations and have certain rights and benefits protected by law. They are represented by the Assembly of First Nations (AFN, 2011). Those Aboriginal peoples not registered are referred to as "non-status" and are represented by the Congress of Aboriginal Peoples (CAP, 2011). Métis are Aboriginal people with mixed ancestry; they are represented by the Métis National Council (MNC, 2011). Inuit live primarily in northern Canada and are represented by the Inuit Tapiriit Kanatami (ITK, 2011).

SOCIAL DETERMINANTS OF HEALTH FOR ABORIGINAL PEOPLES IN CANADA

> We have survived Canada's assault on our identity and our rights.... Our survival is a testament to our determination and will to survive as people. We are prepared to participate in Canada's future—but only on the terms that we believe to be our rightful heritage.
>
> —*Wallace Labillois, Council of Elders, 1996*

Although the general health of the Aboriginal population in Canada is much better than that of many other Indigenous populations around the world, their specific health indices still lag behind those of non-Aboriginal Canadians (HC-SC, 2011). As Figure 17.2 shows, broad health indicators such as life expectancy, infant mortality, and self-reported health status are all worse among Indigenous populations compared to national averages. There is no single cause for the poorer health of Aboriginal peoples; it is the end result of a range of inequities, both historical and contemporary. Identifying and quantifying every variable would be difficult; lower socio-economic standards, lack of self-determination, and the legacy residential school system are just a few of the factors that have had significant adverse health effects. Some of the principal variables influencing the health of Indigenous peoples in Canada are as follows.

Socio-Economic Status

> The first priority is economic development. This is obviously the most essential step to improving the lives of Aboriginal people and their families.
>
> —*Stephen Harper, Canadian prime minister, 2007*

In keeping with Indigenous populations around the world, measures of the socio-economic status of Aboriginal peoples in Canada are all significantly lower than national Canadian averages. Educational attainment and employment rates lag behind those of the general population. Consequently, average income remains at or below two-thirds of the national average (Figure 17.3). Figures are worst for First Nations living on reserve land. The underlying reasons are complex and include unresolved claims to land and natural resources, reduced access to education in remote communities, lower educational levels, and, consequently, reduced job

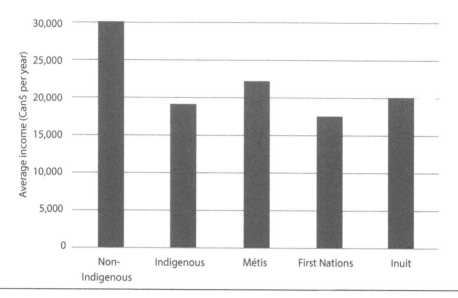

Figure 17.3: Average income for Indigenous and non-Indigenous groups in Canada

Source: Mendelson, M. 2006. Aboriginal peoples and postsecondary education in Canada, Caledon Institute of Social Policy. Retrieved from: www.caledoninst.org/Publications/PDF/595ENG.pdf.

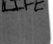

opportunities and income. The Aboriginal population is the youngest and fast-est-growing segment of the population in Canada, so it is an increasing source of workers for a growing economy. The Canadian government recognized this with its 2006 Federal Framework for Aboriginal Economic Development (AANDC, 2009). Since the first initiative in 1989 (Canadian Aboriginal Economic Development Strategy), there have been obvious improvements both in control over land and in education. Things are still far from perfect, but compared to many other groups, there are signs of hope for the future.

Education

With increasing awareness of the importance of higher education and the estab-lishment of various organizations such as the First Nations Education Council, all three Aboriginal groups have made steady progress in school completion rates. In the years since the educational survey by the Canadian Institute for Health Information in 2004, First Nations dropout rates have fallen from 48 percent to 25.8 percent, and Métis rates have fallen from 42 percent to 18.9 percent (StatCan, 2010). Boys reported that the most common obstacles to completion of schooling were boredom and a desire to work. Among girls, the most common reasons were either pregnancy or the need to care for other children in the family. Reasons for not completing post-secondary studies were family responsibilities among women and lack of money for men (O'Donnell et al., 2001). There is clearly a need for more Aboriginal teachers and aides in the classroom to help make the educational experience more culturally relevant and interesting for Aboriginal students.

Effects of Residential Schooling

> While it is not uncommon to hear some former students speak about their positive experiences in these institutions, their stories are overshadowed by disclosures of abuse, criminal convictions of perpetrators and the findings of various studies such as the Royal Commission on Aboriginal Peoples, which tell of the tragic legacy that the residential school system has left with many former students.
>
> —*Indian and Northern Affairs Canada, 2004*

The residential school system officially began in 1892; most were closed by the 1970s. Schools were funded by the federal government and usually operated by the churches (United Church, 2007). Children were forbidden to speak their own language and practise their own traditions and beliefs. The subsequent loss of culture and language weakened the collective identity of Indigenous peoples. Apart from numerous lawsuits and class actions stemming from abuse, the federal government also acknowledged this injustice with an apology in 1998.

The schooling experiment harmed many of the estimated 93,000 former residential students who are still alive today. Specific harmful effects of residential schooling are difficult to disentangle from other socio-economic variables affecting Indigenous populations, but it is widely accepted that it was a significant contributor to current high levels of suicide, substance abuse, and family violence (Smith et al., 2005). These effects also subsequently harm succeeding generations. Residential schooling still runs like a rip through the fabric of Indigenous society.

Housing Standards

Adequate standards of housing and water quality are essential foundations for good health—both these basic necessities are of poorer quality in Indigenous communities (AANDC, 2011). The most recent data show that of the more than 90,000 houses in First Nations communities, 12 percent are overcrowded (more than one person per room), 21.9 percent need major repairs, and 5.7 percent need to be replaced (HC-SC, 2011). The government has responded with a First Nations' housing program that is backed by building loan guarantees. In addition, the growing Aboriginal population means that a steady supply of new houses is also needed. Housing is a particular problem in the North, where 53 percent of Inuit live in crowded conditions. Crowding is a particular risk for the transmission of tuberculosis. Not surprisingly, tuberculosis is many times more common among Inuit than the rest of Canada.

Clean Water and the Environment

Water contamination resulting from inadequate and poorly managed treatment plants can lead to numerous health problems; it is a common problem on First Nations reserves (Rosenberg et al., 1997). In 2005, over 800 people were evacuated from Kasechewan reserve because of health problems associated with poor living standards—fecally contaminated water was only one of many social problems that the community faced. The situation was embarrassing for the Canadian government and prompted urgent action (Eggertson, 2006). In 2006, roughly one in six First Nations reserves had a "boil water" advisory in place.

The North is particularly badly affected. Over the last 40 years, there has been a measurable rise in the temperature in Canada's North, varying from 0.5°C to 1.5°C. This is predicted to continue in the near future and threatens to alter traditional Inuit hunting areas. More immediately, Inuit are also threatened by environmental contaminants that have accumulated in Arctic wildlife. Studies have shown that human exposure to mercury and organic toxins exceeds daily levels set by Health Canada— in some cases, by an order of magnitude (Butler-Walker et al., 2006). Inuit continue to consume traditional hunted food, partly because of the expense of imported food but also because of the importance of hunting within the Inuit social structure.

Aboriginal Languages

Language is an essential part of cultural identity. Partly due to the residential schooling legacy, many Indigenous languages are at risk. The percentage of Indigenous people who can speak an Aboriginal language fell from 20 percent in 1996 to 16 percent in 2001 (O'Donnell et al., 2001). Métis are the least likely to know an Aboriginal language and Inuit are the most likely to have retained a language skill. The Aboriginal Head Start Approach (HSA) is an early childhood development program for Indigenous children and their families. There are currently well over 100 HSA programs throughout Canada (AHSABC, 2011). These and other educational initiatives include Indigenous languages as part of their program. The HSA program began in the US with the aim of supporting early child development for Aboriginal peoples. The Canadian federal government adopted the Head Start Approach in 1985.

Addressing the Determinants of Ill Health for Indigenous Peoples in Canada

> Lack of control over important dimensions of living, in itself contributes to ill health. Aboriginal people want to exercise their own judgment and understanding about what makes people healthy, their own skills in solving health and social problems.
>
> —*Royal Commission on Aboriginal Peoples, 1996*

The influential 1996 Royal Commission on Aboriginal Peoples (RCAP, 1996) included hundreds of recommendations for Indigenous health and social problems. The government's response to the commission was to release *Gathering Strength: Canada's Aboriginal Action Plan*, which has led to many new policy developments since its release. One obvious shift in policy has been to give Aboriginal peoples greater control over their own affairs. The first part of this involves the slow process of land claims and treaty negotiations. The second occurs at a local level and involves a move toward Indigenous control over their own services, particularly health, education, police, and fire services. In a British Columbia study (Chandler et al., 1998), it was found that the suicide rate was 138 per 100,000 population in communities with no control over local services, but there was a steady drop in suicide rate as the number of First Nations-controlled facilities increased. In communities with complete control over their own services, the suicide rate was almost zero.

Several national institutes have also been created, including the National Aboriginal Health Organization, which advocates for the health and well-being of Aboriginal peoples (NAHO, 2011); the Institute of Aboriginal Peoples' Health, which supports Indigenous health research (IAPH, 2011); the Aboriginal Healing Foundation, which supports healing initiatives aimed at reducing the impact of residential schooling (AHF, 2011); and the much-needed First Nations Statistical Institute for the regular collection of Indigenous health and social data (FNSI, 2010). In addition, greater investment has been made in the Head Start program and the housing renovation fund intended to provide water, sewage, and housing upgrades on reserves.

HEALTH STATUS OF INDIGENOUS PEOPLES IN CANADA

> We owe the Aboriginal peoples a debt that is four centuries old. It is their turn to become full partners in developing an even greater Canada. And the reconciliation required may be less a matter of legal texts than of attitudes of the heart.
>
> —*Romeo LeBlanc, governor general of Canada, 1995*

Canadian Aboriginal peoples die earlier than their fellow Canadians and, on average, sustain a disproportionate burden of chronic physical and mental illness
(HC-SC, 2011). Although exact causes are not known in detail, the relatively poor
status of Indigenous health is clearly associated with the unfavourable economic
and social conditions discussed in the previous section. On the bright side, there
have been significant improvements over the last two or three decades. The gap in
life expectancy between Aboriginal groups and the Canadian average is decreasing,
but remains significant. Statistics Canada predicted that by 2017, Inuit males will
still live 15 years less than the national average (Figure 17.4). In Canada, ethnicity
is not recorded on death certificates, so following trends in child mortality indices
is complicated by lack of reliable data. The available research suggests that infant
mortality rates are higher than national averages, particularly in remote rural areas
(Smylie et al., 2010). The following conditions are of particular importance among
Indigenous groups in Canada.

Diseases of Lifestyle

It is widely accepted that the principal risk factors for diabetes, heart attacks,
strokes, and high cholesterol are the so-called lifestyle factors—poor nutrition,
lack of exercise, and smoking. These are not the only causes of vascular disease,

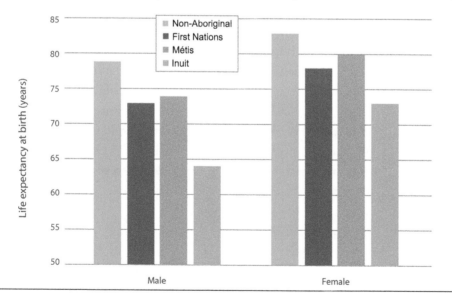

**Figure 17.4: Projected life expectancy at birth by gender and Aboriginal
identity for 2017**

Source: StatCan. 2011b. Projected life expectancy by sex and Aboriginal identity. Retrieved from: www.
statcan.gc.ca/pub/89-645-x/2010001/c-g/c-g013-eng.htm.

but they are the main ones over which people have some control. Unfortunately, Indigenous peoples have high levels of all these risk factors. Smoking rates are two to three times the national average, and obesity has become a major health problem facing First Nations communities, including the children (Caballeros et al., 2003). Compared to Canadian averages, strokes and heart attacks are more common among Aboriginal peoples and have become the leading causes of death in Indigenous adults over 45 years. Type 2 diabetes has now reached epidemic levels, particularly in First Nations communities, where one in five now has diabetes (Young et al., 2000). Type 2 diabetes is also increasingly diagnosed among Aboriginal children. The government has responded with the Aboriginal Diabetes Initiative, which is a collaborative venture between the government and representatives of Indigenous groups.

Infectious Diseases

The most important infectious diseases affecting Indigenous peoples are tuberculosis and HIV/AIDS. Tuberculosis is over five times more common among Aboriginal peoples (Reading, 2009). This is only an average; in some communities, rates are far higher. Wherever there is poverty and poor housing, tuberculosis will not be far behind. Clearly, socio-economic factors are the cause of the high rate of tuberculosis in Indigenous communities. Although rates are much lower than they were during epidemics in early 20th-century Canada (the peak rate was 700 per 100,000), significant improvements in the current rate will require extensive investment in First Nations' housing standards.

In 1992, Indigenous peoples formed 1.7 percent of total HIV/AIDS cases in Canada. By 2001, this had risen to 7.2 percent and is now above 15 percent, (HC-SC, 2010). Ethnicity is not reliably reported on notification forms, so this is certainly an underestimate. Aboriginal communities make up 3.3 percent of the population of Canada. The most common means of transmission is IV drug use (Craib et al., 2003). The HIV epidemic has had a significant effect on Indigenous women. The Canadian national rate of HIV infection among pregnant women is 3.4 per 10,000 population; among Indigenous women, it is 33.3 per 10,000 (PHAC, 2004).

Other infectious risks for Indigenous communities include a higher rate of water-borne diseases, such as hepatitis A and shigellosis, reflecting the poorer water standards in First Nations communities (Rosenberg et al., 1997). There is also evidence that First Nations children are at higher risk of serious chest infection compared to the Canadian average (Seear et al., 1997).

Trauma

Among Indigenous peoples, the potential years of life lost to injury is greater than all other causes of death combined and is also three to four times higher than the average Canadian rate (HC-SC, 2003). Injuries and poisoning combined were the most common causes of death for First Nations people from 1 to 44 years. Suicide and self-injury made up a significant part of this total. Aboriginal peoples are at greater risk of death and injury from a range of sources, including motor accidents, drowning, fire, family violence, and suicide.

Deaths and injuries due to motor vehicle accidents are much higher than national averages (HC-SC, 2003). Contributing factors include high rates of alcohol use, poorer-quality rural roads, and greater use of higher-risk vehicles such as snowmobiles and all-terrain vehicles. The location of First Nations communities near rivers and lakes also increases the risk of drowning. One study showed that only 6 percent of Aboriginal drowning victims had worn a flotation device, and two-thirds of drowning victims over 15 years old had an alcohol level above the legal limit (compared to 27 percent for non-Aboriginal drowning) (Chochinov, 1998). The greatest risk for children was falling into open water. Higher smoking rates, wood-frame housing, lower building standards (particularly lack of smoke detectors), and poorly equipped rural fire services all combine to produce a much greater risk of serious fires on Aboriginal reserves. Almost one-third of all fire deaths in Aboriginal population are between the ages of 1 and 14 years, compared to an average of 16 percent in the total Canadian population.

The high suicide rate noted in many Aboriginal communities tends to be associated with predictable adverse social characteristics (Kirmayer et al., 2007). These include a high number of occupants per household, more single-parent families, fewer elders, lower average income, and lower average education. The Canadian government and Indigenous groups have taken the problem seriously with advisory groups and various reports, but there are no easy solutions for such a complex problem. How are phrases such as "creating strategies for building youth identity, resilience and culture" (HC-SC, 2002), actually translated into action for unemployed Indigenous youth in remote northern communities or on rural reserves across a country as big as Canada? The association between suicide rates and community self-determination, mentioned earlier, offers some hope for interventions that have measurable results (Chandler et al., 1998).

High rates of family violence have been reported in Indigenous communities, but the problem is greatly under-reported. A review of earlier studies by Health Canada quotes abuse rates as high as 50 percent among surveyed Aboriginal women (Bopp et al., 2003). It is suspected that elder abuse is increasing, but no accurate figures exist (PHAC, 2008). Apart from the absence of reliable survey data, a recent review of factors determining Aboriginal maternal and child health did not even mention the subject (HCC, 2011). Family violence is viewed by many First Nations peoples as a social ill that has evolved due to the results of historical injustices and cultural assaults experienced over centuries of colonization; it is clearly a problem with deep roots. An earlier study by the Aboriginal Nurses Association found that the three most common factors behind family violence were poverty, substance abuse, and a history of intergenerational abuse.

The federal government became involved in the 1970s once the scope of the problem became obvious. Programs included the Family Violence Initiative and the Child Sexual Abuse Initiative, as well as the construction of federally funded women's shelters on reserves across Canada. Involvement of the justice system and child-protection agencies is clearly necessary, but prevention through education and community initiatives offers the only long-term solution to this problem (INAC, 2004).

Substance Abuse

Substance abuse, including drug and alcohol abuse, is a common problem and a major issue concerning Indigenous peoples in Canada. Research suggests that fetal alcohol syndrome (FAS) may be more common among Indigenous children, but there is insufficient evidence about the prevalence of fetal alcohol syndrome among the non-Indigenous population to be able to draw firm conclusions. The inhalation of volatile substances, such as glue, gasoline, paint, and dry-cleaning fluids, is also a growing problem among some Indigenous children (Weir, 2001). There is no accurate information, but the problem is common on remote reserves. It has been reported in children as young as four years old.

The issue came to national attention in 2000 when leaders of the Innu community of Davis Inlet on the Labrador coast asked for assistance in dealing with an uncontrollable epidemic of glue sniffing and alcoholism among its children and the highest rate of suicide anywhere in Canada. Children were taken south to detox centres and did well, but ultimately had to be returned to a community that was little better than it had been when they left. No long-term solutions to these terrible social dilemmas can be achieved unless there is widespread improvement in the socio-economic status of remote rural communities. In early 2016, there was a suicide crisis in the Attawapiskat First Nation community in northern Canada, which declared a state of emergency after 11 people attempted to take their own lives in one day (*Globe and Mail*, 2016).

THE HEALTH OF OTHER INDIGENOUS POPULATIONS

> We were all part of a world community of Indigenous Peoples spanning the planet, experiencing the same problems and struggling against the same alienation, marginalization and sense of powerlessness. We had gathered there united by our shared frustration with the dominant systems in our own countries and their consistent failure to deliver justice. We were all looking for, and demanding, justice from a higher authority.
>
> —*Michael Dodson, Australian Aboriginal representative to UN Working Group*
> *on Indigenous Health, 1998*

Within the approximately 300–350 million Indigenous peoples in the world, there are thousands of separate tribal groupings. Despite this enormous social and cultural diversity, these communities face surprisingly similar health challenges. The unifying factor common to most Indigenous peoples is a history of conflict and mistreatment during the period of European expansion, spreading over the last five centuries. Whole tribes, entire cultures, and unknown numbers of lives were lost forever due to violent oppression, slavery, and introduced diseases such as smallpox, measles, and tuberculosis (Coates, 2004).

It is easy to imagine that this is all ancient history—certainly sad, but nothing to do with the modern enlightened world. Nothing could be further from the truth. As recently as the mid-20th century, it was accepted that Aboriginal Australians and New Zealand Maoris would die out as separate races (Kunitz, 2000). Although their numbers are now increasing, general standards of health still lag far behind the averages in these prosperous countries. Guatemala's Supreme Court of Justice calculated that between 100,000 and 200,000 Indigenous Mayan children lost one or both parents from military violence during their civil war (Melville et al., 1992). The war ended in 1996.

The infectious diseases and violence that Indigenous peoples suffered in the past have now largely been replaced by behavioural and psychiatric problems resulting from the common history of discrimination and inequity that many still suffer in their own countries. High rates of suicide can be found from Torres Strait Islanders to Brazilian Amerindians (Loenaars, 2006). Depression, family violence, and alcoholism are all common from the northernmost Indigenous communities of Russia (Fardahl et al., 1997) down to remote Aboriginal reserves in Australia (Ring et al., 2002). In every case where figures are available, the life expectancy of Indigenous populations is always several years below the country's national average (Figure 17.5). *The Lancet* review on Indigenous health is a very useful summary (King et al., 2009).

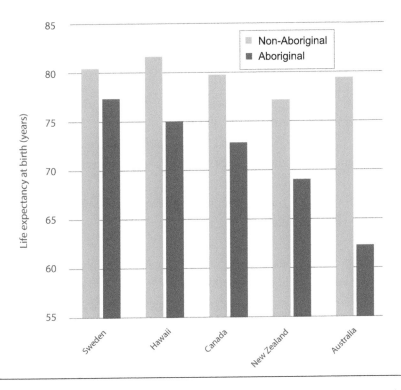

Figure 17.5: Comparative life expectancies at birth for Indigenous populations around the world

Sources: ABS. 2011. Australian Bureau of Statistics. Indigenous population, 2006. Retrieved from: www. abs.gov.au/ausstats/abs@.nsf/Lookup/4713.0Chapter82006; Braun, K., et al. 1996. Life and death in Hawaii: Ethnic variations in life expectancy and mortality, 1980 and 1990. *Hawaii Medical Journal,* 55: 278–283; Hausler, S., et al. 2005. Causes of death in the Sami population of Sweden, 1961–2000. *International Journal of Epidemiology,* 34: 623–629; StatCan. 2011a. Statistics Canada: Aboriginal peoples. Retrieved from: www12.statcan.ca/census-recensement/2006/rt-td/ap-pa-eng.cfm; Bramley, D., et al. 2004. Indigenous disparities in disease-specific mortality, a cross-country comparison: New Zealand, Australia, Canada, and the United States. *New Zealand Medical Journal,* 117: 1215–1223.

This point brings up the topical issue of statistical data. One problem confronting the concept of global Indigenous health is the absence of reliable and easily available health information. In 2002, Australia, Canada, and New Zealand rose to this challenge. All three countries have large Indigenous populations whose health outcomes are significantly poorer than those of the general population. In 2002, all three countries agreed to share their research expertise in Indigenous health and to develop collaborative research projects (Cunningham et al., 2003; WHO, 2010). There are very few comparative studies of Indigenous health in different countries (Bramley et al., 2006; Paradies et al., 2002). However, large reviews of the available literature strongly conclude that there are very obvious similarities between otherwise widely different Indigenous groups (King et al., 2009; Gracy et al., 2009). These common diseases can be grouped under three broad headings:

- *Diseases due to non-traditional lifestyles:* cardiovascular disease, heart attacks, strokes, obesity, and diabetes
- *Diseases due to poverty and poor living conditions:* tuberculosis, exposure to environmental toxins, injuries, and diseases of contaminated water (shigellosis, hepatitis A)
- *Diseases resulting from past injustice and social exclusion:* substance abuse, family violence, suicide

In 2006, the influential medical journal *The Lancet* published a call to action concerning the issue of Indigenous health (Stephens et al., 2006). It is hoped that the international community responds to this challenge so that the future for Indigenous peoples can be a great deal better than their common collective past.

SUMMARY

The current situation of Indigenous peoples remains a global health concern. There are probably well over 300 million people, residing in approximately 90 countries, whose past histories distinguish them as descendants of pre-colonial inhabitants. Traditional Indigenous populations are custodians of an extraordinary range of languages and cultures that form an irreplaceable part of the human race. They make both their own countries and the world a more interesting place to live. In addition, the enormous scientific (particularly pharmaceutical) value of some of their botanical knowledge has only recently been appreciated. Unfortunately, they are among the world's most marginalized and poorest peoples. This influences the health and quality of life of Indigenous peoples. For example, Aboriginal people in Canada die earlier than the average Canadian and sustain a disproportionate burden of chronic physical and mental illness on average. Although exact causes are not known, the relatively poor status of Indigenous health is clearly associated with the unfavourable economic and social conditions that the majority of the population live in. With time, however, the voices of Indigenous populations are slowly being heard, and Indigenous issues are now being given attention by large international agencies. In 2000, the Permanent Forum on Indigenous Issues was established at the United Nations, which led to the creation of the United Nations Declaration on the Rights of Indigenous Peoples. Seven years later, the declaration was adopted by the UN General Assembly.

DISCUSSION QUESTIONS

1. What is the extent and diversity of the world's Indigenous populations?
2. What are some of the historical factors that are behind the current poor health of many Indigenous populations?
3. What are common health problems found among many Indigenous populations? How can they be best addressed?
4. What is the UN Declaration on the Rights of Indigenous People? What is its significance?
5. How do the SDGs relate to Indigenous populations?
6. Indigenous peoples in Canada are divided into which three groups? How do their health outcomes differ from the rest of the population?
7. Why do you think the policies of forced assimilation, through compulsory schooling, have left deep scars on Aboriginal society in Canada? What could have been done differently?
8. The health indices of Indigenous populations in countries such as Canada, Australia, New Zealand, and the United States lag far behind national averages. Why is it still possible to find developing world conditions affecting Aboriginal communities in the reserves, settlements, and downtown cores of all these countries?
9. What is the 1996 Royal Commission on Aboriginal Peoples?
10. Why do Aboriginal peoples in Canada die earlier than the average Canadian and sustain a disproportionate burden of chronic physical and mental illness?

RECOMMENDED READING

Arias, A. 2001. *The Rigoberta Menchu controversy*. Pub: University of Minnesota Press.

Brody, H. 2002. *The other side of Eden: Hunters, farmers, and the shaping of the world*. Pub: North Point Press.

Cardinal, H. 2000. *The unjust society*. Pub: University of Washington Press.

Dean, B., & Levi, J. (Eds.). 2003. *At the risk of being heard: Identity, Indigenous rights, and postcolonial states*. Pub: University of Michigan Press.

Greenwood, M., de Leeuw, S., Lindsay, N. M., & Reading, C. (Eds.). 2015. *Determinants of Indigenous Peoples' Health in Canada*. Pub: Canadian Scholars.

Hall, G. H., & Patrinos, H. 2012. *Indigenous peoples, poverty, and development*. Pub: Cambridge University Press.

Keal, P. 2003. *European conquest and the rights of Indigenous peoples: The moral backwardness of international society*. Pub: Cambridge University Press.

Moore, S. P., et al. 2015. Cancer incidence in indigenous people in Australia, New Zealand, Canada, and the USA: A comparative population-based study. *The Lancet Oncology*, 16: 1483–1492.

Waldram, J., et al. 2006. *Aboriginal health in Canada: Historical, cultural, and epidemiological perspectives.* Pub: University of Toronto Press.

REFERENCES

AANDC. 2009. Aboriginal Affairs and Northern Development Canada: Federal framework for Aboriginal economic development. Retrieved from: www.ainc-inac.gc.ca/ecd/ffaed1-eng.asp.

AANDC. 2011. Aboriginal Affairs and Northern Development Canada. First Nation housing. Retrieved from: www.ainc-inac.gc.ca/ih/fnh/index-eng.asp.

ABS. 2011. Australian Bureau of Statistics. Indigenous population, 2006. Retrieved from: www.abs.gov.au/ausstats/abs@.nsf/Lookup/4713.0Chapter82006.

Adelson, N. 2005. The embodiment of inequity: Health disparities in Aboriginal Canada. *Canadian Journal of Public Health*, 96 (Suppl. 2): S45–S561.

AFN. 2011. Assembly of First Nations. Retrieved from: www.afn.ca.

AHF. 2011. Aboriginal Healing Foundation. Retrieved from: www.ahf.ca/.

AHSABC. 2011. Aboriginal Head Start Association of British Columbia. Retrieved from: www.ahsabc.com.

Alderete, E. 1999. The health of Indigenous peoples. Retrieved from: http://whqlibdoc.who.int/hq/1999/WHO_SDE_HSD_99.1.pdf.

Anderson, I., et al. 2016. Indigenous and tribal peoples' health (*The Lancet*–Lowitja Institute Global Collaboration): A population study. *The Lancet*, 388(10040): 131–157.

Arias, A. 2001. *The Rigoberta Menchu controversy.* Pub: University of Minnesota Press.

Bjerregaard, P., et al. 2004. Indigenous health in the Arctic: An overview of the circumpolar Inuit population. *Scandinavian Journal of Public Health*, 32: 390–395.

Bopp, D., et al. 2003. Aboriginal Healing Foundation. Aboriginal domestic violence in Canada. Retrieved from: www.fourworlds.ca/pdfs/DomesticViolence.pdf.

Bramley, D., et al. 2004. Indigenous disparities in disease-specific mortality, a cross-country comparison: New Zealand, Australia, Canada, and the United States. *New Zealand Medical Journal*, 117: 1215–1223.

Bramley, D., et al. 2006. Disparities in Indigenous health: A cross-country comparison between New Zealand and the United States. *American Journal of Public Health*, 95: 844–850.

Braun, K., et al. 1996. Life and death in Hawaii: Ethnic variations in life expectancy and mortality, 1980 and 1990. *Hawaii Medical Journal*, 55: 278–283.

Brush, S., et al. (Eds.). 1996. *Valuing local knowledge: Indigenous people and intellectual property rights.* Pub: Island Press.

Butler-Walker, J., et al. 2006. Maternal and umbilical cord blood levels of mercury, lead, cadmium, and essential trace elements in Arctic Canada. *Environmental Research*, 100: 295–318.

Caballeros, B., et al. 2003. Body composition and overweight prevalence in 1,704 school children from seven American Indian communities. *American Journal of Clinical Nutrition*, 78: 308–312.

CAP. 2011. Congress of Aboriginal Peoples. Retrieved from: www.abo-peoples.org/.

Chandler, M., et al. 1998. Cultural continuity as a hedge against suicide in Canada's First Nations. *Transcultural Psychiatry*, 35: 191–219.

Chochinov, A. 1998. Alcohol "on board," man overboard—boating fatalities in Canada. *Canadian Medical Association Journal*, 159: 259–260.

CIHI. 2004. Improving the health of Canadians. Chapter 4: Aboriginal Peoples' Health. Retrieved from: http://secure.cihi.ca/cihiweb/products/IHC2004rev_e.pdf.

Coates, K. 2004. *A global history of Indigenous peoples: Struggle and survival.* Pub: Palgrave MacMillan.

Craib, K., et al. 2003. Risk factors for elevated HIV incidence among Aboriginal injection drug users in Vancouver. *Canadian Medical Association Journal*, 168: 19–24.

Cunningham, C., et al. 2003. Health research and Indigenous health. *British Medical Journal*, 327: 445–447.

DESA. 2009. UN Department of Economic and Social Affairs. State of the world's Indigenous peoples. Retrieved from: www.un.org/esa/socdev/unpfii/documents/SOWIP_web.pdf.

DESA. 2015. UN Department of Economic and Social Affairs. State of the world's Indigenous peoples. Volume II. Retrieved from: www.un.org/esa/socdev/unpfii/documents/2015/sowip2volume-ac.pdf.

Durie, M. 2003. The health of Indigenous peoples: Depends on genetics, politics, and socio-economic factors. *British Medical Journal*, 326: 510–511.

Eggertson, L. 2006. Safe drinking water standards for First Nations' communities. *Canadian Medical Association Journal*, 174: 1248.

Fardahl, G., et al. 1997. Indigenous peoples of the Russian North. *Cultural Survival Quarterly*, 21: 30–33.

FNSI. 2010. First Nations' Statistical Institute. Retrieved from: www.fnsi-ispn.com/.

Freemantle J, et al. 2015. Indigenous mortality (revealed): The invisible illuminated. *Am J Public Health*, 105: 644–652.

Glenbow. 2008. The Thule. Retrieved from: www.glenbow.org/thule/?lang=en&p=outside&t=enhanced&s=3-1&mi=1.

The Globe and Mail. 2016. Attawapiskat: Four things to help understand the suicide crisis. Retrieved from: www.theglobeandmail.com/news/national/attawapiskat-four-things-to-help-understand-the-suicidecrisis/article29583059/.

Gracy, M., et al. 2009. Indigenous health part 1: Determinants and disease patterns. *The Lancet*, 374: 65–75.

Hausler, S., et al. 2005. Causes of death in the Sami population of Sweden, 1961–2000. *International Journal of Epidemiology*, 34: 623–629.

HCC. 2011. Health Council of Canada. Understanding and improving Aboriginal maternal and child health in Canada. Retrieved from: www.healthcouncilcanada.ca/docs/rpts/2011/abhealth/HCC_AboriginalHealth_FINAL1.pdf.

HC-SC. 2002. Health Canada. Acting on what we know: Preventing youth suicide in First Nations. Retrieved from: www.hc-sc.gc.ca/fniah-spnia/pubs/promotion/_suicide/prev_youth-jeunes/index-eng.php.

HC-SC. 2003. Health Canada: Unintentional and intentional injury profile for Aboriginal people in Canada. Retrieved from: www.hc-sc.gc.ca/fniah-spnia/pubs/promotion/_injury-bless/2001_trauma/index-eng.php.

HC-SC. 2010. Health Canada, First Nations, Inuit, and Aboriginal health. Retrieved from: www.hc-sc.gc.ca/fniah-spnia/diseases-maladies/index-eng.php.

HC-SC. 2011. Health Canada: First Nations, Inuit, and Aboriginal health. Retrieved from: www.hc-sc.gc.ca/fniah-spnia/index-eng.php.

Hughes, R. 1996. *The fatal shore*. Pub: Harvill Press.

IAPH. 2011. Institute of Aboriginal Peoples' Health. Retrieved from: www.cihr-irsc.gc.ca/e/8668.html.

ICC. 2011. Inuit Circumpolar Conference. Retrieved from: www.inuit.org/.

INAC. 2004. Indian and Northern Affairs Canada. Family violence prevention program: National manual. Retrieved from: http://dsp-psd.pwgsc.gc.ca/Collection/R2-333-2004E.pdf.

ITK. 2011. Inuit Tapiriit Kanatami. Retrieved from: www.itk.ca.

IWGIA. 2010. International Work Group for Indigenous Affairs. Retrieved from: www.iwgia.org/iwgia_files_publications_files/0505_Report2011_eb2.pdf.

King, M., et al. 2009. Indigenous health part 2: The underlying causes of the health gap. *The Lancet*, 374: 76–85.

Kirmayer, L., et al. 2007. Suicide among Aboriginal people. Aboriginal Healing Foundation. Retrieved from: www.ahf.ca/downloads/suicide.pdf.

Kunitz, S. 2000. Globalization, states, and the health of Indigenous peoples. *American Journal of Public Health*, 90: 1531–1539.

Loenaars, A. 2006. Suicide among Indigenous peoples: Introduction and call to action. *Archives of Suicide Research*, 10: 103–115.

Melville, M., et al. 1992. Guatemalan Indian children and the sociocultural effects of government-sponsored terrorism. *Social Science and Medicine*, 34: 533–548.

Mendelson, M. 2006. Aboriginal peoples and postsecondary education in Canada. Caledon Institute of Social Policy. Retrieved from: www.caledoninst.org/Publications/PDF/595ENG.pdf.

MNC. 2011. Métis National Council. Retrieved from: www.metisnation.ca/.

NAHO. 2011. National Aboriginal Health Organization. Retrieved from: www.naho.ca.

Nunavut. 2011a. Government of Nunavut. Retrieved from: www.gov.nu.ca/en/Home.aspx.

Nunavut. 2011b. Legislative Assembly. Retrieved from: www.assembly.nu.ca/.

NZ History. 2011. Treaty of Waitangi. Retrieved from: www.nzhistory.net.nz/category/tid/133.

O'Donnell, V., et al. 2001. Aboriginal peoples survey 2001. Well-being of the non-reserve Aboriginal population. Retrieved from: www.statcan.ca/Daily/English/030924/d030924b. htm.

Osborn, W. 2001. *The wild frontier: Atrocities during the American-Indian war from Jamestown colony to Wounded Knee*. Pub: Random House.

Paradies, Y., et al. 2002. Placing Aboriginal and Torres Strait Islander mortality in an international context. *Australia New Zealand Journal of Public Health*, 26: 11–16.

PHAC. 2004. Public Health Agency of Canada. HIV and AIDS among women in Canada. Retrieved from: www.phac-aspc.gc.ca/publicat/epiu-aepi/epi_update_may_04/5-eng. php.

PHAC. 2008. Public Health Agency of Canada. Aboriginal women and family violence. Retrieved from: www.phac-aspc.gc.ca/ncfv-cnivf/pdfs/fem-abor_e.pdf.

RCAP. 1996. Report of the Royal Commission on Aboriginal Peoples. Retrieved from: www. ainc-inac.gc.ca/ch/rcap/index_e.html.

Ring, I., et al. 2002. Indigenous health: Chronically inadequate responses to damning statistics. *Medical Journal of Australia*, 177: 629–631.

Rosenberg, T., et al. 1997. Shigellosis on Indian reserves in Manitoba, Canada: Its relationship to crowded housing, lack of running water, and inadequate sewage disposal. *American Journal of Public Health*, 87: 1547–1551.

Seear, M., et al. 1997. Chronic cough and wheeze: Do they all have asthma? *European Respiratory Journal*, 10: 342–345.

Smith, D., et al. 2005. Turning around the intergenerational impact of residential schools on Aboriginal people: Implications for health policy and practice. *Canadian Journal of Nursing Research*, 37: 38–60.

Smylie, J., et al. 2010. A review of Aboriginal infant mortality rates in Canada: Striking and persistent Aboriginal/non-Aboriginal inequities. *Canadian Journal of Public Health*, 101: 143–148.

Stannard, D. 1992. *American holocaust: Columbus and the conquest of the New World*. Pub: Oxford University Press.

StatCan. 2010. Statistics Canada: School dropout trends. Retrieved from: www.statcan.gc.ca/ pub/81-004-x/2010004/article/11339-eng.htm.

StatCan. 2011a. Statistics Canada: Aboriginal peoples. Retrieved from: www12.statcan.ca/ census-recensement/2006/rt-td/ap-pa-eng.cfm.

StatCan. 2011b. Statistics Canada: Projected life expectancy by sex and Aboriginal identity. Retrieved from: www.statcan.gc.ca/pub/89-645-x/2010001/c-g/c-g013-eng.htm.

Stephens, C., et al. 2006. Disappearing, displaced, and undervalued: A call to action for Indigenous health worldwide. *The Lancet*, 367: 2019–2028.

Truth and Reconciliation Commission of Canada (TRC). 2015. Honouring the truth, reconciling for the future: Summary of the final report of the Truth and Reconciliation Commission of Canada. Retrieved from: http://nctr.ca/reports.php.

UN. 2016. Indigenous peoples share hopes for the SDGs. Retrieved from: www.un.org/sustainabledevelopment/blog/2016/05/indigenous-peoples-share-hopes-for-the-sdgs/.

United Church. 2007. The history of Indian residential schools. Retrieved from: www.united-church.ca/aboriginal/schools/faq/history.

UNPFII. 2007. UN declaration on the rights of Indigenous peoples. Retrieved from: www.un.org/esa/socdev/unpfii/en/declaration.html.

UNPFII. 2011. UN Permanent Forum on Indigenous Issues. Retrieved from: www.un.org/esa/socdev/unpfii/.

US Census Bureau. 2011. Annual estimates of the population by race alone and Hispanic or Latino origin. Retrieved from: www.census.gov/popest/national/asrh/NC-EST2009/NC-EST2009-03.xls.

USDS. 2011. US Department of State. Guatemala. Retrieved from: www.state.gov/r/pa/ei/bgn/2045.htm.

Weir, E. 2001. Inhalant use and addiction in Canada. *Canadian Medical Association Journal*, 164: 397–400.

WHO. 2010. Indigenous health—Australia, Canada, New Zealand, and the United States—laying claim to a future that embraces health for us all. Retrieved from: www.who.int/healthsystems/topics/financing/healthreport/IHNo33.pdf.

WHO. 2011. World health statistics 2011. Retrieved from: www.who.int/whosis/whostat/2011/en/index.html.

World Bank. 2007. Indigenous peoples policy brief. Retrieved from: siteresources.worldbank.org/EXTINDPEOPLE/Resources/407801-1271860301656/HDNEN_indigenous_clean_0421.pdf.

World Bank. 2015. Indigenous Latin America in the twenty-first century: The first decade. Retrieved from: https://openknowledge.worldbank.org/handle/10986/23751.

Young, T., et al. 2000. Type 2 diabetes mellitus in Canada's First Nations: Status of an epidemic in progress. *Canadian Medical Association Journal*, 163: 561–566.

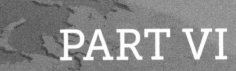

PART VI

WORKING SAFELY AND EFFECTIVELY
IN A DEVELOPING COUNTRY

CHAPTER 18

Planning and Preparing for Safe and Effective Development Work

One of the more enduring myths held by humanitarian workers and soldiers alike is that a truly strong person will experience none of the normal physical responses to a stressful incident or environment. Unfortunately, for aid workers (and soldiers) there is very little substance to this belief.

—John Fawcett, 2003

OBJECTIVES

At some level, the basic aim of any aid project is to improve the lives of others. It doesn't matter if the target is a small family or a large city; this is a serious undertaking. The benefits of a well-run project can be significant for all concerned, but the adverse results of a badly organized project can be equally significant. Teams willing to take on that challenge should be congratulated, but they should understand that they are shouldering a major responsibility. The levels of planning and preparation should reflect the seriousness with which the project team takes that responsibility. After completing this chapter, you should be able to:

- prepare and plan for an overseas development project
- appreciate the ethical problems associated with aid projects
- know how to stay healthy working in a developing country
- understand how to work effectively and co-operatively in a new culture

INTRODUCTION

> He was wearing his favorite T-shirt, which featured a multiple-choice questionnaire for relief workers: (a) Missionary? (b) Mercenary? (c) Misfit? (d) Broken Heart? Henry had ticked (b), which was a joke since his family owned half of northeast England. Me? I was a (c)/(d) hybrid.
>
> —*Helen Fielding, Cause Celeb, 2002*

Apart from the hundreds of thousands of people who work full-time in the aid industry, there are probably 10 times that number who volunteer or spend large amounts of their time and money on short-term aid projects in developing countries. As the interest in the recent debt-relief talks showed, there are many millions more people around the world who have a deep interest in the plight of developing world populations even if they are not actively involved in a project. Surely, this evidence of the good side of human nature should be celebrated and remain beyond criticism? For a long time, this has been the prevailing rose-tinted attitude in articles about aid projects. For the average person, information about life in developing countries comes from fundraising advertisements from large aid agencies, news articles about war and disasters, and short articles that stress happy endings. These may be a good way to raise money, but they don't serve as a reliable source of information concerning the reality of aid projects.

There is a large and apparently growing level of interest worldwide in the broad topic of global health. Many of those people are prepared to take their interest a bit further by investing time and energy working on overseas development projects. For several reasons (including a lack of training courses and underestimation of the seriousness of overseas work), the general levels of project planning and personal preparation are often less than ideal. Apart from showing a lack of respect toward the host population, poor planning will inevitably result in a waste of time and money. At worst, it exposes project participants to significant (and often largely avoidable) personal risks. This does not mean that short-term projects are of no value; they can be of profound value for the team members, but it is best to go into them with a proper appreciation of the seriousness of the task. Clearing away many of the misconceptions about aid will require some straight talk—not gratuitous criticism, but practical, unsentimental advice about development work in the real world.

It is vital that anyone preparing to join a development project is aware of the potential risks associated with overseas work. In 2015, 287 aid workers (109 killed, 110 wounded, and 68 kidnapped) were victims of major attacks across 25 countries (Humanitarian Outcomes, 2016). This was 22 percent fewer attacks compared to 2014, when there were 329 victims across 27 countries (Figure 18.1). For the adventurous types planning to work in war zones, severe injury or even death due to violence should be added to the list. Countries in conflict make up the majority of attacks on civilian aid population globally, with Afghanistan, Somalia, South Sudan, Syria, and Yemen representing the bulk of civilian attacks. The three most dangerous countries are Afghanistan, South Sudan, and Somalia (Figure 18.2). Sheik et al. (2000) studied causes of death among humanitarian workers. They found nearly 380 deaths between 1985 and 1998. International violence was the most pronounced, and

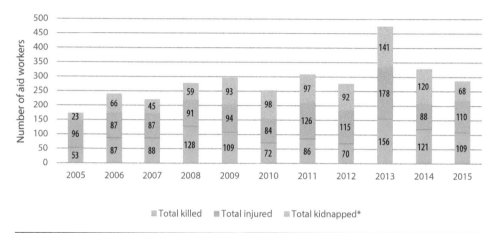

Figure 18.1: Major attacks on aid workers, 2005–2015

Source: Humanitarian Outcomes. 2016. Aid worker security database. Retrieved from: https://aidworkersecurity.org/.

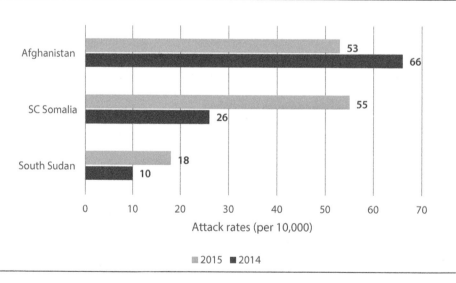

Figure 18.2: Attack rates in the three most dangerous contexts

Source: Humanitarian Outcomes. 2016. Aid worker security database. Retrieved from: https://aidworkersecurity.org/.

motor vehicle accidents was the second-most. Overseas work can be very rewarding, but it has risks. Personal decisions should not be based on a spirit of youthful enthusiasm, but on a clear-headed assessment of the potential problems—ICRC's handbook on the subject of safety is a good starting point (Roberts, 2005).

Risks cannot be entirely avoided, but they can certainly be minimized with careful pre-trip planning aimed, firstly, at the details of the project, and, secondly, at the necessary steps for personal preparation. Adequate preparation is time consuming; at least a year is required to do the job properly. The first job is to plan and prepare your project. Assuming you know what you are going to do, this involves choosing a team, including local people in the planning process, fundraising, and carefully considering the ethical problems associated with the project. The second job is to prepare yourself—really exploring if you have the skills and competencies necessary to do the job, studying local history and culture, gaining a basic knowledge of the language, and knowing how to keep yourself healthy. If you have ever asked any variant of the question, "I just want to get involved—how can I do something to help?" then please read these next two chapters carefully.

OVERSEAS DEVELOPMENT WORK

> Two roads diverged in a wood, and I—
> I took the one less traveled by,
> And that has made all the difference.
>
> —Robert Frost, "The Road Not Taken," 1920

If you have decided to take Robert Frost's advice, that is great, but remember that the results of that decision do not affect just you. Perhaps you are going to do a clinical rotation in a hospital, help build houses, or work as a teacher. No matter what you hope to achieve, a poorly planned and performed project not only reflects badly on you (and, by extension, your country of origin), but also adversely affects the population you choose to work with (Maren, 2002). Quite apart from any problems you might suffer as a result of poor preparation, the effects on your hosts may range from unfairly raising their hopes, all the way to being involved in a medical disaster. Hopefully, it is clear that this is something to be taken very seriously. In the spirit of frank discussion, we may as well start by diving straight into the deep end. The average person has limited access to information about life in very poor countries. The general impression given by news reports of developing countries or by fundraising advertisements for aid agencies is one of hopeless, grinding poverty. While such images may be fair reflections of life in some of the poorest parts of the world, they are not representative of much of the developing world and they certainly aren't accurate pictures of the people living in them; this distinction must be appreciated.

People living in poverty are not helpless or hopeless, they are just unlucky. They do not respond to hardship by huddling in huts, waiting desperately for the next planeload of aid workers to arrive. In essence, their lives are the same as ours. They do the best they can, work hard under terribly difficult circumstances, care for their children, and somehow manage to retain their humanity and dignity under circumstances that would reduce most Canadian residents to tears. They do not want or need religious conversion, pity, or free handouts. What they do want is equal partnerships with hard-working, competent individuals working in well-planned, sustainable assistance projects with clearly defined goals and measured results. They want things to work for them and their kids on a much longer timeframe than that of a typical project. Working this way with people who live in poverty will give you insights into your own life that you might never have gained by staying at home. Under these circumstances, aid projects can truly be life-altering experiences, but you must enter the process understanding that you are the learner and not the teacher.

A small example might help to give a different perspective. Imagine you are sitting with a beer and pizza watching *Hockey Night in Canada*. You answer a knock on the door and find two Ethiopian students who tell you they are part of an East

Box 18.1 History Notes

Catherine and Reginald Hamlin

True heroes are in short supply—the Hamlins are the genuine article. Catherine was born in Australia. She met her New Zealand–born husband, Reginald Hamlin, while they were working together in a London hospital. They travelled to Ethiopia in the 1950s to help start a midwifery school. While the school did not last because of loss of government funding, it did introduce them to the tragedy of women with fistulas, an almost unknown condition in developed countries. Affected women had bowel or bladder fistulas that left them constantly soiled with urine or feces following a prolonged obstructed labour. These women were outcasts and lived lives of utter misery. No local treatment was available, so the Hamlins began what became their life work—providing care for women with this terrible complication of labour. Even learning the operative techniques required extensive research and travel. The necessary building and support staff slowly built up over years despite the most difficult circumstances of recurrent war and civil chaos. By 1974, they were able to open a dedicated fistula hospital, the only one in the world. Reginald Hamlin died in 1993, but Catherine has continued their work. She still operates every week and maintains an active fundraising campaign. Other fistula hospitals have opened in the region, but progress regarding the need for avoidance rather than cure was slower to develop. Finally, their original objective of a midwifery training hospital was realized about 50 years after they first started work in Ethiopia. They have gained awards from around the world, but their greatest achievement was the new life they gave to tens of thousands of young women.

African charity called "Buckets of Tears for Canada." They start giving you advice about eating fresh vegetables, exercising, and not watching so much television. What would your opinion be and what would you do? What if they then decided to hand out some advice about your sexual practices or tried to change your political and religious beliefs? By this point, you would probably be fairly irate, so why should people in developing countries be any different when you arrive at their door? In a more realistic scenario, the students would not have prepared for their trip so would not know your language or have organized an interpreter. Neither side would have understood the other. They would then leave, saying, "He didn't seem to understand a word we were saying," while you would have been left wondering, "What was that all about?"—not a bad analogy for the average aid project.

The success rate of large aid projects is far from perfect. An independent survey of the International Finance Corporation's results over a 10-year period found that only just over half of all projects met their initial goals (IFC, 2008). If all the World Bank's resources can't do much better than 50 percent, then there is no reason that short-term aid projects should fare any better. Although literature does exist showing that short-term projects can lead to measurable benefits (Clemens et al., 2004), that paper's definition of "short term" was four years. Very specialized surgical teams or large-scale immunization campaigns can certainly achieve substantial work in a matter of weeks, but the timeline for most aid projects (education, nutrition, or poverty relief) will be measured in many months and more often in years.

Once a group of people commit to an aid project, their natural response is to get on with the excitement of overseas work as soon as possible. Anyone handing out advice about the need for months of detailed research, planning, and preparation isn't always well received, but without that foundation, the chances of a safe and effective project are slim. Anyone familiar with foreign travel will be aware of the practical difficulties encountered when travelling in a very poor country. The demands of an aid project (customs clearance, work permits, visas, renting offices, hiring interpreters and other local workers, etc.) multiply these problems many times over. When a project has only a few weeks to work with, even small delays and obstructions will become significant. Apart from the disinclination of most humans to be told what to do, human nature will provide you with plenty of other obstacles in the form of personal team dynamics. If you find yourself saying, "He'll behave better when he has some work to do" or "We'll sort this out when we get there," you are probably in for big disappointments.

Given the large number of people who are interested in development work, there is surprisingly little material to meet this educational demand. Degree courses in global health are given by large centres, but for the average student, access to university-level courses in global health is surprisingly limited. Handbooks (Care,

2010) and websites (Aid Workers Network) are available, but affordable university-level training courses are hard to find. Unfortunately, this means that many members of short-term projects will have little or no experience of the history and framework of the aid industry in which they will be working. Apart from making sure the specific skills you need for your project are up to date, it is also important to put a great deal of research into the language, culture, and history of your host country. As a rough rule of thumb, in order to get the best out of a project, it is necessary to start planning and studying at least a year before you are due to leave.

I'LL BE FINE—WHAT COULD POSSIBLY GO WRONG?

> When a thing that cannot possibly go wrong, goes wrong, it usually turns out to be impossible to get at or repair.
>
> —*Douglas Adams, 1978*

Tens of millions of North Americans of all ages travel overseas each year, and only about 5,000 of this number die during travel, most from pre-existing medical conditions (Baker et al., 1992). From a statistical point of view, your chances of dying during a trip are very small (Klein, 1995). However, a study of Peace Corps workers revealed that non-lethal but still significant health problems are quite common (Table 18.1). Overall, the most common cause of a ruined trip is intestinal infection, while the most common cause of mortality or severe injury is

Table 18.1: Most commonly reported health conditions among Peace Corps volunteers, January–October 2015

HEALTH CONDITION	RATE PER 100 VOLUNTEER-TRAINEE YEARS
Gastroenteritis	57.6
Mental health issues	19.6
Dental problems	19.1
Infectious dermatitis	18.7
Unintentional injuries	13.3
Gynecological infections	11.1
Febrile illness	10.1
Ocular conditions	3.3
STDs (non-HIV)	2.5
Malaria, confirmed and presumptive	2.3

Source: Peace Corps. 2015. The health of the volunteer 2015—Annual report of volunteer health. Retrieved from: http://files.peacecorps.gov/documents/open-government/HOV2015.pdf.

traumatic injury (cars, motorbikes, horses, boats, etc.). While it is very important to take professional pre-trip advice concerning immunizations and malaria prophylaxis, it is also necessary to use common sense. Despite all the emphasis placed on infectious risks in developing countries, the danger of road traffic accidents is at least 10 times higher than the mortality from malaria and other infectious diseases (Odero et al., 1997).

The biggest danger facing anyone who travels away from the beaten path is ignorance. At best, poor preparation will result in wasted time and money. At worst, you will be exposed to significant risks that, in most cases, could have been avoided and predicted with adequate pre-trip research. In preparation for this chapter, friends and colleagues with extensive experience in international projects were asked to send in their most memorable examples of what can go wrong. All the extracts given below are true and unedited. They are listed under broad headings with comments and links to further information on the topic.

Drugs and Alcohol

Afterwards, some of the team members told me that the only reason she had come on the project was because of the cheap and easy supply of drugs in that part of the world. I wish they had told me before we left. She would not listen to advice and fell into increasingly bad company. It came to a head when she was admitted to the local psychiatric ward after a bad experience with unknown drugs. We finally managed to get her home by medical evacuation. The expense and worry were considerable.

The dumbest thing I ever did in my life was to accept a friend's teenage son onto a project. I got little work done because I was constantly searching for this boy downtown after dark, where he would go looking for drugs. At the end of the first week, he was brought back to the hospital by two local police, who basically said, "Put him on the plane tomorrow or he'll be cracking rocks in jail for the next 10 years." The boy's parting words at the airport were, "You should have called their bluff; they aren't allowed to arrest foreign citizens."

It is not worth the risk to carry drugs or to use them when travelling overseas. It is important to remember that several countries (including Thailand, Singapore, Indonesia, Malaysia, and Vietnam) have severe penalties for drug offences that include life imprisonment and even the death penalty. Little distinction is made between soft and hard drugs. Travellers in a foreign country are subject to that country's laws. The local consular office has the right to visit you, but cannot override local laws and certainly cannot get you out of jail simply because you are a nice person on an aid project (Foreign Affairs, 2008). Apart from staying away from drugs altogether, the usual common-sense precautions apply. Ensure that any prescription medications you take are not considered illegal, and never leave your bags with a stranger or carry packages for another person. Each year, 2,500 Americans are arrested overseas, one-third of them on drug-related charges (US Department of State, 2010).

Infectious Diseases

It was years ago, during my first trip as a student. Once I got back, I found I had amebiasis and it had spread to my liver. I did not realize how much weight I had lost until my mother burst into tears when she met me at the airport.

I found afterwards that she had not had any of her childhood immunizations. She caught measles from a kid in the clinic that turned into pneumonia a couple of days later. She ended up in the local hospital for several days and took weeks to recover fully, all for an avoidable disease.

Way back when I was a medical student, a group of us went to work in a big hospital outside of Johannesburg. Two of us tested strongly positive for tuberculosis when we got back to Canada and ended up taking isoniazid for six months. It was a disaster—no beer for six months.

Those people directly involved with sick patients will face a variety of risks if they do not take adequate barrier precautions. The greatest of these risks for health workers is tuberculosis (CCDR, 2009). However, for the average aid worker, almost all the significant infectious risks will be carried either by mosquitoes (malaria, dengue, yellow fever, filariasis, viral encephalitis) (Travel Doctor, 2005a) or by contaminated water (gastroenteritis, amebiasis, and giardiasis) (Travel Doctor, 2005b). If the average traveller takes appropriate precautions to avoid mosquito bites, is careful about food and water sources, and follows pre-travel advice about basic immunizations and malaria prophylaxis, then the chances of significant illness will be greatly reduced and more time can be spent worrying about traffic accidents. Whatever else you might leave out before travelling, it is a very good idea to organize traveller's health insurance. Good-quality medical care can be found in most countries as long as you have money. Charges for hospital admission may exceed US$2,000 per day. If surgeons and anaesthetists are involved in your care, those prices will rise rapidly. Repatriation using international medical air ambulance will cost tens of thousands of dollars.

Sex

> We were working so hard in the chaos after the tsunami, social rules were the last things we were thinking of. One of the team members started meeting a married nurse from the ward. In such a small community, this was soon discovered and led to a great deal of trouble. We served out our time, but our relationship with the community was never the same afterwards. The nurse was never seen on the ward again. I don't know what happened to her.

The adventure of exotic travel can make people do things they would never dream of doing at home, particularly if alcohol is added to the mix (ActAlliance, 2007). Sexually transmitted diseases, including HIV, are found everywhere, but are particularly common in some developing countries. Hepatitis B is the only STD for which there is a vaccine. Past infection and treatment for any of the others does not confer immunity. Although several STDs can be treated with antibiotics, widespread resistance to antibiotics is a growing problem (Okeke et al., 2005). Sexual relations between project workers and the target population are ethically highly questionable. The impression of coercion or undue influence will, at the very least, harm relations between the project team and their host. At worst, it can lead to social results that affect people's entire lives. Common sense should guide your actions. It is very unwise to have sex with strangers, casual contacts, or commercial sex workers. If you are going to have sex, follow safe sexual practices and use good-quality latex condoms (Hamlyn et al., 2003).

Traumatic Injury

> One night, four of us crammed into a three-wheeler, heading off for yet another meeting. Halfway round a curve, we met a truck with no lights coming in the other direction. We finished upside down in a drainage ditch—one broken arm and a lot of scratches. With a tiny difference in the roll of the dice we would all have been dead.

> He was unharmed in the crash between his rented motorbike and the ox cart, but required medical treatment for the injuries he received in the fight after the accident when the farmer demanded payment.

The United Nations estimates that 1.25 million people are killed each year in road traffic accidents, and 90 percent of those deaths occur in developing countries (WHO, 2015). Motor vehicle injuries accounted for 9 percent of the unintentional injuries reported among Peace Corps volunteers in January–October 2015 (Peace Corps, 2015). It is also important to note that the majority of victims are not occupants of a motor vehicle but are pedestrians, motorcyclists, or cyclists. Traumatic injury, particularly due to a motor vehicle accident, is the most common cause of serious injury or death during overseas trips (Nantulya, 2002). The US Department of State estimates that over 200 American tourists are killed each year in road traffic accidents (Photo 18.1). There are, of course, many other potential sources of trauma ranging from bungee jumping to horseback riding. It is important to be aware of this problem and to use common sense, particularly when travelling by road.

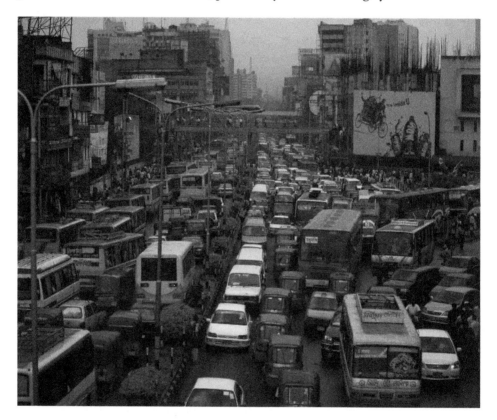

Photo 18.1: It is important to take infectious risks seriously when travelling, but in practice, accidents, particularly traffic accidents, are 10 times more common than infectious diseases. Rented motorbikes, three-wheel taxis, all-night buses, horseback riding, and bungee jumping are common causes of injury among young travellers. The picture shows an average day of smog and traffic in Dhaka, Bangladesh.

Source: Manoocher Deghati/Integrated Regional Information Network photo library (www. irinnews.org/photo).

Psychological Risks

It was my first time on a project, teaching at a village school. I had no training about what to expect and no support when I was there. I was homesick, crying, and unhappy for a couple of weeks. Thought there was something wrong with me because I hated everything about the place. After six months there, it was almost as bad when I got home again. Electric lights, running water, and the supermarket just seemed so excessive. No one understood what I was talking about.

Attention has only very recently been paid to the psychological dangers of aid work. Depression, severe culture shock, chronic fatigue, and post-traumatic stress disorder are now well-recognized risks of aid work (Palmer, 2005). All are minimized with adequate preparation and in-country support from experienced managers. Unfortunately, even the large agencies have taken a long time to improve levels of worker training and in-field support. Psychological problems are still a greatly under-reported problem associated with aid projects, particularly for those working in the most stressful environments, such as large refugee camps and war zones.

Bad Decisions and Odd Behaviour

A group of teachers had come out to work at a local missionary school when I was a government health officer in that area. For unknown reasons, one of these guys decided he wanted to shoot an elephant before going home. As you know, they are as common as rabbits down there—it is about as difficult as shooting a slow-moving bus. His first shot bounced off the elephant's head without killing it. Unfortunately, the missionary could run faster than his wife. When the elephant charged them, his wife was badly injured. The poor woman was brought in to me later that day with fractures of her pelvis and both legs. I don't understand how she wasn't killed.

A Scandinavian teacher who had worked in the area when he was a student brought out a bunch of his schoolchildren to work on a project in a Batonga village in the middle of nowhere. Don't forget that this was during an active guerrilla war! Several children ended up on the ward with dehydration and gastroenteritis, but two of them caught falciparum malaria. I have often wondered if the parents had any clue about the risks this guy was taking with their kids' lives.

I couldn't even begin to describe some of the odd characters that turned up on the east coast of Sri Lanka shortly after the tsunami. Survivors in those early chaotic camps had enough problems without having to deal with scientologists and bands of religious teenagers from all over the world. How do they get there on such short notice? The oddest group I met was a bunch of religious veterinarians who wouldn't treat an animal until the owner had been purified by a religious lecture first. Strange times and some very strange people.

Female Travellers

In the local culture, women who travelled alone without observing dress and behaviour conventions were viewed as either crazy or promiscuous. A single female colleague of mine, who prided herself on her general independence, was in the habit of walking alone at night. Two men molested her one night, claiming later they believed she wanted their attentions. It was only the intervention of some other local men that prevented this from progressing into a severe assault.

In general, women display greater caution than men in new surroundings, which tends to keep them out of trouble. Statistics support this since mortality and morbidity from all causes are both lower for female travellers compared to males.

Unfortunately, in many countries, female travellers are more affected by local religious and cultural beliefs than men. In order to work and travel safely, women may be expected to change the way they dress and behave, particularly in their interactions with men. Women who have grown up in North America or Europe are, quite understandably, unused to accepting imposed limitations on their personal freedoms. Unfortunately, this is a fact of life in many countries and it is not going to change overnight. It is very important for women to research the social and cultural expectations of any country they will be visiting so that decisions about work and personal freedom can be made calmly, long before travelling. The best source of information is women from the local area. This will be much more reliable than any information put out by the country's government. Websites and books specifically aimed at female travellers are also available (Foreign Affairs, 2007).

ETHICAL CONSIDERATIONS IN DEVELOPMENT WORK

Hell is paved with good intentions, not bad ones. All men mean well.

—G. B. Shaw, 1925

For no clear reason, the ethical implications of working in developing countries are rarely discussed. Codes of conduct established by the Sphere Project (Sphere Handbook, 2011) or the Australian Council for International Development (ACFID, 2009) provide guidance for large agencies, but there is little or no material governing personal behaviour. The topic is given little research attention even though almost all overseas workers will face some form of moral ambiguity at some point in their visit (Baratrala et al., 1998).

Although there is a vast literature concerning the ethics of health care in developed countries, ethical analysis of health projects (particularly medical research) in developing countries has only recently gained attention. For example, the first large trials of oral contraceptives were carried out in Puerto Rico because US state laws controlling contraception did not allow the drug to be tested in America. Complaints of side effects among the women in the study group (and also three deaths) attracted little attention at the time (Bernard, 1995).

More recently, attitudes toward the ethics of medical research in developing countries have changed significantly. The testing of anti-HIV drugs in developing countries has raised numerous ethical dilemmas that have attracted attention in the medical press. For example, early research in Africa into drug treatments that might reduce HIV transmission from mother to child attracted a storm of criticism. Study designs often involved treatment of one group with a known active anti-HIV drug while the other group received only an inactive placebo. Numerous commentators felt that this was a highly unethical study approach (Lurie et al., 1997).

The subsequent debate became very heated. Some commentators went so far as to compare this practice to the Tuskegee study of African American men with syphilis who were observed, but not treated, long after penicillin was available. Others argued

---

Box 18.2 Moment of Insight

Number of women dying in labour per 100,000 births in sub-Saharan Africa: 700 In Canada: 5	Average death rate for all climbers attempting K2 in the Himalayas 1954–1994:
Sub-Saharan African woman's lifetime risk of dying while having a baby:	
1 in 25	**1 in 25**
Source: Khan, K., et al. 2006. WHO analysis of causes of maternal deaths: A systematic review. *The Lancet, 367.* 1066–1074.	*Source:* Huey, R., et al. 2000. Supplemental oxygen and death rates on Everest and K2. Journal of the American Medical Association, 284:181.

that when a study is conducted in a country where the standard of care is basically no treatment at all, the use of an inactive placebo is warranted on the grounds of pragmatism (Halsey et al., 1997). The current opinion is that research ethics should not be modified by local circumstances; all populations should have access to the same levels of ethical research standards wherever they are (Eaton, 2005).

Complicated questions concerning medical care and research are an obvious place to start when considering ethical standards of behaviour, but they still form only a small part of a much larger issue. It doesn't matter what broad type of development work you are considering—there will be ethical dilemmas for those thoughtful enough to look for them. Some practical examples will illustrate this point:

- Imagine you are a Canadian obstetric resident who wants to gain experience in surgery by working in a rural African hospital. Local shortages mean that women are often inadequately anaesthetized during Caesarian section, and some of their newborns die because of lack of resuscitation equipment. Do you continue to work, arguing that inadequate care is better than no care, or do you leave, knowing that practising this way could get you sued at home?

- You are an anthropology student staying with a family in a remote part of Indonesia. You are invited to a large family party, but halfway through you realize that this is actually a circumcision ceremony for their youngest daughter. Do you risk offending the whole family by walking out, or do you continue to attend, knowing that such a practice carries a jail sentence at home?

- You are a recent teaching graduate working at a small school in rural Pakistan. Local elders will not allow the girls to go to school. Do you continue to teach the boys, hoping that the elders will eventually relent, or do you try to make a point by flatly refusing? You decide to remain in the village and just teach the boys. After a few months, half of the village insists that their daughters must also attend. The other half is outraged by such an idea. Your excellent intentions have led to threats of violence within the local community. What will you do now?

- After working as a doctor in Sudan for a year, you have gained the trust of local people. One day, senior women come to ask you how to perform female circumcision without causing infection and bleeding. They will not listen to your request that they stop doing the procedure altogether. Do you provide clean instruments and teach them to help reduce side effects, or do you refuse to teach them, knowing they will still continue to do circumcisions without your advice?

There are no clear answers to such questions. The "correct" answer is the one with which you are most comfortable. Whether your problem is personal (accepting significant limitations on dress and behaviour), scientific (use of a placebo control), or social (introducing major reforms such as female education), there are no rules that will help you to reach the best solution. The only advice that can be given is to ensure that ethical topics are confronted openly and thoroughly long before you leave home.

PREPARING YOURSELF FOR TRAVEL

Everyone thinks of changing the world but no one thinks of changing himself.

—Leo Tolstoy, 1900

Why Are You Going?

Before going on a project, it is very important to ask yourself why you wish to put yourself through the expense and hard work of an overseas project. Please examine your motives honestly. The following list of reasons why someone should not go on an aid project will, hopefully, help this process:

- Aid projects are not an opportunity to solve personal problems, particularly if those problems include drug and alcohol abuse.
- The aid industry is not an exotic travel agency designed to provide free trips to interesting places.
- Aid projects are not an opportunity to perform surgical procedures, drug treatments, or medical research that you are not allowed or qualified to perform at home.
- A foreign aid project is not a dating agency.
- Aid projects are not intended to provide a captive audience for religious or political opinions.

If your motives stand up to close scrutiny, then it is time to start planning your trip. To a large extent, the safety and success of your time overseas will depend on the effort you put into the planning stage. Fortunately, there are many excellent sources of information available. Examples include websites and manuals for travellers produced by the Australian government (Smarttraveller, 2011), Canadian government (Travel Health, 2011), the Centers for Disease Control and Prevention (Yellow Book, 2011), and the World Health Organization (WHO, 2011).

What to Pack

The list of things to take will depend on your individual situation, but remember that you do not have to bring the kitchen sink. Most of the items on your list will be available in large towns even though they may be a bit more expensive (another reason to know your country before travelling). Whatever else you pack, do not bring jewellery, expensive watches, or anything that you cannot afford to lose. Taking a backpack, plus a smaller pack for daily use, is a convenient way to travel. If rougher accommodation is likely, you will need a tent, sleeping bag, air mattress, and even a portable stove.

As time passes on a project, there is a tendency to become increasingly casual about avoiding mosquitoes and drinking only clean water—"Local people are fine so I'm sure there'll be no trouble." As a new visitor, you need to maintain a level of caution if you wish to remain healthy. An effective mosquito net needs to be large enough to tuck in under a mattress and should also be treated with long-acting insecticide (NaTHNaC, 2010). Good ones are bulky (particularly if they have a spreader), so it is often better to make this your first purchase when you arrive. The small nets sold in packets at the local camping shop are not adequate defence against a potentially lethal disease like malaria. If you do not have a ceiling hook, you will need some imagination and a ball of string. Obtaining clean water also requires careful planning depending on the circumstances you will be facing (CDC, 2011). Larger organisms such as bacteria and protozoa, including *Giardia*, are effectively removed using 0.2 micron hand-pumped filters. Viruses such as hepatitis A and Norwalk can slip through such a filter, so water will still need further purification (boiling, iodine tablets, carbon filtration disc). Remember that neither procedure removes dissolved chemical pollutants. A wide range of filters and purifiers is available at any camping store.

Clothing will depend on the climate and local custom. Whatever you take should be light and easy to wash. Personal items will depend on the remoteness of the location, but will include personal photographs, camera, flashlight, radio, electric adaptors, and books. Your toilet kit and medical kit will be governed by personal requirements such as asthma and by local malaria recommendations. All should be planned before travel. It is a good idea for a group to carry a standard first aid kit among them.

Whatever corners you are forced to cut due to time or money, it is always worthwhile to obtain good-quality travel insurance that covers medical repatriation. It will provide you (and your parents) with some peace of mind. On arrival in the country, many Canadian aid workers do not bother to register at the local Canadian High Commission or embassy, but it is well worth taking the time to do this (Foreign Affairs,

2010). Obviously, other nationals should follow the same policy. Embassy staff can help in an emergency and, to some extent, are responsible for you, but they have to know that you exist. People at home can also locate you through the High Commission. The following list details the main documents and forms to take with you:

- passport
- tickets
- health insurance and flight insurance
- immunization record
- entry visas
- record of professional qualification
- permit to work or study
- money, credit cards (check expiry dates)
- international driver's licence
- international student card for discounts
- contact information for Canadian embassy or consulate
- specific information about project site

If you lose your passport and need to renew it rapidly, you'll need to have the following papers on hand:

- notarized photocopy of your passport identification page
- notarized photocopy of one other document supporting your identity
- original birth certificate or citizenship certificate
- two recent passport photographs
- contact details of the closest Canadian consulate or embassy

Remember to store these things separately from your passport.

Stress and Culture Shock

The normal physical and psychological responses that result when someone is suddenly immersed in very unfamiliar surroundings are collectively called "culture shock." The term has, to some extent, been trivialized by common usage, but that does not mean that the sensations of culture shock are imaginary. Culture shock is a form of depression and can, for some people and in some circumstances, become disabling (Stewart et al., 1998). Every traveller suffers culture shock to some extent. It is found under any stressful circumstance and is well reported in space crews making long flights (Kanas, 1998).

Attitudes and emotions change in fairly predictable ways as someone moves through the different phases of a project. During the rushed preparation stage before travel, the average person often swings between excitement and anxiety. After arriving in the country, emotions and energy levels may remain high for the first few days, but many people then go through a period of depression, confusion, or anger in response to very unfamiliar customs and practices. The timing and severity of the low phase depends on many variables, including individual variation, prior experience, and pre-departure preparation. Obviously, after a while, most people adapt to their circumstances. Finally, after lengthy visits, there is often a reverse culture shock during the reintegration process at home. Some of the common symptoms of culture shock include:

- irrational anger
- extreme homesickness
- intense feeling of loyalty to one's own culture
- unexplained crying
- loss of ability to work or study effectively
- withdrawal from people who are different from you
- symptomatic complaints such as headache and excessive tiredness

A study by the Canadian Foreign Service Institute found that the following characteristics were predictive of successful adaptation (Foreign Affairs, 2011a):

- respect and sensitivity for local social and cultural realities
- perseverance and confidence when dealing with frustrations
- skill at reading social interactions and flexibility when responding to difficulties

The full list is actually quite a bit longer and may give the impression that superhuman qualities are necessary in order to work overseas. This is not, of course, the case. The absolute requirements are a flexible attitude combined with careful pre-trip preparation so that you will have a good idea of what to expect. Culture shock is the body's response to profoundly unfamiliar surroundings. If that unfamiliarity is minimized by careful preparation, then you will feel more comfortable during the adaptation period. Pre-trip planning should give you a detailed understanding of the country—the CARE handbook is a good source of information (CARE International, 2005). If you know how the buses, taxis, and shops work, and you can make your basic needs understood in the local language, then unpleasant somatic responses to strange surroundings should, under most circumstances, be bearable.

Staying Healthy

There are so many excellent sources of information on travel health that the only problem is deciding which one to choose. Books (Yellow Book, 2011), websites (Travel Health, 2011), and local specialized travel clinics are all valuable resources to help you plan for a healthy stay during your overseas trip. There are no absolute guarantees of safety, but if you avoid mosquitoes, drink clean water, wash your hands, and always behave as if your grandmother were watching, you should be as safe abroad as you are at home.

There is no widely accepted "standard" vaccination schedule, so personal research is necessary. Decisions are also affected by the proposed destination. Although public health authorities differ, most recommend that travellers get boosters for their childhood vaccines (polio, diphtheria, tetanus), plus a full course of hepatitis A and B (PHAC, 2007). There is an ever-growing list of other vaccinations whose use will depend on individual variations and opinions. Examples include vaccines against yellow fever, pneumococcus, typhoid, influenza, Japanese encephalitis, rabies, among others. Obviously, it is important to obtain careful, professional advice that is based on current information about the place you'll be visiting.

Only a few countries require vaccination records prior to entry. A record of yellow fever vaccination is necessary for travel in some African and South American countries. Meningococcal vaccine is necessary for entry to a few Middle Eastern countries during periods of pilgrimage. Obviously, it is important to check before you travel. Remember that your body responds to a vaccine by producing protective antibodies. This process takes time, so make sure that you get any necessary shots early. Apart from immunizations, it is important to determine the malaria risk in the region you will be visiting and also the extent of drug resistance (Travel Doctor, 2011). If regular malaria prophylaxis is recommended, remember to start the drugs before you leave and to continue taking them for a time after you return. Time periods will depend on the medication, so it is important to obtain specialist advice based on current conditions in the country you will be visiting. Drug quality can be unreliable in developing world pharmacies, so ensure that you have a supply of drugs before you travel.

Apart from traumatic accidents, it is worth repeating that the principal risks to health for the average traveller are carried either by contaminated water or by mosquitoes. It takes only one contaminated ice cube or a single mosquito bite to ruin your trip. Just because you have lived in the country for six months does not mean that you are in any way immune. It is important to maintain a regular awareness of basic hygiene and common sense. Avoid mosquitoes by using a treated bed net, plus appropriate repellents and clothing. Drink only treated or commercially bought bottled water and use common sense when eating. Avoid swimming in fresh water in schistosomiasis areas, strongly resist the temptation to nurse sick animals, and do not drink milk unless you are certain it has been pasteurized. If you become sick within a year of return, particularly if you have a high fever, seek urgent medical attention and remember to provide a detailed travel history.

PREPARING YOUR PROJECT

Before anything else, preparation is the key to success.

—Alexander Graham Bell

Finding a Job

Each year, 100,000 people apply for the available 3,000 Peace Corps positions. When it comes to working overseas, there are a lot of talented, well-educated people chasing a limited number of jobs, so it isn't easy for a newcomer to find a place.

Table 18.2: General sources of information about global health, including university courses

Information on university courses:	• GradSchools.com. 2011. Source of information about international development programs given by universities around the world. URL: www.gradschools.com/search-programs/international-development.
Sources of general information:	• Aid Workers Network. 2011. Forum for ideas and information about international aid work. URL: www.aidworkers.net/.
	• AlertNet. 2011. Reuter's humanitarian news site. URL: www.alertnet.org.
	• ReliefWeb. 2011. Source of information about emergencies, plus job listings. URL: http://reliefweb.int/.
	• International Crisis Group. 2011. Excellent information source concerning conflicts. URL: www.crisisgroup.org/.
	• RedR UK. 2009. UK source for international development information. URL: www.redr.org/london/.
	• Health Exchange. 2011. Quarterly online magazine about international development issues. URL: http://healthexchangenews.com/.
	• Stanford Social Innovation Review. 2011. Quarterly print magazine and weekly updates. Articles and views from staff and associates of Stanford Centre on Philanthropy and Civil Society. Good quality, but they charge a fee. URL: www.ssireview.org/about/overview/.
	• IVPA. 2011. International Volunteer Programs Association. An association for NGOs that send volunteers overseas. It is also a source of information for anyone planning to work overseas. URL: www.volunteerinternational.org/volunteer_sites.html.
	• InterAction. 2011. Another good source of current information about crisis areas in the world. URL: www.interaction.org.

For those interested in long-term overseas work or who plan to make their career in global health, the large aid organizations have hiring mechanisms similar to any other big business. Contact them through their websites for information about employment or volunteer opportunities. For short-term projects, word of mouth is the best place to start. As a first step, ask faculty and students who have participated in previous courses for their advice and recommendations.

The first problem facing anyone interested in development work is simply finding easily accessible and reliable sources of information. Every developed country has a variety of international or global health organizations run by students, as well as non-governmental and governmental organizations—quantity isn't a problem, but quality varies widely. As noted earlier, despite all the interest in global health, it is surprisingly difficult to find information about educational courses on the subject. Table 18.2 lists some good starting points. The information on the listed sites is topical, professionally displayed, and the links work. The table also includes a large graduate schools directory.

After learning something about global health, the second problem is finding a job in the industry. Table 18.3 lists some of the larger sites listing jobs; a fee is required for some of them. It is very important to remember that whenever there

Table 18.3: Sources of job listings in global health

Job information:	• Devex. 2011. Development Executive Group. International development news and job source. URL: www.devex.com/en/.
	• DevNetJobs.org. 2011. International development jobs and consulting opportunities. URL: www.devnetjobs.org/.
	• Experience Development. 2011. Information source and job listings. Large site, but they charge a fee. URL: www. experiencedevelopment.org/advertise.php.
	• GoAbroad.com. 2011. Site specializing in finding places for people who wish to volunteer overseas. URL: www.goabroad.com/ volunteer-abroad.
	• IMVA. 2011. International Medical Volunteers Association. Source of information for travellers and also posted job opportunities. URL: www.imva.org/index.html.
Charity watchdogs:	• Charity Intelligence Canada. 2011. A recently formed organization that researches and analyzes the effectiveness of Canadian charities. URL: www.charityintelligence.ca.
	• BBB. 2011. Better Business Bureau, Wise Giving Alliance. Rates charities on their accounting practices and degree of transparency. URL: www.bbb.org/us/charity/.
	• Charity Navigator. 2011. Rates charities using a star scale based on how well donations are used. URL: www.charitynavigator.org/.
	• Charitywatch.org. 2011. Free website, but there is a small fee to receive a larger tri-annual report that has a more complex rating and analysis of charities than simply awarding stars.

is a demand for a product, there will be scams. There is no shortage of stories from people who paid a fee to work on a project, but whose experiences then fell far below their expectations. Do not hand over your money without doing extensive research into the charity organization first. A list of charity watchdog sites is included in Table 18.3. Lastly, there are several books on the subject of working abroad. Jean Marc Hachey's book and associated website, *The Big Guide to Living and Working Overseas*, is very useful and regularly updated (Hachey, 2010). Similar books listed at the end of this chapter provide contact information for agencies and projects abroad and also offer useful travel and preparation advice.

Forming a Project Team

Although some students will find individual positions, many find it better to form a team so they can pool their resources of energy and talent. Most universities have a Student International Health Society. Clearly, this is the best place to start when looking for advice and support for your own team. Peace and harmony among humans does not occur by accident; it must be carefully managed from an early point in the team's formation (please read Chapter 19 carefully). It is very important that the team starts with regular meetings to develop common objectives and goals. Once jointly agreed-upon aims have been clearly established, they tend to act as a "written constitution" for the project and will help to focus future plans and reduce arguments.

Conflicts cannot be avoided, but anticipating the major points of friction will help to keep the peace. Common sources of trouble are money, distribution of work, and failing to stick to the established goals. These and many other problems are best managed by regular meetings, clear communication, and team members who are prepared to be flexible and accommodating. Apart from the information given in the next chapter, there are also several books that give excellent advice on the subject of building and maintaining small teams (Mackin, 2007).

Finances and Fundraising

The major cost facing most small projects will be air travel, but other factors will need to be considered, such as health insurance, visa and licence fees, in-country travel, food, lodging, and project expenses (e.g., translators and local labour). Clearly, a budget is required, both for your own purposes and also to show potential funding sources how much money you need and what you propose to do with it. A well-prepared budget and timeline will show that you have put serious thought into your project. Both are also necessary if you are making a grant application.

Careless money management can be the source of a great deal of trouble, so it is important to choose a treasurer who is competent, responsible, and organized. If you register as a charity, you will have to deal with Canada Revenue Agency's tax laws (or equivalents outside Canada). If you run lotteries, raffles, or bingo games, you will probably be governed by local gambling laws. If you accept significant donations from various people, you will also have to be prepared to answer the obvious question, "What did you do with that money I gave you?" In each case, an accurate record of income and expenditure will be essential.

Fundraising will depend on the ingenuity and energy of each group, but examples include lotteries and raffles, bingo nights, dances, charity runs, Christmas present wrapping at the local mall, snow clearing, and gardening. If your planned project gives you an opportunity to do some research, it is possible to apply for a research grant from funding agencies. Many universities also have travel grants or bursaries for students involved in overseas projects. Many go uncollected each year because they are not advertised; you will not know if they exist unless you ask.

Learning about the Country

Obviously, it is important that you have detailed knowledge about the country you will be working in and its customs. Again, the best place to start is to find people who have worked in that country. Other reliable sources include the Central Intelligence Agency's *World Factbook* (CIA, 2011) and the Lonely Planet websites (Lonely Planet, 2011). Both contain excellent information on just about any country in the world. The Department of Foreign Affairs (or equivalent) of every developed country publishes a website with up-to-date information for its travelling citizens. The website of Canada's Foreign Affairs is a good example (Foreign Affairs, 2011b).

Find out as much as you can about local customs before you travel. Attitudes toward dress, behaviour, drugs, and even corruption may differ sharply from those at home. Your responses to those differences will be an important part of an enjoyable stay. Your efforts to accommodate yourself to local society will likely be noticed and appreciated, particularly if you spend time gaining a basic knowledge of the local language. If you are going to be studying or employed in a new country, it is important to understand very clearly what you are getting yourself into. You should clarify the hours you will be expected to work, your periods of time off, and any expected additional expenses long before you travel.

This is a suitable place to add a few comments about using an interpreter. When working overseas, language will be one of the most difficult barriers to overcome. An effective translator can resolve many of the cross-cultural dilemmas that you

586 PART VI WORKING SAFELY AND EFFECTIVELY IN A DEVELOPING COUNTRY

will initially face, but success depends on careful selection. When recruiting and hiring translators, you must ensure that they are readily available and are also able to navigate well within the numerous racial, ethnic, and economic hierarchies that exist within any culture. In medical projects, avoid asking family members of a patient to translate, particularly if they are emotionally involved. Deception, omission, or just embarrassed confusion will be the result if you unknowingly place a translator in a socially difficult situation. You may require a female translator in order to talk to a woman, and young interpreters may be very uncomfortable asking detailed personal questions of older people. You will have to rely on body language signals to determine if you have unwittingly placed participants in a socially un-acceptable position.

Finally, please always bear in mind the Shona farewell:

Mufambe zvakanaka: Travel safely.

SUMMARY

Planning and preparing for safe and effective development work is critical for impact and sustainability. Before going on a project, it is very important to ask yourself why you wish to put yourself through the expense and hard work of an overseas project. The safety and success of your time overseas will depend on the effort you put into the planning stage. The normal physical and psychological responses that result when someone is suddenly immersed in very unfamiliar surroundings are collectively called "culture shock." Culture shock is a form of depression and can, for some people and in some circumstances, become disabling. It is important to respect and appreciate sensitivity for local social and cultural realities and have perseverance and confidence when dealing with frustrations. Skill at reading social interactions and flexibility when responding to difficulties are critical for a successful trip. It is also important that you have detailed knowledge about the country you will be working in and its customs. Usually, the best place to start is to find people who have worked in that country. Other reliable sources include the Central Intelligence Agency's *World Factbook* and the Lonely Planet websites. Both contain excellent information on just about any country in the world. In addition, the Department of Foreign Affairs (or equivalent) of every developed country publishes a website with up-to-date information for its travelling citizens. It is vital to be knowledgeable about local customs of your destination as attitudes toward dress, behaviour, drugs, social interactions, and so on may differ sharply from those at home.

DISCUSSION QUESTIONS

1. What are the right motives for undertaking development work? Why is it important to have the right motives?
2. Imagine you have been accepted by a major international agency to support a health program in another country. What is the best way to plan for such a development project?
3. What would you consider to be the major ethical problems associated with aid projects? How do you navigate such ethical challenges?
4. How do you plan to stay healthy if working in a developing country? Give some examples.
5. Which countries have the highest attacks on humanitarian workers? Why? Would you consider working in such a country?
6. What are the diseases normally associated with humanitarian work? How do you avoid them?
7. Imagine you have been posted to work on a new project in another country. What are the key ways to working effectively and co-operatively in such a new culture?
8. What is culture shock? How do you deal with culture shock?
9. What is the major cost facing most small aid projects?
10. Where might one find potential job opportunities in global health?

RECOMMENDED READING

Ausenda, F., et al. 2008. *World volunteers: The world guide to humanitarian and development volunteering*. Pub: Universe.

Collins, J., et al. 2004. *How to live your dream of volunteering overseas*. Pub: Penguin.

Ehrenreich, J. 2005. *The humanitarian companion: A guide for international aid, development, and human rights workers*. Pub: Practical Action.

Fielding, H. 2002. *Cause celeb*. Pub: Penguin.

Hachey, J.-M. 2010. *The big guide to living and working overseas*. Earlier print version available. Online updated version only available by subscribing to website at: www.workingoverseas.com/.

Wilson, M. 2009. *The medic's guide to work and electives around the world*. Pub: Hodder Arnold.

Yellow Book. 2010. CDC health information for international travelers. Retrieved from: wwwnc.cdc.gov/travel/page/yellowbook-2012-home.htm.

REFERENCES

ACFID. 2009. Australian Council for International Development Code of Conduct. Retrieved from: www.acfid.asn.au/code-of-conduct/acfid-code-of-conduct.

ActAlliance. 2007. HIV in emergencies and humanitarian work. Retrieved from: www.actalliance.org/resources/policies-and-guidelines/hiv/HIVPolicy_adoptedEmComApril08_ACTAlliance.pdf.

Aid Workers Network. Retrieved from: www.aidworkers.net/?q=advice.

Baker, T., et al. 1992. The uncounted dead: American civilians dying overseas. *Public Health Reports*, 107: 155–159.

Baratrala, N., et al. 1998. Knowing when to say "no" on the student elective: Students going on electives abroad need clinical guidelines. *British Medical Journal*, 316: 1404–1405.

Bernard, A. 1995. *The pill: A biography of the drug that changed the world*. Pub: Random House.

British Columbia Ministry of Health. 2004. Traveller's diarrhea. Retrieved from: www.bchealthguide.org by searching "traveller's diarrhea."

Care. 2010. International emergency toolkit. Retrieved from: www.careemergencytoolkit.org/home/.

CARE International. 2005. Safety and security handbook. Retrieved from: http://coe-dmha.org/care/pdf/EntireBook.pdf.

CCDR. 2009. Canada communicable disease report: Prevention of tuberculosis among travelers. Retrieved from: www.phac-aspc.gc.ca/publicat/ccdr-rmtc/09vol35/acs-dcc-5/index-eng.php.

CDC. 2011. Water treatment methods. Retrieved from: wwwnc.cdc.gov/travel/page/water-treatment.htm.

CIA. 2011. *The world factbook*. Retrieved from: www.cia.gov/cia/publications/factbook.

Clemens, M., et al. 2004. Counting chickens when they hatch: The short-term effect of aid on growth. Center for Global Development working paper no. 44. Retrieved from: www.cgdev.org/files/2744_file_CountingChickensFINAL3.pdf.

Danielli, Y. 2002. *Sharing the front line and the back hills: Peacekeepers, humanitarian aid workers, and the media in the midst of crisis*. Pub: Baywood Publishing Company.

Eaton, L. 2005. Nuffield Council calls for ethical framework for developing world research. *British Medical Journal*, 330: 618.

Fawcett, J. 2003. *Stress and trauma handbook: Strategies for flourishing in demanding environments*. Pub: World Vision International.

Foreign Affairs. 2007. Her own way: A woman's guide to safe and successful travel. Retrieved from: www.voyage.gc.ca/publications/woman-guide_voyager-feminin-eng.asp.

Foreign Affairs. 2008. Drugs and travel: Why they don't mix. Retrieved from: www.voyage.gc.ca/publications/drug-travel_drogue-voyages-eng.asp.

Foreign Affairs. 2010. Directory of Canadian government offices abroad. Retrieved from: www.voyage.gc.ca/contact/offices-list_liste-bureaux-eng.asp.

Foreign Affairs. 2011a. Centre for intercultural learning, Government of Canada. Retrieved from: www.international.gc.ca/cfsi-icse/cil-cai/index-eng.asp.

Foreign Affairs. 2011b. Travel reports and warnings. Retrieved from: www.voyage.gc.ca/index-eng.asp.

Hachey, J.-M. 2010. The big guide to living and working overseas. Retrieved from: www.workingoverseas.com/online.

Halsey, N., et al. 1997. Ethics and international research. *British Medical Journal*, 315: 965–966.

Hamlyn, E., et al. 2003. Sexual health for travelers. *Australian Family Physician*, 32: 981–984.

Health Exchange. 2011. Retrieved from: http://healthexchangenews.com/.

HPA. 2000. Health Protection Agency. Foreign travel-associated illness. Retrieved from: www.hpa.org.uk/web/HPAwebFile/HPAweb_C/1202487132274.

Huey, R., et al. 2000. Supplemental oxygen and death rates on Everest and K2. *Journal of the American Medical Association*, 284: 181.

Humanitarian Outcomes. 2016. Aid worker security database. Retrieved from: https://aidworkersecurity.org/.

IFC. 2008. Independent evaluation of International Finance Corporation's development results 2007. Retrieved from: www.ifc.org/ieg/iedr2007.

Kanas, N. 1998. Psychosocial issues affecting crews during long-duration international space missions. *Acta Astronautica*, 42: 339–361.

Khan, K., et al. 2006. WHO analysis of causes of maternal deaths: A systematic review. *The Lancet*, 367: 1066–1074.

Klein, M. 1995. Deaths of Australian travelers overseas. *Medical Journal of Australia*, 163: 277–280.

Lonely Planet. 2011. Retrieved from: www.lonelyplanet.com.

Lurie, P., et al. 1997. Unethical trials of interventions to reduce perinatal transmission of the human immunodeficiency virus in developing countries. *New England Journal of Medicine*, 337: 853–856.

Mackin, D. 2007. *The team building tool kit: Tips, tactics, and rules for effective work place teams*. Pub: AMACOM.

Maren, M. 2002. *The road to hell: The ravaging effects of foreign aid and international charity*. Pub: Free Press.

Moore, J., et al. 1995. HIV risk behaviour among Peace Corps volunteers. *Aids*, 9: 795–799.

Nantulya, V. 2002. The neglected epidemic: Road traffic injuries in developing countries. *British Medical Journal*, 324: 1139–1141.

NaTHNaC. 2010. National Travel Health Network and Centre. Retrieved from: www.nathnac.org/travel/misc/travellers_mos.htm.

Odero, W., et al. 1997. Road traffic injuries in developing countries: A comprehensive review of epidemiologic studies. *Tropical Medicine and International Health*, 2: 445–460.

Okeke, I., et al. 2005. Antimicrobial resistance in developing countries. *Lancet Infectious Diseases*, 5: 481–493.

Palmer, I. 2005. Psychological aspects of providing medical humanitarian aid. *British Medical Journal*, 331: 152–154.

Peace Corps. 2015. The health of the volunteer 2015—Annual report of volunteer health. Retrieved from: http://files.peacecorps.gov/documents/open-government/HOV2015.pdf.

PHAC. 2007. Public Health Agency of Canada. Travel vaccines. Retrieved from: www.phac-aspc.gc.ca/im/travelvaccines-eng.php.

RedR UK. 2009. Retrieved from: www.redr.org/london/.

Roberts, D. 2005. Safety and security guidelines for humanitarian volunteers. ICRC. Retrieved from: www.icrc.org/eng/assets/files/other/icrc_002_0717.pdf.

Sheik, M., et al. 2000. Deaths among humanitarian workers. *British Medical Journal*, 321: 166–168.

Smarttraveller. 2011. Australian government. Retrieved from: www.smarttraveller.gov.au.

Sphere Handbook. 2011. Humanitarian charter and minimum standards in humanitarian response. Retrieved from: www.sphereproject.org/.

Stewart, L., et al. 1998. Culture shock and travelers. *Journal of Travel Medicine*, 5: 84–88.

Travel Doctor. 2005a. Insect-borne diseases. Retrieved from: www.traveldoctor.co.uk/insects.htm.

Travel Doctor. 2005b. Travellers' diarrhoea. Retrieved from: www.traveldoctor.co.uk/diarrhoea.htm.

Travel Doctor. 2011a. Malaria prophylaxis and vaccination requirements. Retrieved from: www.traveldoctor.co.uk/tables.htm.

Travel Health. 2011b. Public Health Agency of Canada. Retrieved from: www.phac-aspc.gc.ca/tmp-pmv/index-eng.php.

US Department of State. 2010. Drugs abroad. Retrieved from: www.travel.state.gov/travel/living/drugs/drugs_1237.html.

WHO. 2011. International travel and health. Retrieved from: www.who.int/ith/en/.

WHO. 2015. Global status report on road safety 2015. Retrieved from: www.who.int/violence_injury_prevention/road_safety_status/2015/en/.

Yellow Book. 2011. CDC health information for international travelers. Retrieved from: wwwnc.cdc.gov/travel/page/yellowbook-2012-home.htm.

CHAPTER 19

How to Manage a Sustainable Aid Partnership

Good management is the art of making problems so interesting and their solutions so constructive that everyone wants to get to work and deal with them.

—Paul Hawken

OBJECTIVES

It does not matter if you are a medical student planning an attachment to an overseas clinic or a UNICEF official trying to coordinate dozens of agencies for an immunization program—sustainable success requires lots of characters to get along together without fighting. This is fundamentally against human nature, so it doesn't happen without a great deal of careful planning and monitoring. This chapter offers a basic overview of management planning for those interested in getting the most out of their overseas projects. Management jargon, generalizations, and sports metaphors will be kept to a minimum! Whatever your team plans to do, this chapter will help you to do it more efficiently. After completing this chapter, you should be able to:

- appreciate the fundamental importance of true partnering as a basis for successful development projects
- understand the common pitfalls and problems confronting partnerships
- understand the problems of selecting and supporting the people working on the project
- appreciate the specific organizational needs for managing the program itself
- understand how to manage and avoid conflict

INTRODUCTION

All happy families resemble one another, each unhappy family is unhappy in its own way.

—*Leo Tolstoy, Anna Karenina*

Tolstoy may have been right about families, but he was wrong about projects. Unhappy projects are not all unhappy in different ways; the fundamental problem is always the same. No matter what other problems might have occurred, there is usually a common thread of inadequate planning and preparation running through them. From the very start, considerable effort must be devoted to predicting and managing the inevitable problems that occur when humans have to co-operate, particularly when they are working together under difficult circumstances. For the purposes of analyzing this topic, it is convenient to break down a project into three components: (1) the people who do the work, (2) the organizational framework within which they operate, and, finally, (3) the work they produce. Until now, this book has concentrated on the third component (the content of project work). However, this current chapter is concerned only with the first two: the people (selecting and managing people working on the project) and the process (creating an organizational support structure to ensure efficient, trouble-free work).

Box 19.1 History Notes

Florence Nightingale (1820–1910)

Florence Nightingale is often portrayed as a caricature of a starched Victorian nurse. In reality, she was a major scientist who made significant contributions to a variety of disciplines, including nursing, public health, hospital planning, and mathematics. She was an excellent mathematician (she invented pie charts) and was the first woman elected to the Royal Statistical Society. At a time when women from her privileged background were expected to stay at home, she left for Germany to take nursing training. In response to the public outcry over poor conditions for troops in the Crimean War, she was allowed to take a party of 38 nurses to serve in the army hospital in Scutari. She found the patients lying in blood-stained uniforms with no blankets and poor food. Five out of six deaths were due to disease, not wounds. When her attempts at reform were opposed by officers and doctors, she used her society contacts to report the facts through the *Times* newspaper in England. She was subsequently placed in charge of improving hospital standards. Simple hygiene and regular food reduced the death rate dramatically. She returned to England as a national hero. Her work led to the formation of the Army Medical College. She also established the first school for nursing at St. Thomas' Hospital, which laid the foundation for modern nursing. She wrote over 200 books and articles during her life; one of those books, *Notes on Nursing*, is still in print. Go to the reference to learn more: Florence Nightingale Museum (2011).

On first view, this material might seem a bit dry, but anyone who has completed a development project of any form will know that partnership planning and management are the most important factors determining the final outcome. Unfortunately, since each project is different, the partnership and management literature tends to deal in generalizations rather than specifics. This can be off-putting, particularly when management jargon is added. Since all aid projects involve partnerships of one form or another, anyone interested in international development work must understand the basic requirements that make up a successful partnership. There is no shortage of literature in this area, ranging from philosophy to sociology, with stops at psychology and anthropology along the way. The book by Dr. Melville Kerr (1996) is a thoughtful review of partnering based on extensive overseas experience. It is essential reading for anyone involved in project planning.

No team works in isolation. The success of any project depends on the ability of the people involved to get along with each other. Even the smallest overseas initiative will require a fair amount of social interaction between the visitors and other people involved in the project (hosts, student groups, clinic staff, patients, etc.). In larger studies, the involvement of government agencies, university departments, local population representatives, and a host of other professionals who accumulate once a project is planned endlessly multiply the possibilities for disagreement. Once differences in culture, religion, politics, and language are added to the mix, it is easy to see why so many joint international projects fail to meet their initial objectives. The ability to form stable groups for mutual benefit is a basic human quality; we are not solitary animals. It could be argued that many of the dramas of history would have turned out very differently if the groups involved had used peaceful conflict-resolution methods rather than war to solve their differences. What would Alexander have been like if Aristotle had taught him the basics of peaceful partnership management?

A true example will help to illustrate some of the main points of project management:

> Everything started with great enthusiasm. The funding agency would not give money for an initial meeting between the teams, so all contact was maintained by telephone and email, with an occasional video conference. Planning progressed reasonably well, although we were surprised by the slow turnaround time for any letters or decisions. The partners were members of two strong universities and the project certainly looked good on paper. It was awarded a large grant; the various teams set to work.
>
> Unfortunately, there were faults on both sides right from the start. One of the members of the partner team was very unwilling to accept outside assistance and made no secret of these views. One of the joint writing teams failed

to get along and could not agree on the emphasis or content of their material. In another team, there were concerns about the competence of one of the writers and worries that the final material was not good enough. Another problem, which should have been foreseen, was the distribution of money. The partner team was understandably sensitive to any perception of unfairness in the distribution of funding. This was aggravated by the donor agency's unwillingness to support any salaries in the partner country. In addition, our university's financial department was going through a reorganization so there was considerable delay in the transfer of funds on two occasions.

Despite these problems, work progressed fitfully so that an acceptable postgraduate course was developed in the prescribed time. However, our contribution was now fairly small and limited to providing money for work performed—there was no longer any pretense that this was a joint undertaking. Amazingly enough, common sense finally prevailed; both teams included well-meaning, competent staff who organized a face-to-face confrontation that should have happened two or three years earlier. During these very frank exchanges, it became obvious that members in the two countries interpreted even the most basic assumptions in very different ways. There was no common thread amongst participants' motivations (these included altruism, financial gain, career opportunities, religious convictions, and a desire to travel). It was necessary to go back to the absolute basic goals before unequivocal agreement about anything could be found. If we had started with a clearer understanding of the complexities of partnerships, we would all have saved ourselves two or three years of bad feeling and wasted work.

No matter how optimistic and excited everyone feels at the beginning of a project, remember, the honeymoon will end one day. One of the benefits of forming a group is to get different experiences and points of view, but this does have a drawback. Active debate strengthens the final plan, but it is not far from debate to argument. Group members will probably disagree about objectives and how to reach them. When that hurdle is passed, they will certainly disagree again when it comes to division of money and work. Humans argue and debate; that is just their nature. Disagreement should be predicted and managed with clear conflict guidelines, not suppressed because of a worry that the partnership is fragile. Every time you read the example above, you will probably find another mistake the teams made. There were problems with people and problems with the partnership process. Much of that trouble could have been avoided with better planning and leadership at the very first meeting. The broad characteristics of successful and unsuccessful partnerships are given in Table 19.1.

Table 19.1: Characteristics of successful and unsuccessful partnerships

SUCCESSFUL PARTNERSHIPS	UNSUCCESSFUL PARTNERSHIPS
• Respect and trust between people involved	• Manipulative or dominating partner
• Complete agreement that the partnership is necessary	• Lack of clear purpose
• Competent leadership with support of all members	• Unrealistic goals
	• Dishonesty, particularly hidden agendas
• Clearly agreed-upon goals	• Unequal balance of power and control
• Collaborative decision-making process	• Irresolvable differences in philosophy or ways of working
• Regular communications	• Poor communication
• Clearly defined organizational structure	• Poorly trained, unqualified team members
• Fully agreed-upon conflict-resolution procedure	• Money and time commitments that outweigh the potential benefits
• Fully agreed-upon budget	• Poor money management

During the initial excitement and enthusiasm of a new project, it is easy to forget that development projects are the same as any other joint human endeavour—without careful planning, staff selection, and management, the aims are unlikely to be met. In order for an overseas aid initiative to stand the best chance of success, it is important to employ competent, stable, well-trained personnel chosen by a carefully established selection procedure. Potential workers should be briefed and trained adequately before leaving and then fully supported during their overseas assignment. The process should be constantly updated using information gained from regular communications, plus the results of a detailed post-assignment debriefing. Working overseas is a difficult and demanding job that, under some circumstances, involves considerable physical and psychological risks. People who are prepared to take on this challenge deserve the highest levels of preparation and support. Anything less will result in dissatisfaction, poor performance, avoidable ill health, and wasted aid money. Despite the importance of good management, there is surprisingly little evidence-based knowledge in the area of selecting and supporting aid workers. We'll look at the two aspects of people and process separately.

MANAGING THE PROCESS

Management is efficiency in climbing the ladder; leadership determines whether the ladder is leaning against the right wall.

—*Stephen Covey, 2001*

Why Do You Need a Partnership?

No matter how skilful a team might be, they will almost certainly need the help of others at some stage in their project. For example, a visiting surgical team may need hospital beds, operating facilities, and a range of other logistical support, while a nutrition-assessment project might need the support and assistance of local teachers, elders, and parents. The simplest argument in favour of partnerships is that they are almost unavoidable. They are a convenient way to bring all the skills and logistical support needed for an initiative under one roof. A well-organized, broad-based partnership is also more attractive to granting agencies and is much more likely to attract project funding. Once they are established and running, the group also provides mutual support to maintain everyone's enthusiasm when facing inevitable obstacles.

Ensuring that you are committed to a true partnership is particularly important when working directly with a developing world community. Imposed solutions, based on a colonial mindset (no matter how well intentioned), usually lead to passivity and dependence among the targeted population. Active and equal involvement of local people helps to ensure a project's future because there will be committed local staff able to sustain it after the expatriate workers have returned home. The complex, often intangible, variables that exist within any society are also automatically included in the planning process if members of that community are enthusiastically welcomed as planning partners. Finally, partnerships lead to numerous unpredictable benefits that emerge as the project proceeds. Once a community's skills and enthusiasm are harnessed, it is extraordinary what can be achieved.

Types of Partnership

> Good battle is healthy and brings to a marriage the principles of equal partnership.
>
> —*Ann Landers*

In the past, a good deal of lip service has been paid to terms such as "partnership" and "grassroots" involvement. Unfortunately, reality does not always meet the high ideals mentioned in the grant proposal. Recipients of top-down projects may have been referred to as partners, but this is simply an indication of the difficulties of using language to express something as complex as human relationships. Careless choice of definitions can easily give offence in the area of global health. When one half of the team is referred to as the donor university or developed country university and the other half is referred to as the recipient, Third World, or developing university, linguistic battle lines have already been drawn. Whatever definition is chosen to describe a partnership, it should certainly be more than a sterile agreement between two or more groups working together to achieve common aims. Whatever the scale of the project, the key characteristics that make something a true partnership include a feeling of reciprocity where all members feel they are able to gain something from the relationship. There has to be a sense of mutual trust and respect and, of course, an attitude of openness and equality in all the shared dealings. Oxfam Canada's list of basic partnership principles is a good starting point:

- There must be shared vision and values.
- The partnership should have a value-added effect.
- Each partner should have autonomy and independence.
- There should be transparency and mutual accountability in all dealings.
- There should be clarity about roles and responsibilities.
- Joint strategy should be updated regularly based on progress reviews.

The term "partnership" has also been used imprecisely to describe a spectrum of relationships ranging from a true partnership to short-term working arrangements. This does not, of course, mean that partnerships are always necessary. At one end of the spectrum are groups that just happen to be working together on the same project. Through mutual benefit, they might move closer by sharing logistics (transport or accommodation). Once they start sharing information or swapping staff, a closer union is formed until they end up together under a unified set of goals and management. Other arrangements include short-term consultancies or clearly defined subcontracts. While clearly defined rules of engagement will still be necessary for these various degrees of working together, they should not be called partnerships.

A good example of the changing nature of partnerships is the experience of the Onchocerciasis Control Program (OCP). In the late 1980s, an effective drug for control of onchocerciasis (ivermectin) was made available to the OCP (Collins, 2004). In addition to inhibiting the vector insect with insecticides, it became necessary to distribute this drug once or twice a year to large numbers of people living in a high-risk belt running from West Africa across to parts of Central America and South America (Hopkins, 2005). Although the drug administration process was labelled "community-based," it became clear that it was, in reality, a top-down imposed process with little or no real community involvement. Slow progress in onchocerciasis control led to a review of the program in 1994. Poor involvement of local communities was identified as a significant barrier to sustainable distribution, so it was decided to change to a more inclusive partnership with target populations. Based on successful programs in Mali, where a community-based drug delivery system had been practised for several years, communities in other countries were encouraged to take control of their own treatment. Community members collected drugs from supply points, treated eligible members in their community, and referred cases with severe adverse reactions (TDR, 2010).

By 1996, it was already clear that this community-based approach to partnership was working well. Within 10 years of the start of the program, onchoceriasis transmission had been almost eliminated in West Africa. In 2003 alone, 40 million people were treated with ivermectin. The community-based approach was so successful that it has now been adopted as a standard method for involving local communities in their own treatment programs (TDR, 2009). For example, the international eradication program against lymphatic filariasis adopted the same methodology after it was shown to be significantly more efficient than conventional approaches to drug distribution (Gyapong et al., 2001). As a further example of the need for well-planned partnerships, there were initial worries that funds and resources put into a community-based program would divert money and staff away from the existing health care systems. To avoid this problem, local health adminstrators are included as equal planning partners to ensure that the targeted program is well integrated into their various health services. It should also be added that the Special Program for Tropical Disease Research, which developed this partnership method, is itself funded by a joint group consisting of UNICEF, UNDP, the World Bank, and the World Health Organization (TDR, 2010). You cannot avoid partnerships!

Getting Started

Partnering is a co-operative human endeavour, so inevitably there will be problems. Most people feel some apprehension when joining a new group; forming a partnership is no different. The fear of losing a separate identity, lack of trust, and confusion about the nature of involvement are all challenges that face a room full of strangers who decide they are going to work together. Rather than pretending such unworthy emotions do not exist, it is better to be realistic and open in the early discussion phase. These early meetings, during which the various partners get to know each other, are an absolutely basic requirement for any successful partnership. A hurried process that does not allow the development of mutual respect and trust is unlikely to result in a sustainable working relationship. Some team members might want to leave seemingly boring details of organization and management until later and just jump straight to the action. Resist this temptation; forming a firm foundation for the partnership is essential and it takes time. It is also important not to swing too far the other way. Partnerships are important, but they are not an end in themselves. They should always be viewed as a means to an end.

Box 19.2 Moment of Insight

2007 population, Canada and the UK: 93.8 million	2007 population of Africa: 956.8 million
2007 total carbon dioxide production, Canada and the UK:	2007 total carbon dioxide production, all African countries:
1.1 billion metric tons	**1.1 billion metric tons**

Source: US Census Bureau. 2011. International programs. Retrieved from www.census. gov/population/international/data/idb/ informationGateway.php.

Source: EIA. 2011. US Energy Information Administration. Retrieved from: www.eia.gov/.

Once the initial ice has been broken, it is time to start substantive discussions. No matter what you plan to do, there are a few common questions that need to be answered. It is very useful to have someone with experience in partnerships to guide these discussions. Try searching around for groups or partnership committees that seem similar to your own and ask if some of their members would be prepared to help guide you through the process of developing goals and organizing a practical management framework. Larger organizations might consider consulting a professional partnership facilitator. There are many ways of getting a group of strangers to focus on a given question (Mackin, 2007). One approach is to ask participants to write their ideas on a small card. You will need to ask a clear, unambiguous question such as, "What are your goals for this partnership?" After writing down their ideas, cards are pinned to a board and reviewed by all team members. Anyone who disagrees with a statement can move that card to another board. Substituting a new idea on another card is also allowed. After everyone has had a turn, those cards remaining represent the main goals that have support from every member of the group. Of course, if there are no cards left on the board, then you have major problems with this particular partnership.

Whether you come to agreement by open discussion with or without a facilitator, or by using various group activities like the one described above, there are a few essential questions that have to be answered in detail. The Alberta Government Department of Community Development publishes a very useful short guide that helps small groups through those necessary partnership steps (Alberta Community Development, 2001). The major questions that must be answered include the following:

- *Do we need a partnership?* Before embarking on a complex group activity like a partnership program, it is a good idea to decide if you actually need to do it. Would a looser arrangement, such as a formal financial subcontract or information-sharing network, serve the group's goals equally well?

- *What are the goals of the partnership?* The goals or aims of the project should not be viewed as abstract entities that are simply needed to fill in a grant application form. Inevitable disagreements between various team members will be easier to manage if everyone involved is motivated and influenced by an agreed-upon set of objectives, no matter how far in the future these achievements may lie.

- *How do you plan to reach those goals?* Once goals are established, it is time for serious discussions at a "nuts-and-bolts" level. This process should not be rushed, since it is from these discussions that activities, timelines, costs, and an overall budget will emerge. It is always important to maintain a sense of pragmatism so that your plans and budget are grounded in practical, achievable reality. A project of any reasonable size will probably be broken into different tasks, with each requiring a separate subcommittee.

- *How will the project be managed?* During the partnership-building process, plans and ideas will change with each meeting. Until a stable plan has been achieved, it is best to have an interim decision-making process in place. Decide on the final management structure after you have all clearly agreed upon what you want to do and how you plan to do it.

Table 19.2: How to engage with communities in field research

• Focus on trust	• Use the right communication methods
• Engage early	• Get informed consent
• Listen and learn	• Continue communication beyond the end of the research
• Get to know your participants	

Source: Ezezika, O. C. 2014. How do you build trust with communities involved in your research? SciDev.Net's practical guides, Science and Development Network © 2014 SciDev. Net. Retrieved from: www.scidev.net/global/communication/practical-guide/engage-participants-field-research.html.

Running the Project

> It has been said that democracy is the worst form of government, except all the others that have been tried.
>
> —*Winston Churchill, 1947*

Children start saying "You're not the boss of me" in kindergarten and that attitude strengthens as they get older. Humans do not like being told what to do, but they mostly realize that some form of leadership is necessary when group decisions must be made. Given the problems of money, goals, deadlines, and personalities associated with partnership plans, an orderly decision-making process is essential. There is no ideal management structure; it can only be stressed that one will be needed. Each group will find their own solution based on their individual needs. Commonly used decision-making techniques include the following:

- *Election of a leader by the group:* Problems of equal representation are multiplied in large partnerships. In order to keep meetings at a manageable size, it will probably be necessary to elect or appoint representatives from different interest groups onto a steering committee. Under these circumstances, it is important that the voting process is transparent and clearly agreed upon by everyone involved.
- *General group consensus:* This method applies mainly to small groups and is probably the most common one used by student groups. Decision by agreement has the advantage that it is a good test of a group's abilities at getting along. If the group cannot agree in the comfort of their home environment, then they probably should not be working overseas together. Despite this, it is still a good idea to sort out what the group plans to do in the event of major disagreement.
- *Rotating leadership:* This is a rather awkward approach to the need for general equality between large vested interests. For example, regular rotation was used to select new members to the UN Commission on Human Rights. The unelected appearance of Sudan and Zimbabwe on the committee is probably the principal reason behind the collapse of that organization. The method lacks consistency and may bring round a leader no one wants.
- *The biggest partner is the leader:* Control in a partnership is unavoidably influenced by the skills, resources, and money that individual partners bring to the group. For example, votes in the IMF are influenced by the money member states contribute, not by their populations. In the past, partnerships formed between large aid agencies and small developing world communities have certainly suffered from inequality in terms of planning and direction. These problems can be avoided only when the participants (particularly the ones with the money) enter the agreement in a spirit of true respect—not just lip service, but a real understanding that long-term success depends on giving everyone involved an equal voice.

Once the framework has been selected, it is important to maintain clear communication through regular meetings. It should be emphasized that there is no substitute for face-to-face meetings, even when the partners live in different countries. Video conferences, telephone calls, and email are all valuable, but intangible team-building benefits do result from meetings between the main people involved in the project, particularly in the early planning stages. Unfortunately, planning often occurs before grant money has been awarded, so expensive travel might not be an option. A particular point should be made about money. Careful division of any available grants or donations will not be the only worry, but it will probably be the biggest and certainly the most predictable. Again, regular communication and a transparent allocation process are essential. It is important to accept the divisive risks caused by money and to plan accordingly.

Remember that no matter how close the team members are, there will be moments of disagreement as the project progresses. Serious disputes are destructive and they can also be expensive once lawyers and mediators are involved. They can be minimized, but certainly not avoided altogether, by including an agreed-upon conflict-resolution process early in the partnership process. Methods vary, but it can be useful to ask an uninvolved third party, acceptable to both teams, to act as an arbitrator. If the project is funded by a grant agency, then a senior member of that agency is often selected. The Center for Effective Dispute Resolution's website (CEDR, 2011) is a good source of information, and so is the handbook *You're Not Listening to Me!*, published by the National Council of Voluntary Organizations (Laurence et al., 2003).

Evaluation

> I know not any thing more pleasant, or more instructive, than to compare experience with expectation, or to register from time to time the difference between idea and reality. It is by this kind of observation that we grow daily less liable to be disappointed.
>
> —*Samuel Johnson*

The aid industry has a long history of failing to evaluate its initiatives and then being surprised at the last moment by poor results. The approach often taken is to alter the goals so it seems as if the original plan wasn't such a failure after all. The changes follow a progression as each target is missed:

- We will eradicate this disease in 10 years.
- We will halve the incidence of this disease in 10 years.
- We will halve the rate of increase of this disease in 10 years.
- Through the fault of a lot of other people, this disease cannot be controlled; we will practise harm reduction.

The IMF and the World Bank imposed structural-adjustment policies on developing countries for many years before external evaluation finally persuaded them that they had done more harm than good (SAPRIN Report, 2004). Western-style medicine was exported for 20 years before it was finally accepted at Alma Ata that other methods might be worth trying (Venedictov, 1998). In fact, it was not until the MDGs in 2000 that a large project actually published clearly defined and measurable outcomes. They may not all have been met by 2015, but at least it was a good start. Unfortunately, monitoring and evaluation are often viewed as obligations imposed by the granting agency rather than as an essential part of running an efficient project. If outcomes are not measured, then all sorts of fairytale endings can be dreamed up for the annual report. Increasingly, there is a sense that outcomes should be evaluated for the project's sake rather than to complete a quarterly grant report. Even the smallest project needs an evaluation process to ensure that it is achieving something useful.

Global Affairs Canada relies on the widely used Results-Based Monitoring and Evaluation system (GAC, 2016). This, like other evaluation techniques, has a jargon of its own. Once you have mastered the differences between goals and objectives, or impacts and outcomes, results-based management (RBM) is a convenient way to combine planning and evaluation in one package (UNDG, 2016). From the earliest stages, measurable outcomes are included as part of the overall plan. Regular evaluation of each of these measured points gives everyone involved a realistic idea about progress (Kusek et al., 2004). Other agencies use similar approaches. The International Fund for Agricultural Development produces an excellent handbook on management and evaluation that is worth downloading (Lavizzari, 2001). The World Bank also produces a useful evaluation handbook (Baker, 2000). It is aimed more toward assessment in terms of poverty reduction, but still has lessons for the broad field of aid projects.

MANAGING THE PEOPLE

Selecting Project Staff

> Never hire someone who knows less than you do about what he's hired to do.
> —*Malcolm Forbes*

Staff selection is rarely considered for short-term projects. Most student groups seem to choose themselves based on no other criteria than having enough money for the air ticket and enough enthusiasm to attend committee meetings. Given the size of the average student loan and the pressures of course work, these criteria do at least show some degree of commitment, but they are far from complete. The trouble produced by a badly behaved team member can be significant, so some form of selection is worth considering. Unfortunately, this is easier said than done. In an egalitarian society like a university campus, any group that sets up a selection (and rejection) process for membership will be open to a range of criticism. The defence, of course, is that because overseas work is a serious undertaking, it is necessary to choose people with appropriate skills, but the whole process remains a social minefield.

Less confrontational methods are available. Requiring regular attendance at committee meetings will help to weed out the uncommitted, or you might simply choose to approach people on an individual basis to see if they are interested in joining the project. Whatever approach you take to the selection dilemma, this is a nettle that should be grasped. If you do not like or trust someone when you are in your own city, it is very unlikely that the relationship will blossom once you work together in a refugee camp.

Choosing staff for large projects, where they might be spending several years overseas, should be (but often is not) taken very seriously. In the business world, it was realized long ago that the financial costs associated with training, relocation, salary, and accommodation are significant. Early return of such a worker due to dissatisfaction or poor performance is a disaster. It jeopardizes the project and wastes large amounts of money; this is not a minor issue and has great relevance for the aid industry. It has been estimated that nearly 350,000 US nationals work on overseas assignments and the failure rate (measured by early return before job completion) is 25–40 percent (Ashamalla et al., 1997). It has taken quite a while for that lesson to be learned by the aid industry, probably because volunteer workers are a lot cheaper.

This attitude is reflected in the very limited amount of research available on the subject of selecting and supporting overseas project staff, either for non-governmental organizations or for large established agencies—examples include McCall et al. (1999) and Moresky et al. (2001). Both of these studies revealed a surprising lack of standardization. For example, selection techniques by large aid agencies ranged from a single telephone call to a multi-stage process of interviews that lasted all day. Respondents expressed frustration at the lack of a validated interviewing technique or similar instrument that might improve the sensitivity of the selection process. Although there has been plenty of research into the ideal characteristics of an overseas worker, both among aid workers (Vulpe et al., 2001) and business personnel (Ioannou, 1995), it is difficult to apply the results in practice. While it is useful to know that flexibility, communication, and adaptability are important qualities in an applicant, it is difficult to measure and assess these variables during an interview. In practice, selection remains based on ill-defined personal opinion.

Attempts have been made to make the assessment of intercultural effectiveness more of a science than an art. The International Personnel Assessment tool (iPAss), developed by the Centre for Intercultural Learning at Foreign Affairs Canada (Foreign Affairs, 2011), and the work of Langdon and Morrelli (Langdon et al., 2002) are both good examples. However, there is an understandable reluctance to trust measurements of complex variables such as character and behaviour and to feel that one's own intuition about a candidate is superior to a questionnaire. For example, a study of the results of personality testing of astronaut applicants showed no correlation between test results and subsequent selection to the astronaut corps (Musson et al., 2004). It is difficult to tell if this was due to inaccuracy in the personality tests or skepticism of the admission committee, but whatever the reason, it seems likely that selection of aid workers will depend on nothing more than an interview for the foreseeable future.

Pre-Trip Briefing and Training

If you do not know where you are going, any road will get you there.

—*Lewis Carroll, Alice in Wonderland, 1865*

It would seem fairly obvious that after selecting staff for a complex overseas position, it would be a good idea to offer them pre-trip training, as well as support once they start working. Unfortunately, this approach has been very slow to develop among large aid organizations. Sending poorly prepared staff overseas to fend for themselves does not toughen them up—it just leads to failure. Inadequately trained and unqualified overseas staff have a high early return rate, and those who stay may suffer from high stress, poor achievement, and depression (Foyle et al., 1998).

Not surprisingly, McCall's study of relief agencies also showed that standards of pre-trip training for relief workers were much the same as those used for worker selection—highly variable and largely inadequate (McCall et al., 1999). Better standards of training were provided for leaders and managers, but the average worker was simply given a bundle of printed notes. Most organizations had no idea how useful the material was; in fact, they did not bother to ask if the new recruits even read the information. Moresky's study showed that NGOs were no better (Moresky et al., 2001). Training manuals usually provided notes on the worker's job and physical health advice, but there was little or no mention of psychological stress management, conflict resolution, and the unique challenges encountered when working in unfamiliar surroundings.

Perhaps the basic problem is the easy availability of volunteers for overseas work. Early return due to dissatisfaction or stress is not taken seriously if there are many more people willing to fill that empty place. If staff records are not kept, it is hardly even noticed! If aid workers are cheap and easy to find, why bother to invest money training them? As the aid industry becomes more complex (and more dangerous in many places), the selection and training of project staff are both receiving more attention, but there is still a long way to go. The days of the "disposable" aid worker studied by Macnair in 1995 have not passed yet (Macnair, 1995).

Supporting Workers in the Field

Long-term personnel and their families require orientation, training, and regular support to help them adapt and be effective while living and working in unfamiliar countries. These steps all need to be based on a clear knowledge of the experiences of previous workers on the project. The basic requirement is an institutional attitude that values the people who are doing all the hard work. It does not matter if you are an international space crew on a long flight or an aid worker in an unfamiliar country—research has clearly shown that regular support and management are vital to the success of any project and also for the health and well-being of the project workers (Ahmad, 2002; Kealey, 2004; Morphew, 2001).

A Swedish study showed that the aid industry has been slow to learn these lessons (Bjerneld et al., 2004). Interviews of returning relief workers revealed high levels of stress and frustration. The authors concluded that recruiting organizations could improve volunteer performance (and their job satisfaction) by accepting better-trained staff, providing specific preparatory training, and giving better support during the assignment. Similarly, a study of aid workers in complex emergencies found that many did not feel supported or trusted by managers outside the country whom they also felt were out of touch with the practical reality of work in the country (Hearns et al., 2007).

The feeling that aid workers are cheap and easy to find is reflected in the prevailing attitudes toward their mental health. Although it is well established that psychological stress is minimized by training and support, it has taken a long time before attention has been paid to the psychological risks associated with aid work, particularly in disasters and conflict zones. Much of this attention is very recent. The CDC did not publish its own study of depression among relief workers until 2005 (Cardozo et al., 2005). Other research has linked high-stress aid work with a range of disorders, including depression, chronic fatigue syndrome, and post-traumatic stress disorder (Eriksson et al., 2001; Lovell, 1999).

Most of the organizations studied by McCall et al. (1999) admitted that worker-support mechanisms were underdeveloped. One agency asked workers to nominate a few selected people, who were then given extra training in counselling.

Another organization provided in-country mental health support for teams working in high-risk areas, but the general approach was that workers were expected to recognize any problems themselves and then apply for help from senior staff. This system is not likely to work well. Apart from the fact that self-diagnosis of depressive illness is unreliable, many workers will avoid asking for help because of the stigma associated with psychological illness.

In the last few years, specific services have been developed in response to the need for better standards of support for expatriate aid workers and also for the victims of the disaster. Examples include the Center for Humanitarian Psychology (CHP, 2011), and the new WHO guide to psychological first aid for disaster victims (WHO, 2011). By now, there is no doubt that the best way to protect project staff from burnout and depression is to train them well and support them in the field with experienced managers who have had extra training in stress recognition and counselling. Clearly, for many reasons, a development initiative's chances of success are greatly improved if careful attention is paid to the in-country support of that project's staff. Regular communication and assessment of information will improve staff performance and also allow early recognition and treatment of severe stress-related illness.

Post-Trip Debriefing and Evaluation

> Errors using inadequate data are less than those using no data at all.
>
> —*Charles Babbage, 1864*

It is essential that project managers have access to regularly updated information about staff health, staff performance, conditions in the country, and the outcomes of project activities. Detailed, compulsory debriefing of returning health workers is an important part of that process. It is also important to maintain accurate staff records so that retention rates and health problems can be monitored. If there is no mechanism to receive feedback from staff, it is possible to live in a dream world where every worker is happy and every project successful.

It is necessary to be realistic about the potential inaccuracies of self-assessment during debriefing. In a study of Canadian technical advisers, 75 percent expressed high personal satisfaction with their performance, although only 20 percent were rated as being highly effective by their colleagues or superiors (Kealey, 2001). The excitement and novelty of working overseas may give a sense of satisfaction that is out of proportion with the effectiveness of that work. Just because you are having a good time does not necessarily mean you are being effective. Important decisions are based on debrief reports, so the reports should be based on as many information sources as possible.

SUMMARY

All aid projects involve partnerships of one form or another; anyone interested in international development work must understand the basic requirements that make up a successful partnership. Aid partnerships are critical in global health and need to be translated into strategic, intentional, measurable collaboration to create health impacts. Characteristics of successful partnerships include: respect and trust between people involved, complete agreement that the partnership is necessary, competent leadership with support of all members; clearly agreed-upon goals, a collaborative decision-making process, regular communications, clearly defined organizational structure, fully agreed-upon conflict-resolution procedure, and a fully agreed-upon budget. A critical component of partnerships is building trust with partners and the communities the project aims to serve. The elements of unsuccessful partnerships generally include a manipulative or dominating partner, lack of clear purpose, or unrealistic goals. According to Oxfam Canada's Six Core Partnership Principles, there must be shared vision and values; the partnership should have a value-added effect; each partner should have autonomy and independence; there should be transparency and mutual accountability in all dealings; there should be clarity about roles and responsibilities; and joint strategy should be updated regularly based on progress reviews.

Adequate preparation and training is critical before any overseas trip. Sending poorly prepared staff overseas to fend for themselves does not toughen them up—it just leads to failure. The global health community will continually face challenges that will require effective partnerships in order to strengthen health systems, combat individual diseases, and be equipped to deal with disease outbreaks.

DISCUSSION QUESTIONS

1. Is it possible to have successful development projects without partnerships? Why?
2. What would you consider the three most common pitfalls and problems confronting partnerships? Provide examples.
3. You are about to embark on a development project in a developing country. How would you select and support the people working on the project?
4. What are the specific organizational needs for managing international development programs?
5. What structures can you include to manage and avoid conflict on an international development project?
6. What are the Six Core Partnership Principles of Oxfam Canada? Are there other principles you would add to the list?

7. Why does sending poorly prepared staff overseas to fend for themselves lead to failure?

8. Why do inadequately trained and unqualified overseas staff have a high early return rate?

9. In building partnerships, why are early meetings an absolutely basic requirement for any successful partnership?

10. In building partnerships in early planning stages, do you think there are substitutes for face-to-face meetings, such as video conferences, telephone calls, and email? Why or why not?

RECOMMENDED READING

Kerr, M. 1996. *Partnering and health development: The Kathmandu connection.* Pub: University of Calgary Press.

Kusek, J., et al. 2004. Ten steps to a results-based monitoring and evaluation system. Retrieved from: www.oecd.org/dataoecd/23/27/35281194.pdf.

Laurence, L., et al. 2003. *You're not listening to me! Dealing with disputes: Mediation and its benefits for voluntary organizations.* Pub: National Council of Voluntary Organizations.

Mackin, D. 2007. *The team building tool kit: Tips, tactics, and rules for effective work place teams.* Pub: AMACOM.

Roche, C. 2000. *Impact assessment for development agencies: Learning to value change.* Pub: Oxfam Publishing.

Wilson, A., et al. 1997. *Making partnerships work: A practical guide for the public, private, voluntary, and community sectors.* Pub: Joseph Rowntree Foundation.

REFERENCES

Ahmad, M. 2002. Who cares? The personal and professional problems of NGO field workers in Bangladesh. *Development in Practice,* 12: 177–191.

Alberta Community Development. 2001. Working in partnership: Recipes for success. Retrieved from: www.culture.alberta.ca/voluntarysector/partnershipkit/Partnership_Kit.pdf.

Ashamalla, M., et al. 1997. Easing entry and beyond: Preparing expatriates and patriates for foreign assignment success. *International Journal of Commerce and Management,* 7: 106–114.

Baker, J. 2000. *Evaluating the impact of development projects on poverty: A handbook for practitioners.* Pub: World Bank Publications. Retrieved from: http://go.worldbank.org/8E2ZTGBOI0.

Bjerneld, M., et al. 2004. Perception of work in humanitarian assistance: Interviews with returning Swedish health professionals. *Disaster Management Response*, 2: 101–108.

Cardozo, B., et al. 2005. The mental health of expatriate and kosovar Albanian humanitarian aid workers. *Disasters*, 2: 152–170.

CEDR. 2011. Centre for Effective Dispute Resolution. Retrieved from: www.cedr.com/.

CHP. 2011. Center for Humanitarian Psychology. Retrieved from: www.humanitarian-psy.org.

Collins, K. 2004. Profitable gifts: A history of the Merck ivermectin donation program and its implications for international health. *Perspectives in Biology and Medicine*, 47: 100–109.

EIA. 2011. US Energy Information Administration. Retrieved from: www.eia.gov/.

Eriksson, C., et al. 2001. Trauma exposure and PTSD symptoms in international relief and development personnel. *Journal of Traumatic Stress*, 14: 205–212.

Ezezika, O. C., 2014. How do you build trust with communities involved in your research? SciDev.Net's practical guides, Science and Development Network © 2014 SciDev.Net.

Florence Nightingale Museum. 2011. Retrieved from: www.florence-nightingale.co.uk/cms/.

Foreign Affairs. 2011. Centre for Intercultural Learning. IPASS. Retrieved from: www.international.gc.ca/cfsi-icse/cil-cai/ipass-sepi-eng.asp.

Foyle, M., et al. 1998. Expatriate mental health. *Acta Psychiatrica Scandinavica*, 97: 278–283.

GAC. 2016. Results-based management tools at Global Affairs Canada: A how-to guide. Retrieved from: www.international.gc.ca/development-developpement/partners-partenaires/bt-oa/rbm_tools-gar_outils.aspx?lang=eng.

Gyapong, M., et al. 2001. Community-directed treatment: The way forward to eliminating lymphatic filariasis as a public health problem in Ghana. *Annals of Tropical Medicine and Parasitology*, 1: 77–86.

Hearns, A., et al. 2007. The value of support for aid workers in complex emergencies. *Disaster Management Response*, 5: 28–35.

Hopkins, A. 2005. Ivermectin and onchocerciasis: Is it all solved? *Eye*, 19: 1057–1066.

Ioannou, L. 1995. Unnatural selection. *International Business*, 83: 95–99.

Kealey, D. 2001. Cross-cultural effectiveness: A study of Canadian technical advisors overseas. Government of Canada, Department of Foreign Affairs. Retrieved from: www.international.gc.ca/cfsi-icse/cil-cai/pubpap-pubdoc-eng.asp.

Kealey, D. 2004. Research on intercultural effectiveness and its relevance to multicultural crews in space. *Aviation, Space, and Environmental Medicine*, 75 (Suppl. 1): C58–C64.

Kerr, M. 1996. *Partnering and health development: The Kathmandu connection.* Pub: University of Calgary Press.

Kusek, J., et al. 2004. Ten steps to a result-based monitoring and evaluation system. Retrieved from: www.oecd.org/dataoecd/23/27/35281194.pdf.

Langdon, D., et al. 2002. A new model for systematic competency identification. *Performance Improvement*, 41: 16–23.

Laurence, L., et al. 2003. *You're not listening to me! Dealing with disputes: Mediation and its benefits for voluntary organizations.* Pub: National Council of Voluntary Organizations.

Lavizzari, L. 2001. A guide for project management and evaluation: Managing for impact in rural development. Retrieved from: www.ifad.org/evaluation/guide/.

Lovell, D. 1999. Chronic fatigue syndrome among overseas development workers: A qualitative study. *Journal of Travel Medicine,* 6: 16–23.

Mackin, D. 2007. *The team building tool kit: Tips, tactics, and rules for effective work place teams.* Pub: AMACOM.

Macnair, R. 1995. Room for improvement: The management and support of relief and development workers. Retrieved from: http://repository.forcedmigration.org/show_metadata.jsp?pid=fmo:3623.

Mango. 2011. Financial management for NGOs. Retrieved from: www.mango.org.uk/Guide/FinancialGovernance.

McCall, M., et al. 1999. Selection, training, and support of relief workers: An occupational health issue. *British Medical Journal,* 318: 113–116.

Moresky, R., et al. 2001. Preparing international relief workers for health care in the field: An evaluation of organizational practices. *Pre-hospital Disaster Medicine,* 16: 257–262.

Morphew, M. 2001. Psychological and human factors in long duration space flight. *McGill Journal of Medicine,* 6: 74–80.

Musson, D., et al. 2004. Personality characteristics and trait clusters in final stage astronaut selection. *Aviation, Space, and Environmental Medicine,* 75: 342–349.

Oxfam. 2011. Oxfam Canada partnership policy. Retrieved from: www.oxfam.ca/node/2973.

SAPRIN Report. 2004. *The policy roots of economic crisis, poverty, and inequality.* Pub: Zed Books.

TDR. 2009. Integrated community-based interventions. Retrieved from: http://apps.who.int/tdr/publications/about-tdr/annual-reports/bl11-annual-report/pdf/bl11-annual-report-2009.pdf.

TDR. 2010. Special programme for research and training in tropical diseases (onchocerciasis). Retrieved from: http://apps.who.int/tdr/svc/diseases/onchocerciasis.

UNDG. 2016. Results-based management. Retrieved from: https://undg.org/home/guidance-policies/country-programming-principles/results-based-management-rbm/.

US Census Bureau. 2011. International programs. Retrieved from: www.census.gov/population/international/data/idb/informationGateway.php.

Venedictov, D. 1998. Alma Ata and after. *World Health Forum,* 19: 79–86.

Vulpe, T., et al. 2001. A profile of the interculturally effective person. Retrieved from: www.sietar.eu/about_us/Newsletter/Mar04/Aprofileoftheinterculturallyeffectiveper.html.

WHO. 2011. Psychological first aid: Guide for field workers. Retrieved from: http://whqlibdoc.who.int/publications/2011/9789241548205_eng.pdf.

COPYRIGHT ACKNOWLEDGEMENTS

Figures

Figure 11.2: OECD. 2016. *Development Co-operation Report 2016: The Sustainable Development Goals as Business Opportunities*, OECD Publishing, Paris. Retrieved from: http://dx.doi.org/10.1787/dcr-2016-14-en. Used by permission of the OECD.

Figure 11.6: OECD. 2015. *Multilateral Aid 2015: Better Partnerships for a Post-2015 World*, OECD Publishing, Paris. Retrieved from: http://dx.doi.org/10.1787/9789264235212-en. Used by permission of the OECD.

Figure 16.4: United Nations High Commissioner for Refugees, *Global Trends: Forced Displacements in 2015*. Retrieved from:

http://www.unhcr.org/statistics/unhcrstats/576408cd7/unhcr-global-trends-2015.html. Used by permission of the UNHCR.

Figure 16.5: United Nations High Commissioner for Refugees, *Global Trends: Forced Displacements in 2015*. Retrieved from:

http://www.unhcr.org/statistics/unhcrstats/576408cd7/unhcr-global-trends-2015.html. Used by permission of the UNHCR.

Photos

Photo 1.2: Photo by Cia Pak, used by permission of the UN Photo Library (www.unmultimedia.org/photo).

Photo 1.5: Photo by F. Charton, used by permission of the UN Photo Library (www.unmultimedia.org/photo).

Photo 1.6: Photo by Mark Garten, used by permission of the UN Photo Library (www.unmultimedia.org/photo).

Photo 2.3: Photo by Eskinde Debebe, used by permission of the UN Photo Library (www.unmultimedia.org/photo).

Photo 4.2: Photo by Eric Kanalstein, used by permission of the UN Photo Library (www.unmultimedia.org/photo).

Photo 5.2: Photo by McGlynn, used by permission of the UN Photo Library (www.unmultimedia.org/photo).

Photo 6.2: Photo by Logan Abassi, used by permission of the UN Photo Library (www.unmultimedia.org/photo).

INDEX